ADVANCES IN NEUROLOGY

Volume 58

Advances in Neurology

Advances in Neurology
Volume 58

Tourette Syndrome
Genetics, Neurobiology, and Treatment

Editors

Thomas N. Chase, M.D.
Chief, Experimental Therapeutics Branch
National Institute of Neurological Diseases
and Stroke
National Institutes of Health
Bethesda, Maryland

Arnold J. Friedhoff, M.D.
Director, Millhauser Laboratories
Department of Psychiatry
New York University Medical Center
New York, New York

Donald J. Cohen, M.D.
Director, Child Study Center
Yale University School of Medicine
New Haven, Connecticut

Raven Press ⟐ New York

Raven Press, Ltd., 1185 Avenue of the Americas, New York, New York 10036

Made in the United States of America

ISBN 0-88167-922-4

ISSN 0091-3952

The material contained in this volume was submitted as previously unpublished material, except in the instances in which some of the illustrative material was derived.

Great care has been taken to maintain the accuracy of the information contained in the volume. However, neither Raven Press nor the editors can be held responsible for errors or for any consequences arising from the use of the information contained herein.

9 8 7 6 5 4 3 2 1

Advances in Neurology Series

Vol. 58: Tourette Syndrome: Genetics, Neurobiology, and Treatment: *T. N. Chase, A. J. Friedhoff, and D. J. Cohen, editors.* 400 pp., 1992.

Vol. 57: Frontal Lobe Seizures and Epilepsies: *P. Chauvel, A. V. Delgado-Escueta, E. Halgren, and J. Bancaud, editors.* 752 pp., 1992.

Vol. 56: Amyotrophic Lateral Sclerosis and Other Motor Neuron Diseases: *L. P. Rowland, editor.* 592 pp., 1991.

Vol. 55: Neurobehavioral Problems in Epilepsy: *D. B. Smith, D. Treiman, and M. Trimble, editors.* 512 pp., 1990.

Vol. 54: Magnetoencephalography: *S. Sato, editor.* 284 pp., 1990.

Vol. 53: Parkinson's Disease: Anatomy, Pathology, and Therapy: *M. B. Streifler, A. D. Korczyn, E. Melamed, and M. B. H. Youdim, editors.* 640 pp., 1990.

Vol. 52: Brain Edema: Pathogenesis, Imaging, and Therapy: *D. Long, editor.* 640 pp., 1990.

Vol. 51: Alzheimer's Disease: *R. J. Wurtman, S. Corkin, J. H. Growdon, and E. Ritter-Walker, editors.* 308 pp., 1990.

*Vol. 50: Dystonia 2: *S. Fahn, C. D. Marsden, and D. B. Calne, editors.* 688 pp., 1988.

*Vol. 49: Facial Dyskinesias: *J. Jankovic and E. Tolosa, editors.* 560 pp., 1988

Vol. 48: Molecular Genetics of Neurological and Neuromuscular Disease: *S. DiDonato, S. DiMauro, A. Mamoli, and L. P. Rowland, editors.* 288 pp., 1987.

Vol. 47: Functional Recovery in Neurological Disease: *Stephen G. Waxman, editor.* 640 pp., 1987.

Vol. 46: Intensive Neurodiagnostic Monitoring: *R. J. Gumnit, editor.* 336 pp., 1987.

Vol. 45: Parkinson's Disease: *M. D. Yahr and K. J. Bergmann, editors.* 640 pp., 1986.

Vol. 44: Basic Mechanisms of the Epilepsies: Molecular and Cellular Approaches: *A. V. Delgado-Escueta, A. A. Ward, Jr., D. M. Woodbury, and R. J. Porter, editors.* 1,120 pp., 1986.

Vol. 43: Myoclonus: *S. Fahn, C. D. Marsden, and M. H. Van Woert, editors.* 752 pp., 1986.

Vol. 42: Progress in Aphasiology: *F. Clifford Rose, editor.* 384 pp., 1984.

Vol. 41: The Olivopontocerebellar Atrophies: *R. C. Duvoisin and A. Plaitakis, editors.* 304 pp., 1984.

Vol. 40: Parkinson-Specific Motor and Mental Disorders, Role of Pallidum: Pathophysiological, Biochemical, and Therapeutic Aspects: *R. G. Hassler and J. F. Christ, editors.* 601 pp., 1984.

*Vol. 39: Motor Control Mechanisms in Health and Disease: *J. E. Desmedt, editor.* 1,224 pp., 1983.

Vol. 38: The Dementias: *R. Mayeux and W. G. Rosen, editors.* 288 pp., 1983.

Vol. 37: Experimental Therapeutics of Movement Disorders; *S. Fahn, D. B. Calne, and I. Shoulson, editors.* 339 pp., 1983.

Vol. 36: Human Motor Neuron Diseases: *L. P. Rowland, editor.* 592 pp., 1982.

Vol. 35: Gilles de la Tourette Syndrome: *A. J. Friedhoff and T. N. Chase, editors.* 476 pp., 1982.

Vol. 34: Status Epilepticus: Mechanisms of Brain Damage and Treatment: *A. V. Delgado-Escueta, C. G. Wasterlain, D. M. Treiman, and R. J. Porter, editors.* 579 pp., 1983.

*Vol. 33: Headache: Physiopathological and Clinical Concepts: *M. Critchley, A. Friedman, S. Gorini, and F. Sicuteri, editors.* 417 pp., 1982.

*Vol. 32: Clinical Applications of Evoked Potentials in Neurology: *J. Courjon, F. Mauguiere, and M. Revol, editors.* 592 pp., 1982.

Vol. 31: Demyelinating Diseases: Basic and Clinical Electrophysiology: *S. Waxman and J. Murdoch Ritchie, editors.* 544 pp., 1981.

Vol. 30: Diagnosis and Treatment of Brain Ischemia: *A. L. Carney and E. M. Anderson, editors.* 424 pp., 1981.

*Vol. 29: Neurofibromatosis: *V. M. Riccardi and J. J. Mulvihill, editors.* 288 pp., 1981.

Vol. 28: Brain Edema: *J. Cervós-Navarro and R. Ferszt, editors.* 539 pp., 1980.

*Vol. 27: Antiepileptic Drugs: Mechanisms of Action: *G. H. Glaser, J. K. Penry, and D. M. Woodbury, editors.* 728 pp., 1980.

*Vol. 26: Cerebral Hypoxia and Its Consequences: *S. Fahn, J. N. Davis, and L. P. Rowland, editors.* 454 pp., 1979.

*Vol. 25: Cerebrovascular Disorders and Stroke: *M. Goldstein, L. Bolis, C. Fieschi, S. Gorini, and C. H. Millikan, editors.* 412 pp., 1979.

*Vol. 24: The Extrapyramidal System and Its Disorders: *L. J. Poirier, T. L. Sourkes, and P. Bédard, editors.* 552 pp., 1979.

*Vol. 23: Huntington's Chorea: *T. N. Chase, N. S. Wexler, and A. Barbeau, editors.* 864 pp., 1979.

Vol. 22: Complications of Nervous System Trauma: *R. A. Thompson and J. R. Green, editors.* 454 pp., 1979.

*Vol. 21: The Inherited Ataxia: Biochemical, Viral, and Pathological Studies: *R. A. Kark, R. Rosenberg, and L. Schut, editors.* 450 pp., 1978.

Vol. 20: Pathology of Cerebrospinal Microcirculation: *J. Cervós-Navarro, E. Betz, G. Ebhardt, R. Ferszt, and R. Wüllenweber, editors.* 636 pp., 1978.

*Vol. 19: Neurological Epidemiology: Principles and Clinical Applications: *B. S. Schoenberg, editor.* 672 pp., 1978.

*Vol. 18: Hemi-Inattention and Hemisphere Specialization: *E. A. Weinstein and R. P. Friedland, editors.* 176 pp., 1977.

*Vol. 17: Treatment of Neuromuscular Diseases: *R. C. Griggs and R. T. Moxley, editors.* 370 pp., 1977.

Vol. 16: Stroke: *R. A. Thompson and J. R. Green, editors.* 250 pp., 1977.

*Vol. 15: Neoplasia in the Central Nervous System: *R. A. Thompson and J. R. Green, editors.* 394 pp., 1976.

*Vol. 14: Dystonia: *R. Eldridge and S. Fahn, editors.* 510 pp., 1976.

Vol. 13: Current Reviews: *W. J. Friedlander, editor.* 400 pp., 1975.

Vol. 12: Physiology and Pathology of Dendrites: *G. W. Kreutzberg, editor.* 524 pp., 1975.

*Vol. 11: Complex Partial Seizures and Their Treatment: *J. K. Penry and D. D. Daly, editors.* 486 pp., 1975.

*Vol. 10: Private Models of Neurological Disorders: *B. S. Meldrum and C. D. Marsden, editors.* 270 pp., 1975.

*Vol. 9: Dopaminergic Mechanisms: *D. B. Calne, T. N. Chase, and A. Barbeau, editors.* 452 pp., 1975.

*Vol. 8: Neurosurgical Management of Epilepsies: *D. P. Purpura, J. K. Penry, and R. D. Walter, editors.* 370 pp., 1975.

Vol. 7: Current Reviews of Higher Nervous System Dysfunction: *W. J. Friedlander, editor.* 202 pp., 1975.

Vol. 6: Infectious Diseases of the Central Nervous System: *R. A. Thompson and J. R. Green, editors.* 402 pp., 1974.

*Vol. 5: Second Canadian-American Conference on Parkinson's Disease: *F. McDowell and A. Barbeau, editors.* 526 pp., 1974.

*Vol. 4: International Symposium on Pain: *J. J. Bonica, editor.* 858 pp., 1974.

*Vol. 3: Progress in the Treatment of Parkinsonism: *D. B. Calne, editor.* 402 pp., 1973.

*Vol. 2: The Treatment of Parkinsonism—The Role of DOPA Decarboxylase Inhibitors: *M. D. Yahr, editor.* 304 pp., 1973.

Vol. 1: Huntington's Chorea, 1872–1972: *A. Barbeau, T. N. Chase, and G. W. Paulson, editors.* 902 pp., 1973.

---

*Asterisk books are out of print.

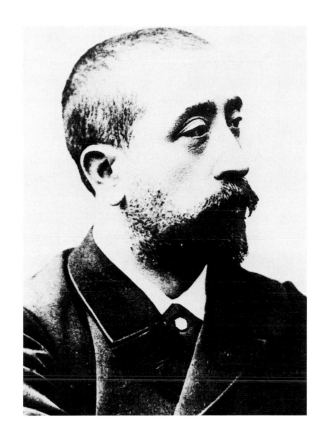

Gilles de la Tourette

Contents

Contributing Authors xiii

Preface xv

Acknowledgments xix

Clinical Phenomenology

1. The Natural History of Tourette Syndrome 1
   Ruth Dowling Bruun and Cathy L. Budman

2. Diagnosis and Classification of Tics and Tourette Syndrome 7
   Joseph Jankovic

3. Pathogenesis of Tourette Syndrome: Clues from the Clinical
   Phenotype and Natural History 15
   James F. Leckman, David L. Pauls, Bradley S. Peterson,
   Mark A. Riddle, George M. Anderson, and Donald J. Cohen

4. Clinical Phenomenology of Tic Disorders: Selected Aspects 25
   Anthony E. Lang

5. Tourette Syndrome and Obsessive-Compulsive Disorder: An
   Analysis of Associated Phenomena 33
   Danielle C. Cath, C. A. L. Hoogduin, B. J. M. van de Wetering,
   T. C. A. M. van Woerkom, R. A. C. Roos, and H. G. M. Rooymans

Epidemiology

6. Methodology of Epidemiological Studies of Tic Disorders and
   Comorbid Psychopathology 43
   Theodore Fallon, Jr. and Mary Schwab-Stone

7. Psychosocial Factors in Tourette Syndrome 55
   Felton Earls

8. A Population-Based Epidemiological Study of Tourette Syndrome
   Among Adolescents in Israel 61
   Alan Apter, David L. Pauls, Avi Bleich, Ada H. Zohar,
   Shmuel Kron, Gidi Ratzoni, Anat Dycian, Moshe Kotler,
   Avi Weizman, and Donald J. Cohen

9. Epidemiology and Comorbidity: The North Dakota Prevalence
   Studies of Tourette Syndrome and other Developmental
   Disorders 67
   Jacob Kerbeshian and Larry Burd

10. Tourette Syndrome in a Special Education Population: Hypotheses 75
Roger Kurlan

Comorbid Conditions

11. Tourette Syndrome and Obsessive-Compulsive Disorder 83
Henrietta L. Leonard, Susan E. Swedo, Judith L. Rapoport,
Kenneth C. Rickler, Deborah Topol, Stephen Lee, and David Rettew

12. Comorbidity, Tourette Syndrome, and Anxiety Disorders 95
Barbara Coffey, Jean Frazier, and Stephen Chen

13. Self-Injurious Behavior and Tourette Syndrome 105
Mary M. Robertson

Neurochemistry and Neuropathology

14. Immunohistochemical Study of the Basal Ganglia in Normal and Parkinsonian Monkeys 115
Brigitte Lavoie, Pierre-Yves Côté, and André Parent

15. Postmortem Analysis of Subcortical Monoamines and Amino Acids in Tourette Syndrome 123
George M. Anderson, Eleanor S. Pollak, Diptendu Chatterjee,
James F. Leckman, Mark A. Riddle, and Donald J. Cohen

16. Neurochemical Analysis of Postmortem Cortical and Striatal Brain Tissue in Patients with Tourette Syndrome 135
Harvey S. Singer

17. Basal Ganglia Peptidergic Staining in Tourette Syndrome: A Follow- up Study 145
Suzanne N. Haber and D. Wolfer

Genetics

18. Issues in Genetic Linkage Studies of Tourette Syndrome: Phenotypic Spectrum and Genetic Model Parameters 151
David L. Pauls

19. Tourette Symptoms in 161 Related Family Members 159
William M. McMahon, Mark Leppert, Francis Filloux,
Ben J. M. van de Wetering, and Sandra Hasstedt

20. Genetic Study on Tourette Syndrome in The Netherlands 167
Peter Heutink, B. J. M. van de Wetering, G. J. Breedveld, and
B. A. Oostra

21. Application of Microsatellite DNA Polymorphisms to Linkage Mapping of Tourette Syndrome Gene(s) 173
Patricia J. Wilkie, Peter A. Ahmann, Jeff Hardacre,
Robert J. LaPlant, Bradley C. Hiner, and James L. Weber

22. Linkage Studies in 16 St. Louis Families: Present Status and Pursuit of an Adjunct Strategy 181
    Eric J. Devor

23. Alternative Hypotheses on the Inheritance of Tourette Syndrome ... 189
    David E. Comings and Brenda G. Comings

Neuroimaging

24. Structural Imaging in Tourette Syndrome 201
    Steven Demeter

25. SPECT Imaging of Cerebral Blood Flow in Tourette Syndrome 207
    Mark A. Riddle, Ann M. Rasmusson, Scott W. Woods, and Paul B. Hoffer

26. Functional Neuroanatomy of Tourette Syndrome: Limbic-Motor Interactions Studied with FDG PET 213
    Brigitte Stoetter, Allen R. Braun, Christopher Randolph, Jeffrey Gernert, Richard E. Carson, Peter Herscovitch, and Thomas N. Chase

27. PET Studies on the Integrity of the Pre and Postsynaptic Dopaminergic System in Tourette Syndrome 227
    David J. Brooks, N. Turjanski, G. V Sawle, E. D. Playford, and A. J. Lees

28. Positron Emission Tomography Evaluation of Dopamine D-2 Receptors in Adults with Tourette Syndrome 233
    Harvey S. Singer, Dean F. Wong, Janice E. Brown, Jason Brandt, Laura Krafft, Elias Shaya, Robert F. Dannals, and Henry N. Wagner, Jr.

Pharmacological Treatments

29. Treatment of Tourette Syndrome with Neuroleptic Drugs 241
    Gerald Erenberg

30. Clonidine and Clonazepam in Tourette Syndrome 245
    Christopher G. Goetz

31. Neuroendocrine and Behavioral Effects of Naloxone in Tourette Syndrome 253
    Phillip B. Chappell, James F. Leckman, Mark A. Riddle, George M. Anderson, S. J. Listwack, S. I. Ort, M. T. Hardin, L. D. Scahill, and Donald J. Cohen

32. Therapeutics of Tourette Syndrome: New Medication Approaches 263
    Peter A. LeWitt

33. Methylphenidate in Hyperactive Boys with Comorbid Tic
    Disorder: I. Clinic Evaluations 271
    Jeffrey Sverd, Kenneth D. Gadow, Edith E. Nolan, Joyce Sprafkin,
    and Stacy N. Ezor

34. Psychopharmacology of Obsessive-Compulsive Disorder in Tourette
    Syndrome 283
    Robert A. King, Mark A. Riddle, and Wayne K. Goodman

35. Effects of Foods on the Brain: Possible Implications for
    Understanding and Treating Tourette Syndrome 293
    Richard J. Wurtman

36. Is There a Role for Megavitamin Therapy in the Treatment of
    Attention Deficit Hyperactivity Disorder? 303
    Robert H. A. Haslam

Non-Pharmacological Interventions

37. Educational Management of Children with Tourette Syndrome 311
    Larry Burd and Jacob Kerbeshian

38. The Family in Tourette Syndrome 319
    Gordon Harper

39. Social Adaptation of Tourette Syndrome Families in Japan 323
    Yoshiko Nomura, Michiko Kita, and Masaya Segawa

40. Behavior Therapy for Obsessive-Compulsive Disorder and
    Trichotillomania: Implications for Tourette Syndrome 333
    Lee Baer

Perspectives: Research and Treatment

41. Tourette Syndrome: Extending Basic Research to Clinical Care 341
    Donald J. Cohen, Arnold J. Friedhoff, James F. Leckman, and
    Thomas N. Chase

Subject Index 363

Contributing Authors

George M. Anderson, 15, 123,253

Peter A. Ahmann, 173

Alan Apter, 61

Lee Baer, 333

Avi Bleich, 61

Jason Brandt, 233

G. J. Breedveld, 167

Allen R. Braun, 213

David J. Brooks, 227

Janice E. Brown, 233

Ruth Dowling Bruun, 1

Cathy Budman, 1

Larry Burd, 67,311

Richard E. Carson, 213

Danielle C. Cath, 33

Phillip B. Chappel, 253

Thomas N. Chase, 213, 341

Diptendu Chatterjee, 123

Stephen Chen, 95

Barbara Coffey, 95

Donald J. Cohen, 15,61,123,253,341

Brenda G. Comings, 189

David E. Comings, 189

Pierre-Yves Côté, 115

Robert F. Dannals, 233

Steven Demeter, 201

Eric J. Devor, 181

Anat Dycian, 61

Felton Earls, 55

Gerald Erenberg, 241

Stacy N. Ezor, 271

Theodore Fallon, Jr., 43

Francis Filloux, 159

Jean Frazier, 95

Arnold J. Friedhoff, 341

Kenneth D. Gadow, 271

Jeffrey Gernert, 213

Christopher G. Goetz, 245

Wayne K. Goodman, 283

Suzanne N. Haber, 145

Jeff Hardacre, 173

M. T. Hardin, 253

Gordon Harper, 319

Robert H. A. Haslam, 303

Sandra Hasstedt, 159

Peter Herscovitch, 213

Peter Heutink, 167

Bradley C. Hiner 173

C. A. L. Hoogduin, 33

Paul B. Hoffer, 207

Joseph Jankovic, 7

Jacob Kerbeshian, 67,311

Robert A. King, 283

Michiko Kita, 323

Moshe Kotler, 61

Laura Krafft, 233

Shmuel Kron, 61

Roger Kurlan, 75

Anthony E. Lang, 25

Robert J. LaPlant, 173

Brigitte Lavoie, 115

James F. Leckman, 15, 123,253,341

Stephen Lee, 83

A. J. Lees, 227,341

Henrietta L. Leonard, 83

Mark Leppert, 159

Peter LeWitt, 263

S. J. Listwack, 253

William M. McMahon, 159

Edith E. Nolan, 271

Yoskiko Nomura, 323

S. I. Ort, 253

B. A. Oostra, 167

André Parent, 115

David L. Pauls, 15,61,151

Bradley S. Peterson, 15

E. D. Playford, 227

Eleanor S. Pollak, 123

Christopher Randolph, 213

Judith L. Rapoport, 83

Ann M. Rasmusson, 207

Gidi Ratzoni, 61

David Rettew, 83

Kenneth C. Rickler, 83

Mark A. Riddle, 15,123, 207,253,283

Mary M. Robertson, 105

R. A. C. Roos, 33

H. G. M. Rooymans, 33

G. V. Sawle, 227

L. D. Scahill, 253

Mary Schwab-Stone, 43

Masaya Segawa, 323

Elias Shaya, 233

Harvey S. Singer, 135,233

Brigitte Stoetter, 213

Joyce Sprafkin, 271

Jeffrey Sverd, 271

Susan E. Swedo, 83

Deborah Topol, 83

N. Turjanski, 227

Ben J. M. van de Wetering, 33,159,167

T. C. A. M. van Woerkom, 33

Henry N. Wagner, Jr., 233

James L. Weber, 173

Avi Weizman, 61

Patricia J. Wilkie, 173

D. Wolfer, 145

Scott W. Woods, 207

Dean F. Wong, 233

Richard J. Wurtman, 293

Ada H. Zohar, 61

Preface

Gilles de la Tourette's syndrome is a familial, childhood onset and often lifelong neuropsychiatric disorder with a distinctive range of neurological and behavioral symptoms. Since its first description in Charcot's clinic over one century ago, it has fascinated neurologists and psychiatrists and has bridged the disciplines concerned with brain and behavior. This volume describes the remarkable advances in the study and care of individuals with Tourette's syndrome during the past decade.

Tourette's syndrome has served, throughout its history, as a testing ground for new ideas about the relations between mind and body in neurological and developmental psychopathological conditions. Explanatory paradigms have shifted along with advances in understanding neurological and psychiatric disorders. Early in its history, Tourette's syndrome was included among the hysterical disorders and choreas. It then was approached as a manifestation of emotional and unconscious conflicts. With the advent of neuroleptic treatment and the pioneering work of Drs. Arthur Shapiro and Elaine Shapiro in the 1960s, neurochemical models achieved major emphasis in pathogenesis. During the past decade, new paradigms have beem based on genetic evidence for the transmission of the vulncrability to the cardinal tic symptoms and on associated behavioral manifestations. Today, Tourette's syndrome has emerged as an exemplary model disorder for the application of the full range of neuroscience and behavioral methodologies on an important clinical condition which engages the clinical concern of psychiatrists, neurologists, pediatricians, psychologists, educators, social workers, and others.

This volume describes a decade of advances in the understanding of Tourette's syndrome and associated conditions. The forerunner of this volume, *Gilles de la Tourette Syndrome*, published in 1982 as volume 35 in the *Advances in Neurology* series, was based on the First International Scientific Symposium on Tourette syndrome held in New York in 1981. That meeting brought together the leaders in the study of Tourette's syndrome with basic scientists working in relevant fields of research. Tourette's syndrome was no longer a "rare and curious disorder" but one of importance in its own right as well as a very useful model condition that could provide information about other serious developmental, neurobehavioral conditions. However, many of the contributions to the 1982 volume were speculative; although there were many suggestions for further research, there was relatively little hard data.

This volume documents the burgeoning of knowledge and the recruitment of a number of major research groups. As a result, new fields of investigation and treatment have opened up. Advances in understanding the genetics of Tourette's syndrome, and the search for the underlying genetic vulnerability, have profoundly influenced both the conceptualization and research on the disorder. A number of chapters in this volume describe the advances in defining the mode of transmission and the varied molecular biological approaches that are now being applied. Along with the genetic research, there is now far greater interest in the relationship between Tourette's syndrome and associated behavioral and psychiatric disorders, particularly obsessive-compulsive disorder, which may represent an alternate manifestation of the underlying genetic diathesis. Only quite recently have investigators been able to perform neurochemical research on post-mortem brains from patients with Tourette's syndrome and begin to test neurochemical hypotheses.

Brain imaging techniques have been applied to Tourette's syndrome and are beginning to bring together structural, functional, and neurochemical concepts in pathogenesis. Rigorous epidemiological studies are now providing data about incidence and associated features in various groups of patients and in larger populations. The clinical investigation of individuals with Tourette's syndrome over long periods has increased understanding of the natural history, phenomenology, and clinical manifestations of Tourette's syndrome and associated disorders. And, perhaps most importantly, there have been advances in therapy which have provided immediate benefit for many patients.

Progress in the study of Tourette's syndrome has resulted from new methodologies and advances in basic and clinical sciences. It also reflects the emergence of successful, interdisciplinary collaborations, and a new, international network of investigators, as well as the existence of teams of clinical and basic researchers who have made Tourette's syndrome a major emphasis of their research and clinical work. The contributions to this volume exemplify all of these achievements—scientific and institutional—to a degree that could not have been predicted a decade ago.

Along with scientific progress there have remained many areas of continuing controversy and uncertainty. These issues are reflected in this volume and sugggest areas for future research. Among the controversies are some fundamental issues, including the very basic question, How broadly should the clinical spectrum be defined? Some investigators emphasize the cardinal tic features while others explore how far to extend the boundaries of the condition, based on epidemiological, clinical and genetic data, to include other manifestations. There are important differences in the interpretation of basic areas of research, such as genetic mechanisms, brain imaging studies, neurochemical findings, and pharmacological approaches. Debate within the field is rigorous. As editors, we have not attempted to smooth out the differences in viewpoint but rather allowed the authors to argue for their ideas as they wished. We hope these will inspire further empirical research.

This volume remains, as did its earlier companion, still very much a book about work in progress. The location and cloning of the gene or genes involved in Tourette's syndrome, and the clarification of the pathogenic pathways between genetic vulnerability and clinical disorder, will require years of further work that will mark a new era in research on gene-environment interactions and clinical care. Clarification of biology will also be accompanied by increased understanding of how an individual's clinical course is modified by various types of psychosocial factors within the individual, family, and community.

Advances in other areas of neuroscience, including brain imaging, molecular neurochemistry, and neuroendocrinology, as well as behavioral research on developmental disorders and fields such as psychiatric epidemiology, will continue to enrich the understanding of Tourette's syndrome as a developmental, neuropsychiatric syndrome. As more is learned about the underlying neurobiology, we can look forward to the application of new knowledge to the field of therapeutics. Just as it has for the past century, we anticipate that Tourette's syndrome will continue to serve as a testing ground for new hypotheses about brain-behavior relations. As such, the findings of research in relation to Tourette's syndrome may help illuminate other complex clinical disorders, such as obsessive-compulsive disorder, attentional disorders, and learning disturbances.

One continuing controversy concerns the name of the syndrome. Probably *Gilles de la Tourette's Syndrome* would be most correct. Yet, *Tourette's syndrome* has achieved some popularity and we felt comfortable in using it throughout this Preface. In 1982, we opted for *Tourette syndrome* with some anxiety and received suitable letters of reprimand. However, this designation is concise and has a solid track record. Therefore, with apology to our French colleagues, and after soul searching, we will continue to use it in this volume.

A future volume in this series, in a decade or so from now, will no doubt provide an even more fascinating and deeper account of the neurobiology, natural history, and clinical care of individuals with Tourette syndrome. Those individuals and their families have been the true advocates of research in the field. They have supported the work of investigators, have volunteered for scientific studies, and have brought the needs of patients with Tourette syndrome to the attention of the scientific world. The research described in this volume is testimony to the remarkable achievements which can be realized when there is sustained, interdisciplinary and international collaboration among clinical and basic researchers and those most concerned about the care of individual patients.

Thomas N. Chase
Arnold J. Friedhoff
Donald J. Cohen

Acknowledgments

This volume is based on the Second International Scientific Symposium on Tourette Syndrome (TS) held in Boston, Massachusetts, in June, 1991. The Symposium was organized by an interdisciplinary committee that conceptualized the scope and nature of presentations (Drs. J. Coyle, G. Golden, R. Kurlan, M. Conneally, G. Erenberg, S. Koslow, A. Young and ourselves).

Far-sighted and generous funding was provided by the National Institute for Neurological Diseases and Stroke (NINDS), the National Institute of Mental Health (NIMH), and the Gateposts Foundation, Inc. The overall organization of the Symposium was under the administration of the Permanent Research Fund, Inc., of the Tourette Syndrome Association (TSA), which also provided direct financial support and motivation for the meeting as it has for many of the major advances reported in this volume.

We wish to offer special recognition for their participation in planning and supporting the Symposium to Susan Cimini of the TSA, Florence Diamond (New York University), Peter Jensen, M.D., and Eleanor D. Dibble, D. S. W. (NIMH), and Philip H. Sheridan, M. D. and Karen Skinner, Ph.D. (NINDS).

The history of research on Tourette's syndrome has been shaped by the powerful, positive influence of the major advocacy organization, the Tourette Syndrome Association. The Symposium and this volume are among the products of TSA's sustained efforts to merge advanced scientific research with clinical concerns. One individual stands out as the champion of this effort, Ms. Sue Levi-Pearl, TSA Liaison for Scientific and Medical programs. Among her many contributions to the field of Tourette syndrome research, she envisioned and coordinated the International Symposium.

ADVANCES IN NEUROLOGY

Volume 58

Advances in Neurology, Vol. 58, edited
by T. N. Chase, A. J. Friedhoff, and
D. J. Cohen. Raven Press, Ltd.,
New York © 1992.

1

The Natural History of Tourette Syndrome

Ruth Dowling Bruun and Cathy L. Budman

*Department of Psychiatry, North Shore University Hospital-Cornell Medical
Center, Manhasset, New York 11030*

Although Tourette syndrome (TS) was originally described more than a century ago, physicians took little interest in this disorder until the past 20 years. Previously, patients afflicted with TS were rarely diagnosed. They either managed to conceal most of their symptoms and got by, perhaps being considered nervous or eccentric, or they were subjected to a host of different but unproven treatments. Some of the more severely afflicted patients languished in chronic wards of mental hospitals for most of their lives. A few case histories were published describing the effects of varied psychiatric treatments.

In the 1960s the discovery that haloperidol could be an effective treatment for TS symptoms led to an increasing curiosity about the nature of this baffling condition. As neurologists and psychiatrists became interested in collecting scientific data on TS patients, the diagnosis was made more frequently. Still, by the early 1970s, few cases had been identified. Tourette syndrome (then still known as Gilles de la Tourette syndrome) was considered to be an extremely rare, esoteric condition. The largest sample at that time was a group of 34 patients, described extensively by A.K. and E.S. Shapiro et al. (1,2). While much was learned about TS from this early study, there was little awareness then that these

patients were representative of the more severe end of the TS spectrum. Consequently, the conclusion that this was a "chronic, lifelong illness" was not seriously questioned until the end of the 1970s (2,3).

In the 1980s, more rigorous scientific investigation provided a new perspective. Although there are still few studies on the natural course of TS over a long period of time, it is now clear that in many cases tic symptoms either remit completely or are considerably ameliorated when patients reach maturity.

In addition, there has been an increasing awareness of the existence of "associated symptoms" in TS patients. These non-tic symptoms may include other neuropsychiatric conditions such as obsessive–compulsive disorder (OCD), attention deficit hyperactivity disorder (ADHD), learning disabilities, and a variety of conduct and impulse control disorders. It remains to be clarified which of these associated problems are intrinsic to TS and which merely have a frequent comorbidity. Nonetheless, it is apparent that a comprehensive examination of the natural history of TS must include a consideration of these conditions as well as of simple and complex tics.

TICS

The onset and early progression of tics have been well studied. Large international patient studies are generally consistent in their description of the onset and evolution of these symptoms during childhood and adolescence. While the age of onset may occur anywhere between infancy and age 21 (even later in rare cases), the symptoms usually appear before the early teens, and the mean age of onset is 7 years (4). Simple tics are the most common first symptoms (50–70%), eye blinking being the most common of all (2,5). In a review of several large studies comprising a total of approximately 2,400 patients, 66% reported facial tics as their first symptom. Other motor tics were initial symptoms in 22%, the upper body being involved more often than the legs and trunk. Vocal tics occurred as initial symptoms in only 13%, and usually consisted of noises such as throat clearing, sniffing, grunting, and squeaking. Words were less common, and coprolalia was the presenting symptom in only 1.4% (4).

As the syndrome progresses, new symptoms will appear while previous ones may disappear. The condition spontaneously waxes and wanes; there may be periods, lasting from days to months, when all symptoms will remit. There will certainly be periods of tic amelioration, alternating with exacerbations.

On an hour to hour or even minute to minute basis stress produces an increased tendency to tic, while absorbed concentration causes an alleviation of tics. Relaxation may have a paradoxical effect. For example, when patients have been controlling their tics for a period of time and then are able to relax at home or in privacy, tics may actually increase in both frequency and intensity.

Physical stresses may also cause an increase in tic symptomatology. Premenstrual stress and exogenous stimulants such as caffeine, methylphenidate, and amphetamines have been implicated in tic exacerbation (4,6,7). As the syndrome progresses, complex tics become common occurrences. These may include complicated actions such as squatting and touching the ground or stereotypic, repetitive sequences of tics (e.g., touch nose, grimace, and whistle).

Coprolalia is generally a later occurring symptom appearing, on the average, 4–7 years after the onset of the syndrome and only in one-third or less of patients (1,4,8). There is some evidence that this symptom may be culturally influenced since studies from Japan indicate a far lower incidence of coprolalia (only 4% have "true coprolalia") than other countries (5).

Other symptoms such as dystonic movements, echokinesis, copropraxia, echolalia, palilalia, and other speech irregularities are fairly common as the syndrome develops into its fullest form. Symptoms such as coprographia and self-injurious tics are less common. A variety of subjective symptoms, which may not be reported by patients unless specifically asked about, may also occur. These include sensory tics (internal sensations that are premonitory to, or causative of, a motor or vocal tic), mental coprolalia, and mental palilalia (2,4,8,9).

During adolescence, although the symptoms may not be worse, they tend to be more unpredictable from day to day. Symptoms may be more problematic at this age, since this is a developmental phase when patients are particularly sensitive to peer acceptance. Consequently, teenagers may deny their symptoms or be less compliant about medication. Emotional lability may cause exacerbations of tic symptomatology, and coping difficulties may result in outbursts of anger, social withdrawal, or other problems that make treatment far more challenging for the physician.

Because relatively few patients have been followed for long periods of time and patients tend to be lost to follow-up as they improve, good data on the later course of tics has been difficult to collect. In 1987 Erenberg et al. (10) reported on anonymous questionnaire replies obtained from 58 patients (ages 15–25 years). Of this group 26% reported that their tics had almost disappeared, 47% felt that their tics were considerably lessened, 14% had remained essentially unchanged, and only 14% had experienced a worsening. The average age of the respondents was 18. The degree of maximum tic severity did not correlate with the degree of improvement.

A study done on Bruun's patients in 1988 also indicated a better prognosis than had been anticipated. Of 136 patients who had been followed from 5 to 15 years, 59% had been rated as mild to moderate (with respect to tics) when first evaluated. At follow-up, 91% were now rated in these categories. More than a quarter of these patients had discontinued medication and most others were on lower doses than they had originally required. As part of the same study 121 patients were questioned retrospectively about the course of their tics. Fifty-two percent stated that they had spontaneously improved, not because of treatment with medication. Thirty-six percent of these had first experienced improvement in their late teenage years, 9% in their early 20s, and another 5% in their late 20s or early 30s. Three patients noted significant remissions when they were in their 50s (4).

Nee and colleagues (11) also reported on a retrospective study of 30 adult TS patients. Forty percent of these patients rated their symptoms as worst during the first decade after their onset. Sixty-seven percent experienced improvement during the second decade and there was a gradual continuing improvement throughout life, with the exception of a slight worsening during the fourth decade.

Singer reviewed the courses of 120 of his patients. All patients initially rated as mild continued in this category. Seventy-one percent of those patients initially rated as moderate, 44% of those initially rated as moderately severe, and 18% of those initially rated as severe were now in the mild category. This would seem to indicate that milder symptoms lead to a better prognosis (Presentation to Clinical Symposium, Tourette Syndrome Association, 1985).

A demographic study done by Burd et al. (12) in North Dakota (1986) also indicates

that many patients must improve with maturity. An extensive study was undertaken in order to identify all cases of TS in the state. The prevalence rate of the disorder was found to be far greater in children (under age 19) than in adults. Projecting from their figures, these investigators estimated that there were approximately 33,000 children and only 8,000 adults in the United States who had TS by *Diagnostic and Statistical Manual*, 3rd ed. (DSM-III) criteria.

A review of these and other studies has led to a recent estimate that, considering the tic symptoms of TS, 30–40% of cases will remit completely by late adolescence; an additional 30% will show significant improvement in both frequency and severity of tics; and the remaining third will continue to be symptomatic in adulthood (8).

There are very little data on how symptomatology may change, if at all, as TS patients reach the geriatric age period. In a group of more than 700 of Bruun's patients, only 9 are over 70 years of age and only one of these is significantly symptomatic. Anecdotal reports indicate that elderly TS patients rarely exhibit anything but mild symptoms. This impression is supported by the notable dearth of reports in the literature on elderly TS patients. However, more investigation needs to be done in order to ascertain how old age affects the course of tics.

ASSOCIATED SYMPTOMATOLOGY

While the association of TS with obsessive–compulsive behaviors, ADHD learning disabilities, and a variety of conduct, impulse control, and affective disorders has received considerable attention in the past 10–15 years, there continues to be disagreement on the exact relationship these problems bear to TS. The natural history of these "associated symptoms" has not been studied systematically and is less well defined than the course of the tic disorder.

The relationship between ADHD and TS

has been studied extensively by Comings and Comings (7,13,14). They state that ADHD symptoms will precede the onset of tics by an average of 2.5 years, will reach a maximum severity at about 10 years of age, and will gradually recede through the teenage years and early 20s. Unfortunately, in most cases it is extremely difficult to pinpoint the onset of ADHD symptoms. However, there is a general consensus that 50% or more of TS patients will have symptoms of attention deficit disorder (6,8,15–17). These are often associated with so-called soft signs suggesting neuromaturational problems and, with more severe tics, predispose toward greater morbidity and more social impairment (2,8,14,16).

There is mounting evidence that obsessive–compulsive symptoms and/or OCD may be genetically related to Tourette syndrome and chronic tic disorder and may, in fact, represent alternative expressions of the same genetic vulnerability (18,19). While there is still some disagreement on the incidence of OCD in Tourette patients (reports vary between 11% and 90%), most investigators agree that the incidence is significantly higher than in the general population (11,20–25). The wide variations of incidence found by different investigators may have been caused by ambiguities in the distinctions between OCD and obsessive-compulsive symptoms and between complex tics and compulsions. The inclusion of varying age groups in different study samples may also have contributed to the differences in incidence (22).

Obsessive–compulsive symptomatology may begin in early childhood. One study by Singer and Rosenberg (23) found OC behavior in more than 40% of TS patients in the 6–10-year age group. However, as a rule in TS patients, OC symptoms begin somewhat later than tic symptoms and continue to progress at least into early adulthood (6,7, 13,24,25). There are some reports suggesting that OC symptoms may differ qualitatively in TS patients, being more commonly concerned with "evening-up" (especially both sides of the body), symmetry and arithromania (counting games), checking, and arranging than with other typical OCD concerns (22). There is also some evidence that OC symptoms in TS patients change in character with age, younger patients being more concerned with impulse control rituals while older patients are more concerned with checking, arranging, and a fear of contamination (26).

A diversity of other problems such as conduct disorders, aggressivity, depression, panic attacks and anxiety, withdrawal, inappropriate sexual behaviors, self-injurious behaviors, sleep disorders, and learning disabilities have been reported by various TS investigators (6,13,21–23,25, 27–31). However, there is a considerable controversy on the true incidence of these problems, and whether they can be meaningfully linked with TS. For example, while some investigators have found a correlation between tic severity and behavior problems, others have not (4,13,21,23,25).

In Erenberg et al.'s (10) follow-up study the patients themselves reported a fairly high incidence of associated problems. Sixty-two percent reported that they had experienced learning difficulties (evidenced by the need for extra help in school, the repetition of a grade, or the need for home tutoring), and 57% reported troubles with concentration. Severe mood swings were reported by 52%, extreme anxiety by 45%, severe temper outbursts by 41%, and obsessive–compulsive behaviors by 32%. These patients were, on the average, around the age when their tics had become less of a problem. Of the patients who reported both tics and behavioral/learning problems, 45% felt that the associated problems were causing greater interference in their lives than the tics.

Singer and Rosenberg (23) compared the incidence of behavioral/social problems in two groups of TS patients at different periods (6–11 and 12–16 years of age). They found that abnormal ratings on the Child Behavior Checklist were more common in the older group. While it has been suggested that associated ADHD rather than TS itself might be etiologically related to behavioral problems, this study found no higher rate of behavioral difficulties in a group of hyperactive children than in the TS children without hyperactivity.

Comings and Comings (6,7,13), who have written extensively on behavioral problems associated with TS, state that while tics tend to improve with age, associated problems arise in adolescence or later and tend to persist through adulthood. The Comings's studies described associated problems such as OCD, conduct disorders, inappropriate sexual behaviors, panic attacks and agoraphobia, alcoholism in males, and obesity due to compulsive eating in females.

Robertson et al. (21) and Trimble (25) have also reported significantly higher levels of depression, aggression, hostility and self-mutilating behavior in Tourette patients when compared with controls who had other movement disorders. Aggression, hostility, and obsessionality were found to be significantly associated with coprolalia, copropraxia, and echophenomena as well as with a family history of tics or TS. However, these investigators have repeatedly pointed to the likelihood of an ascertainment bias inherent in their patient samples.

In Bruun's patient group a large number of patients were referred for symptoms of aggression, hostility, and conduct disorders, more than 86% (74 of 86) being under the age of 20. Since these patients were selectively referred for their symptoms, no meaningful conclusions can be drawn regarding the incidence of these behaviors in the TS population. However, there was no apparent selection for age. While no systematic testing was done on these patients, clinical experience with their treatment indicates that there is definite improvement in their behavior when they become adults. While patients may continue to have hostile thoughts and impulses, as adults they are able to control these impulses far better.

Surprisingly, few of the adult patients seen by Bruun over the past 20 years have demonstrated serious problems with alcohol or drug abuse.

On the other hand, self-abusive behaviors, although fairly rare in this patient sample, appear to remain constant or even worsen as patients mature from adolescence into adulthood.

In conclusion, as more prospective studies are performed examining patients with milder forms of TS, a clearer profile of this disorder may become available. To date, the study of the natural history of TS has been severely compromised by the selective attention to more symptomatic and dysfunctional cases, which require ongoing, aggressive treatment. Milder cases, which may constitute the majority of TS patients, rarely present for psychiatric intervention. Thus, future efforts should involve larger studies of the course of symptoms in more mildly affected individuals.

Furthermore, the relationship and course of associated disorders such as OCD, ADHD, conduct disorders, and affective disturbances in TS patients remain to be defined. It appears that, while in most cases tic disorders per se improve over time, a significant number of patients continue to suffer profoundly from associated disorders as well as from the social sequelae of their childhood tics. In addition, potential physiological effects of medications used to treat TS may play an important role in altering or modifying the expression and evolution of TS symptoms.

New and important information about TS has accumulated over the past decades, yet its natural history remains enigmatic. Clearly, in many patients earlier symptoms of TS do not become chronic in nature. On the other hand, there appears to be at least a subpopulation of adult TS patients who retain many of their earlier symptoms or who acquire new and different symptoms over time. Identifying the evolution of TS symptoms, the precise relationship of related disorders, and the environmental influences that may modify the course of this illness pose exciting challenges for scientists and clinicians in this field.

REFERENCES

1. Shapiro AK, Shapiro ES, Wayne H, Clarkin J, Bruun RD. Tourette's syndrome: summary of data on 34 patients. *Psychosom Med* 193;5:419–35.
2. Shapiro AK, Shapiro ES, Bruun RD, Sweet RD. *Gilles de la Tourette syndrome.* New York: Raven Press, 1978.
3. Shapiro AK, Shapiro ES, Bruun RD, Sweet RD, Wayne H, and Solomon G. Gilles de la Tourette's syndrome: summary of clinical experience with 250 patients and suggested nomenclature for tic syndromes. In: Eldridge R, Fahn S, eds. *Advances in neurology*, vol 14. New York: Raven Press, 1976;277–83.
4. Bruun RD. The natural history of Tourette's syndrome. In: Cohen DJ, Bruun RD, Leckman JF, eds. *Tourette's syndrome and tic disorders: clinical understanding and treatment.* New York: John Wiley & Sons, 1988.
5. Nomura Y, Segawa M. Tourette syndrome in Oriental children: clinical and pathophysiological considerations. In: Friedhoff AJ, Chase TN, eds. *Gilles de la Tourette syndrome.* New York: Raven Press, 1982;277–80.
6. Comings DE, Comings BG. Tourette syndrome: clinical and psychological aspects of 250 cases. *Am J Hum Genet* 1985;37:435–50.
7. Comings DE. *Tourette syndrome and human behavior.* Duarte, CA: Hope Press, 1990.
8. Singer HS, Walkup JT. Tourette syndrome and other tic disorders. *Medicine* 1991;70:15–32.
9. Kurlan R, Lichter D, Hewitt D. Sensory tics in Tourette's syndrome. *Neurology* 1989;39:731–33.
10. Erenberg G, Cruse RP, Rothner AD. The natural history of Tourette syndrome. A follow-up study. *Ann Neurol* 1987;22:383–5.
11. Nee LE, Polinsky RJ, Ebert MH. Tourette syndrome: clinical and family studies. In: Friedhoff AJ, Chase TN, eds. *Gilles de la Tourette syndrome.* New York: Raven Press, 1982.
12. Burd L, Kerbeshian J, Wilkenheiser M, Fisher W. Prevalence of Gilles de la Tourette syndrome in North Dakota adults. *Am J Psychiatry* 1986; 143:787–8.
13. Comings DE, Comings BG. A controlled study of Tourette syndrome I–VII. *Am J Hum Gen* 1987; 41:701–866.
14. Comings DE, Comings BG. Tourette syndrome and attention deficit disorder. In: Cohen DJ, Bruun RD, Leckman JF, eds. *Tourette syndrome and tic disorders.* New York: John Wiley & Sons, 1988; 19–35.
15. Pauls DL, Hurst CR, Kruger SD, Leckman JF, Kidd KK, Cohen DJ. Gilles de la Tourette syndrome and attention deficit disorder with hyperactivity: evidence against a genetic relationship. *Arch Gen Psychiatry* 1986;43:1177–9.
16. Shapiro AK, Shapiro E, Young JG, Feinberg TE. *Gilles de la tourette syndrome*, 2nd ed. New York: Raven Press, 1988.
17. Nee LE, Caine ED, Plursky RJ, Eldridge R, Ebert MH. Gilles de la Tourette's syndrome. clinical and family study of 50 cases. *Ann Neurol* 1980;7:41–9.
18. Pauls DL, Leckman JF. The inheritance of Gilles de la Tourette's syndrome and associated behaviors. Evidence for autosomal dominant transmission. *N Engl J Med* 1886;315:993–7.
19. Pauls DC, Pakstis A, Kurlan R, et al. Segregation and linkage analysis of Tourette's syndrome and related disorders. *J Am Acad Child Adolesc Psychiatry* 1990;29:195–203.
20. Kelman DH. Gilles de la Tourette's disease in children: a review of the literature. *J Child Psychol Psychiatry* 1965;6:219–26.
21. Robertson M, Trimble MR, Lees AJ. The psychopathology of the Gilles de la Tourette syndrome: a phenomenological analysis. *Br J Psychiatry* 1988; 152:383–90.
22. Robertson MM. The Gilles de la Tourette syndrome: the current status. *Br J Psychiatry* 1989; 154:147–69.
23. Singer HS, Rosenberg LA. The development of behavioral and emotional problems in Tourette syndrome. *Pediatr Neurol* 1989;5:41–4.
24. Pitman RK, Gren RC, Jenicke MA, Mesullam MM. Clinical comparison of Tourette's disorder and obsessive-compulsive disorder. *Am J Psychiatry* 1987;144:1166–71.
25. Trimble M. Psychopathology and movement disorders: a new perspective on the Gilles de la Tourette syndrome. *J Neurol Neurosurg Psychiatry [Suppl]* 1989;90–5.
26. Frankel M, Cummings JL, Robetson MM, et al. Obsessions and compulsions in Gilles de la Tourette's syndrome. *Neurology* 1986;36:378–82.
27. Barabass G, Mathew WS, Ferrari M. Somnabulism in children with treatments in children with Tourette's Disorder. *Dev Med Child Neurol* 1984; 26:457–60.
28. Singer HS, Allan R, Brown J, Salam M, Hahn IH. Sleep disorders in Tourette syndrome: a primary or unrelated problem? (abstract) *Ann Neurol* 1990; 28:424.
29. Incagnoli T, Kane R. Neuropsychological functioning in Tourette syndrome. In: Friedhoff AJ, Chase TN, eds. *Gilles de la Tourette syndrome.* New York: Raven Press, 1982.
30. Hagin RA, Beecher R, Pagano G, Kreeger H. Effects of Tourette syndrome on learning. In: Friedhoff AJ, Chase TN, eds. *Gilles de la Tourette syndrome.* New York: Raven Press, 1982.
31. Hagin RA, Kugler J. School problems associated with Tourette's syndrome. In: Cohen DJ, Bruun RD, Leckman JF, eds. *Tourette's syndrome and tic disorders: clinical understanding and treatment.* New York: John Wiley & Sons, 1988.

Advances in Neurology, Vol. 58, edited
by T. N. Chase, A. J. Friedhoff, and
D. J. Cohen. Raven Press, Ltd.,
New York © 1992.

2

Diagnosis and Classification of Tics and Tourette Syndrome

Joseph Jankovic

Department of Neurology, Baylor College of Medicine, Houston, Texas 77030

Once considered a rare psychiatric curiosity, Tourette syndrome (TS) is now recognized as a relatively common neurologic disorder characterized by unwanted movements and noises and by a variety of behavioral abnormalities, including obsessive–compulsive behavior (OCD) and attention deficit hyperactivity disorder (ADHD). As a result of mounting evidence in support of a neurologic origin for the disorder, the attitude toward patients with TS has changed, and their symptoms are becoming more acceptable in school and work environments. Despite this remarkable progress, both in terms of scientific knowledge and social adaptation, the diagnosis is still frequently missed and made not by physicians, but by patients, parents, and teachers who learn about TS from the lay media. The purpose of this review is to provide a

framework for a better understanding of this complex neurobehavioral disorder and to facilitate early diagnosis and proper treatment. In the absence of a disease-specific biological marker, the diagnosis rests on the recognition of typical symptoms and signs. Therefore, recognizing the full spectrum of phenomenology is critical to making a correct diagnosis, selecting the most appropriate therapy, and encouraging a more compassionate attitude toward those with TS.

CLASSIFICATION OF MOVEMENTS

To understand better the categorization of tics and how they fit into the general schema of movement disorders, it is helpful to begin with a simple classification of movements (Table 1). Most movements in the repertoire of normal human behavior occur without any conscious effort and can be classified as *automatic*. They consist of learned motor acts, such as walking, speaking, and chewing. Extracellular recordings from the globus pallidus of monkeys suggest that this portion of the basal ganglia is involved in generating internal cues for automatic movements (1). The pallidal output is directed via thalamus to the supplementary motor area (SMA), which seems to be primarily concerned with the programming of sequences of movements. In contrast, the

TABLE 1. *Movements*

Automatic
  Learned, performed without conscious effort
Voluntary
  Intentional (planned, self-initiated)
  Responsive (induced by external stimulus)
Unvoluntary (semivoluntary)
  Induced by an inner sensory stimulus
  Induced by an unwanted feeling/compulsion
Involuntary
  Nonsuppressible (reflexes, seizures, myoclonus)
  Suppressible (tics, tremor, dystonia, chorea, stereotypy)

premotor area (PMA) appears to be involved with the selection of a movement plan based on external cues. Thus the motor system is organized according to the nature of the movement; the pallidum (and possibly the cerebellum) seems to be involved in motor learning and execution of automatic movements. *Voluntary* movements can be classified as either intentional (planned and self-induced) or responsive (generated in response to an external stimulus). A quick turn of the head in the direction of a sudden loud noise, closing the eyes to shut out bright light or withdrawing a hand from hot water are examples of externally induced voluntary movements. Papa et al. (2), studied these two types of voluntary movement using a back-averaging technique to record the readiness potential or Bereitschaftpotential (BP) in 12 normal volunteers. A surface-negative, slow wave potential was recorded an average of 1.3 ± 0.2 seconds before the onset of self-initiated movement in all subjects. When the same movements were triggered by external stimuli, such as electrical stimulation of the index finger, a brief flash of a light-emitting diode, and a click, the BP was not seen. This finding suggests that the BP represents a neurophysiologic correlate of cognitive processes, possibly originating in the SMA, associated with self-induced voluntary movements. *Unvoluntary* or *semivoluntary* movements are those that occur in response to some irresistable internal sensory stimulus, such as the need to "stretch" the neck or arm. Unvoluntary movements may also occur in response to unwanted feelings or compulsions. These are usually more complex and include compulsive, repetitive touching or smelling. *Involuntary* movements are categorized as either nonsuppressible (e.g., reflexes, seizures, and myoclonus) or suppressible (e.g., tics, tremor, dystonia, chorea, and stereotypies). Some tics are clearly involuntary, more or less suppressible, while others, particularly certain complex tics, seem semipurposeful (unvoluntary); yet others are voluntary. In addition, some patients utilize voluntary ("pseudovoluntary") movements to "camouflage" their tics or to incorporate tics into a seemingly purposeful activity ("parakinesia").

PHENOMENOLOGY AND DIFFERENTIAL DIAGNOSIS

Tics are relatively brief and intermittent movements (motor tics) or sounds (vocal tics) (3). While currently accepted criteria require both types of tics to be present for the diagnosis of TS (4–6), this division into motor and vocal tics seems artificial. Vocal tics are actually motor tics involving respiratory, laryngeal, pharyngeal, oral, and nasal musculature. Contractions of these muscles may produce sounds by moving air through the nose, mouth, or throat. The sudden occurrence of movements and sounds out of a background of normal activity helps differentiate tics from other hyperkinesias such as chorea and dystonia, which are continual. Paroxysmal dyskinesias are intermittent, usually consisting of brief episodes of chorea, dystonia, or both and hence are easily distinguishable from tics (7). Exaggerated startle response (hyperekplexia) rarely presents a diagnostic problem, because this myoclonic movement occurs in response to some stimulus that is often specific for that affected individual (8).

Tics can be classified as either *simple* or *complex* (Table 2). Simple tics involve only one group of muscles, causing a brief, iso-

TABLE 2. *Differential diagnosis of tics*

Classification	Differential diagnosis
Simple tics	
Clonic	Myoclonus
	Chorea
	Seizures
Tonic or dystonic	Dystonia
	Athetosis
Complex tics	Mannerisms
	Stereotypies
	Restless legs
	Seizures

lated, jerk-like movement or a single, meaningless sound. Examples of simple motor tics include an eyeblink, nose twitch, head jerk, and shoulder shrug. Simple vocal tics typically consist of sniffing, throat clearing, grunting, squeaking, screaming, coughing, blowing, and sucking sounds. *Complex motor tics* consist of coordinated, sequenced movements resembling normal motor acts or gestures that are inappropriately intense and timed. They may be seemingly nonpurposeful, such as head shaking or trunk bending, or they may seem purposeful, such as touching, throwing, hitting, jumping, and kicking. Additional examples of complex motor tics include gesturing "the finger" and grabbing or exposing one's genitalia (copropraxia) or imitating gestures (echopraxia). Complex vocal tics include linguistically meaningful utterances and verbalization, such as shouting of obscenities or profanities (coprolalia), repetition of someone else's words or phrases (echolalia) and repetition of one's own utterances or phrases (palilalia). Complex motor tics may resemble mannerisms which are complex motor acts or sounds that are peculiar to the individual and are habitually and automatically performed in certain situations. Examples of mannerisms include ritualistic self-touching by a baseball pitcher before throwing the ball, tongue protruding and lip biting during physical exertion, facial grimacing when singing, abducting–adducting leg movements, repetitive dangling of crossed legs, and habitual finger or foot tapping. Mannerisms should be differentiated from gestures that are normal, culturally determined expressive movements, such as hand gesticulations used to add emphasis to speaking.

Tics may be classified according to their duration and movement characteristics into *clonic*, *tonic*, or *dystonic* (Table 2). Clonic tics are produced by abrupt and brief (<100 msec) muscle contractions, whereas tonic and dystonic tics represent more sustained (>300 msec) contractions. Tonic tics consist of isometric contractions of muscles without accompanying movement, such as limb or abdominal muscle tensing. Dystonic tics are manifested by twisting, squeezing, or other movements and abnormal postures. Examples of dystonic tics include oculogyric deviations, blepharospasm, bruxism, sustained mouth opening, torticollis, and rotatory movements of the shoulder. To characterize clonic and dystonic tics further, we studied 156 patients with TS; 89 (57%) exhibited dystonic tics, including oculogyric deviations (28%), blepharospasm (15%), and dystonic neck movements (7%) (9). Since patients with dystonic tics did not significantly differ in any clinical variables from those with only clonic tics, we concluded that, despite previous reports, the presence of dystonic tics should not be considered atypical or unusual. We have treated some of these patients (with disabling, repetitive, dystonic tics) successfully with botulinum toxin injections in the eyebrows, eyelids, and facial and neck muscles (Table 3) (10).

Dystonic tics should be distinguished from persistent dystonia, typically seen in patients with idiopathic torsion dystonia. Intermittent ocular deviations, phenomenologically similar to ocular tics, have been

TABLE 3. *Botulinum toxin injections for tics*

Pt. no./sex/age	Site of injection[a]	Dosage/session (mouse units)	Peak effect (0–4)	Duration (weeks)
1/M/16	B, L	40	3.2	17
2/M/20	C	82	3.8	16
3/M/53	B, F	45	4.0	20

[a] B, eyebrow; C, cervical muscles; F, frontalis; L, eyelid; M, male.
[b] Peak effect: 0 to 4 rating; 0, no response; 4, marked or complete resolution of spasms (10).

reported in patients with encephalitis lethargica and tardive dyskinesia (11). The presence of clonic or dystonic tics in patients with torsion dystonia is relatively rare, but may occur more frequently than in the general population. We reported nine patients, and have studied many additional cases, with coexistent TS and persistent dystonia (12). Tics began at an average age of 9 years, and dystonia followed the onset of tics by an average of 22 (10–38) years. Several other studies have suggested that tics and persistent dystonia coexist with higher than expected frequency (13,14). However, because tics are relatively common, properly designed epidemiologic studies will be needed before it can be concluded that the two disorders are in some way pathogenically related.

When complex tics become repetitive and patterned, they may resemble stereotypies (15). These repetitive, coordinated, seemingly purposeful or ritualistic movements, postures, or utterances are more typically seen in mentally retarded and autistic children (16), schizophrenics (even before they are exposed to neuroleptics), and patients with tardive dyskinesia. Stereotypies, such as continuous orofacial chewing or body rocking movements, represent the most frequent type of hyperkinesia in tardive dyskinesia (17). The term *akathisia* is used to describe stereotypic movements associated with an inner feeling of restlessness and an inability to be still (18). Stereotypic movements are also characteristically present in patients with restless legs syndrome, who are forced to move constantly in order to relieve unpleasant sensations in their legs and other body parts (19).

Tics are characteristically associated with feelings or sensations that immediately precede the movement or sound and are typically relieved, albeit temporarily, by their execution (Table 3). These *premonitory symptoms* may be localized sensations or discomforts, such as "burning feeling" in the eye before an eye blink, a "tension or crick in the neck" relieved by stretching of the neck or jerking of the head, "feeling of tightness or constriction" relieved by arm or leg extension, "nasal stuffiness" before a sniff, "dry or sore throat" before a grunt, "itching" before a shoulder shrug, and others. Alternatively, the premonitory phenomenon may be a nonlocalized and poorly characterized feeling, such as an urge, anxiety, anger, or other psychic sensations. The observed movements or sounds sometimes occur in response to these premonitory phenomena and have been previously referred to as sensory tics (2–22). Because they are not purely voluntary (wanted, planned, or intended) and are often suppressible, they are sometimes regarded as voluntary (intentionally produced), semivoluntary, or unvoluntary (22). In one study of 60 patients with tic disorders, 41 (68%) thought that all their tics were intentionally produced, and 15 (25%) additional patients had both voluntary and involuntary movements; thus 93% of the tics were perceived to be "irresistibly but purposefully executed" (22). Although this is probably an overestimate, the "intentional" component of the movement may be a useful feature differentiating tics from other hyperkinetic movement disorders. Complex motor tics may be difficult to differentiate from compulsions, which frequently accompany tics, particularly in TS. We consider a complex, repetitive movement a compulsion when it is preceded or accompanied by a feeling of anxiety or panic. This anxious feeling may be associated with an irresistible urge to perform the movement or sound and a fear of something "bad" happening if it is not promptly or properly executed. In contrast to tics, the performance of a compulsive act is neither satisfying nor pleasurable. However, the distinction between a complex tic and a compulsion is not always possible, particularly when the patient is unable to describe the premonitory or associated feelings.

Tics are more suppressible than the other hyperkinetic movement disorders (23,24) (Table 4). They are also characterized by suggestibility and exacerbation by stress

TABLE 4. *Differential diagnosis of tics*

Characteristics of tics	Differential diagnosis
Abrupt	Myoclonus
	Chorea
	Hyperekplexia
	Paroxysmal dyskinesia
	Seizures
Premonitory	Stereotypy (akathisia)
symptoms (urge →	Restless legs
relief)	Dystonia
Suppressibility	All hyperkinesias (most
	typical in tics)
Decrease with	Akathisia
distraction *and*	Psychogenic
concentration	hyperkinesias
Decrease during	Chorea
skilled tasks	
Increase with stress	Most hyperkinesias
Increase with	(Parkinsonian tremor)
relaxation after a	
period stress	
Multifocal, migratory	Chorea
	Myoclonus
Fluctuate	Paroxysmal dyskinesias
spontaneously	Seizures
Present during sleep	Myoclonus (segmental)
	Periodic movements
	Painful legs/moving toes
	Other hyperkinesias
	Seizures

and during poststress relaxation. Many patients note a reduction in their tics when they are distracted by concentrating on mental or physical tasks, while others have increased frequency and intensity of their tics when distracted (particularly when they no longer have the need to suppress). Fluctuation in frequency, intensity, and distribution is another typical feature of tics. Although most hyperkinetic movement disorders decrease or completely disappear during sleep (25), tics have been demonstrated to persist during all stages of sleep (26). In 34 polysomnographic studies, we documented motor tics in 23 and vocal tics in 4 patients during all stages of sleep (27).

PATHOPHYSIOLOGY

Although the pathophysiologic mechanisms of tics and TS are still unknown, the weight of evidence supports an organic rather than psychogenic origin. Despite the observation that some tics may be voluntary, physiologic studies suggest that tics are not generally mediated through normal motor pathways utilized for willed movements. Using back-averaging techniques, Obeso et al. (28) observed a normal BP in six subjects who voluntarily simulated tic-like movements, but no such premovement electroencephalographic potential was noted in association with an actual tic. This finding has been interpreted as evidence for the involuntary nature of tics. Some authors contend, however, that certain tics may start as voluntary movements and if they are performed repeatedly they eventually become automatic and generated through subcortical pathways; hence they are not preceded by BP (1,21). Further studies are needed to resolve the question of the degree to which tics are voluntary versus involuntary. In addition to exploring the physiological mechanisms of motor tics, further studies are needed to improve our understanding of the premonitory symptoms and to unravel the complex relationships between motor and behavioral expressions of the genetic defect.

One of the major concerns with genetic linkage studies, which have already excluded over 80% of the genome, has been the lack of specificity of the current clinical criteria for diagnosis of TS (Table 5). The boundaries of neurologic and behavioral manifestations of TS have not been clearly defined. Some investigators believe that the spectrum of behavioral expression of the TS gene is quite broad, encompassing (in addition to ADHD and OCD) such diverse symptoms as conduct disorders, stuttering, dyslexia, panic attacks, phobias, depression, mania, and severe anxiety (29,30). Others argue that more restrictive criteria are needed, particularly for genetic linkage studies (31). Pauls et al. (32), studying 338 biological relatives of 86 TS probands and comparing them with 21 biologically unrelated relatives of adopted TS probands, recently confirmed their earlier observations

TABLE 5. *Diagnostic criteria for tic disorders[a]*

A-1. Definite Tourette syndrome
1. Both multiple motor and one or more phonic tics have been present at some time during the illness, although not necessarily concurrently
2. The tics occur many times a day, nearly every day, or intermittently throughout a period of more than one year
3. The anatomic location, number, frequency, type, complexity, or severity of tics change over time
4. Onset before age 21
5. Involuntary movements and noises cannot be explained by other medical conditions
6. Motor and/or phonic tics must be witnessed by a reliable examiner directly at some point during the illness or be recorded by videotape or cinematography

A-2. Tourette syndrome by history
1.–5. Same as A-1.
6. Tics were not witnessed by a reliable examiner, but tics were witnessed by a reliable family member or a close friend, and description of tics as demonstrated is acceptable by a reliable examiner

B-1. Definite chronic multiple motor (phonic) tic disorder
1. Either multiple motor or phonic tics, but not both, have been present at some time during illness
2.–6. Same as A-1

B-2. Chronic multiple motor (phonic) tic disorder by history
1.–5. Same as B-1
6. Tics were not witnessed by a reliable examiner, but tics were witnessed by a reliable family member or a close friend, and description of tics as demonstrated is acceptable by a reliable examiner

C. Chronic single tic disorder
1. Same as B-1 and B-2, but with a single motor or phonic tic

D-1. Definitie transient tic disorder
1. Single or multiple motor and/or phonic tics
2. The tics occur many times a day, nearly every day for at least 2 weeks, but for no longer than 12 consecutive months
3. The anatomic location, number, frequency, complexity, and severity of tics change over time
4. No history of Tourette syndrome or chronic or phonic tic disorders
5. Onset before age 21
6. Motor and/or phonic tics must be witnessed by a reliable examiner directly at some time during the illness or by videotape or cinematography

D-2. Transient tic disorder by history
1.–5. Same as D-1
6. Tics were not witnessed by a reliable examiner, but tics were witnessed by a reliable family member or a close friend, and description of tics as demonstrated is acceptable by a reliable examiner

E-1. Definite nonspecific tic disorder

E-2. Nonspecific tic disorder by history

F. Definite tic disorder, diagnosis deferred

G. Probable Tourette syndrome
Type 1. Meets all criteria for A-1, except 3 and/or 4
Type 2. Meets all criteria for A-1, except 1; includes either single motor tic with phonic tics or multiple motor tics with possible phonic tic(s)

[a] The Tourette's Syndrome Study Group, 1989.

that TS and OCD are etiologically related. Other family studies also provided evidence that transient and chronic tic disorders are etiologically related to TS (33). The debate whether TS is genetically related to OCD and ADHD, or whether these or some other comorbid behavioral disorders can be the sole manifestations of TS, will not be resolved until a TS-specific genetic marker is found. In order to facilitate the genetic link-age studies the full spectrum of tics has to be recognized and precise criteria must be defined.

Finding a genetic marker and ultimately the gene will be helpful not only in improving our understanding of this complex neurobehavioral disorder, but also in clarifying the epidemiology of TS. Because the clinical criteria are not well defined, the reported prevalence rates for TS range between 1/

TABLE 6. *Classification of tics*

I. Physiologic tics
   A. Mannerisms
   B. Gestures
II. Pathologic tics
   A. Primary (idiopathic)
      1. Chronic motor *or* vocal tics
      2. Transient motor *or* vocal tics
   B. Inherited
      1. Tourette syndrome
      2. Huntington's disease
      3. Torsion dystonia
      4. Neuroacanthocytosis
      5. Other
   C. Secondary tics or "Tourettism"
      1. Infections: encephalitis, Creutzfeldt-Jakob disease, Sydenham's chorea
      2. Drugs: stimulants, levodopa, anticonvulsants, dopamine receptor blocking drugs
      3. Toxins: carbon monoxide
      4. Static encephalopathy and mental and developmental retardation
      5. Other: head trauma, stroke, neurocutaneous syndromes, chromosomal abnormalities, schizophrenia, degenerative disorders

100 and 1/10,000 (5). Since about a third of patients with tics do not even recognize their presence (34), it is difficult to derive more accurate prevalence figures for TS without a well-designed door-to-door survey. While TS is the most frequent cause of tics, there are many other neurologic disorders manifested by tics (Table 6) (35).

REFERENCES

1. Brotchie P, Iansek R, Horne MK. Motor function of the monkey globus pallidus. 2. Cognitive aspects of movement and phasic neuronal activity. *Brain* 1990;114:1685–702.
2. Papa SM, Artieda J, Obeso JA. Cortical activity preceeding self-initiated and externally triggered voluntary movement. *Mov Disord* 1991;6:217–24.
3. Jankovic J, Fahn S. The phenomenology of tics. *Mov Disord* 1986;1:17–26.
4. Robertson MM. The Gilles de la Tourette syndrome: the current status. *Br J Psychiatry* 1989;154:147–69.
5. Golden GS. Tourette syndrome: recent advances. *Neurol Clin* 1990;8:705–14.
6. Singer HS, Walkup JT. Tourette syndrome and other tic disorders. Diagnosis, pathophysiology, and treatment. *Medicine* 1991;70:15–32.
7. Fahn S. Paroxysmal dyskinesias. In: Marsden CD, Fahn S, eds. *Movement disorders*, vol 3. London: Butterworth Scientific, 1992 (in press).
8. Brown P, Rothwell JC, Thompson PD, et al. The hyperekplexias and their relationship to the normal startle reflex. *Brain* 1991;114:1903–28.
9. Jankovic J, Stone L. Dystonic tics in patients with Tourette's syndrome. *Mov Disord* 1991;6:248–52.
10. Jankovic J, Brin MF. Therapeutic uses of botulinum toxin. *N Engl J Med* 1991;324:1186–94.
11. FitzGerald P, Jankovic J. Tardive oculogyric crises. *Neurology* 1989;39:1434–37.
12. Stone L, Jankovic J. The coexistence of tics and dystonia. *Arch Neurol* 1991;48:862–5.
13. Lees AJ, Robertson M, Trimble MR, Murray NMF. A clinical study of Gilles de la Tourette syndrome in the United Kingdom. *J Neurol Neurosurg Psychiatry* 1984;47:1–8.
14. Elston JS, Granje FC, Lees AJ. The relationship between eye-winking tics, frequent eye blinking and blepharospasm. *J Neurol Neurosurg Psychiatry* 1989;52:477–80.
15. Jankovic J. Stereotypies. In: Marsden CD, Fahn S, eds. *Movement disorders*, vol 3. London: Butterworth Scientific, 1992 (in press).
16. FitzGerald PM, Jankovic J, Glaze DG, Schultz R, Percy AK. Extrapyramidal involvement in Rett's syndrome. *Neurology* 1990;40:293–5.
17. Stacy M, Jankovic J. Tardive stereotypy. (in press).
18. Burke RE, Kang UJ, Jankovic J, Miller LG, Fahn S. Tardive akathisia: an analysis of clinical features and response to open therapeutic trials. *Mov Disord* 1989;4:157–75.
19. Walters AS, Hening WA, Chokroverty S. Review and videotape recognition of idiopathic restless legs syndrome. *Mov Disord* 1991;6:105–10.
20. Kurlan R, Lichter D, Hewitt D. Sensory tics in Tourette's syndrome. *Neurology* 1989;39:731–4.
21. Lang AE. Clinical phenomenology of tic disorders: selected aspects. In: Chase T, Friedhoff A, Cohen DJ, eds. Tourette's syndrome. Advances in Neurology, vol 58. New York: Raven Press, 1992.
22. Lang A. Patient perception of tics and other movement disorders. *Neurology* 1991;41:223–8.
23. Koller WC, Biary NM. Volitional control of involuntary movements. *Mov Disord* 1989;4:153–6.
24. Walters AS, McHale D, Sage JI, et al. A blinded study of the suppressibility of involuntary movements in Huntington's chorea, tardive dyskinesia, and L-dopa-induced chorea. *Clin Neuropharmacol* 1990;13:236–40.
25. Fish DR, Sawyers D, Allen PJ, et al. The effect of sleep on the dyskinetic movements of Parkinson's disease, Gilles de la Tourette syndrome, Huntington's disease, and torsion dystonia. *Arch Neurol* 1991;48:210–4.
26. Glaze DG, Frost JD, Jankovic J. Sleep in Gilles de la Tourette's syndrome: disorder of arousal. *Neurology* 1983;33:586–92.
27. Jankovic J, Rohaidy H. Motor, behavioral and pharmacologic findings in Tourette's syndrome. *Can J Neurol Sci* 1987;14:541–6.

28. Obeso JA, Rothwell JC, Marsden CD. The neurophysiology of Tourette syndrome. *Adv Neurol* 1982;35:105–14.

29. Comings DE. A controlled study of Tourette syndrome, VII. Summary: a common genetic disorder causing disinhibition of the limbic system. *Am J Hum Genet* 1987;41:839–66.

30. Comings DE, Comings BG. A controlled study of Tourette syndrome—revisited. *Am J Hum Genet* 1988;43:209–17.

31. Pauls DL, Cohen DJ, Kidd KK, Leckman JF. Tourette syndrome and neuropsychiatric disorders: is there a genetic relationship? *Am J Hum Genet* 1988;43:206–9.

32. Pauls DL, Raymond CL, Stevenson JM, Leckman JF. A family study of Gilles de la Tourette syndrome. *Am J Hum Genet* 1991;48:154–63.

33. Kurlan R, Behr J, Medved L, Como P. Transient tic disorder and the clinical spectrum of Tourette's syndrome. *Arch Neurol* 1988;45:1200–1.

34. Kurlan R, Behr J, Medved L, et al. Severity of Tourette's syndrome in one large kindred: implications for determination of disease prevalence rate. *Arch Neurol* 1987;44:268–9.

35. Jankovic J. Tics in other neurologic disorders. In: Kurlan R, ed. *Handbook of Tourette's syndrome and related tic and behavioral disorders*. New York: Marcel Dekker, 1992 (in press).

Advances in Neurology, Vol. 58, edited by T. N. Chase, A. J. Friedhoff, and D. J. Cohen. Raven Press, Ltd., New York © 1992.

3

Pathogenesis of Tourette Syndrome

Clues from the Clinical Phenotype and Natural History

James F. Leckman, David L. Pauls, Bradley S. Peterson, Mark A. Riddle, George M. Anderson, and Donald J. Cohen

Child Study Center, Yale University School of Medicine, New Haven, Connecticut 06510

A decade ago Cohen et al. (1982) (1) described Tourette syndrome as an "exemplary neuropsychiatric disorder of childhood," and pointed to the likely etiological importance of interactions among genetic, neurophysiological, mental, behavioral, and environmental factors over the course of central nervous system (CNS) development. Although the precise pathogenic mechanisms responsible for the development of Tourette syndrome and other tic disorders remain unknown, advances of the past decade have served to reinforce the need to incorporate these factors in any explanatory model.

In this chapter, a model of the pathogenesis of Tourette syndrome and etiologically related disorders is presented and discussed with reference to current knowledge. Beyond this, the chapter focuses on the value of closely examining the phenomenology and natural history of Tourette syndrome, using the premonitory urges and the marked gender differences in phenotypic expression as examples, in order to generate questions that can be addressed by interdisciplinary studies in the context of this model of pathogenesis.

A MODEL OF PATHOGENESIS

The proposed model consists of four interrelated areas: phenomenology and natural history, genetic factors; epigenetic and environmental factors; and neurobiological substrates. Figure 1 depicts these areas and their interactions. This model provides a heuristic framework for understanding much of the ongoing research in this field.

Phenomenology and Natural History

Tourette syndrome is a chronic neuropsychiatric disorder of childhood onset characterized by tics that wax and wane in severity and an array of behavioral problems including some forms of obsessive–compulsive disorder (2). The range of symptoms is enormous and includes motor and phonic tics (sudden repetitive movements, gestures, or utterances that typically mimic some aspect of the normal behavioral repertoire) and obsessions and compulsions (sudden repetitive thoughts, images or urges to action that are intrusive and difficult to resist). Less well appreciated are the sensorimotor phenomena that frequently accompany tics

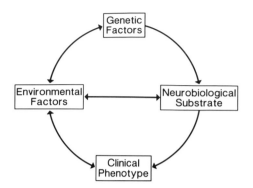

FIG. 1. Pathogenesis of tic disorders. Interactions among genetic factors, neurobiological substrates, and environmental factors in the production of the clinical phenotypes. The genetic vulnerability factor(s) that underlie Tourette syndrome and other tic disorders undoubtedly influence(s) the structure and function of the brain, which in turn produces clinical symptoms. Available evidence (see text) indicates that a range of epigenetic or environmental factors are also critically involved in the pathogenesis of these disorders. In addition, symptoms of the disorder can affect and alter aspects of the microenvironment of the brain, which in turn may alter the expression of the genetic factor(s).

(3–5) and compulsions. These experiences include premonitory feelings or urges that are relieved with the performance of the act, and a "need" to perform tics or compulsions until they are felt to be "just right."

A significant proportion of individuals with Tourette syndrome within clinic populations also present with attentional difficulties and impulsive and disruptive behaviors that often overshadow the tic symptoms as sources of impairment for the child and distress for the family (6–9). Epidemiologically based natural history studies are needed to describe better the longitudinal course of Tourette syndrome and to explore fully the relationship between Tourette syndrome and a range of possible comorbid conditions such as attention deficit hyperactivity disorder.

In their most extreme forms, Tourette syndrome and obsessive–compulsive disorder are lifelong conditions that are chroni-

cally disabling. Once thought to be a rare condition, the prevalence of Tourette syndrome is now estimated to be between one and six cases/1,000 boys; milder variants of the syndrome are likely to occur in 2–10% of the population (10–12). Clinically significant obsessive–compulsive disorder is also a relatively common condition in children and adolescents, affecting at a minimum 1 in 200 teenagers (13). A recent study also suggests that obsessive–compulsive disorder may affect as many as 2–3% of adults at some point in their lifetime (14).

Genetic Factors

Twin studies indicate that genetic factors play an important role in the transmission and expression of Tourette syndrome and related phenotypes (15,16). Specifically, monozygotic (MZ) twin pairs have been found to be highly concordant for Tourette syndrome (53%), and if other tic disorders are included, the overall concordance for the MZ pairs is substantially higher (>75%) (16). The concordance of same-sex dizygotic twin pairs is much lower (8% for Tourette syndrome or 23% if other tic disorders are included). These concordance figures are consistent with a genetic etiology with variable phenotypic expression. Twin and family studies also provide evidence that some forms of obsessive–compulsive disorder may be etiologically related to Tourette syndrome (15–18).

Using mathematical models of genetic transmission, the distribution of affected individuals within families follows a pattern consistent with an autosomal dominant form of transmission using either a broad or narrow definition of the affected phenotype (17). This finding, coupled with recent advances in human genetics, has led directly to the initiation of genetic linkage studies and eventually to the formation of an international collaboration, all in an effort to identify the chromosomal location of the putative Tourette syndrome gene.

The potential benefits of detecting linkage to a chromosomal region are many and include improved diagnostic capability, the identification of high-risk individuals, and the potential for using molecular genetic techniques to identify the Tourette syndrome vulnerability gene itself and to unravel the pathophysiology of these related disorders from their source. Thus far, more than 80% of the genome has been excluded (19,20), and the search continues.

Advances in molecular neurobiology also make this a propitious time to search for the putative Tourette syndrome vulnerability gene. Numerous candidate genes, such as the family of dopamine receptors, are being characterized (21). In addition, it is now possible to use highly efficient polymerase chain reaction (PCR) techniques to generate linkage data (22).

Epigenetic or Environmental Factors

Studies of monozygotic twins in which one member of the twin pair has been found to have more severe tic or obsessive–compulsive symptoms than the genetically identical cotwin also indicate that epigenetic or environmental factors play an important role in mediating the extent to which the genetic vulnerability to Tourette syndrome and related disorders is expressed (15,16). Apart from gender (males are three to four times more likely than females to develop Tourette syndrome), other epigenetic factors that mediate expression have not been unequivocally identified. Possible candidates include adverse perinatal events (23–25); exposure to chronic intermittent psychosocial stress (24); exposure to thermal stress (26); exposure to androgenic steroids (27); and exposure to cocaine (28) or other CNS stimulants (29).

The prospects for being able to identify specific or nonspecific risk and/or protective factors will be greatly enhanced when the Tourette syndrome vulnerability gene has been mapped. By selecting biologically homogenous high-risk carriers, investigators will be able to control for a significant portion of the biological variance so that detecting effects of a risk or protective factor will be more readily accomplished. It should also be noted that the successful identification of risk and/or protective factors may lead directly to early interventions that will limit, if not prevent, clinically significant forms of Tourette syndrome and obsessive–compulsive disorder.

Neurobiological Substrates

There is a substantial body of data that implicates the basal ganglia and related cortical and thalamic structures in the pathobiology of Tourette syndrome and obsessive–compulsive disorder (30). These data include the ameliorative effects on tic behaviors following neurosurgical lesions to thalamic nuclei (31–33) and following procedures that isolate regions of the prefrontal cortex (34–36).

Recent positron emission tomography (PET) studies have demonstrated decreased regional metabolic activity in frontal, cingulate, and insular cortices in Tourette syndrome subjects (37). In contrast, subjects with obsessive–compulsive disorder appear to have increased regional metabolic activity in the caudate nuclei (38,39) and a variety of cortical areas (orbital, prefrontal, cingulate, and sensorimotor) (38–41). Magnetic resonance imaging (MRI) studies are now being conducted with Tourette syndrome and obsessive–compulsive disorder subjects, and the preliminary data are suggestive of volume differences in the basal ganglia (Denkla, personal communication, 1991; Peterson, personal communication, 1992).

Functionally, the basal ganglia are composed of pathways that contribute to the multiple parallel cortico-striato-thalamo-cortical (CSTC) circuits that concurrently subserve a wide variety of sensorimotor, motor, oculomotor, cognitive and ''limbic'' processes (42,43). We have hypothesized that Tourette syndrome and etiologically related forms of obsessive–compulsive disorder are associated with a failure to inhibit subsets of CSTC minicircuits (44). Based on this hypothesis, we anticipate that the frequently encountered tics involving the face would be associated with a failure of inhibition of those minicircuits that include the ventromedian areas of the caudate and putamen that receive topographic projections from the orofacial regions of the primary motor and premotor cortex. Using similar logic, we and others (45) anticipate that obsessions with aggressive and sexual themes would be associated with a failure to inhibit portions of the limbic minicircuits, while the counting obsessions and the obsessive need for symmetry and exactness result from a failure to inhibit prefrontal minicircuits.

Although the neurophysiologic defect that underlies Tourette syndrome and etiologically related conditions remains unknown, a more complete understanding of these disorders may well illuminate some of the mechanisms that regulate the activity of the multiple parallel CSTC circuits that subserve much of our normal cognitive, behavioral, and emotive repertoire.

Among the most remarkable developments in the neurobiology of the basal ganglia and related structures over the past decade are the extensive immunohistochemical studies that have demonstrated the presence of a wide spectrum of classic neurotransmitters, neuromodulators, and neuropeptides (46,47). The functional status of a number of these systems has been evaluated in Tourette syndrome (30). Some of the most compelling evidence has focused attention on the endogenous opioid projections from the striatum to the palladium and substantia nigra that form one portion of the CSTC circuits (48). In addition, mesencephalic monoaminergic (dopaminergic, noradrenergic, and serotonergic) projections that modulate the activity of the CSTC circuits have also been repeatedly implicated in both Tourette syndrome and obsessive–compulsive disorder.

POTENTIAL CONTRIBUTIONS FROM NATURAL HISTORY DATA

Table 1 presents some of the features of the phenomenology and natural history that may serve as clues to understanding the pathogenetic mechanisms underlying the development of Tourette syndrome and related conditions. Conversely, any thoroughgoing account of Tourette syndrome will need to address these features. For the purposes of discussion, two of these topics, the presence of premonitory urges and the

TABLE 1. *Pathogenesis of Tourette syndrome and related disorders: clues from the natural history*

Developmental continuities and discontinuities: What developmental events account for the emergence of tic disorders in the first two decades of life? Why do most patients experience a marked reduction in tic symptoms in late adolescence and early adulthood?

Premonitory urges: What neurobiological factors underlie the existence of premonitory urges and how do they relate to the mechanisms responsible for tic behaviors? Is Tourette syndrome better characterized as a sensorimotor disorder as opposed to a hyperkinetic movement disorder?

Anatomic distribution: What structural features of the basal ganglia and related structures account for the particular anatomic distribution of motor tics and the premonitory urges that can precede them?

Timing of symptoms: What are the neurophysiological events that govern the timing of tic behaviors? Given the bout-like occurrence of tics, is it possible that nonlinear (fractal) dynamics are at work in this systems?

Alteration in symptoms secondary to changes in CNS state: Why do symptoms increase during periods of fatigue and diminish during sleep? Why does distraction associated with complex motor activity usually lead to a transient reduction in symptoms?

Gender differences: What is the biological basis for the variations in clinical presentation of males and females?

marked gender differences in phenotype expression, will serve as examples.

Premonitory Urges

Clinical Description

As noted above, the inner experience of tics is frequently characterized by the presence of premonitory urges. A majority of patients with Tourette syndrome (73–94%) report that they regularly have unpleasant sensory perceptions or mental awarenesses that precede some of their tic behaviors and that are momentarily relieved by the performance of the tics (4,5,49). These sensations contribute to the perception by many Tourette sufferers that their tics are a voluntary motor or vocal response to these urges and that were it possible to reduce or eliminate these urges, they would not tic (5).

Data from a survey of 135 individuals with Tourette syndrome indicate that many children with tics are unaware of these sensory phenomena and that there is often a lag, lasting several years, between the onset of the tics and the individual's first awareness of these urges (49).

These sensory perceptions are often focal in character so that they can be discretely localized and described as being experienced in a muscle or in a joint or, more rarely, in the skin. The anatomic distribution of these urges is similar to but distinct from the anatomic distribution of tics. As shown in Fig. 2, the shoulder girdle, the palms of the hands, the throat, the eyes, the midline of the abdomen, and the dorsum of the hands and feet have the highest density of premonitory urges (49). In contrast, the areas with the highest density of tics are the eyes, mouth, face, head, and shoulders.

These premonitory urges may precede either simple or complex motor tics or dystonic tics. They are less commonly associ-

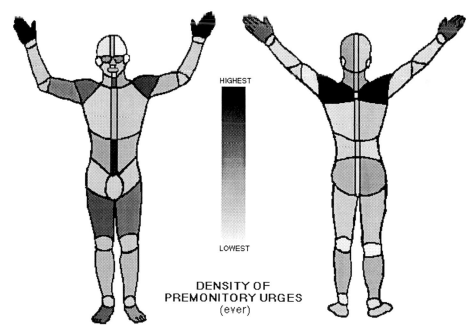

FIG. 2. Density of premonitory urges. The densities of premonitory urges for each of 89 anatomical regions are depicted. The highest density on the scale represents .40 total premonitory urges/region/person, the lowest 0 urges/region/person, and the midpoint .20 urges/region/person. Data based on any premonitory urges ever experienced as assessed in a self-report questionnaire (N = 101). See Leckman et al. (49) for details.

ated with rapid, more automatic, behaviors such as eyeblinking. They can be unilateral or, more commonly, distributed with precise bilateral symmetry.

Possible Neurobiological Origins

The combination of somatosensory urges and fragmentary motor behaviors is consistent with the involvement of the motor CSTC circuits described above that channel and subchannel information involved in the anticipation and performance of motor behaviors. As depicted in Fig. 3, these circuits are somatotopically organized, with the orofacial regions of the striatum occupying the most ventral areas of the putamen (50). Intriguingly, information from the somatosensory cortex is also processed in parallel by these same structures with roughly the same somatotopic distribution (Fig. 3). The existence of contiguous, if not overlapping, projection areas within the striatum from both

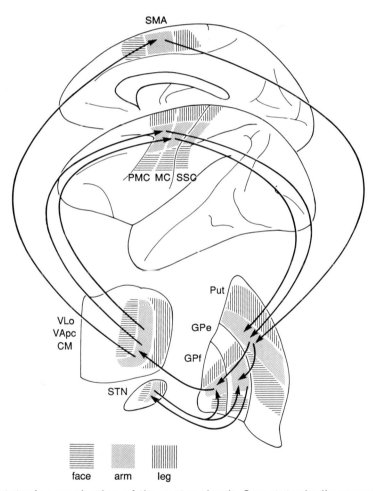

FIG. 3. Somatotopic organization of the motor circuit. Somatotopically organized pathways connecting functionally related brain regions. *CM*, centromedian nucleus; *GPe*, external segment of globus pallidus; *GPi*, internal segment of globus pallidus; *MC*, primary motor cortex; *PMC*, premotor cortex exclusive of the arcuate premotor area; *Put*, putamen; *SMA*, supplementary motor area; *SSC*, somatosensory cortex; *VApc*, nucleus ventralis anterior pars parvocellularis; *VLo*, nucleus ventralis lateralis pars oralis. Adapted from Alexander and Crutcher (50).

the motor and sensorimotor cortical areas is provocative and suggests that these projections may be critically involved in the neurobiology of Tourette syndrome.

Adding further complexity is the presence of projections from the intralaminar nuclei of the thalamus to the somatotopically organized areas of the striatum (51). These thalamostriatal projections arise in part from collaterals of thalamocortical fibers (52) and could contribute to activating both cortical and striatal areas. The view that the intralaminar thalamic nuclei play an important mediating role is reinforced by the limited neurosurgical data that stimulation of these areas can generate premonitory urges while ablation can ameliorate tic symptoms (31–33).

Gender Differences

Clinical Description

The importance of gender differences in the expression of tic disorders and associated phenotypes is clear given the observations that boys and men are more likely to present with tic disorders (53) and that women are more likely than men to display obsessive–compulsive symptoms without concomitant tics (18). These observations are particularly noteworthy given the results of genetic studies suggesting that the vulnerability to Tourette syndrome is transmitted within families as an autosomal dominant trait in which males and females should be at equal risk to receive the putative vulnerability gene (17).

Possible Neurobiological Origins

The gender-dependent expression of the vulnerability to Tourette syndrome has led us to hypothesize that androgenic steroids act at key developmental periods to influence the natural history of Tourette syndrome and related disorders (2,63). These key developmental periods include the pre-

natal period when the brain is being formed, adrenarche when adrenal androgens first appear at age 5–7 years, and puberty. The androgenic steroids may act directly or through their conversion to estradiol, which is formed in key brain regions by the aromatization of testosterone.

Surges in testosterone and other androgenic steroids during critical periods in fetal development are known to be involved in the production of long-term functional augmentation of subsequent hormonal challenges (as in adrenarche and during puberty) and in the formation of structural CNS dimorphisms (54). In recent years several sexually dimorphic brain regions have been described, including portions of the amygdala (and related limbic areas) and the hypothalamus (including the medial preoptic area that mediates the body's response to thermal stress) (55). These regions contain high levels of androgen and estrogen receptors and are known to influence activity in the basal ganglia both directly and indirectly (56). It is also of note that some of the neurochemical and neuropeptidergic systems implicated in Tourette syndrome and related disorders, such as dopamine, serotonin, and the opioids, are involved with these regions and appear to be regulated by sex-specific factors.

Further support for a role of androgens comes from open trials of antiandrogens for the treatment of patients with severe obsessive–compulsive disorder (57) in which all the subjects reported a remission in their symptoms while on medication and an exacerbation when the medication was withdrawn. In addition, two boys with obsessive–compulsive disorder who were treated with spironolactone, a peripheral antitestosterone agent, and testolactone, a peripheral antiestrogen agent, experienced a reduction of their symptoms that lasted for 3–4 months (58).

Complementary evidence comes from our observation of athletes with a history of Tourette syndrome who have experienced exacerbations of tics while using androgenic steroids (27). In addition, we have observed positive responses to the antiandrogen flutamide in three Tourette syndrome patients who had not responded to conventional therapies (Peterson et al., unpublished data).

Other aspects of the circuitry of the basal ganglia may provide important clues concerning gender differences, as well as the anatomic distribution of motor tics and the "choice" of obsessive themes frequently encountered in forms of obsessive–compulsive disorder related to Tourette syndrome. Of special interest is the unidirectional input from the amygdala to widespread areas of the nucleus accumbens and ventral portions of the caudate and putamen. These striatal areas are among the brain areas most likely to be affected in Tourette's syndrome and obsessive–compulsive disorder (61–64).

In addition, reciprocal connections between midbrain sites (periaqueductal gray, substantia nigra, and the ventral tegmental area), portions of the hypothalamus, and structures in the basal ganglia and amygdala are likely to play a critical role in the genesis and maintenance of the symptoms of Tourette syndrome. These connections may also contribute to the stress sensitivity (including sensitivity to thermal stress observed in a limited number of subjects) and to the more frequent expression of Tourette syndrome in males than females (many of these structures contain receptors for gonadal steroids and are responsive to alterations in their hormonal environment).

PROSPECTS FOR THE NEXT DECADE

Tourette syndrome and related disorders are likely to be associated with detectable alterations in brain function. Systematic and sustained investigation of possible pathobiological mechanisms, guided in part by clinical investigations of the phenomenology and natural history of these disorders, has led to promising new lines of inquiry that may in turn lead to new and more effective treatment strategies. Although the enormous complexity of the neurochemical, neuroendocrine, and neuropharmacological data in Tourette syndrome and obsessive–compulsive disorder does not yield readily to simplistic explanations focused on a single neurotransmitter or neuromodulatory systems, it is likely that significant progress will be made over the next decade with regard to understanding the biological causes and determinants of Tourette syndrome and related disorders and the development of safe and effective treatments.

REFERENCES

1. Cohen DJ, Detlor J, Shaywitz BA, Leckman JF. Interaction of biological and psychological factors in the natural history of Tourette syndrome: a paradigm for childhood neuropsychiatric disorders. In: Friedhoff AJ, Chase TN, eds. *Advances in neurology: Gilles de la Tourette syndrome*, vol 35. New York: Raven Press, 1982;31–40.
2. Leckman JF, Walkup JT, Riddle MA, Towbin KE, Cohen DJ. Tic disorders. In: Meltzer HY, ed. *Psychopharmacology: the third generation of progress*. New York: Raven Press, 1987.
3. Bliss J. Sensory experiences of Gilles de la Tourette syndrome. *Arch Gen Psychiatry* 1980; 37:1343–7.
4. Kurlan R, Lichter D, Hewitt D. Sensory tics in Tourette's syndrome. Neurology 1989;39:731–4.
5. Lang A: Patient perception of tics and other movement disorders. *Neurology* 1991;41:223–8.
6. Cohen DJ, Leckman JF, Shaywitz BA: Tourette's syndrome and other tic disorders. In: Shaffer D, Ehrhardt AA, Greenhill L, eds. *A clinical guide to child psychiatry*. New York: MacMillan Free, 1983.
7. Comings DE, Comings BG. A controlled study of Tourette syndrome. I. Attention-deficit disorder, learning disorders, and school problems. *Am J Hum Genet* 1987;41:701–41.
8. Comings DE, Comings BG. A controlled study of Tourette syndrome. II. Conduct. *Am J Hum Genet* 1987;41:742–60.
9. Stefl ME. Mental health needs associated with Tourette syndrome. *Am J Public Health* 1984; 74:1310–3.
10. Burd L, Kerbeshian L, Wikenheiser M, Fisher W. Prevalence of Gilles de la Tourette's syndrome in North Dakota adults. *Am J Psychiatry* 1986; 143:787.
11. Comings DE, Himes JA, Comings BG. An epidemiological study of Tourette's syndrome in a single school district. *J Clin Psychiatry* 1990;51:463–9.
12. Zahner GEP, Clubb MM, Leckman JF, Pauls DL. The epidemiology of Tourette's syndrome. In: Cohen DJ, Bruun RD, Leckman JF, eds. *Tour-*

ette's syndrome and tic disorders. New York: John Wiley & Sons, 1988.

13. Flament MF, Whitaker A, Rapoport JL, et al. Obsessive-compulsive disorder in adolescence: an epidemiological study. *J Am Acad Child Adolesc Psychiatry* 1988;27:764–71.

14. Karno M, Golding JM, Sorenson SB, et al. The epidemiology of obsessive-compulsive disorder in five US communities. *Arch Gen Psychiatry* 1988; 45:1094–9.

15. Price AR, Leckman JF, Pauls DL. A twin study of Tourette syndrome. *Arch Gen Psychiatry* 1985; 42:815–22.

16. Walkup JT, Leckman JF, Price AR, et al. The relationship between obsessive compulsive disorder and Tourette's syndrome. *Psychopharmacol Bull* 1988;24:375–9.

17. Pauls DL, Leckman JF. The inheritance of Gilles de la Tourette syndrome and associated behaviors: evidence for autosomal dominant transmission. *N Engl J Med* 1986;315:993–7.

18. Pauls DL, Raymond CL, Stevenson JF, Leckman JF. A family study of Gilles de la Tourette. *Am J Hum Genet* 1991;48:154–63.

19. Pauls DL, Pakstis AJ, Kurlan R, et al. Segregation and linkage analysis of Gilles de la Tourette's syndrome and related disorders. *J Am Acad Child Ad olesc Psychiatry* 1990;29:195–203.

20. Pakstis AJ, Heutinik P, Pauls DL, et al. Progress in the search of genetic linkage with Tourette syndrome: an exclusion map covering more than 50% of the autosomal genome. *Am J Hum Genet* 1991; 48:281–94.

21. Gelernter J, Pakstis AJ, Pauls DL, et al. Gilles de la Tourette syndrome not linked to D2-dopamine receptor. *Arch Gen Psychiatry* 1990;47:1073–7.

22. Weber JL, May PE. Abundant class of human DNA polymorphisms which can be typed using polymerase chain reaction. *Am J Hum Genet* 1989; 44:388–96.

23. Pasamanick B, Kawi A. A study of the association of prenatal and paranatal factors in the development of tics in children. *J Pediatr* 1956;48:596.

24. Leckman JF, Cohen DJ, Price RA, Mindera RB, Anderson GM, Pauls DL. The pathogenesis of Gilles de la Tourette's syndrome: a review of data and hypothesis. In: Shah AB, Shah NS, Donald AG, eds. *Movement Disorders*. New York: Plenum Press, 1984.

25. Leckman JF, Dolnansky ES, Hardin MT, et al. Perinatal factors in the expression of Tourette's syndrome: an exploratory study. *J Am Acad Child Adolesc Psychiatry* 1990;29:220–6.

26. Lombroso PJ, Mack G, Scahill L, et al. Exacerbation of Tourette's syndrome associated with thermal stress: a family study. *Neurology* 1992; 41:1984.

27. Leckman JF, Scahill L. Possible exacerbation of tics by androgenic steroids. *N Engl J Med* 1990; 322:1674.

28. Mesulam MM. Cocaine and Tourette's syndrome. *N Engl J Med* 1986;315:398.

29. Price AR, Leckman JF, Pauls DL, Cohen DJ, Kidd KK. Tics and central nervous system stimulants

30. Chappell P, Leckman JF, Pauls D, Cohen DJ. Biochemical and genetic studies of Tourette's syndrome. Implications for treatment and future research. In: Deutsch S, Weizmar A, Weizmar R, eds. *Application of basic neuroscience to child psychiatry*. New York: Plenum, 1990;241–60.

31. Cooper IS. *Involuntary movement disorders*. New York: Hoeber Medical Division, Harper & Row, 1969.

32. Hassler R, Diekmann G. Traitement stéréotaxique des tics et cris inarticulés ou coprolaliques considerés comme phénomène d'obsession motrice au cours de la maladie de Gilles de la Tourette. *Rev Neurol (Paris)* 1970;123:89–100.

33. Mansfield L. No more apologies. *Tulane* 1991; Spring:12–5.

34. Baker EFW. Gilles de la Tourette syndrome treated by biomedical frontal leukotomy. *Can Med Assoc J* 1962;86:746–7.

35. Kurlan R, Kersun J, Ballantine HT, et al. Neurosurgical treatment of severe obsessive-compulsive disorder associated with Tourette's syndrome. *Move Disord* 1990;5:152–5.

36. Stevens H. The syndrome of Gilles de la Tourette and its treatment. *Med Ann District Columbia* 1964;33:27–9.

37. Chase TN, Geoffrey V, Gillespie M, et al. Structural and functional studies of Gilles de la Tourette's syndrome. *Rev Neurol (Paris)* 1986; 142:851–5.

38. Baxter LR, Phelps ME, Mazzlota JC, et al. Local cerebral glucose metabolic rates in obsessive compulsive disorder. *Arch Gen Psychiatry* 1987; 44:211.

39. Baxter LR, Schwartz JM, Mazziota JC, et al. Cerebral glucose metabolic rates in obsessive-compulsive disorder. *Arch Gen Psychiatry* 1988; 145:1560–3.

40. Nordahl TE, Benkalfat C, Semple WE, et al. Cerebral glucose metabolic rates in obsessive compulsive disorder. *Neuropsychopharamacology* 1989; 2:23–8.

41. Swedo SE, Shapiro ME, Grady CL, et al. Cerebral glucose metabolism in childhood-onset obsessive compulsive disorder. *Arch Gen Psychiatry* 1990; 46:518–23.

42. Alexander GE, DeLong MR, Strick PL. Parallel organization of functionally segregated circuits linking basal ganglia and cortex. *Annu Rev Neurosci* 1986;9:357–81.

43. Goldman-Rakic PS, Selemon DL. New frontiers in basal ganglia research. *Trends Neurosci* 1990; 13:244–5.

44. Leckman JF, Hardin MT, Riddle MA, Stevenson J, Ort SI, Cohen DJ. Clonidine treatment of Gilles de la Tourette's syndrome. *Arch Gen Psychiatry* 1991;48:324–8.

45. Laplane D, Levasseur M, Pillon B, et al. Obsessive-compulsive and other behavioral changes with bilateral basal ganglia lesions. *Brain* 1989; 112:699–725.

46. Graybiel AM. Neurotransmitters and neuromodu-

lators in the basal ganglia. *Trends Neurosci* 1984;
13:244–54.

47. Parent A. *Comparative neurobiology of basal ganglia.* New York: John Wiley & Sons, 1986.

48. Chappell PB, Leckman JF, Riddle MA, et al. Neuroendocrine and behavioral effects of naloxone in Tourette's syndrome. *Life Sci* (in press).

49. Leckman JF, Walker DE, Cohen DJ. Premonitory urges in Tourette's syndrome. *Am J Psychiatry*, (in press).

50. Alexander GE, Crutcher MD. Functional architecture of basal ganglia circuits: neural substrates of parallel processing. *Trends Neurosci* 1990; 13:266–71.

51. Berendse HW, Groenewegen HJ. Organization of the thalamostriatal projections in the rat, with special emphasis on the ventral striatum. *J Comp Neurol* 1990;299:187–228.

52. Cesaro P, Nguyen-Legros J, Pollin B, Laplante S. Single intralaminar thalamic neurons project to cerebral cortex, striatum and nucleus reticularis thalami: a retrograde anatomical tracing study in the rat. *Brain Res* 1985;325:29–37.

53. Shapiro AK, Shapiro ES, Young JG, Feinberg TE, eds. *Gilles de la Tourette syndrome*, 2nd ed. New York: Raven Press, 1988.

54. Sikich L, Todd RD. Are neurodevelopmental effects of gonadal hormones related to sex differences in psychiatric illness? *Psychiatr Dev* 1988; 6:277–310.

55. Boulant JA. Hypothalamic mechanisms in thermoregulation. *Fed Proc* 1981;40:2843–50.

56. Fehrbach SE, Morell JI, Pfaff DW. Identification of medial preoptic neurons that concentrate estradiol and project to the midbrain in the rat. *J Comp Neurol* 1985;247:364–82.

57. Casas M, Alvarez E, Duro P, et al. Antiandrogenic treatment of obsessive-compulsive neurosis. *Acta Psychiatr Scand* 1986;73:221–2.

58. Swedo SE, Rapoport JL. Neurochemical and neuroendocrine considerations of obsessive compulsive disorders in childhood. In: Deutsch SI, Weizman A, Weizman R, eds. *Application of basic neuroscience to child psychiatry.* New York: Plenum, 1990;275–84.

59. Nauta WJH. In: Friedhoff AJ, Chase TN, eds. *Advances in neurology, vol 58, Gilles de la Tourette syndrome.* New York: Raven Press, 1982.

60. Russchen FT, Bakst I, Amaral DG, et al. The amygdalostriatal projections in the monkey: an anterograde tracing study. *Brain Res* 1985; 329:241–57.

61. McLean P, Delgado J. Electrical and chemical stimulation of frontotemporal portion of limbic system in the waking animal. *EEG Clin Neurophysiol* 1953;5:91–100.

62. Baldwin M, Frost LL, Wodd CD. Investigation of primate amygdala. *Neurology* 1954;4:586–98.

63. Peterson BS, Leckman JF, Scahill L, et al. Hypothesis: steroid hormones and sexual dimorphisms modulate symptom expression in Tourette's syndrome. *Psychoneuroendocrinology*, (in press.)

64. Peterson BS, Leckman JF, Scahill L, et al. Steroid hormones and Tourette's syndrome: early experience with antiandrogen therapy. *Psychoneuroendocrinology*, (in press.)

Advances in Neurology, Vol. 58, edited by T. N. Chase, A. J. Friedhoff, and D. J. Cohen. Raven Press, Ltd., New York © 1992.

4

Clinical Phenomenology of Tic Disorders Selected Aspects

Anthony E. Lang

Movement Disorders Clinic, Toronto Western Hospital, Toronto, Ontario M5T 2S8, Canada

The clinical aspects of tic disorders encompass a broad range of motor, phonic, and behavioral signs and symptoms. Several recent reviews have detailed the clinical phenomenology of tic disorders with additional definitions of other dyskinetic or hyperkinetic movement disorders and clues to the differentiation of tics from these other conditions. For this reason, I do not propose to describe the previously emphasized classical features of tic disorders or Tourette syndrome (TS) or to provide general descriptions of other movement disorders with which they can be confused. Instead, I hope to highlight certain selected clinical aspects, many of which have not been emphasized in previous reviews of the topic.

SENSORY TICS

Despite almost a century of writings dealing with TS, possibly the first report to emphasize the significance of sensory experiences was the personal account of Bliss in 1980 (1). He emphasized the importance of distinct and discrete sensations, which then triggered or invoked the tics as intentional movements comparable to scratching in order to relieve an itch. Subsequently, Bullen and Hemsley (2) described another patient with an uncomfortable sensation akin to an itch, which triggered the tics. Shapiro

and his colleagues (3) first coined the term *sensory tics* to describe the tics that occurred in a small proportion of patients who experienced "involuntary" localizable sensations. These then invoked a *voluntary* tic response, which could either be a movement or a vocalization. The authors emphasized that the movements typically differed from rapid or sudden tics. Instead, patients demonstrated tonic, tightening, or stretching movements ("dystonic" tics). They claimed that the vocalizations also differed, usually being more prolonged lower pitched humming sounds. Their earlier surveys of Tourette patients found sensory tics alone to be present in 4.1% and the combination of both typical and sensory tics in 4.4%. They emphasized that these figures were almost certainly underestimates since their questionnaires were not attuned to the presence of sensory tics originally.

In 1989, Kurlan and his colleagues (4) carried out a telephone questionnaire survey of 34 TS patients. Forty-one percent of these individuals experienced focal sensory phenomena preceding tics. The nature of the tics, however, was not specific or different from that found in individuals not experiencing premonitory sensory symptoms; however, the authors did emphasize that "dystonic" tics may be more common. Some patients both with and without these focal sensations also described either somatic or psychic generalized sensations including a poorly defined urge preceding the tics. Interestingly, 96% with sensory antecedents reported an ability to suppress tics voluntarily, while only 63% of those without sensory phenomena noted the feature. Since both sensory tics and more typical motor and phonic tics respond equally well to medical therapy, the authors suggested the existence of a common pathophysiology for these symptoms. In contrast to the earlier descriptions of these sensory experiences, Kurlan and colleagues commented that patients "have difficulty stating that the movements are truly voluntary. We suspect that the distinction between sensory tics and more typical tics based on voluntary versus involuntary nature of the movement . . . is inaccurate." In general, my experience agrees with their criticism of Shapiro et al.'s distinction. However, a recent study of patients' perception of their movements provides information that contrasts somewhat with the views of Kurlan et al.

SUBJECTIVE PERCEPTION OF TICS

I have recently reported a study (5) in which patients with a variety of different types of abnormal movements were asked to chose whether their abnormal movement or vocalization was completely "involuntary," as if the body part affected had a mind of its own that was beyond their control or whether the movements and/or vocalizations were "voluntary" in the sense that the patient was aware of consciously performing the act but in response to an inner need or urge that caused them to do it. In other words, the patient was asked "is the affected body part making the movement/sound on its own or are you actually causing the body part to move on purpose?" One hundred and two of 110 patients with nontic movement disorders stated that all the movements were "involuntary." Those who felt that the movements were com-

pletely "voluntary" all had akathisia. These latter patients had other movement disorders as well (e.g., spasmodic torticollis, tardive dyskinesia) and in all cases, patients appreciated the akathitic movements as voluntary and the other abnormal movements as involuntary. In contrast to the nontic group, 41 of the 60 tic patients felt that all of their tics were "voluntary" or intentionally produced. Fifteen others had both voluntary and involuntary components, usually with the former predominating. The occasional patient with the combination of tics and another movement disorder (e.g., spasmodic torticollis, parkinsonian tremor) always easily distinguished a subjective difference between the tics and these other abnormal movements, the former being "voluntary" and the latter "involuntary." When the referral diagnostic category (tic versus nontic) was incorrect, a "voluntary" response could have been used to predict the correct diagnostic category in 8 of 9 patients. In this survey, patients were not asked about the occurrence or nature of a preceding focal or generalized sensory phenomena and so it is not possible to provide a definite correlation between the occurrence of perceived sensory experiences and the appreciation of tics as purposefully executed. It is my impression that most, if not all patients with this perception have some preceding subjective experience, while those without such an experience usually perceive the tics as involuntary. However, the premonitory sensory experience is often not focal and thus does not fulfill previously proposed diagnostic criteria for sensory tics (4). It is important to point out that it is not uncommon for patients to describe the combination of both "voluntary" and "involuntary" tics or to state that all of their tics are voluntary but to demonstrate certain tics that they seem to be unaware that they are making.

We can conclude from this experience that patients often recognize tics as intentionally produced or irresistibly but purposefully executed. This would place tics into the "intentional unvoluntary action" category of Culver and Gert (6), in contrast to the "nonintentional action" of most other forms of abnormal involuntary movements such as tremors, dystonia, chorea, myoclonus, etc. Patients frequently perceive that the tic is produced in response to either a nonlocalizable or difficult to define urge or generalized sensation (somatic or psychic) or to a specific localizable sensation affecting the body part involved in the tic. Both of these ill-defined and well-localized sensations are usually relieved or dampened temporarily by the performance of the tic. Clinically, the nature of the movements or phonations and the additional clinical features (e.g., presence and severity of obsessive–compulsive features, degree of waxing and waning of symptoms, family history) demonstrated by the patient with this perception of tics are similar to those without. Given this clinical perception of tics, I would question the need to distinguish "sensory tics" as a separate or distinct category. Questioning patients about the subjective perceptions of their movements can be extremely helpful in the differential diagnosis of patients presenting with movement disorders (Table 1). Finally, this subjective perception of abnormal movements experienced by the majority of tic patients aligns their motor and phonic symptoms closer to compulsions than to other "involuntary" hyperkinesias with which they are commonly discussed.

CLINICAL DIFFERENTIATION BETWEEN TICS AND OTHER DYSKINESIAS

As indicated in the introduction, it is not my purpose to list all of the clinical points that help distinguish between tics and other movement disorders. The **personal, past, and family histories** as well as **associated be-**

TABLE 1. *Responses of selected movement disorders to questions regarding subjective perception, distraction maneuvers, voluntary suppressability, and effects of selected motor activities[a]*

	Subjective perception	Distraction	Suppression	Effect of selected movements (e.g., writing)
Tics	Vol	↓	+++	Usually ↓
Akathitic movements	Vol	↓	++	↓
Psychogenic movements	Inv	↓[b]	±	Usually ↓[b]
Tremors	Inv	0 or ↑	PD tremor ++ Others 0	May ↑
Chorea	Inv	0 or ↑	±	Variable
Orofacial tardive dyskinesia (also L-dopa dyskinesia)	Inv	↑	++	Often ↑
Dystonia	Inv	0 or ↑	±	Commonly ↑
Myoclonus	Inv	0 or ↑	0	Commonly ↑ (e.g., essential myoclonus)

[a] "Vol" refers to the patient's appreciation of the movements (and/or phonations) as purposefully executed. "Inv" refers to the patient's appreciation of the movements as completely involuntary. Downward arrows refer to a reduction of the movements, while upward arrows refer to an increase. The size of the arrow indicates the degree of change, the largest downward arrows often indicating complete suppression, while the largest upward arrows indicate marked exacerbation of the movements. 0, no change; ±, a variable change; +, ++, +++, mild, moderate, marked suppressibility, respectively.

[b] When psychogenic movements are not fully suppressed by these activities the characteristics of the abnormal movements often change or become quite variable.

havioral disturbances are often extremely helpful in this regard. However, given the high prevalence of tic disorders, it is not uncommon to recognize their coincidental presence in patients presenting with other neurological diseases including those with movement disorders. The pronounced **variability** in both the presence and nature of the movements and phonations are characteristic of tics. Their **intermittency** also distinguishes them from most other movement disorders. Other intermittent dyskinesias that might be confused with this feature are the paroxysmal dyskinesias and isolated action-induced movement disorders, especially certain forms of dystonia. However, in practice, it is extremely rare for these disorders to present a significant problem in differential diagnosis with tics. A feature that has been regularly emphasized as characteristic of tics is **voluntary suppressibility**. Although tics remain the most suppressible of movement disorders, many patients with other forms of dyskinesias demonstrate this feature to a lesser degree (7). This is especially the case for parkinsonian tremor, tardive dyskinesia, and levodopa-induced dyskinesias (7,8). Another clinical feature that is often overlooked or not emphasized but that can be extremely useful in clinical practice is the effect of distraction maneuvers or motor/cognitive challenges. Most forms of dyskinesia will be aggravated by such tasks as mental arithmetic (e.g., serial 7s) or the performance of rapid alternating movements in the hands or some other more complex manual task. A task that I have found particularly useful is thumb opposition to fingers designating each finger (index to small finger) with a number 1–4. After the patient has performed the usual order of 1–4, he/she is then asked to tap out a different numerical sequence (e.g., 1, 3, 2, 4; 1, 4, 2, 3; etc.) with continued pressure by the examiner to complete the task as accurately and as quickly as possible. Once the sequence is mastered, a new one is given. In some cases, for example with orofacial tardive dyskinesia or levodopa-induced dyski-nesia, the increase in abnormal movements brought about by these tasks can be quite marked and striking. In contrast, tics will almost always diminish or subside completely although they may return during brief periods of rest (e.g., immediately after giving one mathematical answer before going on to calculating the next). This response to distraction is similar for akathitic movements and most forms of psychogenic abnormal movements. In contrast to tics and akathitic movements, when psychogenic abnormal movements are not fully suppressed by distraction they usually change in character (e.g., distribution, frequency, rhythmicity, etc.) and become quite inconsistent or incongruous with organic dyskinesias. In assessing the movement disorder patient the response of the abnormal movements to **selected motor tasks** is particularly important. Possibly the best example is writing. Just as less specific motor tasks will diminish tics, one usually sees a suppression of tics during the act of writing with a recurrence during pauses or breaks between words. In contrast, certain other disorders such as task-specific dystonias and essential myoclonus are particularly aggravated by writing. Table 1 provides the characteristics of tics and other movement disorders in the categories of subjective perception, suppressibility, and the effects of distraction and selected motor tasks. As can be seen, tics share similar features with akathitic movements as well as movements of the restless leg syndrome (not listed in the table). Others have also drawn attention to these similarities in the past (9,10).

DYSTONIA AND TICS: RELATIONSHIP AND CONFUSION

One common source of diagnostic confusion, somewhat underemphasized by the dissimilarities listed in Table 1, is the differentiation of dystonia from dystonic tics. It is important to emphasize that although the more tonic or prolonged movements of dystonic tics could be easily mistaken for dystonia, these movements share all of the features listed in Table 1 with the more common rapid or clonic tics and complex tics. However, there may be other causes for this confusion. Occasionally patients presenting with tics may also be found to have dystonia and vice versa. For example, in one study of Tourette syndrome from the United Kingdom by Lees et al. (11), 4 of 53 patients were also found to have forms of focal dystonia. Other authors have also questioned the possibility of a greater than expected association between tics and idiopathic dystonia (12); however, this connection remains to be proved with a properly designed epidemiological survey. As mentioned previously, the high prevalence of tics in the general population makes a simple coincidental occurrence of the two disorders in the same patient a strong possibility. Another interesting relationship between dystonia and tics has been reported by Elston and his colleagues (13), who described a family in which the three generations were affected by eyeblinking tics and/or dystonic blepharospasm. They also reported five patients with adult-onset blepharospasm or Meige's syndrome who had had excessive eyeblinking dating back to childhood. These authors suggested that eyeblinking tics, frequent blinking, and blepharospasm may share common pathophysiological mechanisms and that the clinical expression of these disorders may be age-related. Three additional sources of overlap between dystonia and tic syndromes are the occurrence of pain, the use of various forms of geste antagoniste, and the potential successful use of botulinum toxin. Each of these will be discussed briefly below.

PAIN IN TIC DISORDERS

Little has been written regarding the varied and common complaints of pain in tic patients. We described a series of cases and

TABLE 2. *Classification of pain in relation to tic disorders*

Pain caused by tics or compulsions
  Exertional
    Muscular pain due to excessive contraction
    Skeletal or joint pain
    Neuropathic pain (due to spinal cord, radicular or peripheral nerve compression)
  Traumatic
    Pain in a body part struck by a moving limb
    Pain in a moving body part striking something nearby
    Self-mutilation (including biting)
    Pain from compulsive touching of hot or sharp objects
    Pain inflicted on others from tics or compulsions
Premonitory sensation ("sensory tics") perceived as painful
Pain caused by suppression of tics
Pain-relieving tics

attempted to provide a preliminary classification scheme for these disorders (14). Table 2 outlines an altered version of this classification. It has been my experience that 15–20% of tic patients spontaneously volunteer a history of pain related to the tics. Some 50% of these have been greatly bothered by the pain, and this occasionally represents their chief complaint. In some patients the pain may result in a delay in diagnosis or a series of unnecessary investigations. Certainly the commonest source of pain is exertional, simply related to excessive muscle contraction. However, some patients have more than one type or source of the pain. For example, a patient may experience muscular pain secondary to tics but also discomfort described as painful on attempting to voluntarily suppress the abnormal movements or a painful sensation preceding the tic ("sensory tic"). We have also seen unusual patients who find that painful experiences tend to lessen or relieve the tics. Our patient 7 was an example of this:

A 31 year old man, with a history of multiple motor and vocal tics dating from the age of 4 years noted that his tics would subside for a brief period if he experienced pain. He stated that the sensation of pain in a certain body part would reduce the tendency of that area to perform a tic. Consequently he deliberately induced pain by excessive muscle contraction of the body part affected by frequent tics to produce a respite from his tics. In retrospect, he stated that the previous tendency to bite his lips, tongue or the inside of his cheeks was a similar attempt to provoke pain to reduce the frequency of his orolingual tics (14).

Thus it can be also appreciated that pain related to tics may be an additional source of diagnostic confusion regarding the nature of the demonstrated motor behavior. In this case, the deliberate induction of pain to relieve tics could easily have been misinterpreted as purposeless self-mutilation.

GESTE ANTAGONISTE

The use of "sensory-tricks" is typically linked to dystonic syndromes. Indeed, most movement disorder specialists search for these features in the history, and their diagnosis tends to be influenced by the presence of an antagonistic gesture. On the other hand, occasional patients with tic disorders use similar maneuvers to lessen the production of their abnormal movements. For example, Samuel Johnson was said commonly to bring his left hand across his chest to support his chin in order to dampen head movements (15). It is not certain whether this was to suppress a dystonic tic or true spasmodic torticollis. On the other hand, patient "O" of Meige and Fiendel (16) definitely had dystonic neck tics. These authors described a variety of peculiar "para tics" with the utilization of a curved handle of a cane in putting on his hat, the common tendency of supporting the chin on the cane and pressing down as well as the tendency to place the cane between the jacket and the overcoat. These maneuvers resulted in the development of corns on the bridge of the nose and chin.

I have seen a small number of patients who utilize various forms of geste antagoniste. It is not known how common this phenomenon is, and I am currently in the process of carrying out a study assessing the feature. Those patients who have described the use of geste maneuvers have usually noted an increase in suppressibility or some relief of the "urge" or "tension" that precedes their execution of the tics. For the most part, these patients have predominantly had tics involving the eyelids and head. In the case of excessive blinking, patients have pressed their hand to their forehead or worn a tight cap. In a similar fashion to the gestes antagoniste of spasmodic torticollis, patients with head rotation tics have tended to hold their chin or place the head against the back of a high chair. Patients with both clonic and dystonic types of tics seem to utilize these maneuvers; however, they may be more common in the latter group.

BOTULINUM TOXIN IN TIC DISORDERS

A final source of overlap between dystonia and tics is the potential efficacy of botulinum toxin. As indicated above, pain is not uncommonly associated with tics. Indeed, dystonia and tics differ from almost all other forms of hyperkinesia in terms of the common occurrence of pain. The selective injections of specific muscles with botulinum toxin may effectively lessen the abnormal movements as well as relieve the pain when it is due to excessive muscle contraction. Another unique effect of botulinum toxin seen in one patient (D. Hobson, personal communication) has been both the resolution of the movements in the short term due to muscle weakness but also in the long term due to a resolution of the urge to perform the movements in that location. This patient had experienced long-standing (>15 years) frequent frontalis and scalp contractions (invariant tics), which had become a significant source of discomfort. These were usually followed by head-nodding tics. Botulinum toxin injections sufficient to paralyze the frontalis muscle eliminated both urge and tics including the head nodding as well as the ability to elevate the forehead voluntarily. Importantly, as power returned to the frontalis, the patient no longer experienced the urge in this location. While his other long-standing tics remained unchanged and no new tics developed, the resolution of the tics of the forehead, scalp, and head persisted for over a year of follow up. This experience suggests an important role for peripheral feedback mechanisms to the persistence of tics and possibly to the development of more automatic forms of the tics with the loss of a perception of the movements as purposefully executed. This phenomenon clearly requires further study.

SIGNING TICS

Finally, I would like to describe an unusual form of tic behavior that further emphasizes the complex, purposeful, but automatic nature of the motor tic symptomatology. We (with Dr. E. Consky and P. Sandor, unpublished observations) have seen an extremely interesting young woman with Tourette syndrome who demonstrated heretofore unreported motor disturbances. This normally hearing and speaking individual became proficient in the use of sign language in her midteens and eventually taught it professionally. Early on, extensive use of signing seemed to lessen her tics. However, subsequently she noted that "my signs started as tics" and signing became incorporated into tic behavior. Coprolalia only began after she was fluent in sign language. Initially she would combine the vocalization of shortened forms (e.g., "sh" or "fu") with the complete sign for the obscenity. Later, the signing of swear words occurred in isolation without associated vocalizations. She also utilized sign language to echo what others said or what she had said, read, or thought. Initially the signing always had meaning or was related to what she was thinking; how-

ever, with time the signs were often not associated with the thought or word coming to mind, especially when the sign was only partially or incompletely performed. Given the use of an action or movement (praxis) in the performance of such complex "phonic" tics as coprolalia, echolalia, and palilalia, we suggest the descriptive terms of *coprolaliopraxia*, *echolaliopraxia*, and *palilaliopraxia* to denote these unique symptoms.

The incorporation of such complex and learned motor behavior into the repertoire of abnormal movements is unique but characteristic of tics in contrast to other dyskinesias. It might be argued that this phenomenon, as well as the subjective appreciation of tics as purposefully executed, is difficult to reconcile with certain other features such as the presence of tics in all stages of sleep (17), the absence of a normal premovement electroencephalographic (EEG) potential preceding simple tics (18), and a lack of awareness of the presence of tics by some patients. Differences between tics and other dyskinesias discussed in the preceding sections emphasize that subcortical pathways principally involved in the *generation* of many other dyskinesias (e.g., dystonia, chorea), most notably the dorsal basal ganglia, cannot be the sole site of origin of tics. Possibly the strongest candidate for this origin is an alternation of limbic function that could serve as a driver or stimulus (alternatively, a source of disinhibition), which then results in the disturbances of motor as well as psychic behavior. Often patients will experience some premonitory "sensation" at a conscious ("cortical") level, which may be followed by the purposeful execution of the movement or the voluntary suppression of the "urge." Alternatively, it is likely that repeated intended or learned motor actions can eventually become automatically executed through participation of subcortical motor pathways not originally involved in their genesis. This may be why Obeso and his colleagues (18) were unable to demonstrate a normal Bereitschafts readiness potential in advance of spontaneous tics, whereas such potentials did occur when the patients performed simulated tics. It could also account for the observation that 30% of affected individuals in one large pedigree were completely unaware of their tics (19). Despite the striking and at times disabling nature of the abnormal movements and phonations, it is likely that a more definitive understanding of tic disorders will not come from the study of these motor phenomena but from greater insight into the disturbed neural function that evokes or generates the abnormal behavior either through stimulation or disinhibition of various motor centers that are probably not involved in the primary pathological process.

REFERENCES

1. Bliss J. Sensory experiences of Gilles de la Tourette syndrome. *Arch Gen Psychiatry* 1980; 37:1343–7.
2. Bullen JG, Hemsley DR. Sensory experience as a trigger in Gilles de la Tourette syndrome. *J Behav Ther Exp Psychiatry* 1983;14:197–201.
3. Shapiro AK, Shapiro ES, Young JG, Feinberg TE. *Gilles de la Tourette syndrome.* New York: Raven Press, 1988.
4. Kurlan R, Lichter D, Hewitt D. Sensory tics in Tourette's syndrome. *Neurology* 1989;39:731–4.
5. Lang A. Patient perception of tics and other movement disorders. *Neurology* 1991;41:223 8.
6. Culver GM, Gert B. Philosophy in Medicine. London: Oxford University Press, 1982.
7. Koller WC, Bairy NM. Volitional control of involuntary movements. *Mov Disord* 1989;4:153–6.
8. Walters AS, McHale D, Sage JI, Hening WA, Bergen M. A blinded study of the suppressibility of involuntary movements in Hungtington's chorea, tardive dyskinesia and L-dopa-induced chorea. *Clin Neuropharmacol* 1990;13:236–40.
9. Fahn S. The clinical spectrum of motor tics. In: Friedhoff AJ, Chase TN, eds. *Gilles de la Tourette syndrome.* New York: Raven Press, 1982;341–4.
10. Fahn S, Erenberg G. Differential diagnosis of tic phenomena: a neurologic perspective. In Cohen DJ, Bruun RD, Leckman JF, eds. *Tourette's syndrome and tic disorders, clinical understanding and treatment.* New York: John Wiley & Sons, 1988;41–54.
11. Lees AJ, Robertson M, Trimble MR, Murray NMF. A clinical study of Gilles de la Tourette syndrome in the United Kingdom. *J Neurol Neurosurg Psychiatry* 1984;47:1–8.
12. Shale HM, Truong DD, Fahn S. Tics in patients with other movement disorders. *Neurology* 1986; 36 (suppl 1):118.
13. Elston JS, Granje FC, Lees AJ. The relationship between eye-winking tics, frequent eye blinking and blepharospasm. *J Neurol Neurosurg Psychiatry* 1989;52:477–80.
14. Riley DE, Lang AE. Pain in Gilles de la Tourette syndrome and related tic disorders. *Can J Neurol Sci* 1989;16:439–41.
15. Lees AJ. *Tics and related disorders.* New York: Churchill Livingstone, 1985.
16. Meige H, Feindel E. Tics and their treatment. Wilson SAK, ed and trans. New York: William Wood, 1907.
17. Glaze DG, Frost JD Jr, Jankovic J. Sleep in Gilles de la Tourette's syndrome: disorder of arousal. *Neurology* 1983;33:586–92.
18. Obeso JA, Rothwell JC, Marsden CD. Simple tics in Gilles de la Tourette syndrome are not prefaced by a normal premovement potential. *J Neurol Neurosurg Psychiatry* 1981;44:735–8.
19. Kurlan R, Behr J, Medved L, Shoulson I, Pauls D, Kidd KK. Severity of Tourette's syndrome in one large kindred: implication for determination of disease prevalence rate. *Arch Neurol* 1987;44:268–9.

Advances in Neurology, Vol. 58, edited by T. N. Chase, A. J. Friedhoff, and D. J. Cohen. Raven Press, Ltd., New York © 1992.

5

Tourette Syndrome and Obsessive–Compulsive Disorder

An Analysis of Associated Phenomena

*Danielle C. Cath, †C. A. L. Hoogduin, ‡Ben J. M. van de Wetering, §T. C. A. M. van Woerkom, ‖R. A. C. Roos, and ¶H. G. M. Rooymans

Endegeest Psychiatric Hospital, Outpatient Clinic, 2342 AJ Oegstgeest, The Netherlands, †Department of Psychiatry, Reinier de Graaf Gasthuis, Delft, Delft, The Netherlands, ‡Department of Psychiatry, Dijkzigt University Hospital Rotterdam, Rotterdam, The Netherlands, §Department of Neurology, Leyenburg Hospital, Gravenhage, The Netherlands, ‖Department of Neurology, Leiden University Hospital, Leiden, The Netherlands and ¶Department of Psychiatry, Leiden University Hospital, Leiden, The Netherlands

Since George Gilles de la Tourette described the tic syndrome (1), the relationship between Tourette syndrome (TS), obsessive–compulsive phenomena, and obsessive–compulsive disorder (OCD) has been a focus of discussion (2–6). Whether OCD should be regarded as an integral part of TS, is debatable. Frankel et al. (2), and Pitman et al. (5) find a high (up to 63%) incidence of OCD in TS patients. On the basis of their family studies, Pauls et al. (3,4) suggest that obsessive–compulsive behavior is associated with TS. They support the hypothesis of genetic linkage between TS and OCD.

Shapiro et al. (6) argue that the obsessive–compulsive-like symptoms found in TS patients are in fact impulsions. They state that obsessive–compulsive symptoms, obsessive–compulsive personality traits, impulsions, and impulse control pathology should be seen as separate diagnostic entities. Hoogduin (7) stresses the necessity to differentiate between OCD and impulse control disorders. In his opinion, the difference lies primarily in the fact that the patient with an impulsion experiences some form of pleasure from the deed; feelings of guilt and regret arise later. The patient with obsessions or compulsions experiences anxiety and tension.

The first aim of the pilot study that is presented in this paper was to compare the associated behaviors of TS and OCD patients, especially regarding obsessions, compulsions, and impulsions. The second aim was to compare the two groups on the basis of their depressive states; depressive states are found in both disorders (7,8). The third aim of this study was to compare personality characteristics in both disorders. We hypothesized that specific psychopathology in TS patients, if associated with aggression and hostility (8), could be manifest in extravert or impulsive personality traits. Recent studies on OCD (9,10) reveal a high prevalence of personality disorder (>50%), the majority of diagnoses showing anxious or fearful traits. We speculated that the OCD patients would present a higher frequency of personality disorders, with more inhibited and anxious traits than TS patients.

Associated phenomena of obsessions, compulsions, and OCD were defined in accordance with *Diagnostic and Statistical Manual*, 3rd ed., revised (DSM-III-R) criteria (11). Impulsions and impulse control pathology were defined according to Shapiro et al. (6), since we regarded the DSM-III-R criteria for impulse control disorder inappropriate for the impulsions and impulse control pathology to be investigated in our study. All definitions are summarized in Appendix A.

Ten adult patients with TS from the neurology outpatient clinic of Leiden University Hospital, and ten adult patients with OCD from the psychiatry outpatient clinic of the Reinier de Graaf Hospital in Delft were invited consecutively to take part in the study. The patients who responded to the invitation were selected on the basis of scheduling convenience. It was explained to all patients that the aim of the study was to gain more insight into the symptomatology of their ailment, but not that the relationship between TS and OCD would be explored. All had been diagnosed according to DSM-III-R criteria, and written informed consent was obtained after the procedure had been explained. Patients with previous or current psychosis, affective disorder, substance abuse, or mental deficiency were excluded from the study. On the basis of these criteria, one TS patient and one OCD patient were excluded. The TS patient had a manic psychotic episode in his medical history, and the OCD patient was excluded because he suffered from epilepsy. One OCD patient withdrew from the study at the last moment without giving a reason.

The groups were not matched for age, sex, education, or duration of illness. The TS group (8 males, 1 female) had a mean age of 26 years (SD 6.7). The OCD group (2 males, 6 females) had a mean age of 44.5 (SD 16.9). The differences in age and sex

between patients with TS and OCD were both significant ($p < 0.05$).

Each patient was interviewed using a semistructured interview (constructed for the study, available on request), which was recorded on videotape. The interview included specific detailed items on frequency, characteristics, and subjective experiences of tics, obsessions, impulsions, other repetitive thoughts and compulsions, other repetitive actions, auto- and heteromutilative behavior, avoidance, and reckless behavior throughout the patient's life. All videotapes were systematically evaluated by two of the authors (D. C. C. and T. C. A. M. v. W.) using a checklist. The results were subsequently discussed until consensus was reached. The occurrence of the various associated phenomena over the past year, as well as the emotional implications of each phenomenon was evaluated for both groups. Emotional implications were evaluated using the parameters "pleasant/unpleasant," "suffering," "accompanying fear," and "accompanying tension." Scores ranged from "yes" to "neutral/sometimes" to "no." Other variables involved were: "goal of the phenomenon," "amount of time per day spent on each phenomenon," "interconnection with other phenomena," and "onset of the phenomenon in relation to life events." Concerning the goal of the various phenomena, inquiries were made as to whether the behavior was intended to neutralize or suppress a fearful thought or impulse, whether it was intended as a pastime, or whether it had no other goal than to discharge an impulse or give effect to a thought.

All the patients subsequently completed the following self-administered instruments: the Zung depression rating scale [20 items 1989 Dutch revised version (12)], the Dutch revised version of the Leyton Obsessive–Compulsive Inventory [1976; Kraaimaat and van Dam-Baggen, (13,14)], and the Eysenck Personality Questionnaire (EPQ) [1988 Sandeman, Eysenck, and Arrindell Dutch revised version (15)]. Finally, each patient was interviewed by an independent psychiatrist using the SCID II [1987, Spitzer et al., Dutch version (16)].

At the end of the interview we assessed all patients on an adult version of the Global Assessment of Functioning Scale (A-GAS) (11), in order to get an impression of the disruption of their daily lives caused by the ailment.

The results of the Zung, the LOI, and the EPQ were analyzed for significance, and *p* values were calculated using two-tailed Student's *t* tests.

SYMPTOMATOLOGY

Table 1 summarizes the associated phenomena (as reported by the TS and OCD patients) that occurred in the year before the study.

Some phenomena, namely "echophenomena in thinking"—defined as repetitive thoughts with neutral affective content (without the character of playful pastime)—and "mental play"—defined as repetitive seemingly useless thoughts or images, mostly not unpleasant in nature, and intended as a pastime—occurred only among TS patients. Mental play includes visual, auditive, word, and number games, and will be described in detail elsewhere (Cath et al., 22). Smelling, taking up/putting down objects, symmetry behavior, touching, echo-, pali-, and coprophenomena, and auto- and heteromutilative and reckless behavior occurred only, or much more often, in TS patients. Other phenomena, such as doubting and ruminating, putting away/taking out objects, cleaning, repetitive questions from which to derive comfort, and slow and explicit behavior, occurred only, or much more often, in OCD patients. Some phenomena, such as counting, aggressive repetitive thoughts, dressing/undressing, turning lights and/or gas on and off, rearranging objects, fixed sequences, checking, reading/writing repetitions, and avoidance behavior occurred in both groups.

TABLE 1. *Phenomena reported by Tourette syndrome (TS) and obsessive–compulsive disorder (OCD) patients*

	TS (n = 9)	OCD (n = 8)
Repetitive thoughts, images, impulses		
Neutral content		
Echophenomena	1	0
Counting	4	6
"Mental play"	5	0
Aggressive content		
Repetitive thoughts "as such"	6	7
Frightening content		
Doubting	2	6
Ruminating	1	7
Praying	0	1
Repetitive actions		
Smelling objects, self, others	3	0
Touching objects, self, others	7	0
Picking up/putting down objects	3	0
Symmetry behavior	2	0
Putting away/taking out objects	0	2
Dressing/undressing	0	3
Switching light on/off	2	4
Switching gas on/off	1	3
Rearranging objects	2	1
Fixed sequences and rituals	1	4
Checking	4	8
Washing/cleaning	0	5
Reading/writing	2	2
Verbal repetitions		
Echolalia, palilalia	3	0
Coprolalia	4	0
Repetitive questions (for reassurance)	0	2
Echopraxia, copropraxia	4	0
Hoarding	0	1
Slow and explicit behaviours	0	3
Other repetitions	1	1
Self-mutilation	5	0
Mutilation of others	1	0
Reckless behavior	5	1
Avoidance behavior	3	6

EMOTIONAL IMPLICATIONS AND OTHER VARIABLES OF THE ASSOCIATED PHENOMENA

The TS group experienced the various phenomena in different ways, ranging from "pleasant" to "unpleasant." The intensity of suffering varied from "no suffering" to "explicit suffering." If fear was reported, it was usually not experienced concurrent with the associated behaviors, but was secondary to it: for example, fear caused by the consequences of auto- and heteromutilative behavior, or fear of social disapproval as a consequence of coprolalia. However, one patient had aggressive repetitive thoughts about family members dying in terrible car accidents that provoked accompanying fear, but no compulsions. Another patient reported fearful thoughts about his own death. Another exception was found in the checkers (n = 4), who all experienced some accompanying fear while checking. All patients experienced accompanying tension while performing the various associated phenomena.

The repetitive phenomena in the TS group were aimed at realizing an impulse or thought, or at releasing tension that was sometimes produced by some sensory precursor. Sometimes their behavior resulted in the mutilation of themselves or others. For example, a patient reported touching her cheeks with a lit cigarette until she felt a burning sensation on her skin. An exception was found in the TS patients (n = 4) who checked. The checking was in all cases aimed at preventing some dreaded event. The other exception was provided by a TS patient who reported counting behavior (that could be interpreted as) aimed at the reduction of anxiety.

The amount of time/day spent on associated behaviors by the TS group ranged from episodes of seconds (just once more), to hours uninterrupted. Four TS patients spent more than 1 hour/day on associated behaviors; two patients spent up to 2 hours/day on "mental play," one patient up to 7 hours/day on "echophenomena in thinking," and one of the patients with checking behavior (n = 4) checked and rearranged objects for several hours a day. The patients with mental play regarded their thoughts as pleasant and voluntary, and had no resistance to it, except for one patient who sometimes had

difficulty falling asleep due to the inability "to stop playing." The patient with the echophenomena in thinking regarded his symptoms, although purposeless and senseless and no cause of anxiety to him when suppressed, as unsuppressable and therefore the cause of much distress. The patient who checked several hours a day regarded his checking as the purposeful consequence of his punctuality, a personality trait of which he was proud! It was notable that the various symptoms were not interconnected, but arose separately. We found no clear relationship between the onset of various symptoms and specific life events in the TS group.

In the OCD group, all obsessions and compulsions were experienced as unpleasant, and the cause of much suffering. One exception was found in a patient who reported that he sometimes revelled in aggressive and fearful thoughts concerning the death of family members, imagining what a pitiful and desperate object he would be, and how he would be consoled by his friends. He experienced these obsessions as pleasant, to some extent.

All patients experienced accompanying fear and tension while performing their repetitive behaviors. In most cases the compulsions were aimed at neutralizing a fearful thought or warding off a dreaded event. An exception was found in a patient who moved clothes in and out of her wardrobe, experiencing it as a senseless, non-goal-directed impulse. The same patient had an aimless writing ritual, which made her write everything 20 times "until it was alright," sometimes destroying the paper she wrote on; in that respect her behavior was destructive.

The amount of time per day spent on the various repetitive behaviors ranged from 30 minutes to 12 hours. Repetitions were performed in uninterrupted episodes. In the OCD group, most repetitive symptoms were interrelated, with all sorts of neutralizing and fear-evoking connections. Furthermore, many repetitive behaviors in the OCD group had a tendency to extend from one isolated activity to all daily activities. In the OCD group, three patients reported a relationship between the onset of obsessive–compulsive behavior and a life event.

PSYCHOMETRIC TESTS

The results of the various tests are presented in Table 2. Analyses of the Zung depression scale and of the Leyton Obsessional Inventory revealed significantly lower scores in the TS group. In the TS group, scores on both tests were within the normal range, whereas the scores in the OCD group indicated pathology (12,17).

With regard to the personality tests, the EPQ revealed significant differences on the psychoticism and sociability subscales; the TS group scored higher on psychoticism and lower on sociability. The results of the

SCID II revealed more personality pathology in the OCD group. The TS group showed one personality disorder and four personality traits, spread over three patients. The OCD patients showed two personality disorders in two patients, and eight personality traits, spread over six patients.

COMPARISON OF PHENOMENA IN TS AND OCD

As described above, differences were reported concerning the symptomatology, as well as the emotional implications of the associated phenomena in both groups. No TS patient met the criteria for OCD, and no OCD patient met the criteria for a tic disorder or for impulse control disturbances. Although many associated symptoms were found among the TS patients, only 1 TS

TABLE 2. *Test results*

	Score				Differences between groups (TS vs. OCD)	
	TS (n = 9)		OCD (n = 8)			
Test	Mean	SD	Mean	SD	t	$p <$
Zung	38.3	9.1	50.1	9.0	2.68	<0.05
LOI	80.8	22.3	99.1	13.3	1.99	<0.05
A-GAS	65.5	—	57.5	—	—	—
EPQ						
Psychoticism	4.1	2.3	1.0	1.3	3.9	<0.05
Extraversion	12.0	4.6	9.0	4.6	1.9	n.s.
Neuroticism	13.0	5.6	16.0	4.0	1.3	n.s.
Social desirability	7.0	5.0	15.0	2.5	4.2	<0.05
SCID II	Disorder	Trait	Disorder	Trait		
Avoidant	1		1	2		
Dependent		1				
Obsessive compulsive		1	1	4		
Passively aggressive				1		
Paranoid				1		
Self-defeating		1				
Schizotypal						
Schizoid		1				
Histrionic						
Narcissistic						
Borderline						
Antisocial						

A-GAS, adult Global Assessment of Functioning Scale; EPQ, Eysenck Personality Questionnaire; LOI, Leyton Obsessive–Compulsive Inventory; OCD, obsessive–compulsive disorder; SCID II, structured clinical interview for DSM-III; TS, Tourette syndrome.

patient exhibited associated symptoms (namely, echophenomena in thought) to such an extent that he fulfilled the criteria of a disorder. However, his phenomenology pointed the direction of impulse control disturbances; the echophenomena were not fear-evoking, had no aggressive or repugnant content, and served no special goal. Another patient reported checking behavior for up to 8 hours a day. Nevertheless, he regarded it as purposeful, and felt hardly any resistance to it, although it interfered with his daily life. Therefore, he was not diagnosed as having an OCD. Outcome of SCID II in this patient revealed an avoidant personality disorder, as well as obsessive–compulsive traits.

Although some "normal" obsessions and compulsions were found in TS patients, most of the symptoms were diagnosed as impulsions, as opposed to the obsessions and compulsions found in OCD patients. In the OCD group, one patient exhibited impulsions. Comparison of these data with data from the comparative study by Pitman et al. (5) calls for discussion. In both studies, comparable results are found with regard to a higher incidence of "compulsive" touching, self-mutilative behaviors, and echophenomena in patients with Tourette syndrome. Furthermore, our study revealed results comparable to theirs with regard to the psychometric testing. However, in their study, a 63% incidence of OCD was found in TS patients, and a 6% incidence of TS was found in the patients with OCD. Although we have no clear-cut explanation for these divergent results, several remarks can be made. Age and sex differences between the groups in the two studies are significant. Differences in gender in particular could partly account for the lower incidence of obsessive–compulsive symptomatology in our group of TS patients; family studies have reported less obsessive–compulsive behavior in male TS patients than in females (3,4). Furthermore, in Pitman's study, although the criterion of purpose was investigated to distinguish compulsions from tics, no mention was made of clear differentiation between obsessions, compulsions, and impulsions. In our opinion, in line with Shapiro et al. (6), this differentiation is essential for an adequate interpretation of the various associated symptoms in TS and OCD.

Another explanation for the reported differences could be an overdiagnosis of OCD, due to insufficient strictness in diagnosing OCD as opposed to obsessive–compulsive symptoms in Pitman's study. Furthermore, according to the literature (18), there is an incidence of up to 80% of "normal" obsessions and compulsions in normal populations. Normal and abnormal obsessions seem to be similar in form and content, but differ in frequency, intensity, and consequences (more distress, and more discomfort reducing actions). This means that one may assume that obsessions and compulsions are also to be found in TS populations that do not justify the diagnosis of OCD. On the incidence of impulsions in normal populations no information is available to our knowledge. Finally, we do not exclude theoretically the occurrence of obsessive–compulsive behaviors in TS populations, resulting from a secondary adaptation mechanism to the occurrence of disabling tics and impulsions.

The results of the depression scale and the obsessive–compulsive inventory (Table 2) showed significant differences between the two groups, thus supporting our opinion that TS and OCD patients don't reflect much conformity in symptomatology. However, the relevance of these findings is debatable, since sex and age differences could partly account for these differences. Although differences in scores between TS and OCD were not all significant, the results obtained from the EPQ gave modest support to the hypothesis that TS personality traits indicate impulsivity. Higher neuroticism scores in OCD could indicate more inhibited or anxious traits in OCD. However, the results of the SCID II indicated that personality disorders in the two groups, although differing quantitatively, did not differ qualitatively.

Associated symptoms in TS patients seem to rise from enhanced reaction to inner or outer environmental stimuli, urging the TS patient to respond. Sensory experiences (19,20) as well as auditive, visual, or tactile "provocative irregularities" cause a strong impulse to react. Inner stimuli can also provoke a direct urge to respond. In our opinion, most repetitive thoughts have the characteristics of tics, in accordance with DSM-III-R criteria (11). We would like to introduce the terminology *cognitive tics* for the following repetitive thoughts in TS patients: echophenomena in thought, mental play, counting behavior, and those repetitive thoughts with aggressive content that provoke no fear or neutralizing actions. They differ from obsessions in that they produce no accompanying fear, and therefore no attempt is made to suppress or neutralize the thoughts.

The behavior of the TS patient that seems to be based in impulse control disturbances contrasts with the behavior of the anxious OCD patient. Any unexpected evocative stimulus makes him respond with increased anxiety and fearful obsessions that trigger repetitive and neutralizing actions to ward off dreaded events. As a consequence, in OCD obsessions and compulsions are almost always associated (7,20).

The limitations of the methods used in this pilot study require attention. The groups of patients were small, and age and sex differences between the groups were significant. Difference in gender in particular could affect the results obtained from both groups. The patients were recruited from specialist outpatient clinics, so the population may have reflected different pathology from a general TS and OCD population. Another important bias may be caused by the fact that the interviews were not performed and scored by interviewers unaware of the diagnoses of the individual patients. Definite conclusions should not be drawn from this pilot study, but it should be seen as an attempt to establish a concept in differentiating associated phenomena in TS

patients from those in OCD patients, thus paving the way for a comparative study with larger groups of patients. Also, we did not systematically compare the course of the various repetitive phenomena in both groups. The waxing and waning course of TS-associated symptoms (1,6), in contrast to the mainly uninterrupted course of obsessive–compulsive phenomena (21), as reported in the literature, could be of use in differentiating between the various symptoms in both groups of patients. Moreover, it might be important to study the course of the obsessive–compulsive symptoms that are reported in children and adolescents with TS as they reach adulthood. It is our clinical impression, that some compulsions of TS children wane after adolescence. For obvious reasons, conclusions drawn from studies of the associated phenomena in children and adolescents with TS or OCD should not be applied to adults without great restriction.

As TS as well as OCD reflect heterogeneous disorders, the results of this study seem to indicate that the associated so-called obsessive–compulsive symptoms in adult TS patients differ from the symptoms in adult OCD patients. The associated symptoms in TS patients seem to be more related to impulse control pathology, in contrast to the anxiety-related obsessive–compulsive phenomena in OCD patients. In line with Shapiro et al. (6), we suggest that a clinical differentiation be made between impulsions, obsessions, and compulsions in TS patients.

Further research, including studies implying double-blind comparative phenomenological analysis with pharmacological and neurophysiological correlates, matched patient groups, and controlled treatment studies, is indicated to delineate the various dysregulations responsible for the phenomena in both groups.

REFERENCES

1. Gilles de la Tourette G. Etude sur une affection nerveuse characterisée par l'incoordination mo-

trice accompagnée d'echolalie et coprolalie. *Arch Neurol* 1886;9:19–42.

2. Frankel M, Cummings JL, Robertson MM, et al. Obsessions and compulsions in Gilles de la Tourette's syndrome. *Neurology* 1986;36:378–82.

3. Pauls DL, Towbin KE, Leckman JF, et al. Gilles de la Tourette's syndrome and obsessive-compulsive disorder. *Arch Gen Psychiatry* 1986; 43:1180–2.

4. Pauls DL, Leckman JF. The inheritance of Gilles de la Tourette syndrome and associated behaviors. *N Engl J Med* 1986;16:993–7.

5. Pitman RK, Green RC, Jenike MA, et al. Clinical comparison of Tourette's disorder and obsessive-compulsive disorder. *Am J Psychiatry* 1987; 144:1166–71.

6. Shapiro AK, Shapiro ES, Young JG, et al. *Gilles de la Tourette syndrome*, 2nd ed. New York: Raven Press, 1988.

7. Hoogduin CAL. On the diagnosis of obsessive-compulsive disorder. *Am J Psychother* XL: 1986:36–51.

8. Robertson MM, Trimble MM, Lees AJ. The psychopathology of the Gilles de la Tourette syndrome: a phenomenological analysis. *Br J Psychiatry* 1988;152:383–90.

9. Jenike MA, Baer L, Minichiello WE. *Obsessive-compulsive disorders: theory and management*, 2nd ed. Chicago: Year Book Medical Publishers, 1990;80–81.

10. Joffe RT, Swinson RP, Regan JJ. Personality features of obsessive compulsive disorder. *Am J Psychiatry*, 1988;145:1127–9.

11. Williams JBW, Spitzer RL. American Psychiatric Association, *Diagnostic and statistical manual of mental disorders, Third revised edition*. Washington, D.C.: 1987;78,245,335,321.

12. Mook J, Kleyn W, van der Ploeg HM. Depression as disposition measured with the Zung scale. *Nederlands tijdshrift psychol* 1989;44:328–40.

13. Kraaimaat FW, van Dam-Baggen CMJ. Development of a self rating scale for obsessive-compulsive behaviour. *Nederlands tijdschrift pschol.* 1976;31:201–11.12.

14. Cooper J. The Leyton Obsessional Inventory *Psychol Med* 1970;1:48–64.

15. Eysenck JH, Eysenck SBG. *Manual of the Eysenck personality questionnaire*, London: Hodder and Stroughton Educational, 1975.

16. Spitzer RL, Williams JBW. *Structured clinical interview for DSM-III-R personality disorders (SCID II)*. New York: New York State Psychiatric Institute, 1985.

17. Arts W, Severijns R, Hoogduin CAL, et al. The IDB (LOI): a replication study on reliability and validity. *Gedragstherapie* 1990;23:17–27.

18. Rachman S, de Silva P. Abnormal and normal obsessions. *Behav Res Ther* 1978;16:233–48.

19. Bliss J. Sensory experiences of Gilles de la Tourette syndrome. *Arch Gen Psychiatry* 1990; 37:1343–7.

20. Kurlan R, Lichter D, Hewitt D. Sensory tics in Tourette's syndrome. *Arch Gen Psychiatry* 1989; 43:1180–2.

21. Rasmussen SA, Tsuang MT. Clinical characteristics and family history in DSM-III obsessive compulsive disorder. *Am J Psychiatry* 1986; 143:317–22.

22. Cath DC, Wetering van de BJM, Hoogduin CAL, et al. Mental play in Gilles de la Tourette syndrome and obsessive-compulsive disorder. *Br J Psychiatry* 1992; in press.

APPENDIX A. Definitions

Obsessions

recurrent and persistent ideas, thoughts, impulses, or images, that are experienced, at least initially, as intrusive and senseless.

The person attempts to ignore or suppress such thoughts or images, or to neutralize them with some other thought or action.

Compulsions

repetitive, purposeful, and intentional actions performed in response to an obsession, or according to certain rules or in a stereotyped fashion.

The behavior is designed to neutralize or prevent discomfort or some dreaded event or situation.

The activity is not connected realistically with what it is designed to prevent, or it is excessive.

The person recognizes the behavior as being excessive or unreasonable.

Impulsions   repetitive and intentional actions performed according to certain rules, or in a stereotyped fashion.

> The behavior is either performed automatically, without purpose, or as the consequence of the failure to resist an impulse or temptation to perform some act that is harmful to the individual or to others.
>
> Either pleasure, gratification or relief at the time of committing the act.
>
> The person recognizes the behavior as being unrealistic and/or excessive.

Obsessive–compulsive disorder (OCD)   the obsessions and compulsions

> cause distress,
>
> are time-consuming (>1 hour a day), or significantly interfere with the person's life and/or relationships.

Impulse control pathology   the impulsions

> cause distress,
>
> are time-consuming (>1 hour a day), or significantly interfere with the person's life and/or relationships.

Advances in Neurology, Vol. 58, edited by T. N. Chase, A. J. Friedhoff, and D. J. Cohen. Raven Press, Ltd., New York © 1992.

6

Methodology of Epidemiological Studies of Tic Disorders and Comorbid Psychopathology

Theodore Fallon, Jr, and Mary Schwab-Stone

Child Study Center, Yale University School of Medicine, New Haven, Connecticut 06510

Over the past century since the description of Tourette syndrome (TS) by Gilles de la Tourette (1), fundamental questions about the nature of this disorder have been posed: How many people have TS and how severely are people in the general population affected? How do we know if someone has TS or not? This question can sometimes be difficult to answer because of problems in defining a threshold for diagnosis and because of the waxing and waning nature of TS. What are the associated features and what is their relationship to TS? Are they causative, predisposing, a result of TS, or manifestations of TS itself? While partial answers to these questions have been found, definitive answers will come from studies yet to be done utilizing different strategies of inquiry. One such line of inquiry is epidemiology.

Epidemiological methods have been used for centuries as tools to study biomedical diseases; however, these methods also have the potential for the study of behavioral disorders. For TS, these epidemiological techniques have the potential to provide prevalence estimates of TS, thereby clarifying its public health significance; to elucidate the full range of clinical expression and natural history of the symptoms of TS, thereby

contributing to the definition of TS; and to help explicate the relationships between these symptoms and associated conditions, thereby clarifying the role of environmental, genetic, protective, and risk factors as they affect the expression of these symptoms.

This chapter will consider how these epidemiological methods can assist in answering these questions about TS. It will first focus on a key concept at the foundation of epidemiology, the disease definition. This discussion will consider differences between TS and other biomedical diseases and will explore the implications of these differences for the study of TS. Then, epidemiological work on TS will be reviewed, considering the methodological strengths and weaknesses of this research. This chapter will conclude by anticipating future work in the epidemiological research of TS and the methodological elements that will be important in this work.

THE FOUNDATION OF EPIDEMIOLOGY IN TS RESEARCH

For a study of any disease, a clear definition is imperative, to discriminate consistently between those who have the disease and those who do not. However, definitions of disease may be used quite differently in clinical versus research situations, and these discrepancies may be particularly problematic in TS because the disease has indistinct boundaries. For instance, in clinical practice, a disease is diagnosed by taking into account the situation in which the presentation is made. For example, a father brings his 7-year-old son to a clinic because of concerns about disruptive behavior and multiple motor and vocal tics. The father is observed to have a single motor tic but has no other history for TS. Clearly, the child has TS, but one could argue the clinical utility of giving a diagnosis of TS to the father. In research, however, the outcome and conclusions of a study may depend on whether or not a diagnosis of TS is given to this father. Because he may be a carrier, failure to make the diagnosis in a family genetic study would decrease the power of the analysis of genetic linkage. On the other hand, to diagnose the father if he is not a carrier would seriously distort the results of the analysis (see Pauls et al., *this volume*). For the purposes of research, it is critical that the definition be clear, precise, and accurate.

Biomedical diseases are generally defined by physical processes that can be measured by laboratory tests to identify those who have a disease and those who do not. For example, infections are defined by bacterial growth with tissue damage and are measured by bacterial cultures. With the present state of knowledge about TS, however, identification of those who have TS is more of a problem than for other biomedical diseases. The difficulty stems largely from the variability of the behavioral expression of TS across time and place. In the example of the father of the 7-year-old boy cited above, there is no clear measure to determine whether or not the father has TS. At present, a true definition of TS can only be approximated using criteria that one hopes will include most of those who have the disease and exclude most who do not have the disease.

Also involved in the definition of a disease is an implicit assumption that there is utility in calling attention to the group of attributes named in the disease. The purposes of calling a group of attributes by a single name include a known *natural history* for this set of attributes, a common *etiology*, and effective *treatment*. This point can be illustrated by an example in which there is no utility in naming a set of attributes. Everyone with red hair and blue eyes could be said to have "dichromatic pigment disease." Although the etiology is clear (genetic inheritance of particular pigmentation), there is no utility in making this distinction from the point of view of natural history, or treatment. In the biomedical example of infection, the utility of this definition is to name a common etiology (bacterial growth), an expected natural history (progression of bacterial growth and tissue damage), mechanisms of pathology (bacterial toxins), and effective treatment.

The original definition of TS derived from observations of a clinical population and used features of the natural history as criteria; a rare, severe, life-long, debilitating disease with distinctive symptoms that included multiple motor and vocal tics, compulsions, and echo phenomena (1). It is likely that Gilles de la Tourette was motivated to call TS a syndrome because of the unusual and particular set of behaviors that seemed to be associated with it. Additionally, his clinic patients with the disorder seemed to have a poor prognosis.

At the core of Gilles de la Tourette's description is the hypothesis that the symptoms of TS are etiologically related. The nature of these etiological relationships is, however, quite complex, as genetic, biochemical, developmental, behavioral, and social phenomena are all involved (2). When considering a disease that spans phenomena from the molecular to the social realm, one needs to be clear about what is meant by "etiologically related." At what level on this hierarchy between molecular and behavioral do phenomena need to be related and what is the nature of that relationship in order to consider behaviors "etiologically related"? It may be that the idea of a single etiology of TS may be too simplistic. As well as no clear etiology, at present there is no known pathognomonic mechanism of pathology that can be targeted for treatment such as there is with infections. One way to conceptualize such a complex state is to consider a multifactorial model (such as is done with cardiovascular disease) in which there are many conditions necessary, in combination over time, for the disease to prevail.

An example will illustrate this point about etiology. Tics and compulsions are descriptions of two behaviors considered to be part of TS. Although it is unclear how these behaviors are related, Pauls et al. (3) suggest that the same genetic locus conveys risk for both of these behaviors. If the identical genetic lesion is shown to convey risk for both behaviors, however, it will still remain to be seen whether or not these behaviors share the same neurostructural, biochemical, developmental, or psychological processes. When it is known which processes these behaviors share and which processes are not shared, the question of etiology will become a matter of semantics.

When the processes at each of these levels can be measured, the methods of epidemiology can begin to delineate the relationships between these processes, thereby placing these processes in the context of normal functioning in the general population. Before beginning a discourse on how this might be done, let us examine what has been learned from past epidemiological studies of TS.

The first task of epidemiology is to determine how frequently a disease can be identified in a population. In the past 100 years there have been a number of efforts to estimate prevalence rates of TS and to determine which conditions are commonly associated with it. Table 1 lists these studies.

As can be seen from this table, the prevalence rates have varied considerably across studies. Early studies used clinic and referred populations. For example, Koester (4), in reviewing admissions to a clinic, found an estimated rate of 8 in 10,000, while Feild's (5) review of case records yielded an estimate of 5 per million. Koester's study had as a denominator all patients in a clinic population while Feild's denominator was the entire population of a county.

Although these prevalence estimates vary by orders of magnitude, it is unlikely that the actual rates varied so dramatically in these populations. Instead, it is likely that this variability reflects methodological inconsistencies across these studies. The history of the epidemiology of TS underscores the need to examine a set of methodological issues that affect the interpretation of results from existing studies and that can guide future research efforts.

METHODOLOGICAL PROBLEMS

Three potential sources of methodological error may account for the differences in rates seen in Table 1: sample selection bias, variability in case identification, and problems in syndrome definition.

Sample selection bias affects both prevalence estimates of TS and estimates of the degree of association between TS and other features such as risk factors and comorbid psychopathology. Early studies of TS were conducted on clinic patients, not people from a general community; however, it is well known that patients in treatment for any disease do not represent the general population of those with the disorder. Patients who come for treatment have illnesses that concern them in some way. They are usually more impaired and have been ill for a longer time than those with the same disease processes who do not ask for treatment. Trying to generalize about a disease from a clinical setting to a general population will therefore be misleading. Using the clinical setting as the basis for understanding a disease will lead to an overesti-

TABLE 1. *Prevalence of Tourette syndrome reported in studies*

Study	Site	Sample characteristics	Sample size	No.	Prevalence/ thousand
Koester, 1899 (4)	Leipzig	Admissions, Universitats Poliklnik	2,500	2	0.8
Ascher, 1948 (24)	Baltimore	Hospitalized and outpatients, Johns Hopkins	590,000	4	0.007
Salmi, 1961 (25)	Finland	Educational Guidance Clinic	5,300	1	0.19
Feild et al., 1966 (5)	Minnesota	Mayo Clinic Admissions, 1935–1965	1,500,000	7	0.005
Caine et al., 1985 (9)	New York	Survey of referred 5–18-year-old children	142,000	41	0.29
Burd et al., 1986 (7)	North Dakota	Survey of 6–18-year-old children			
		Males	71,640	67	0.935
		Females	60,910	6	0.099
		Total	140,580	73	0.519
Burd et al., 1986 (8)	North Dakota	Survey of adults over 18 years of age			
		Males	223,537	17	0.076
		Females	224,999	5	0.022
		Total	448,556	22	0.049
Comings et al., 1991 (23)	California	Examination of 6th–8th grade school children			
		Males	1,517	21	10.5
		Females	1,517	2	1.3
		Total	3,034	23	5.9
Apter et al., 1991 (this volume)	Israel	Examination of children 16–17 years of age			
		Males	18,364	9	0.49
		Females	9,673	3	0.31
		Total	28,037	12	0.43

Adapted from Shapiro et al., ref. 26.

mate of the severity and chronicity of this disease in the general population. Cohen and Cohen (6) have described this phenomenon as the *clinician's illusion*. Therefore, studies using clinic patients will overestimate severity and chronicity of TS by selecting and studying only those more severe cases who present themselves to a clinic and missing those less severe cases in the general population who do not present themselves to a clinic. Failing to count the less severe cases will also lead to decreased prevalence estimates if the population served by the clinic is taken as the denominator.

Epidemiological studies of TS done in the past 5 years have attempted to circumvent this selection bias by using community-based, as opposed to clinically based, case ascertainment. Burd et al. (7,8) surveyed the whole state of North Dakota for TS. This was done by using many different types of care providers as informants, including primary care practitioners and nonmedical facilities to identify possible TS cases. The multiplicity of the referral sources increased the likelihood that nonclinic cases might be detected. Burd et al., however, only recorded people who had contact with these informants. It is unknown how many people did not have contact with his informants. Thus, it is quite likely that the derived prevalence rate of 5.2/10,000 children is low and biased in severity toward a clinic population.

Caine et al. (9) endeavored to survey the entire population of school children in Monroe County, New York for TS. This study attempted to compensate for selection bias by using mass media advertisements to recruit individuals from the general community. This method of recruitment, however, introduced its own ascertainment bias. As with the study by Burd et al., Caine et al. derived a prevalence rate by assuming that every child in the county that had TS had been found. Caine et al. indicated that after their study had ended they continued to find additional cases in this population. They concluded that the prevalence rate estimate of 2.8/10,000 was low. However, even with these disclaimers, this study found that in comparison with their community data, ". . . studies based on clinical patient populations tend to overrepresent the frequency of severe behavior disorders in their samples. Our results indicate that TS in the school age population is a much milder disorder than most clinicians and investigators would assume based on impressions gained from patients coming for treatment." Here, then, is evidence of the clinician's illusion.

The Israel Defense Force study of TS (Apter et al., *this volume*) surveyed an entire population, which is the most effective way of avoiding selection bias. This study still has a possible bias, however—a reporting bias. There may be considerable pressure not to report symptoms because of the stigma that may result from being found unfit to serve in the Israel military.

These last three studies have derived more consistent prevalence rates than did earlier studies. As we know from the natural history of TS, these estimates will vary according to the age of the population studied.

Selection bias using clinic populations affects not only the estimates of prevalence and severity of the disease, it can also give a distorted view of associated features. Selection bias that distorts estimates of associated features is known as *Berkson's bias* (10). Berkson's bias derives from the observation that clinical samples disproportionately represent individuals who have multiple conditions. This disproportionate representation of multiple conditions results from the increased likelihood that people with two disorders will seek help more readily than people with only one of these two disorders. This situation will lead to the appearance of comorbidity in clinic populations, which is not substantiated in general population samples.

A classic example of Berkson's bias from chronic disease epidemiology is coronary heart disease and ulcer disease. Patients with comorbid coronary heart disease and ulcer disease present more often to hospitals than by chance alone given the prevalence of each of these disorders in the general population. These clinical data in isolation would lead to the conclusion that heart disease and ulcer disease are related. However, in the general population, these two diseases are not found together more often than would be suggested by their independent rates. Knowledge of the pathophysiology of these two diseases further confirms their nonassociation.

Patients with TS who have a second unrelated form of psychopathology are probably more likely to present to clinics than those who have TS alone. When clinic-based case control studies are conducted to look for psychopathology associated with TS, it may erroneously be concluded that a particular disorder is related to TS when in fact the disorder is only related to TS in the clinic population and not in the general population. Similarly, the risk factors associated with these second psychopathologies will also seem related to TS when they are not.

Numerous studies using clinical populations have explored the association of TS and other comorbid psychopathology, and have suggested a myriad of associated symptoms including attention deficit disorder (11), conduct disorder (12), phobias and panic attacks (13), obsessions and compulsions, schizoid behaviors (14), depression, and mania (15). However, Berkson's bias suggests that studies of clinic populations which have found associations between TS and other pathology are suspect. Other data that explore associations between TS and some of these symptoms will be briefly examined. At present, the most hotly debated features associated with TS are attention deficit, hyperactivity, and obsessive–compulsive symptoms.

Probably the least controversy exists concerning the co-occurrence of TS and obsessive compulsive symptoms. Obsessive compulsive symptomatology has long been noted to co-occur in clinic patients with TS. Family genetic studies by Pauls et al. (3), which are free of the effects of Berkson's bias, independently support an etiological link between obsessive compulsive symptoms and TS. These studies show that tics and obsessive compulsive symptoms co-occur within families of TS probands whether or not the TS proband has obsessive compulsive symptoms. Pauls's studies also found increased rates of obsessive compulsive symptoms without TS or tics in families with a TS proband. These findings further support the interpretation that TS and at least some form of obsessive compulsive symptoms are etiologically related. In the case of TS and obsessive compulsive symptoms, observations from separate lines of inquiry, clinical observation and family genetic studies are in agreement. The conclusion is that obsessive compulsive symptoms may represent an alternate expression of factors, presumably genetic, that are responsible for TS.

Unlike obsessive compulsive symptomatology, it is less clear whether there is an association between attention-deficit hyperactivity symptoms and TS. While the rate of attention-deficit hyperactivity symptoms in the general population of children is between 5% and 10%, in patients with TS, rates of attention-deficit hyperactivity symptoms from 25% to 60% have been reported. However, family studies by Pauls et al. (16) appear to contradict these results by showing that the two disorders segregate independently in family pedigrees. Pauls' data suggest that TS and attention-deficit

hyperactivity symptoms are genetically independent disorders. Can Berkson's bias be invoked to explain the contradictory results between these clinical and family studies?

To answer this question, a community study using unbiased sampling methods is needed. The study by Burd et al. (7,8) attempted to obtain a sample that was independent of being defined as a patient with TS by soliciting primary care providers to identify people with TS. Although this method simulates a community sample more closely than taking patients from a neurological clinic, Burd's subjects were still not independent of patient status since clinicians were providing information about their patients; it is uncertain how much bias is introduced with Burd's method. There is also a second, perhaps more important, problem with Burd's study regarding comorbidity. There was a poor response rate (43%) when those people identified with TS were surveyed for associated features, thus reducing accuracy of data interpretation.

The study by Caine et al. (9) also made a valiant attempt to gather a community sample by using mass media to recruit subjects. This study found lower rates of comorbidity between TS and obsessive compulsive symptoms and attention deficit hyperactivity symptoms than have been found in clinic populations, demonstrating the effects of Berkson's bias in clinic-based studies. Caine et al. (9), however, still conclude that attention-deficit hyperactivity symptoms and obsessive compulsive symptoms are associated with TS. The rates of comorbidity identified in this study are difficult to interpret since there is no comparison with a control population. It is also difficult to estimate the effect of the mass media on selection bias: people who respond to mass media solicitations most certainly will not be a simple random sample of the general population.

Summarizing across studies of comorbid behaviors, different research techniques collectively suggest that obsessive compulsive symptoms and TS are etiologically related, presumably in a genetic manner. However, data are contradictory with respect to the association between TS and attention-deficit hyperactivity symptoms. It is likely that Berkson's bias has some role in contributing to this contradiction. A community-based study of TS and comorbid conditions would provide definitive information about these associations and would indicate the extent to which clinic samples can legitimately be used to study TS. Most likely, however, Berkson's bias does not account for all of the association between TS and attention-deficit hyperactivity symptoms in clinical and community settings. Presuming there is an association between TS and attention-deficit hyperactivity symptoms, the nature of this relationship is unclear. How do TS symptoms interact with attention-deficit hyperactivity symptoms, or are they both etiologically related to a third agent? To answer this question, a prospective longitudinal study is necessary.

Protective and risk factors are other areas in which the tools of epidemiology are helpful. Clinical studies have suggested a host of risk factors that are associated with TS and that are involved in the pathogenesis, expression, and course of the disease. Leckman et al. (17) examined the prenatal histories of mothers of TS children and found that maternal prenatal stress was associated with severity of TS. Leckman et al. have also suggested that the onset of adrenarche may be an important factor in the development of TS. Intramorbid environmental stress seems to exacerbate tics, at least in the short run (18). Caine et al. (9) assessed risk factors including prenatal, developmental, and drug exposure, yet the small number of subjects with each risk factor prevented conclusions regarding risk factors.

Although there have been few studies of possible protective factors, clinical experience suggests that certain healthy family dynamics can provide some insulation from the effects that tics may have on a child interpersonally. Additionally, Mahler (19) in her psychoanalytic study of individuals with tics, suggests that although psychoanalysis does not prevent or cure tic behavior, it considerably improves a patient's long-term adjustment. Thus certain features of the psychotherapeutic process may protect against concomitant problems. Information about protective and risk factors is derived from clinical observation, which may or may not have employed case-control comparisons. These factors, however, have not been explored in the larger context of nonclinical populations. As such, we do not know to what extent knowledge of these factors is distorted by selection bias. Here again, a community study would help to understand this distortion.

Another source of methodological error involves problems in case identification. For example, Bornstein et al. (20) examined two Ohio surveys and found that between 1983 and 1987, the mean time from initial appearance of symptoms to time of diagnosis dropped from 2.9 years to 1.9 years for children less than 10 years of age. During these same years, the Tourette's Syndrome Association (TSA) membership in Ohio approximately doubled. Based on Ohio TSA membership, the estimate of TS prevalence would appear to have doubled over 4 years. However, since the time from onset of symptoms to diagnosis had also dropped by over 30%, it is more likely that the prevalence rate did not change; rather, many more people were made aware of their diagnosis of TS. Increased awareness of TS by both the lay population and physicians is most likely due to education of the general public and professional community. Thus, education in Ohio had a profound effect on prevalence estimates, mediated by what is called case identification.

In epidemiological studies, case identification is dependent on an informant, and the informant's awareness about TS symptoms. The North Dakota study by Burd et al. (7,8) controlled for TS awareness by educating physicians about TS as they conducted their survey. This ensured that all informants shared a certain minimal under-standing of the primary features of the disorder. Education of the informant clearly has a major effect on identification of individuals with TS.

Informant misinformation is another potential source of methodological error in case identification bias. This misinformation is found in distorted predetermined notions that informants, as well as diagnostic instruments, bring to the process of identifying cases. Pauls et al. (3), in their family study of the association of obsessive compulsive symptoms and TS, elegantly demonstrated how to test for this bias using blind diagnostic rating procedures, multiple diagnostic assessments by different raters, and specific hypothesis testing for distorted relationships.

Case identification bias is clearly important in epidemiological work with TS as demonstrated by Bornstein's study (20). Biases introduced in case identification will have the same potential effects as selection bias on estimates of prevalence, severity of disease, and degree of association with other factors. Thus, thorough education of informants and careful scrutiny of the instruments and assessment procedures are critical methodological requirements in epidemiological research in TS.

The third potential source of bias involves problems in disease definition, the critical element in epidemiological methods with which this chapter began. Sample selection bias can implicitly affect disease definition by selecting individuals in a way that restricts the range of disease seen. The disease definition can also be altered directly by altering the formal criteria (such as is delineated in DSM-III-R) that is used to make the diagnosis. Both of these methods will influence who is identified as having disease.

Gilles de la Tourette used clinical and historical criteria to define TS operationally. Even today the definition of TS relies mostly on clinical observation. Recent data, however, suggest that a broader concep-tualization of TS is necessary that includes etiology and the complete natural history of the disease. Clinical study has revealed that the presence of motor and vocal tics does not necessarily confer such a grave prognosis as was once thought. Family pedigree and genetic studies suggest that there is an underlying genetic vulnerability, the expression of which may be transient tics (21), chronic motor tics (22), obsessive compulsive symptoms (3), or full-blown TS. The study by Caine et al. (9) suggests that TS may not always be disabling; almost half of the subjects identified in this study were from nonclinician sources, and even after they were identified, most of these individuals were free of socially troubling behavioral disturbances. The studies by Burd et al. (7,8) suggest that the intensity of the disease peaks in childhood, and then wanes throughout life; ten times as many children as adults had TS, as identified by health care workers. Considered together, results from these studies demonstrate the variability in the expression of TS.

As more is learned about physiological and genetic features associated with the clinical syndrome, however, the boundaries for defining the disease are often challenged. There may be a demand to redefine TS in terms of genetic and physical parameters, resulting in a potential deemphasis of the clinical features and in a less distinctive, more ambiguous clinical picture. An example of this ambiguity can be noted in the work by Comings et al. (1990 and *this volume*). This group has noted prevalence rates of TS in school children four to ten times higher than other recent epidemiological studies. Although not clearly delineated in this work, one might suspect that the disease definition used by Comings et al. differs from work by other researchers.

Thus, an agreement between researchers on the criteria used for the definition of TS is needed. This agreement will require consideration of TS criteria and the interrelationships between these criteria and the associated features. Epidemiology can assist in this process by delineating the full range of tic and other psychopathological symptomatology and by explicating their interrelationships in the natural setting, the community. This information can inform decisions regarding criteria used to define TS for clinical and research purposes.

FUTURE RESEARCH EFFORTS

Let us summarize what a review of the methodology has told us about studies in epidemiology. Recent epidemiological studies of TS have demonstrated that it is possible to identify TS consistently in community populations, despite lingering problems in identifying all cases. Community-based studies are needed to avoid selection biases and to survey the full range and frequency of the manifestations of TS as they occur in nature. These manifestations include the entire spectrum of the disorder, from those with severe impairment to those who are completely asymptomatic. Survey methods need to adopt standardized assessment procedures that control for informant biases and that use widely accepted criteria for TS. The sensitivity, specificity, reliability, and validity of these assessment procedures also need to be clearly established.

Additionally, informants in community surveys of TS will need to be standardized. It is important to educate informants about tic behaviors, particularly when surveying a general population in which, as a rule, informants may have little or no prior knowledge of tic behavior.

Finally, to understand how preventive and risk factors relate to TS, longitudinal studies are necessary. Cross-sectional studies cannot identify whether factors associated with TS are causes or effects of TS. A longitudinal design, however, allows for assessment of premorbid functioning and detailed examination of the occurrence of risk factors in relation to symptoms.

An epidemiological study of TS with all of the above requirements is not likely to be done, as it requires resources and circumstances beyond reach. For example, perhaps 100 children with TS from a community sample would be needed for such a study. With liberal estimates that 1 in 1,000 children develop TS, 100,000 children from a community would need to be followed for a period of perhaps 20 years with extensive, frequent, and detailed evaluation. Even if such an ambitious study were done, the information might ultimately be outdated as the definition of TS may change to incorporate new genetic or physiological findings.

A more reasonable and alternative approach to this problem would be a longitudinal community study of the major symptoms of TS, motor and phonic tics. Tic behavior is the salient feature of TS, and as such shares many attributes with TS. However, tic behavior is a relatively common occurrence. In a second-stage sample of a recent survey of Eastern Connecticut, teachers identified 10% of children between the ages of 6 and 12 years as having tic behavior (T. Fallon—M. Schwab-Stone, unpublished data). Therefore, a study of tic behavior would only need to survey 2,000–4,000 children.

This methodological compromise would yield important information about the full range of symptoms of TS and tics and would provide an opportunity to explore relationships between tics and associated features. A longitudinal component in such a study would provide needed information on phenocopies of TS, and yield critical information about the natural history of tics through a salient developmental period for contrast to the natural history of TS. Additionally, such a study would permit exploration of cause and effect relationships with respect to risk and preventive factors as well as associated features of tic behavior. Thus, a community study of tic behavior in children would provide information needed to discriminate TS syndrome and its spectrum manifestations from unrelated forms of tic behavior.

Another useful methodological compromise would be a longitudinal study of children at high risk for developing TS, as is presently being done by Pauls and his group. This study is recruiting young children prior to the average age of onset of TS (7 years) from families in which there is a proband with TS. Many of these children have the familial predisposition to TS, and some of them will indeed develop TS. Following these children longitudinally will provide important information regarding cause and effect of associated features of TS, as well as a clearer delineation of the natural history of TS.

Although there is considerable potential yield from epidemiologic research of TS, both methodological and logistical obstacles exist. It is possible to guard against methodological hazards of selection bias, poor syndrome definition, and imperfect case identification through awareness, careful study design, and case ascertainment. The major logistical limitation for epidemiologic research on TS involves the low base rate of this disorder in the population. However, methodological compromises make it possible to conduct studies needed to further our understanding of TS. Such studies promise to yield valuable information on the prevalence and full range of symptoms of tic behavior and TS, patterns of comorbidity, and preventive and risk factors. In these respects, results from epidemiological research will contribute to efforts to prevent and treat those afflicted with this disorder.

REFERENCES

1. Gilles de la Tourette G. Etude sur une affection nerveuse caracterisée par de l'incoordination motrice accompagnée d'echolalie et de copralalie. *Arch Neurol* 1885;9:19–42.
2. Cohen DJ, Detlor J, Shaywitz BA, Leckman JF. Interaction of biological and psychological factors in the natural history of Tourette syndrome: a paradigm for child neuropsychiatric disorders. In: Friedhoff AJ, Chase TN, eds. *Advances in Neurology: Gilles de la Tourette Syndrome*, vol 35. New York: Raven Press, 1982;31–40.
3. Pauls DL, Towbin KE, Leckman JF, Zahner GEP, Cohen DJ. Gilles de la Tourette's syndrome and obsessive-compulsive disorder: evidence supporting a genetic relationship. *Arch Gen Psychiatry* 1986;43:1180–2.
4. Koester G. Uber die Maladie des Tics impulsifs (mimische Krampfneurose). *Dtsch Z Nervenkr* 1899;1:147–59.
5. Feild JR, Corbin KB, Goldstein NP, Klass DW. Gilles de la Tourette's syndrome. *Neurology* 1965; 453–62.
6. Cohen P, Cohen J. The clinician's illusion. *Arch Gen Psychiatry* 1984;41:1178–82.
7. Burd L, Kerbeshian J, Wikenheiser M, Fisher W. A prevalence study of Gilles de la Tourette syndrome in North Dakota school-age children. *J Am Acad Child Adolesc Psychiatry* 1986;25:552–3.
8. Burd L, Kerbeshian J, Wikensheiser M, Fisher W. Prevalence of Gilles de la Tourette's syndrome in North Dakota adults. *Am J Psychiatry* 1986; 143:787–8.
9. Caine Ed, McBride MC, Chiverton P, Bamford KA, Rediess S, Shiao J. Tourette's syndrome in Monroe county school children. *Neurology* 1988; 38:472–5.
10. Berkson J. Limitations of the application of fourfold table analysis to hospital data. *Biomet Bull* 1946;2:47–53.
11. Comings DE, Comings BG. A controlled study of Tourette's syndrome I. Attention deficit disorder, learning disorders and school problems. *Am J Hum Genet* 1987;451:701–41.
12. Comings DE, Comings BG. A controlled study of Tourette's syndrome II. Conduct. *Am J Hum Genet* 1987;41:742–60.
13. Comings DE, Comings BG. A controlled study of Tourette's syndrome III. Phobias and panic attacks. *Am J Hum Genet* 1987;41:761–81.
14. Comings DE, Comings BG. A controlled study of Tourette's syndrome IV: Obsessions and compulsions and schizoic behavior. *Am J Hum Genet* 1987;41:782–803.
15. Comings DE, Comings BG. A controlled study of Tourette's syndrome V: depression and mania. *Am J Hum Genet* 1987;41:804–21.
16. Pauls DL. Towbin KE, Leckman JF, Zahner GEP, Cohen DJ. Gilles de la Tourette's syndrome and attention deficit disorder with hyperactivity: evidence against a genetic relationship. *Arch Gen Psychiatry* 1986;43:1177–9.
17. Leckman JF, Dolnansky ES, Hardin MT, et al. Perinatal factors in the expression of Tourette's syndrome: an exploratory study. *J Am Acad Child Adolesc Psychiatry* 1990;29:220–6.
18. Jagger J, Prusoff BS, Cohen DJ, Kidd KK, Carbonario CM, John K. The epidemiology of Tourette's syndrome: a pilot study. *Schizoph Bull* 1982; 8:267–78.
19. Mahler MS, Luke JA. Outcome of the tic syndrome. *J Nerv Ment Dis* 1949;103:433–45.
20. Bornstein RA, Stefl ME, Hammond L. A survey of Tourette syndrome patients and their families: the 1987 Ohio Tourette Survey. Presented at American Academy of Neurology Meeting, Cincinnati OH, April 21, 1988.
21. Kurlan R, Behr J, Medved L, Como P. Transient tic disorder and the spectrum of Tourette's syndrome. *Arch Neurol* 1988;45:1200–1.

22. Pauls DL, Kruger SD, Leckman JF, Cohen DJ, Kidd KK. The risk of Tourette's syndrome and chronic multiple tics among relatives of Tourette's syndrome patients obtained by direct interview. *J Am Acad Child Psychiatry* 1984;23:134–7.

23. Comings DE, Himes JA, Comings BG. An epidemiological study of Tourette's syndrome in a single school district. *Neurology* 1991;51:463–9.

24. Ascher E. Psychodynamic considerations of Gilles de la Tourette's disease (*maladie des tics*): with a report of five cases and discussion of the literature. *Am J Psychiatri* 1948;105:267–76.

25. Salmi K. Gilles de la Tourette's syndrome: the report of a case and its treatment. *Acta Psychiatr Scand* 1961;36:156–62.

26. Shapiro A, Shapiro E, Young JG, Feinberg TE. *Gilles de la Tourette syndrome*, 2nd ed. New York: Raven Press, 1988;57.

Advances in Neurology, Vol. 58, edited by T. N. Chase, A. J. Friedhoff, and D. J. Cohen. Raven Press, Ltd., New York © 1992.

7

Psychosocial Factors in Tourette Syndrome

Felton Earls

Department of Maternal and Child Health, Harvard School of Public Health and Department of Child Psychiatry, Harvard Medical School, Boston, Massachusetts 02115

Just about a decade ago I had a remarkable clinical encounter. The incident involved an 11-year-old girl hospitalized at the Shangai Psychiatric Institute. At the time I was spending several months at the Institute as part of a World Health Organization fellowship to study cross-national diagnostic practices in child psychiatry (1). China represented an especially interesting case study because at the time child psychiatry was just being resurrected following the excesses of the Cultural Revolution. The Institute had a small child inpatient unit of ten beds. It was the only unit for this metropolis of over 10 million inhabitants. This fact alone was reason enough to wonder how serious the psychopathology of a child must be to warrant admission.

The reasons for this child's hospitalization were not well delineated for me during the case presentation by the staff. I was told that she had exhibited bizarre behavior of a seizure-like quality that was refractory to the interventions of both traditional and western medical approaches. Her behavior problems, which had progressively worsened since age 7, were a nuisance to her parents, and her shrill vocalizations were a particular annoyance to neighbors. The parents had become quite embarrassed over

their inability to control this child. Perhaps the shame they experienced was especially acute since the child was female. It appeared that her hospitalization in a psychiatry unit was requested to relieve the parents of severe disciplinary problems and to see if separation might improve her condition.

The description of this child's symptoms were of textbook quality for the diagnosis of Tourette syndrome, with one possible exception. The content of her vocalization was difficult for her doctors to describe. My question as to whether or not they were equivalent to foul language was met with curiosity and initial silence. I was reminded that Mao Tse Tung had abolished such words from the language over 30 years ago. After some discussion it was decided that the best description for her vocalizations was that they represented the shouting out of "reactionary political slogans." A full disclosure of the content was never revealed to me, but they had roughly the character of saying "down with Chou En-lai." Chou, a veteran of the revolution, was still highly revered in this post-Cultural Revolution era. It was these boisterous statements that had the parents exhausted and the neighbors outraged. A consensus was reached on the diagnosis and the child started on haloperidol. Within 48 hours, her tics had diminished and within 1 week she was discharged.

This single case is enticing because it illustrates how a set of social and cultural factors can influence what we now suspect to be a genetically determined disorder. While this example appears to remove psychosocial influences from the sphere of causal factors, it is useful to keep in mind that such influences had obscured the nature of the child's illness. My colleagues engaged in a momentary debate on whether or not Tourette syndrome occurred in Chinese populations. Once that matter was resolved, we saw several other children with the syndrome during the next few months of my visit.

A recent chapter in a new textbook on child and adolescent psychiatry adequately summarizes what we know about the psychosocial factors in Tourette syndrome in not much more than 300 words (2). These authors note the following characteristics: (a) symptoms may worsen during periods of stress, even when the events are perceived in a positive light; (b) the content of symptoms may be linked to important developmental transitions and life events; and (c) abusive relationships may become established between the patient and other intimates because of a misunderstanding of the involuntary nature of symptom occurrence.

It is against this background that the two major points of this chapter are presented. First, it is instructive to consider the various uses of the term *psychosocial factor*. Suggestions are made on promising approaches to adopt as well as ones to avoid in studying psychosocial factors. These may not only assist researchers interested in understanding the mechanisms that bring about the onset of this disorder and contribute to its persistence over the years, but may help family members better care for persons with Tourette syndrome (3). The second issue concerns recommendations on how to study psychosocial factors in a way that is most likely to advance our understanding of their role in a disorder such as this one.

DEFINITION

There are at least four ways in which psychosocial factors have been defined. The most conventional use relates to the actual experiences of an individual, especially those of an adverse nature. A second use of the term relates to conditions that appear to be linked to the waxing and waning of symptoms. Periods of stress are commonly thought to exacerbate the clinical picture (4). The family environment and specifically the nature of the parent–child or parent–adolescent relationship is often looked to in explaining stress in children. While other sources of stress related to peer acceptance and school achievement are influential, the most intimate relationships in a person's life may represent the greatest sources of stress and, by contrast, of emotional support. Just as parental overinvolvement and hostility are likely to influence the course of schizophrenia negatively (5), this factor may create an environment in which the patient with a tic disorder may also do poorly. A third way in which the term psychosocial factor may be used relates to the consequences of a disorder. For instance, physical abuse, lowered self-esteem, and academic failure may all be social consequences of a tic disorder.

Finally, and perhaps paradoxically, a psychosocial factor may serve a protective function. That is, in the presence of a familial risk, some as yet unexplained factor or set of factors may inhibit or suppress the expression of a disorder in some individuals. It is feasible that such protective factors are far more common than risk factors since even among monozygotic twins the occurrence of the syndrome in both members of a pair is only about 50%. Of course, protective factors need not be strictly psychosocial in nature. Neither should the concept of a protective factor be restricted to nonoccurrence of the disorder. It is plausible that we will yet uncover mechanisms that improve the course of the disorder or encourage remission. It may be that highly structured settings (both family and school) or certain types of diets exert a protective influence in preventing or delaying onset, or in ameliorating the course of the disorder once it is established.

HOW TO STUDY PSYCHOSOCIAL FACTORS

Three areas in which research on the role of psychosocial factors in Tourette syndrome may be particularly productive, and two ways that I deem unproductive are proposed. The first area represents the most intriguing and is derived from one of the most consistently found differences noted in studies of Tourette syndrome: the excess of males over females. Sex differences represent a useful beginning for psychiatric epidemiological detective work, because they occur so consistently as population markers for disease entities (6). Conceivably, they might represent differences in biological make-up, socialization experiences, or lifestyle. As an indicator of differential risk, this characteristic should elicit more scientific scrutiny than it currently receives. In conceptualizing the possible roles that sex can assume in various mechanisms of transmission, it is appropriate to distinguish the concepts of sex and gender. The former is reserved for reasoning about biological distinctions, the latter about psychosocial experiences. Boys may be subject to harsher punishment during the preschool period, while girls are more likely to have a particularly difficult time encountering the early adolescent years (7,8). The criticism that is experienced either in the context of strained family interactions or difficult peer relationships may plausibly have a role in the genesis of psychopathology.

While there are numerous ways to measure interpersonal relationship (using questionnaires, interviews, and observational methods), a technique involving spontaneous descriptions by a parent of a child, or by a child of a parent has particular merit because of its simplicity and wide applicability. It is termed the Five Minute Speech Sample (9). Originally designed in England as a method to measure the emotional climate in families of schizophrenic patients and the relationships that contributed to relapse (10), the approach has been revised by American researchers and recently has been applied to studies of childhood disorders (11). It is plausible that the variables of warmth, criticism, and overinvolvement measured with this method might be used productively in work related both to the onset of tics and their progression and maintenance. It is important to emphasize that such interpersonal experiences may not be specific to any particular chronic disease, but may simply be a general indicator of family adversity that disrupts and stresses vulnerable individuals.

A second area of work that has the potential to uncover risk mechanisms related to the disorder regards the developmental tasks surrounding school performance. Cognitive and socialization demands intensify for most children at the time of school entry, and the impact of such demands on both brain function and behavioral control may be linked, as suggested over half a century ago by Mahler and Rangell (12), to an onset of symptoms. Yet the educational experiences of most children have changed quite markedly in the past 25 years. Two or three years of preschool experience before entering elementary school has become commonplace, and many children have even greater lengths of time in "out of the home" caretaking. Such a secular change in the normative experiences of young children should result in a less stressful transition to elementary school for many children. Alternatively, exposure to school structure at an early age, especially for children who are maturing at a relatively slow rate, may result in greater levels of overall stress than experienced by children remaining in the home. Such early experience could bring about the onset of tics at a younger age. Epidemiologists have documented trends showing a decreasing age of onset for many psychiatric problems, including depression, anorexia nervosa, substance abuse, and suicide (13). It is worth investigating this phenomenon in Tourette syndrome.

There is insufficient documentation in the literature to explore confidently the influences of culture and socioeconomic class on the prevalence and natural history of Tourette syndrome. International comparisons, especially in non-Western and developing countries, are still rare. It is in this connection that my account of the case of the 11-year-old in Shanghai is important. A recent note in the *British Journal of Psychiatry* describes a single case of Tourette's in a 13-year-old girl in Saudi Arabia (14) with a similar history of the syndrome. Although there are very few cases described in the literature from other non-Western countries, little reason exists to believe that the disorder has any different diagnostic features, prevalence, or course in such settings. Cross-national and cross-cultural studies are of great interest because they offer an approach to investigate socialization and cultural pressures on children that may increase our understanding of the role of psychosocial factors (15). There is ample evidence that girls are subject to harsher and more rejecting rearing experiences than boys in many societies (16). It is worth exploring in detail the implications of such sex role reversals cross-culturally for disorders such as Tourette syndrome.

Within industrialized societies it is also important to investigate the impact of economic and psychosocial disadvantages on the prevalence and course of Tourette syndrome. It should be expected that access to health services is reduced for poor individuals with this disorder, and that this fact alone results in delayed recognition and treatment for the disorder, with a concomitant increase in the burden of suffering.

There are two areas of research into psychosocial factors that I consider nonproductive. They are investigations on the timing and content of life events and personality characteristics. Both these areas have their intrinsic interest, but I doubt that there will be much payoff in including them in studies on the causes, course, or response to treatment in Tourette syndrome. Admittedly, this is a bias, which can be partly attributed to my monitoring the contribution that these much studied areas have made to our understanding of psychopathology generally.

CONCLUSION

This paper has examined the concept of psychosocial factors broadly, considering both the intimate environment of family life and the broader social and economic conditions that define how populations live. The significance of carefully considering the role of this range of factors in clinical and epidemiological studies is bolstered by the fact that we are much closer to the ''hereditary taint'' suggested by Charcot over a century ago. Knowledge of the biological basis of this disorder should make it easier to delineate the psychosocial factors that contribute to its onset and waxing and waning over time. As yet, there is not much of a clue to the protective factors that may play a role in offsetting the risk in genetically vulnerable individuals.

Of great immediate concern are those psychosocial conditions that result from lack of awareness and bias. The suffering and stigmatization that emanate from such conditions include harsh punishment and abuse, social ostracism, and the labeling effects of being considered mentally incompetent (17). Because the vast majority of children likely to have Tourette syndrome live in non-Western countries and in socially and economically disadvantaged sectors of the industrialized nations of the West, it is crucial that efforts be made to increase membership from these parts of the world in the Tourette Syndrome Association. My guess is that this will make a more substantial contribution to relief of suffering than increased knowledge of the role that psychosocial factors play in understanding the disease's etiology.

REFERENCES

1. Earls F. Child psychiatry in an international context: with remarks on the current status of child psychiatry in China. In: Super CM ed. *The role of culture in developmental disorder.* San Diego: Academic Press, 1987.

2. Leckman JF, Cohen DJ. Tic disorders. In: Lewis M, ed. *Child and adolescent psychiatry: a comprehensive textbook.* Baltimore: Williams & Wilkins, 1991;613–31.

3. Cohen DJ, Ort SI, Leckman JF. Family functioning and Tourette's Syndrome. In: Cohen DJ, Brunn D, Leckman JF, eds. *Tourette's syndrome and disorders.* New York: John Wiley & Sons, 1988;129–55.

4. Michultka DM, Blanchard EB, Rosenblum EL. Stress management and Gilles de la Tourette's syndrome. *Biofeedback Self Regul* 1989;14:115–23.

5. Vaughn CE, Synder KS, Jones S, Freeman WB, Falloon IRH. Family factors in schizophrenic relapse: a California replication of the British research on expressed emotion. *Arch Gen Psychiatry* 1984;41:1169–77.

6. Earls F. Sex differences in psychiatric disorders: origins and developmental influences. *Psychiatr Dev* 1987,3.1–23.

7. Earls F, Jung KG. Temperament and home environment characteristics on causal factors in the early development of childhood psychopathology. *J Am Acad Child Adolesc Psychiatry* 1987; 26:491–8.

8. Brooks-Gunn J, Reiter EO. The role of pubertal processes. In: Elliott GR, Feldman SS, eds. *At the threshold: the developing adolescent.* Cambridge, MA: Harvard University Press, 1990;16–53.

9. Magana AB, Goldstein MJ, Karno M, Miklowitz DJ, Jenkins J, Falloon IRH. A brief method for assessing expressed emotion in relatives of psychiatric patients. *Psychiatry Res* 1986;17:203–12.

10. Brown GW, Birley JLT, Wing JF. Influence of family life on the course of schizophrenic illness. *Br J Prevent Soc Med* 1962;16:55–68.

11. Hibbs ED, Hamburger MS, Lenane M, et al. Determinants of expressed emotion in families of disturbed and normal children. *J Child Psychol Psychiatry* 1991;32:758–70.

12. Mahler MS, Rangell L. A psychosomatic study of maladie des tics (Gilles de la Tourette's disease). *Psychiatr Q* 1943;17:579–602.

13. Earls F. Epidemiology and child psychiatry: entering the second phase. *Am J Orthopsychiatry* 1989; 59:279–83.

14. El-Assra A. A case of Gilles de la Tourette's syndrome in Saudi Arabia. *Br J Psychiatry* 1987; 151:397–8.

15. Earls F. Cultural and national differences in the epidemiology of behavior problems of preschool children. *Culture Med Psychiatry* 1982;6:45–56.

16. Earls F, Eisenberg L. International perspectives in child psychiatry. In: Lewis M, (ed). *Child and adolescent psychiatry: a comprehensive textbook.* Baltimore: Williams & Wilkins, 1991;1189–96.

17. Edell-Fisher BH, Motta RW. Tourette syndrome: relation to children's and parent's self-concepts. *Psychol Rep* 1990;66:539–45.

Advances in Neurology, Vol. 58, edited by T. N. Chase, A. J. Friedhoff, and D. J. Cohen. Raven Press, Ltd., New York © 1992.

8

A Population-Based Epidemiological Study of Tourette Syndrome Among Adolescents in Israel

*†‡Alan Apter, §‖David L. Pauls, *†Avi Bleich, §Ada H. Zohar, *Shmuel Kron, *†‡Gidi Ratzoni, *Anat Dycian, ¶Moshe Kotler, ‡Avi Weizman, and §Donald J. Cohen

Israel Defense Force, †Department of Psychiatry, Sackler School of Medicine, Tel Aviv University, Ramat Aviv, ‡Geha Psychiatric Hospital, Department of Child and Adolescent Psychiatry, Sackler School of Medicine, Tel Aviv University, Petah Tikva, Israel, §Child Study Center, Yale University School of Medicine, New Haven, Connecticut, ‖Department of Genetics, Yale University School of Medicine, New Haven, Connecticut, ¶Department of Psychiatry, Albert Einstein College of Medicine, New York, New York

Few epidemiological studies have been conducted to establish the prevalence of Tourette syndrome (TS) in the general population. In 1986 Burd et al. (1) conducted a survey of all physicians in North Dakota for ascertainment of TS patients. They reported prevalence rates of 0.77/10,000 males and 0.22/10,000 females. One shortcoming of this study was the fact that there was no population screening for TS. Thus it might be hypothesized that these prevalence data would underestimate the true population prevalence. This shortcoming was addressed in a study done by Caine et al. (2), who conducted a survey of school children in Monroe County, New York. This study relied on referrals from public announcements, contact with the public and private schools, and mailings to physicians and other treating health professionals for screening of prospective cases. A total of 41 cases was identified, yielding a prevalence of 2.87/10,000. These findings may also represent an underestimate since this method of ascertainment could have biased the sample towards the more severe previously diagnosed cases of TS in the population.

Comings et al. (3) conducted a survey of selected classrooms in southern California. In this study, a school psychologist screened over 3,000 school children during a period of 2 years. There was an overrepresentation of full-day special education classes in the sample, and the number of girls and boys in the sample was estimated rather than reported. These problems with the survey may partially explain the elevated rates reported by these investigators: 105.05/10,000 boys and 13.18/10,000 girls.

As suggested, all three of these recent studies have specific shortcomings. Burd et al. (1) relied on physician-identified cases; Caine et al. (2) relied primarily on cases identified by physicians and other health care workers; and Comings et al. (3) oversampled special education classrooms. None of the studies personally screened all individuals in a population for tics. By not screening all members of a given population, several different biases could effect the estimated prevalences for TS.

Israel provides a unique opportunity for population-based studies of developmental psychopathology in adolescence. Between the ages of 16 and 17, all Jewish and Druze adolescents are evaluated for physical, psychological, and cognitive fitness, in preparation for army service. The only exceptions are some religious girls. Thus it is possible to screen all 16- and 17-year-old boys and the majority of girls for the occurrence of any symptomatology including TS and tics. In this paper we report the findings from the first phase of an ongoing study of most 16–17-year-old individuals in Israel.

EPIDEMIOLOGY OF TS IN THE ISRAEL DEFENSE FORCE

The sample consisted of a cohort of 16–17-year-old Jewish individuals in the catchment area of an Israel Defense Force (IDF) induction center in Israel. Some institutionalized individuals on whom information was available from other sources were not screened, but extensive information on them was available from medical records. Girls who claimed exemption from the military on religious grounds were not included in the study. The subjects were screened at the time of preliminary induction evaluations for lifetime occurrence of motor and/or phonic tics. Altogether, over 28,000 16–17-year-old individuals were screened in a 1-year period.

Three groups emerged from the sample: (a) a group of subjects diagnosed with Tourette syndrome, (b) a group of subjects with motor tics, and (c) a group who endorsed at least one item on the initial screen, but were later found to be free of TS or tics.

For each group, controls were matched for date of birth, place of residence, sex, ethnicity, and date of conscription. In this report we present preliminary findings for the TS group only.

There was a three-stage procedure for the diagnosis of affected individuals. The initial screening stage utilized a four-item self-report questionnaire extracted from the Yale Schedule for Tourette's Syndrome and Other Behavioral Syndromes (Yale-STSOBS) (4), which asked about the lifetime occurrence of tics. After completion of the questionnaire, each subject was examined by a physician especially trained for the recognition of tics and TS for this research project who specifically asked the same four questions and reviewed the written responses. For quality assurance each physician signed the questionnaire after the physical examination. In the next screening stage, all individuals who responded positively to at least one screening question were examined by a board-certified child psychiatrist with special research interest and training for the diagnosis of tic disorders. All individuals who received a diagnosis of possible, probable, or definite TS were included in the third stage of the ascertainment process. These individuals were formally administered the Yale-STSOBS (4) by a board-certified child psychiatrist.

In addition, all of these individuals were administered the standard assessment given by the IDF. These measures have been described in detail by Gal (5). The assessments included:

1. The *Physicians Global Assessment Scale* (*P-GAS*). Known in IDF as the medical screening "profile" (5, p. 77), this score is assigned on the basis of a two-stage assessment of overall medical status determined by direct physical examination, a review of laboratory tests, and the medical history. The P-GAS takes into account both psychiatric and medical illnesses. The first stage of P-GAS evaluation involves assigning a categorical International Classification of Disease (ICD) diagnosis where appropriate. The second stage involves determining the severity of the diagnosis as expressed in impairment of functioning.

2. The *IDF Composite Competence Index* (*CCI*). The CCI comprises measured IQ, academic achievement batteries ("Scholastic Ability"), and a test of Hebrew Language Proficiency ("Hebrew"), as well as semistructured interviews that determined personality and motivation, adaptive skills, and ability to cope with adversity and stress ("Combat Suitability"). This is the primary battery used for guiding decisions used for placement in suitable military units (combat versus noncombat) by the IDF. The CCI has demonstrated high reliability and predictive validity for military performance under combat conditions (5, p. 83).

3. *Scholastic Ability* or the *Primary Psychotechnical Rating*, ("Dapar" in Hebrew acronym). This score includes a measure of IQ (the IDF Revised Otis and the Raven Progressive Matrices) and academic achievement scores. The scholastic ability scores are a component of the CCI, and are reported here for comparability to IQ.

4. The *Hebrew Language Proficiency* test. This instrument measures fluency in reading, writing, and speaking Hebrew.

5. The *Combat Suitability Index*. This score reflects a motivation to serve in the IDF. It is determined from a semistructured interview similar to that used in the CCI. Six traits are assessed for Combat Suitability: initiative, motivation to serve in a combat unit, sociability, responsibility, independence, and punctuality (5, p. 79).

In addition to these measures, individuals who had any indication of emotional, behavioral, or psychiatric problems on the basis of their initial induction evaluations were introduced into the standard multistage psychiatric evaluation process. These individuals were evaluated by a team consisting of a psychometric technician, psychologist, and psychiatric social worker.

Individuals who were considered to have a possible psychiatric diagnosis were subsequently evaluated by at least one psychiatrist who assigned a formal Diagnostic and Statistic Manual (DSM) diagnosis if appropriate.

The TS group was compared with matched control. Since the groups were small, the traits measured did not have normal distributions, or equal variances. Thus, the nonparametric U-Mann Whitney (M-W) test was used in these comparisons. The M-W orders the values in both groups and ranks them from smallest to largest. It then calculates the mean rank of the values in each group, and reports the significance of the difference in the mean ranks.

A total of 18,364 boys and 9,673 girls between the ages of 16 and 17 were screened. Nine boys and three girls were diagnosed with TS. Thus the prevalence for boys is 4.90/10,000 and for girls 3.10/10,000, giving a total of 4.28/10,000 and a male to female ratio of 1.58 to 1.

The comparison between the TS subjects and their matched controls on cognitive traits and measures of overall functioning is presented in Table 1. The means of the control group were higher for all the measures, so that a sign test shows a significant group difference. The values of the differences between the means of the groups for the individual measures were not significant except for the P-GAS ($p < 0.01$).

TABLE 1. *Tourette syndrome (TS) patients and matched controls*

	Comparison of mean ranks	
	TS subjects	Matched controls
CCI	11.3	16.5
Scholastic ability	12.2	16.2
Combat suitability	6.7	10.7
Hebrew	13.5	15.6
P-GAS	8.1	17.6*

CCI, Composite Competence Index; P-GAS, Physicians Global Assessment Scale.
* $p < 0.01$.

IMPLICATIONS OF FINDINGS FOR FUTURE STUDIES

This is the first population-based study that has systematically screened for the presence of TS. The prevalence estimates obtained from this study are consistent with previous estimates. The overall prevalence was estimated at 4.28/10,000. The sex-specific prevalences were 4.90/10,000 for boys and 3.10/10,000 for girls. The overall prevalence rates are slightly higher but are comparable with Caine et al. (2). They are, however, higher by about an order of magnitude than those reported by Burd et al. (1) but considerably lower than those reported by Comings et al. (3).

Of interest is the lower than expected male to female ratio. In all previous studies the rate for boys has been significantly higher than girls. The usual reported rate for boys has been at least three to four times higher than the rate for girls. It is not clear why the rates in this study are closer to 1:1. It could be due to underreporting by boys. To determine if this is true, a sample of individuals who denied having any history of tics on the initial screen should be interviewed to determine the false-negative rate. In such a study it should be possible to assess whether there is a difference in reporting among boys and girls that could account for this observed sex ratio. This diminished sex ratio could also be due to a difference in remission between boys and girls. Boys might be more likely to recover spontaneously by late adolescence than girls. Prospective longitudinal studies of younger children would be necessary to determine if this is actually the case.

The first-stage screening for TS was a self-administered questionnaire, especially devised for this study, asking about tics and TS. The subject's answers were subsequently confirmed by the induction center examining physician. While this two-stage procedure should result in a fairly specific ascertainment of tics and TS, it is necessary to estimate the specificity and sensitivity of this screen empirically. Until such a study is completed, the results reported here should be interpreted with caution. If a large number of individuals are missed in the initial screen, the population prevalences reported here would be significantly too low.

One advantage of conducting an epidemiological study through the IDF induction center is that it is possible to screen a large representative sample from a cohort, which can then be followed over time. Most of the individuals identified as having TS have already been drafted into the IDF. Thus it will be possible to follow them and evaluate their functioning over the next 3 years. There is a wealth of information collected during the course of training and service in all IDF units so that it will be possible to assess the effects of the specific environments in which each individual has been placed. The army is a highly comprehensive environment, since soldiers work, eat, and sleep together. Since we have the preinduction clinical status of the individuals with TS, it will be possible to examine the effects of these specific environments on the course of TS. Furthermore, since all men in Israel serve in the military reserves until they are at least 50 years of age, it will be possible to follow up each boy in this study annually. It will also be possible to compare army service functioning and the development over the life span of TS individuals with their matched controls selected at the same preinduction time that the TS individuals were identified. This follow-up information should be invaluable in the understanding of the life span course of this syndrome.

Furthermore, a family study of individuals identified in an epidemiological study would provide an opportunity to examine whether the patterns in families are related to severity of TS. Since it is more likely for more severe cases to be seen in clinics and it is more likely for individuals seen in TS clinics to be enrolled in family studies, the reported familial findings could be an artifact of such a bias. By studying a sample of probands identified through an epidemiological study, it would be possible to determine if the patterns in these families are similar to those observed in families of clinically ascertained TS probands. By examining both types of families it will be possible to learn more about the underlying genetic mechanisms for TS as well as the relationship between TS and other possibly related conditions [e.g., obsessive–compulsive disorder (OCD) and attention deficit hyperactivity disorder (ADHD)]. Individuals ascertained through clinics are more likely to have associated conditions (6), and the patterns in families might be skewed because of this ascertainment bias. By studying families of individuals identified through a true epidemiological study, it should be possible to examine more carefully the relationship between the familiality of TS and other disorders.

REFERENCES

1. Burd L, Kerbeshian J, Wikenheiser M, Fisher W. Prevalence of Gilles de la Tourette's syndrome in North Dakota adults. *Am J Psychiatry* 1986; 143:787–8.
2. Caine ED McBride MC, Chiverton P, Bamford KA, Rediess S, Shiao J. Tourette's syndrome in Monroe County school children. *Neurology* 1988;38:472–5.
3. Comings DE, Himes JA, Comings BG. An epidemiologic study of Tourette's syndrome in a single school district. *J Clin Psychiatry* 1990;51:463–9.
4. Pauls DL, Hurst CR. *Schedule for Tourette's syndrome and other behavioral syndromes.* New Haven: Yale University Child Study Center, 1987.
5. Gal R. *A portrait of the Israeli soldier.* New York: Greenwood Press, 1986.
6. Berkson J. Limitations of the application of fourfold table analysis to hospital data. *Biometrics* 1946; 2:47–51.

Advances in Neurology, Vol. 58, edited by T. N. Chase, A. J. Friedhoff, and D. J. Cohen. Raven Press, Ltd., New York © 1992.

9

Epidemiology and Comorbidity

The North Dakota Prevalence Studies of Tourette Syndrome and other Developmental Disorders

*Jacob Kerbeshian and †Larry Burd

*Department of Neuroscience, University of North Dakota School of Medicine, Grand Forks, North Dakota 58202, †Departments of Neuroscience and Pediatrics, University of North Dakota School of Medicine, Center for Teaching and Learning, University of North Dakota, Grand Forks, North Dakota 58202

As a neurological condition, Tourette syndrome (TS) is characterized by multiple motor and vocal tics of over 1 year's duration, emanating from subcortical central nervous system substrates (1). As a neuropsychiatric condition, TS has associated with it behavioral, emotional, and cognitive manifestations that reverberate through different levels of biopsychosocial organization. As a developmental disorder, TS influences and in turn is influenced by the unfolding sequences of transactions across various developmental lines. TS appears to be heritable, and that heritability is manifested also in at least the expression of obsessive–compulsive disorder (2–5). Although a candidate gene has been hypothesized for TS, there is the distinct possibility of genetic heterogeneity (6). Although TS was once felt to be a rare syndrome, recent prevalence estimates indicate otherwise (7–9).

Epidemiological investigations estimate the frequency of a specified condition in a distinct population group. The incidence of a condition is the number of new cases coming to light during a defined time period. The prevalence of a condition is the total number of cases present in that population group at a certain point in time. Our North Dakota (ND) study group has conducted a number of investigations of the prevalence of TS and of other developmental disorders. North Dakota is amply suited to such work. The population subgroups are well defined, and the census has been fairly stable over decades at about 640,000. Medical and mental health care are centralized for the most part in larger group entities in the larger cities. The health care professionals are readily identifiable. At the time of our studies, there were a limited number of professionals receiving referrals and providing care to individuals with developmental disorders. In the case of TS, there is an active TS Association that has been quite cooperative in providing data for studies. We have seen most of our cases at a statewide developmental center with a multidisciplinary orientation. Table 1 summarizes results from two of our prevalence studies on TS and one on pervasive developmental disorders (PDD) (7,8,

10,11). PDD as defined in the Diagnostic and Statistical Manual, 3rd ed., revised (DSM-III-R) is characterized by severe delays and distortions in social, communicative, and volitional capabilities (1). Subsets of the condition are autistic disorder (AutDis) and a nonspecific category (PDDNOS). The DSM-III has a more restrictive set of criteria for PDD (12,13). Subsets include infantile autism (IA), atypical PDD (APDD), and childhood-onset PDD (COPDD). Our findings are consistent with studies done by Caine et al. (9), and by Ritvo and his group (14–17). Included in Table 1 are the numbers of patients with TS personally evaluated by the authors for the prevalence study, and the numbers outside of and since the study with ages corrected to 1991. A preponderance of males to females was as expected. In school-age children and adolescents the male to female ratio was three times that in adults. Our school-age male to female ratio is consistent with the 37/4 ratio reported by Caine et al. (9). Additionally, the prevalence rate for TS in school-agers is ten times that in adults. Based on this data, the expression of TS is influenced by sex, the condition becomes less evident or improves by adulthood for both males and females, and the degree of improvement is proportionately greater for males than for females.

Sabshin (18) has emphasized the increasing importance of comorbidity and its implications for research and treatment. He offers one definition of comorbidity as the "increased likelihood of higher prevalence of a discrete disorder in the presence of another disorder." We have had a particular interest in our epidemiologic studies in the comorbidity of TS with other developmental disorders, and with PDD in particular. Table 2 lists the comorbidities present in our PDD prevalence study, with particular reference to the presence of TS, other tic disorders, a family history of tics, and a family history of PDD. The expected chance cooccurrence of TS and PDD based on ND prevalence data would be 1.66/ 10,000,000. Twelve cases of TS + PDD were found in a school-age population of 180,986, for a cooccurrence of 660/ 10,000,000. The cooccurrence of these conditions is close to 400 times that expected by chance alone. Cohen et al. (19) observed that some children with infantile autism may express symptoms of TS as they emerge from their autistic stance. The particular characteristics of the TS + PDD group in the prevalence study are revealing (11). The

TABLE 1. *North Dakota prevalence studies*

	TS		PDD child & adolescent	IA child & adolescent	APDD child & adolescent
	Adult	School age			
Date completed	1985	1984	1986		
Professionals responding (%)	72 or 97[a]	97	>99%		
Total patients	22	73	59	21	36
Male:female	3.4:1	9.3:1	2.7:1	2.5:1	2.7:1
Prevalence/10,000	0.5	5.2	3.3	1.2	2.0
No. authors' patients in prevalence study	15	54			
No. authors' other patients	42	72			

[a] 72% includes the state's family physicians (300 plus); 97% includes pediatricians, psychiatrists, and neurologists, and state agencies.

APDD, atypical PDD; IA, infantile autism; PDD, pervasive developmental disorders; TS, Tourette syndrome.

TABLE 2. *North Dakota prevalence studies*

	IA		APDD		COPDD	
	No.	%	No.	%	No.	%
Total	21		36		2	
TS	2	10	10	28	0	0
Tic	1	5	2	6	0	0
Family history of tics	1	5	1	3	0	0
Family history of PDD	3	15	1	3	0	0
Asperger syndrome	0	0	4	11	0	0
Hyperlexia	1	5	3	8	0	0
Bipolar symptoms	2	10	0	0	0	0

APDD, atypical PDD; COPDD, childhood-onset PDD; IA, infantile autism; PDD, pervasive developmental disorders; TS, Tourette syndrome.

proportions of the parameters for the TS + PDD group to the PDD alone group are as follows: mean IQ, 70/40; mean receptive language quotient, 59/31; mean expressive language quotient, 56/29. As measured by intelligence and language capability, the TS + PDD group exhibits a better developmental outcome than the PDD without TS group. Cases of exception to this association with positive outcome have been reported (6,20,21). Fisher et al. (22) described four patients with PDD, a tic disorder, and a characteristic speech and language impairment. Diminution in tics with haloperidol treatment led to marked improvement in language, strengthening the association of TS and positive outcome in PDD. The influence of comorbid TS on PDD outcome must be viewed against the backdrop of the usual course of intelligence and language function in individuals with PDD. Of 59 children and adolescents in the North Dakota PDD prevalence study, IQ and receptive and expressive language scores were inversely correlated with age for individuals with infantile autism, and remained stable for individuals with other PDD (11). That study indicated that of the 12 individuals with TS + PDD, 2 had IA while 10 had APDD, consistent with a clustering of TS, nonautistic better outcome PDD, and improved IQ and language skills.

The association of TS, better outcome PDD, higher intelligence, and higher language functioning is shown in two subgroups of individuals with comorbid TS and PDD: persons with Asperger syndrome (AS) and persons with hyperlexia. Individuals with AS exhibit developmental aberrations with pedantic, lengthy, stereotyped, aprosodic speech, and impaired nonverbal communication. There is peculiarity in social interaction and a lack of empathy for others. Hypertrophied interests, repetitive activities, resistance to change, and clumsy or stereotyped movements are further hallmarks of the condition. The preponderance of opinion is that AS is part of the autistic spectrum, although the issue has not yet been settled (23–25). Individuals with hyperlexia have highly developed reading recognition skills acquired before age 5, inconsistent with their general level of cognition (26). In the North Dakota PDD prevalence study AS clustered with APDD. In a later work, of six individuals with AS, three developed TS and a fourth had a vocal tic, strengthening the association of TS as a marker for a better outcome PDD (23). Hyperlexia clustered with APDD in three of four children and adolescents with PDD. The prevalence rate of hyperlexia in ND children and adolescents with PDD is 6.6/100 (26). These children experienced improvement in IQ and language scores with age (27). In North Dakota there were five children and adolescents with a "triple" comorbidity for PDD, TS, and hyperlexia. Of these, two were from the same family. The chance cooccurrence of such an association is 3/trillion (27–29). The association of TS with better outcome PDD is further strengthened. This association is of some importance as our data indicate that as many as 20% of younger children with a PDD later develop the symptoms of TS (30).

Comings and Comings (6) and Sverd (21) have also looked at the relationship between TS and PDD in comorbid individuals, inferring that the presence of TS in family members of index individuals with comorbid TS and PDD points to a common underlying genetic cause. Table 3 summarizes data we extracted from their case reports and pedigrees. The trend toward higher functioning PDD is present. There is no evidence of PDD in family members, whereas the ND prevalence data would have predicted by chance a total of 0.5–2.4 in the Comingses' cases and 0.3–1.5 in Sverd's cases. As the expected numbers are small, the meaning of the absence of PDD in family members is far from clear. In the Comingses' cases the proportion of comorbid probands with a family history of tics is 0.4, in Sverd's 1.0.

The question as to whether there might be in our ND PDD prevalence individuals a common genetic diathesis with TS is intriguing. Paraphrasing Crowe (31), if TS is a direct cause of PDD, the rate of PDD will be elevated in families of probands with TS and with TS + PDD. Moreover, the increased incidence of PDD will only occur in relatives who have TS, creating a strong association between the two in the family members. If probands with PDD alone have a familial disorder, then the rate of PDD will be increased in these families, and otherwise it will not. If both TS and PDD are the result of the same underlying disorder, the rate of each will be increased in the relatives of all three groups of probands compared with the population rates. Moreover, an association between the two may or may not exist among relatives, since the underlying trait may produce either TS or PDD independently, or the two together. Another possibility for the association would, of course, be ascertainment bias. Ascertainment bias is likely not operating in our prevalence studies due to our methodology. In our caseload we have one possible and admittedly isolated example of a common genetic etiology for both TS and PDD, namely fragile X (32,33).

FAMILY HISTORY STUDY

In an attempt to understand better the factors involved in the manifestations of TS + PDD comorbidity, we undertook a family history inquiry of our study group cases. We hoped that such a study might also clarify the question of whether there is a causal genetic association between TS and PDD.

Our chart review sample included 69 school-age and adult individuals whom we had seen personally as part of the ND TS prevalence study. This also included every patient in the study diagnosed with comorbid TS + PDD. There was an additional

TABLE 3. *Comings and Comings: Tourette syndrome (TS) + pervasive developmental disorders (PDD cooccurrence (ref.6)*

	Total	FAMwTIC	FAMwTIC/TOTAL	FAMwPDD/TOTAL
TS + all PDD	16	7	0.4	0
TS + bad prognosis PDD	3	1	0.3	0
TS + better prognosis PDD	13	6	0.5	0
SVERD (ref. 21):				
TS + AutDis cooccurrence				
TS + all AutDis	10	10	1.0	0
TS + poor IQ AutDis	1	1	1.0	0
TS + better IQ AutDis	9	9	1.0	0

PDD, pervasive developmental disorder; AutDis, autistic disorder.

group of 114 TS individuals of all ages either from outside of ND, younger than school age, or seen by us subsequent to the prevalence study. Our total sample was 183 TS individuals. AutDis, PDDNOS, and TS were diagnosed by DSM-III-R criteria. IA was diagnosed according to DSM-III. All individuals diagnosed with IA also met criteria for AutDis. AS was diagnosed clinically (24).

We culled from the ND TS prevalence subgroup 40 school-age children and adolescents with TS not occurring with mental retardation, PDD, or bipolar symptomatology. A number of our cases had attention deficit hyperactivity disorder (ADHD), or obsessive–compulsive symptoms (OCS). We excluded two individuals as being siblings, in two a family history was not available, and four were adopted without a reliable family history. We designated these 32 individuals our control group, presumably reflecting the most common expression of TS. We felt that a school-age TS control group might provide expectable TS family history data that could be more meaningfully compared with expectable PDD family history data as predicted by our child and adolescent PDD study. A negative aspect is that the use of school-age controls might have the effect of giving a less precise estimate of expectable TS in families as applied to adult index individuals. As we were seeking trends and comparability with our PDD data, rather than statistical soundness, we decided on school-age controls. From our total study pool, we also extracted a subgroup of 22 individuals of all ages comorbid for TS + PDD. We excluded the boy with fragile X syndrome as being perhaps a unique example of a common factor leading to the emergence of TS and/or PDD. Among the 21 remaining, there were then 7 of the ND TS prevalence study school-agers comorbid for TS + PDD. (The ND PDD prevalence study was published 2 years later. By then we had accumulated 12 individuals with comorbid TS + PDD.)

Using a family history method, we tabulated the number of control probands with at least one first- or second-degree relative with tics or OCS (34). We interpreted the presence of tics or OCS in family members as indicative of hereditary factors responsible for the expression of TS in the proband (3–5). We were in no way attempting to establish an accurate estimate of tics or OCS in these families. Instead, given our method of data gathering, which remained fairly constant across all individuals in our study, we hoped to define a threshold value indicative of the heritability of TS in our probands. From our ND PDD prevalence study we took estimates of proband individuals with a family history of PDD. These estimates are consistent with values discovered by Ritvo et al. (15). Next, with our ND prevalence school-age TS + PDD individuals, we tabulated the number with at least one first- or second-degree relative with tics or OCS, and the number with at least one first- or second-degree relative with PDD, all as a function of subtype of PDD. Finally we performed the same operation on our subgroup of 21 TS + PDD individuals of all ages.

Our results are given in Table 4. We are presenting this data as indicative of trends, rather than asserting statistical validity. The proportions from the controls are listed, as are the proportions from the ND PDD prevalence study. There was no PDD in first- or second-degree relatives of controls. The numbers comprising the PDD subtypes of school-agers with TS + PDD are small, but the proportions are similar to those present in the TS + PDD cases of all ages. We will discuss the trends evident in this latter group. Our cases with IA and/or AutDis had no tics, OCS, or PDD in first- or second-degree relatives. One would have expected about three families with tics/OCS, and one family with PDD. Our cases with AS, and with PDDNOS both including and excluding AS, had families with tics/OCS similar to our controls. There was no PDD in the families of our PDDNOS without AS group. The expected number would be 0.2. The

TABLE 4. *North Dakota prevalence studies*

Proband (no.)	FAM: Tics, OCS/TOTProband	FAM: PDD/TOTProband
Child and Adolescent[a]		
TS no BPL, no MR, no PDD (32)	0.4	0.0
IA (21)		0.15
APPD (36)		0.03
TS +		
IA (1)	0.0	0.0
AutDis (3)	0.0	0.0
PDDNOS(−)ASP (2)	0.5	0.0
Asperger syndrome (2)	0.5	0.0
PDDNOS (4)	0.5	0.0
PDD all (7)	0.3	0.0
All patients[b]		
TS +		
IA (7)	0.0	0.0
AutDis (9)	0.0	0.0
PDDNOS(−)ASP (5)	0.4	0.0
Asperger syndrome (8[c])	0.4	0.12 (1 ASP)
PDDNOS (12)	0.4	0.08 (1 ASP)
PDD all (21)	0.2	0.05 (1 ASP)

[a] Cooccurrence of TS + PDD, not FraX, child and adolescent <18 years old. FAM, proband with first and/or second degree relative with the condition.
[b] Cooccurrence of TS + PDD, not FraX, all age groups.
[c] One patient once also met criteria for autistic disorder.
OCS, obsessive–compulsive symptoms; TOTProband, pervasive developmental disorder; TS, Tourette syndrome; BPL, bipolar symptoms; MR, mental retardation; IA, infantile autism; APPD, atypical PDD; AutDis, autistic disorder; PDDNOS, nonspecific PDD; ASP, Asperger syndrome; FraX, fragile X syndrome.

PDD in the families of our AS group and in our PDDNOS including AS group was accounted for by one AS relative who also had tics. This pattern of the presence of AS in family members of higher functioning PDD individuals is consistent with that described by DeLong and Dwyer (35). Our results suggest that the TS evident in our TS + PDD cases with IA and/or AutDis does not have the familial pattern evident in our controls, whereas the TS in our AS and PDDNOS cases does. It is more difficult to generalize regarding the trend of PDD in their families.

TS AND PDD

As has been stated, the presence of TS in individuals with PDD is generally a marker for improved outcome. Our family history study indicates that there may be at least two patterns of the familial presence of a tic diathesis in individuals comorbid for TS +

PDD. In our cases with PDD somewhat divergent from classical IA the familial pattern is similar to that of controls with TS. There may be no increased incidence of PDD in these families, and we found only one case of comorbid TS + AS. In these individuals the PDD may be secondary to TS or the PDD may be a phenocopy epiphenomenal to the primary symptoms of TS. The apparent absence of a tic diathesis in the families of our more classically autistic cases is provocative. As a group, these individuals experienced greater developmental gains than expected. It may be useful in this group to view TS more in functional terms than in genetic/etiologic terms. For our comorbid TS + PDD individuals with a more classically autistic presentation, and perhaps for other developmental and neuropsychiatric syndromes as well, TS may be primarily an expression of process. TS may be a neurodevelopmental and perhaps a neurochemical point of confluence through which a number of neuropsychiatric and neurodevelopmental processes must pass on the pathway from either a common or multibiologic potentiality, to a common or multipotential phenotypic outcome. This point of confluence may be more determined by the canalization of neurodevelopmental process, than by the genetic starting point or by the phenotypic end point.

Our inquiry suggests that a multicenter study is needed to elucidate further the status of individuals comorbid for TS + PDD. Required would be direct study of family members, comparable diagnostic instruments across centers, and ideally genetic, biologic, or behavioral markers. Prior to initiating such a study, additional pilot studies would be desirable. How does one operationalize meaningful subsets of PDD? What is the spectrum of PDD-related disorders in family members? How does one define good prognosis, or positive outcome? What is the place of chronic motor or vocal tic disorders in the investigation? How does medication as a variable affect outcome?

We would like to reiterate the following points. The prevalence of TS is ten times greater in children and adolescents compared with adults. TS stabilizes and/or improves throughout development. The male:female ratio of TS is about three times greater in children compared with adults. More males are afflicted throughout development, but with a comparatively better prognosis than females. The expression and course of TS are influenced by other genetic conditions, i.e., gender. TS and PDD cooccur at rates much higher than expected by chance. TS + PDD individuals as a group have a better outcome than PDD individuals without TS. Individuals with comorbid hyperlexia + PDD have as a group a better prognosis than those with PDD alone. The cooccurrence of hyperlexia + TS + PDD is much higher than expected by chance. There is a higher than chance expectation of tic/OCS in families of individuals with comorbid TS + PDD. This may be more evident in individuals less classically autistic.

The following not necessarily mutually exclusive hypotheses require affirmation, or refutation. TS is a homogeneous condition with a single genetic etiology. TS is a heterogeneous condition with a single genetic or a polygenetic etiology. TS may be a canalized neurodevelopmental point of confluence in a variety of genetically heterogeneous disorders with a variety of outcomes. Some cases of PDD are phenocopies caused by TS. Some cases of TS, PDD, and TS + PDD are caused by the same etiology.

Further work using epidemiologic methods in conjunction with well-orchestrated direct interview family studies is bound to increase our understanding of TS further, and add to the findings of the bedside, the laboratory, and the imaging room. The benefit will be not only to our scientific data base, but also to those who are afflicted with and struggle with the burdens of TS.

REFERENCES

1. American Psychiatric Association. *Diagnostic and statistical manual of mental disorders*, 3rd ed, revised. Washington, DC: American Psychiatric Association, 1987.
2. Comings DE. A controlled study of Tourette syndrome. VII. Summary: a common genetic disorder causing disinhibition of the limbic system. *Am J Hum Genet* 1987;41:839–66.
3. Pauls DL, Leckman JF. The inheritance of Gilles de la Tourette's syndrome and associated behaviors. *N Engl J Med* 1986;315:993–8.
4. Pauls DL, Leckman JF, Towbin KE, Zhaner GEP, Cohen DJ. A possible genetic relationship exists between Tourette's syndrome and obsessive–compulsive disorder. *Psychopharmacol Bull* 1986;22:730–3.
5. Pauls DL, Towbin KE, Leckman JF, Zahner GEP, Cohen DJ. Gilles de la Tourette's syndrome and obsessive–compulsive disorder. *Arch Gen Psychiatry* 1986;43:1180–2.
6. Comings DE, Comings BG. Clinical and genetic relationships between autism—pervasive developmental disorder and Tourette syndrome: a study of 19 cases. *Am J Hum Genet* 1991;39:180–91.
7. Burd L, Kerbeshian J, Wikenheiser M, Fisher W. Prevalence of Gilles de la Tourette's syndrome in North Dakota adults. *Am J Psychiatry* 1986; 143:787–8.
8. Burd L, Kerbeshian J, Wikenheiser M, Fisher W. A prevalence study of Gilles de la Tourette syndrome in North Dakota school-age children. *J Am Acad Child Psychiatry* 1986;25:552–3.

9. Caine ED, McBride MC, Chiverton P, Bamford KA, Rediess S, Shiao J. Tourette's syndrome in Monroe County school children. *Neurology* 1988; 38:472–5.

10. Burd L, Fisher W, Kerbeshian J. A prevalence study of pervasive developmental disorders in North Dakota. *J Am Acad Child Adolesc Psychiatry* 1987;26:700–3.

11. Fisher W, Burd L, Kerbeshian J. Comparisons of DSM-III defined pervasive developmental disorders in North Dakota children. *J Am Acad Child Adolesc Psychiatry* 1987;26:704–10.

12. American Psychiatric Association. *Diagnostic and Statistical Manual of Mental Disorders,* 3rd ed. Washington, DC: American Psychiatric Association, 1980.

13. Volkmar F, Bregman J, Cohen D, Cicchetti D. DSM-III and DSM-III-R diagnosis of autism. *Am J Psychiatry* 1988;145:1404–8.

14. Ritvo ER, Freeman BJ, Pingree C, et al. The UCLA-University of Utah epidemiological survey of autism: prevalence. *Am J Psychiatry* 1989; 146:194–9.

15. Ritvo ER, Jorde LB, Mason-Brothers A, et al. The UCLA-University of Utah epidemiologic survey of autism: recurrence risk estimates and genetic counseling. *Am J Psychiatry* 1989;146:1032–6.

16. Ritvo ER, Mason-Brothers A, Freeman BJ, et al. The UCLA-University of Utah epidemiologic survey of autism: the etiologic role of rare diseases. *Am J Psychiatry* 1990;147:1614–21.

17. Jorde LB, Mason-Brothers A, Waldmann R, et al. The UCLA-University of Utah epidemiologic survey of autism: genealogical analysis of familial aggregation. *Am J Med Genet* 1990;36:85–8.

18. Sabshin M. Comorbidity: a central concern of psychiatry in the 1990s. *Hosp Community Psychiatry* 1991;42:345.

19. Cohen DJ, Leckman JF, Shaywitz BA. The Tourette syndrome and other tics. In: Shaffer D, Ehrhardt AA, Greenhill L, eds. *A clinician's guide to child psychiatry.* New York: Macmillan, 1984.

20. Kano Y, Ohta M, Nagai Y. Two case reports of autistic boys developing Tourette's disorder: indications of improvement? *J Am Acad Child Adolesc Psychiatry* 1987;26:937–8.

21. Sverd J. Tourette syndrome and autistic disorder: a significant relationship. *Am J Hum Genet* 1991; 39:173–9.

22. Fisher W, Kerbeshian J, Burd L. A treatable language disorder: pharmacological treatment of pervasive developmental disorder. *J Dev Behav Pediatr* 1986;7:73–5.

23. Kerbeshian J, Burd L. Asperger's syndrome and Tourette syndrome: the case of the pinball wizard. *Br J Psychiatry* 1986;148:731–6.

24. Kerbeshian J, Burd L, Fisher W. Asperger's syndrome: to be or not to be? *Br J Psychiatry* 1990; 156:721–5.

25. Szatmari P, Bartolucci G, Bremner R. Asperger's syndrome and autism: comparison of early history and outcome. *Dev Med Child Neurol* 1989; 31:709–20.

26. Burd L, Kerbeshian J, Fisher W. Inquiry into the incidence of hyperlexia in a statewide population of children with pervasive developmental disorder. *Psychol Rep* 1985;57:236–8.

27. Fisher W, Burd L, Kerbeshian J. Markers for improvement in children with pervasive developmental disorders. *J Men Defic Res* 1988; 32:357–69.

28. Burd L, Fisher W, Knowlton D, Kerbeshian J. Hyperlexia: a marker for improvement in children with pervasive developmental disorder? *J Am Acad Child Adolesc Psychiatry* 1987;26:407–12.

29. Burd L, Kerbeshian J. Familial pervasive developmental disorder, Tourette disorder and hyperlexia. *Neurosci Biobehav Rev* 1988;12:233–4.

30. Burd L, Fisher W, Kerbeshian J, Arnold M. Is development of Tourette disorder a marker for improvement in patients with autism and other pervasive developmental disorders? *J Am Acad Child Adolesc Psychiatry* 1987;26:162–5.

31. Crowe R. The application of genetic methods to the study of disease associations in psychiatry. *Psychiatr Clin North Am* 1990;13:585–96.

32. Kerbeshian J, Burd L, Martsolf J. Fragile X syndrome associated with Tourette symptomatology in a male with moderate mental retardation and autism. *J Dev Behav Pediatr* 1984;5:201–3.

33. Kerbeshian J, Burd L, Martsolf J. A family with fragile-X syndrome. *J Nerv Ment Dis* 1984; 172:549–51.

34. Andreasen N, Rice J, Endicott J, Reich T, Coryell W. The family history approach to diagnosis. *Arch Gen Psychiatry* 1987;43:421–9.

35. DeLong GR, Dwyer JT. Correlation of family history with specific autistic subgroups: Asperger's syndrome and bipolar affective disease. *J Autism Dev Disord* 1988;18:593–600.

Advances in Neurology, Vol. 58, edited by T. N. Chase, A. J. Friedhoff, and D. J. Cohen. Raven Press, Ltd., New York © 1992.

10

Tourette Syndrome in a Special Education Population

Hypotheses

Roger Kurlan

Department of Neurology, University of Rochester School of Medicine and Dentistry, Rochester, New York 14642

Tourette syndrome (TS) can be considered to represent a clinical spectrum disorder, including both motor and behavioral features (1). Although the boundaries of the TS behavioral spectrum remain to be clearly delineated, it is clear that a variety of clinical features associated with TS may impair learning skills and contribute to academic failure for children with the disorder. Since TS has traditionally been considered a rare condition, its possible contribution to the large population of learning disabled children has not received serious consideration. However, mounting evidence indicates that TS and related tic disorders are much more common than generally appreciated. Based on these considerations, I hypothesize that TS is a common, misdiagnosed, and often overlooked disorder that is an important contributor to school problems in the childhood population at large. The presence of tics is suspected of being associated with academic failure and signifying an underlying dysfunction of neurological development. Thus children requiring special educational services are expected to represent a high-risk population for identifying TS. This notion is important since many of the major clinical features of TS [i.e., tics, obses-sive–compulsive disorder (OCD), attention deficit hyperactivity disorder (ADHD)] are treatable, and prompt recognition of the diagnosis and institution of appropriate therapy could have a favorable impact on school performance.

TOURETTE SYNDROME AND SCHOOL PROBLEMS

Clinicians caring for TS children are keenly aware that both the motor and the behavioral aspects of the illness present a variety of barriers to successful academic achievement. In fact, schooling probably represents the most significant focus of clinical management for children with TS. A survey of 200 child and adolescent cases of TS found that 36% of the population experienced learning problems, including learning disability (22%), needing to repeat a grade (12%), poor grades (18%), full-time special education classes (8%), the part-time special education classes (12%) (2). Another study revealed that the percentages of children with TS functioning below educational expectancy for several academic skills were as follows: oral reading (16%), individual reading comprehension (40%), group reading comprehension (68%), spelling (52%), and mathematics (56%) (3). Comings (4) has found that children with TS are five times more likely to require special educational services than the general childhood population.

The school performance of a child with TS may be impaired by various combinations of several problems (Table 1). Direct effects of motor and vocal tics upon the performance of specific learning tasks are apparent with such school activities as public speaking or handwriting (3). Fine motor tasks may be difficult to perform when a tic can cause a writing utensil, scissors, etc. to fly out the child's grasp. Slowed writing can result in incomplete note taking, missed details in homework assignments, or failure to finish tests within time limits. Vocal tics may interfere with oral expression, and the stress of speaking to an audience may exacerbate all forms of tics so that active participation in class discussions is avoided. Attempts by the child to suppress tics voluntarily in the classroom may redirect "mental energy" more appropriately needed for attending to classroom activities, and the increasing inner tension that results from attempts to suppress tics may

take a heavy emotional toll. The occurrence of active tic suppression in the classroom by TS children has been confirmed by the finding that the mean number of tics observed during a clinical interview outside the classroom was 9 in contrast to the mean of 2.5 tics counted by an anonymous classroom observer during a similar time period (3). School performance may be impaired by medications used to treat tics due to a variety of associated side effects, including drowsiness, cognitive blunting, anxiety, school-phobic reactions (5), and depression.

Children with TS and associated OCD may be so preoccupied by intrusive thoughts or rituals that they are unable to concentrate on classroom tasks at hand or to complete homework assignments in a timely fashion. Investigators studying children with OCD have identified cognitive differences between obsessive–compulsive and control subjects, including a slightly decreased performance IQ score, occasional wide verbal-performance differences, and a subgroup with marked impulsivity (6). A specific information-processing deficit in adolescents with OCD has been reported (7), and selected neuropsychological tests have demonstrated significant dysfunction in this group when compared with controls (8).

ADHD, present in nearly half of TS patients, is one of the more commonly recognized neuropsychiatric disorders of childhood that contributes to school and behavior problems (9). Although the full extent of the TS behavioral disorder remains to be accurately delineated, a variety of other behavioral problems, such as conduct disorder, school phobia, test anxiety, and depression, have been linked to the disorder and may contribute to academic difficulties as well (10).

Studies of higher cerebral function in patients with TS have revealed a variety of neuropsychologic abnormalities that might interfere with learning skills (11). Normal

TABLE 1. *Causes of school problems in Tourette syndrome (TS)*

Primary TS symptoms
  Motor tics (including excessive touching)
  Vocal tics (including echolalia, coprolalia)
  Mental "energy" expended in suppressing tics
Obsessive–compulsive behavior
Attention deficit hyperactivity disorder
Other behavioral disturbances
  Primary school and other phobias
  Testing anxiety
  Conduct disorder
  Anxiety disorder
  Depression
  Short temper, argumentative personality traits
Neuropsychological/cognitive disturbances
Poor socialization skills
Low self-esteem
Medication side effects (including sedation, depression)

intelligence has been confirmed by several investigators (11,12). However, various batteries of neuropsychologic tests when administered to TS patients have been reported to reveal evidence of "encephalopathy" (13), learning disorder (13), "organic dysfunction" (14), "brain damage" (15), left or right hemispheric dysfunction (16), and impaired motor skills (16). Several authors have observed significant discrepancies between verbal and performance IQ scores (12,19). Some studies have identified impaired language skills associated with TS, including decreased verbal fluency (17), impaired immediate recall of a verbally presented story (17), deficient verbal expressive skills (18), and difficulties in immediate auditory–verbal memory, phoneme–grapheme matching, and oral arithmetic (18). Golden found that TS patients demonstrated confusion in the interpretation of complex linguistic cues involving spatial and temporal concepts or inverted grammar (12). A number of investigators have documented deficits in visuospatial skills that include block design (14), coding (16,19), digit symbol (17,20), problems in adapting to changes in speed on a road tracking test (20), and deficits in copying and drawing from memory (17). Hagins et al. (21) reported that TS patients show a number of deficits in visuopractic abilities, including impaired performance on the Bender Gestalt and the Purdue Pegboard Tests, difficulties with finger schema, and poor figure–ground discrimination (21). Deficient arithmetic scores have been observed by three groups of investigators (12,18,19).

The results of the reviewed neuropsychologic studies are confounded by inclusion of subjects with ADHD, learning, and other neurological disorders, and also those receiving drug therapy. Nevertheless, specific deficits in higher cerebral function appear to be present for at least a portion of TS patients and may thereby contribute to academic difficulties. In addition to the specific psychopathological and neuropsychological problems outlined above that may accompany TS and impair school functioning, patients with the disorder may experience a variety of psychosocial problems related to living with and adapting to the condition (22). These problems, including depression, conduct disorder, lack of self-confidence, and social isolation, may also contribute to academic failure. Taken together, it is clear that TS is associated with a wide-ranging number of factors that may interfere with appropriate classroom participation and effective completion of learning tasks.

TOURETTE SYNDROME AS A COMMON DISORDER

Traditionally, TS has been viewed as a rare disorder so that its possible contribution to the large population of learning disabled children has not been considered. However, recent evidence suggests that it is much more common than generally appreciated. An accurate lifetime prevalence rate for TS has not been established. Past estimates, ranging from 0.03% to 1.6% (23–26), have been based largely on case series of patients referred for medical evaluation or on data obtained from questionnaires without direct clinical examinations (27). For example, in estimating the prevalence of TS in North Dakota adults and children, Burd and colleagues (24,25) included only subjects on a statewide list of medical diagnoses. Caine et al.'s epidemiologic survey of TS in Monore County, New York involved only children referred by school and health personnel following an extensive informational campaign in the local news media (26). Several lines of recent evidence suggest that these approaches are likely to be inaccurate and lead to gross underestimates of disease prevalence. We have shown that systematic examination of all available members of large TS kindreds indicates that most cases of TS are mild and do not come to medical attention and that the disorder is often unrecognized and misdiagnosed by physicians (27). Furthermore, studies of TS prevalence have been restricted to an analysis of the tic disorder, while mounting evidence indicates that behavioral disorders, including OCD and ADHD, may be the only clinical manifestations of illness for some individuals (1,28). Thus the prevalence of the disorder may be much higher than current estimates, especially if behavioral manifestations are included. Comings (10) has estimated that if one accepts TS as a broadly based behavioral disorder, up to 1 in 100 individuals may manifest one or more clinical aspects of the TS genetic trait, making it one of the most common neurobehavioral disorders affecting humans. This conclusion has been challenged (29), and Cohen et al. (30) estimate that TS may affect up to 1 person in every 2,500 in its full-blown form and perhaps a single person in several 100 in its milder variants (30).

Further support for a high prevalence for tic disorders comes from epidemiologic surveys of school-age children. The first survey, conducted by Boncour in 1910 (31) on 1,759 French children aged 2–13 years, demonstrated an overall prevalence of 24% with an unexplained peak frequency in the 54 12-year-old boys of 50%. In the British National Child Development study, examination of 7,970 healthy 7-year-olds revealed tics in 4% (32). The same frequency of 4% was found in a large American study, published in 1954, with a peak incidence of 10% in 6- and 7-year-olds (33). Twelve percent of a randomly selected group of 482 children living in Buffalo, New York, aged 6–12 years, were found to have tics (34). A slightly higher frequency of 18% was found in the 63 black children (34). A lower prevalence of 8.7/1,000 was found by Debray-Ritzen and Dubois in a 1980 study (35), following examination of 4,258 children attending 15 schools in the Paris suburbs. To date, no study has examined the possibility that the

appearance of tics in childhood is associated with learning problems, perhaps signifying underlying dysfunction in neurological development.

In a recent epidemiologic study, Comings et al. (36) used a school psychologist to monitor a single school district encompassing about 3,000 students over a 2-year period. The selection and assessment methods were not systematic or well standardized. The frequency of definite TS was found to be 1 in 95 for boys and 1 in 759 for girls. These figures did not include an additional ten boys diagnosed as having definite transient tic disorder, two boys diagnosed as having probable TS, and ten boys diagnosed as having possible TS. Seventy percent of the students with definite TS were in special education classes, and the investigators reported that a remarkable 12% of all children in special education classes had definite TS and that a total of 28% fell within a tic disorder diagnostic category. In addition to adding support to the notion that TS is a common, often overlooked and misdiagnosed disorder, this study also suggests that children receiving special education may represent a high-risk population with a particularly high prevalence of tic disorders (Table 2). Even this study, which is based on cases referred for psychoeducational assessment, could represent an underestimate for dis-

TABLE 2. *Tourette syndrome prevalence estimates*

Estimate (per 10,000)	Population	Reference
0.7	All	Ascher, 1948 (37)
1.9	All	Salmi, 1961 (38)
0.07	All	Feild, 1966 (39)
0.05	All	Lucas, 1982 (23)
0.22	Women	Burd, 1986 (24)
0.77	Men	Burd, 1986 (24)
1.0	Girls	Burd, 1986 (25)
9.3	Boys	Burd, 1986 (25)
2.9	Children	Caine, 1988 (26)
105	Boys	Comings, 1990 (36)
13	Girls	Comings, 1990 (36)
1,200	Special education	Comings, 1990 (36)

ease prevalence for the entire population of children in special education.

Based on the foregoing evidence, the following hypotheses can be drawn:

1. TS is associated with numerous clinical factors that may impair school performance
2. TS is a common, misdiagnosed and overlooked disorder
3. TS is an important contributor to school problems in the childhood population at large
4. Children requiring special education represent a high-risk population for identifying TS

A community-based epidemiological survey, including direct interviews and assessments for the presence of tics, of a randomly selected sample of students requiring special education and a matched control population of children attending a regular classroom program would serve to determine whether or not the special education population indeed represents a high-risk group for TS. Our hypotheses would predict that a significantly higher prevalence for TS and related tic disorders would be found for the special education population when compared with the regular classroom control group. Direct face-to-face evaluations are required since current evidence strongly indicates that indirect interviews, based on questionnaires or historical information obtained from subjects, parents, or teachers, or methods that rely on subjects referred by school personnel or physicians, grossly underestimate the true prevalence of tic disorders (27). Subject matching for age and sex between the special education and regular classroom populations is important since the prevalence of tics appears to differ across different ages (33,34), and it has been recognized that boys are more commonly affected by TS (1). With such a matching scheme, however, it must be recognized that the observed prevalence rate for tic disorders in the matched control population might differ somewhat from that in a general regular classroom population, largely related to the expected greater proportion of boys in the matched sample.

This type of epidemiological survey should also prove valuable in addressing some other important scientific issues relevant to TS. For example, by using a randomly selected representative sample of an entire population of interest, rather than subjects referred for evaluation, a community-based study of children requiring special education should overcome the problem of ascertainment bias and provide an excellent method for determining the true limits of the TS behavioral disorder (40). Thus a comparison of special education subjects with or without tics for the prevalence of behavioral disorders reported in association with TS (e.g., OCD, ADHD, conduct disorder, mood disorders, anxiety disorders) should clarify current controversies regarding which specific psychopathologies are etiologically related to TS (1,28,41). Furthermore, an examination of family members of children in the epidemiological survey diagnosed with tics for evidence of TS might clarify the role of genetic factors in the etiology of childhood tic disorders. For example, as reviewed above, at least transient tics are observed commonly over the course of childhood development (31–34); however, it remains unknown what proportion of these cases are etiologically related to TS and occur on a hereditary basis (42). The possibility that TS, a hereditary and potentially treatable disorder, is responsible for a substantial fraction of learning problems in the childhood population at large might have profound educational, medical, and socioeconomic implications.

REFERENCES

1. Kurlan R. Tourette's syndrome: current concepts. *Neurology* 1989;39:1625–30.
2. Erenberg G, Cruse PR, Rothner AD. Tourette syndrome: an analysis of 200 pediatric and adolescent cases. *Cleve Clin Q* 1986;53:127–31.
3. Hagin RA, Kugler J. School problems associated with Tourette's syndrome. In: Cohen DJ, Bruun

RD, Leckman JF, eds. *Tourette's syndrome and tic disorders.* New York: John Wiley & Sons, 1988;223–36.

4. Comings DE, Comings BG. A controlled study of Tourette syndrome. I. Attention-deficit disorder, learning disorders and school problems. *Am J Hum Genet* 1987;41:701–4.

5. Mikkelsen EJ, Detlor J, Cohen DJ. School avoidance and social phobia triggered by haloperidol in patients with Tourette's disorder. *Am J Psychiatry* 1981;138:1572–5.

6. Keller BB. Cognitive assessment of obsessive-compulsive children. In: Rapoport JL, ed. *Obsessive-compulsive disorder in children and adolescents.* Washington, DC: American Psychiatric Press, 1989;33–9.

7. Ludlow CL, Bassaich CJ, Connor NP, Rapoport JL. Psycholinguistics testing in obsessive-compulsive adolescents. In: Rapoport JL, ed. *Obsessive-compulsive disorder in children and adolescents.* Washington, DC: American Psychiatric Press, 1989;87–106.

8. Cox CS, Fedio P, Rapoport JL. Neuropsychological testing of obsessive-compulsive adolescents. In: Rapoport JL, ed. *Obsessive-compulsive disorder in children and adolescents.* Washington, DC: American Psychiatric Press,, 1989;73–85.

9. Wender PH. *The hyperactive child, adolescent and adult.* New York: Oxford University Press, 1987.

10. Comings DE. A controlled study of Tourette syndrome VII. Summary: a common genetic disorder causing disinhibition of the limbic system. *Am J Hum Genet* 1987;41:839–66.

11. Shapiro AK, Shapiro ES, Young JG, Feinberg TE, eds. *Gilles de la Tourette syndrome. 2nd ed.* New York: Raven Press, 1988;241–51.

12. Golden GS. Psychologic and neuropsychologic aspects of Tourette's syndrome. *Neurol Clin* 1984; 2:91–102.

13. Lucas AR, Kauffman PE, Morris EM. Gilles de la Tourette's disease, a clinical study of 15 cases. *J Am Acad Child Psychiatry* 1967;6:700–22.

14. Shapiro AK, Shapiro ES, Bruun RD, et al. *Gilles de la Tourette syndrome.* New York: Raven Press, 1978.

15. deleted in proof.

16. Sutherland RJ, Kolb B, Schoel WM, et al. Neuropsychological assessment of children and adults with Tourette syndrome: a comparison with learning disabilities and schizophrenia. *Adv Neurol* 1982;35:311–22.

17. Thompson RJ, O'Quinn AN, Logue PE. Gilles de la Tourette's syndrome: a review and neuropsychological aspects of four cases. *J Pediatr Psychol* 1979;4:371.

18. Joschko M, Rourke BP. Neuropsychological dimensions of Tourette syndrome: test-retest stability and implications for intervention. *Adv Neurol* 1982;35:297–304.

19. Incagnoli T, Kane R. Neuropsychological functioning in Gilles de la Tourette's syndrome. *J Clin Neuropsychol* 1981;3:165.

20. Harcherik DF, Carbonari CM, Shaywitz SE, et al. Attentional and perceptual disturbances in children with Tourette's syndrome, attention deficit disorder, and epilepsy. *Schizophr Bull* 1982; 8:356–59.

21. Hagins RA, Beecher R, Pagano G, et al. Effects of Tourette syndrome on learning. *Adv Neurol.* 1982; 35:323–8.

22. Riddle MA, Hardin MT, Ort SI, Leckman JF, Cohen DJ. Behavioral symptoms in Tourette's syndrome. In: Cohen DJ, Bruun RD, Leckman JF, eds. *Tourette's syndrome and tic disorders.* New York: John Wiley & Sons, 1988;151–62.

23. Lucas AR, Beard CM, Rajput AH, et al. Tourette syndrome in Rochester, Minnesota. *Adv Neurol* 1982;35:267–9.

24. Burd L, Kerbeshian J, Wikenheiser M, et al. Prevalence of Gilles de la Tourette's syndrome in North Dakota adults. *Am J Psychiatry* 1986;143:787–8.

25. Burd L, Kerbeshian J, Wikenheiser M, Fisher W. A prevalence study of Gilles de la Tourette syndrome in North Dakota school-age children. *J Am Acad Child Psychiatry* 1986;4:552–5.

26. Caine ED, McBride MC, Chiverton P, Bamford KA, Redress S, Shiao J. Tourette's syndrome in Monroe County School children. *Neurology* 1988; 38:472–5.

27. Kurlan R, Behr J, Medved L, Shoulson I, Pauls D, Kidd KK. Severity of Tourette's syndrome in one large kindred: implication for determination of disease prevalence rate. *Arch Neurol* 1987;44:268–9.

28. Kurlan R. The spectrum of Tourette's syndrome. *Curr Opin Neurol Neurosurg* 1988;1:294–8.

29. Pauls DL, Cohen DJ, Kidd KK, Leckman JF. Tourette syndrome and neuropsychiatric disorders: is there a genetic relationship? [Letter] *Am J Hum Genet* 1988;43:206–9.

30. Cohen DJ, Bruun RD, Leckman JR. *Tourette's syndrome and tic disorders.* New York: John Wiley & Sons, 1988;xiii.

31. Boncour GP, Les tics chez l'ecolier et leur interpretation. *Prog Med* 1910;26:495–6.

32. Kellmer Pringle ML, Butler NR, Davie R. 1st report of national child development study. In: *11,000 seven-year-olds.* National Bureau for Co-Operation in Child Care, Long, 1967;185.

33. MacFarlane JW, Honzik MP, Allen L. In: *Behavior problems in normal children.* University of California Publications in Child Development, 1954.

34. Lapouse R, Monk M. Behavior deviations in a representative sample of children: variation by sex, age, race, social class and family size. *Am J Orthopsychiatry* 1964;34:436–46.

35. Debray-Ritzen P, Dubois H. Maladies des tics de l'enfant. *Rev Neurol (Paris)* 1980;136:15–18.

36. Comings DE, Himes JA, Comings BG. An epidemiologic study of Tourette's syndrome in a single school district. *J Clin Psychiatry* 1990;51:463–9.

37. Ascher E. Psychodynamic considerations in Gilles de la Tourette's disease (maladie des tics): with a report of 5 cases and discussion of the literature. *Am J Psychiatry* 1948;105:267–76.

38. Salmi K. Gilles de la Tourette's syndrome: the report of a case and its treatment. *Acta Psychiatr Scand* 1961;36:156–62.

39. Feild JR, Corbin KB, Goldstein NP, Klass DW. Gilles de la Tourette's syndrome. *Neurology* 1966; 16:453–62.

40. Como PG, Kurlan R. Neuropsychological testing in Tourette's syndrome: a comparison of clinic and family populations. *Neurology* 1989;39(Suppl 1):342.

41. Pauls DL, Cohen DJ, Kidd KK, Leckman JF. Tourette syndrome and neuropsychiatric disorders: is there a genetic relationship? *Am J Hum Genet* 1988;43:206–9.

42. Kurlan R, Behr J, Medved L, Como P. Transient tic disorder and the clinical spectrum of Tourette's syndrome. *Arch Neurol* 1988;45:1200–1.

Advances in Neurology, Vol. 58, edited by T. N. Chase, A. J. Friedhoff, and D. J. Cohen. Raven Press, Ltd., New York 1992.

11

Tourette Syndrome and Obsessive–Compulsive Disorder

Henrietta L. Leonard, Susan E. Swedo, Judith L. Rapoport, Kenneth C. Rickler, Deborah Topol, Stephen Lee, and David Rettew

Child Psychiatry Branch, National Institute of Mental Health, Bethesda, Maryland 20892

Historically, tics have been reported in obsessive–compulsive patients, as well as obsessive–compulsive symptomatology in Tourette syndrome (TS) patients. Despite this observation, until very recently, there has been no systematic study of this relationship. This chapter will review the literature on the relationships between the two disorders and will present recent findings from a large cohort of children and adolescents with obsessive–compulsive disorder (OCD).

OVERVIEW OF OBSESSIVE–COMPULSIVE DISORDER

OCD is characterized by recurrent obsessions and/or compulsions that are distressing and interfere in one's social or occupational functioning (1). The disorder is far more common than initially thought, with prevalence estimated to be 2% of the adult (2) and 0.8% (3) of the adolescent population. One-third to one-half of adult OCD patients had their onset in childhood (4), and cases have been reported to develop in individuals as young as 2 years of age. In childhood OCD, boys predominate (at a 2:1 ratio) and have an earlier age of onset (5), while in adulthood, women are more frequently afflicted (6).

Most OCD patients report a combination of both obsessions (persistent thoughts or worries) and compulsions (rituals). A ritual is a repetitive behavior that is performed in response to an obsession, typically in order to prevent discomfort or a feared event or to "undo a bad thought." Rituals are distinguished from motor tics in that they are purposeful, intentional, and in response to a cognition, for example, "my mother may die if I don't retrace my steps." Motor tics, although they can be complex and may dispel an "urge" or a build-up of tension, are not instigated by a thought and not typically accompanied by anxiety. Complex motor tics preceded by a sensation or urge sometimes may resemble rituals, thus making the distinction difficult. Touching behavior may be either a compulsive ritual or a motor tic depending on its character and the accompanying cognition. Similarly, tapping, spitting, and licking are most frequently tics, although they may be rituals if they are complex and specifically directed against an obsessive thought. Although sometimes difficult, it is important to make the distinction between a complex motor tic and a compulsive ritual, as each would require different treatment.

In 70 child and adolescent OCD patients studied at the National Institute of Mental

Health (NIMH) (5), the most common ritual was excessive cleaning (handwashing, showering, bathing, or tooth brushing), which occurred at some point in 85% of the patients. Repeating rituals, such as getting up/down from chairs, retracing steps, rereading, restarting phases, going in/out doors, etc., were reported by 51% of the patients. Checking rituals, such as making sure that appliances were turned off, that windows and doors were locked, or that homework was done "just right" were seen in 46%. Counting, ordering/arranging, and hoarding were also common. Obsessions most commonly centered on either fears that harm might come to themselves or loved ones or on contamination thoughts. Scrupulosity (the excessive concern that one might have done something wrong) and the somatic preoccupation that one might have an illness, were less common. Characteristically, the specific content of the obsessions and rituals changes over time, and symptoms typically wax and wane.

The etiology of OCD is unknown; however, strong evidence supports a neurobiologic model. Neurotransmitter abnormalities have been implicated by a number of studies, and the "serotonin hypothesis of OCD" has been based on the findings of controlled treatment studies demonstrating that the serotonin reuptake blockers clomipramine (7), fluoxetine (8), and fluvoxamine (9) are selectively effective. Neuroanatomical, neurophysiologic, and neuroimmunological evidence supports a theory of frontal lobe–basal ganglia dysfunction. Luxenberg et al. (10) reported a decreased left caudate size on computerized tomography (CT) in OCD patients compared with controls. Positron emission tomographic (PET) studies have reported orbital frontal regional hypermetabolism (11–14) and alterations in metabolism in the left anterior cingulate (14) and caudate nucleus (11). There is an increased rate of OCD in several illnesses of the basal ganglia, specifically TS (which is discussed in detail later) (15), postencephalitic Parkinson's disease (16), and Huntington's chorea (S. Folstein, personal commu-

nication). Brain injuries resulting in basal ganglia damage, for example carbon monoxide poisoning (17), also have been reported to cause OCD. Swedo et al. (18) reported an increased incidence of OCD in pediatric patients with Sydenham's chorea (an autoimmune inflammation of the basal ganglia caused by a streptococcal infection) when compared with nonchronic rheumatic fever patients. Although the neuroanatomic localization of the dysfunction in TS is unknown, areas (frontal cortex, limbic system, basal ganglia) similar to those hypothesized for OCD have been proposed (19).

Genetic susceptibility for OCD and TS has been reported in TS families by Pauls et al. (15). Lenane et al. (20) reported that 20% of personally interviewed first-degree relatives of OCD probands (100% of all those over the age of 6 years of age were evaluated) met criteria for a lifetime diagnosis of OCD. Interestingly, the principal OCD symptom in the family member was different from that of the proband, which suggests that the "inheritance" of OCD is genetic rather than modeled (20).

TICS IN OCD PATIENTS

Early reports noted the presence of tics in OCD patients. Pierre Janet's (21) report Obsessions and Psychasthenia," published in 1907, described repetitive "forced agitations" that included motor tics; additionally, he writes of the difficulty in distinguishing complex motor tics from repetitive rituals. Subsequently, Schilder (22) in 1937 and Grimshaw (23) in 1964 each reported one case of such an association, and Robinson and Vitale (24) described an obsessive child with "circumscribed interest patterns" who cleared his throat and barked.

Until recently, the studies of tics in OCD patients were limited by the lack of standardized diagnostic criteria and the absence of structured assessment measures. Table 1 reviews the more recent and systematic studies. Rasmussen and Tsuang (25) found 2 cases (5%) of TS in 44 OCD patients, al-

TABLE 1. *Reports of tics in OCD patients*

Authors	OCD subjects	Structured interview/or rating scales	DSM-III-(R)/ICD-9 diagnosis for OCD	OCD OCP OCB OCS	Tics distinguished from rituals?	Results
Rasmusen and Tsuang, 1986	N = 44 16 women, 26.3 ± 11.4 yr 28 men, 31.2 ± 10.6 yr	Semistructured interview	DSM-III	OCD	?	n = 2 (5%) TS
Pitman, et al., 1987 (26)	N = 16 8 women 8 men 40 ± 12.1 yr	Yale Schedule for TS, Maudsley OC Inventory	15 of 16 met DSM-III criteria	OCD	Yes	n = 6 (37%) with tics, 5 men, 1 woman; 3, CMT; 2, transient tics; 1, TS
Swedo, et al. 1989 (18)	N = 70 47 boys 23 girls 13.7 ± 2.67 yr	DICA NIMH-OCD	DSM-III	OCD	Yes	20% (n = 14) had a tic disorder at baseline; (TS initial exclusionary criteria)
Riddle, et al., 1990 (27)	N = 21 9 boys 12 girls 12.2 ± 3.1 (7.8–16.9) yr	CBCL YOCDQ	DSM-III-R	OCD	?	5 patients (24%) had observable tics (TS initial exclusionary criteria)

CBCL, Child Behavior Checklist; CMT, chronic motor tics; DICA, Diagnostic Interview for Child; DIS, Diagnostic Interview Schedule; DSM-III, *Diagnostic and Statistical Manual*, 3rd ed.; ICD9, International Classification of Diseases, 9th ed.; LOI, Leyton Obsessional Inventory; NIMH-OCD, National Institute of Mental Health Global OCD Scale; OC, obsessive–compulsive; OCB, obsessive–compulsive behavior; OCD, obsessive–compulsive disorder; OCP, obsessive–compulsive personality; OCS, obsessive–compulsive symptoms; TS, Tourette syndrome; YOCDQ, Yale Obsessive–Compulsive Disorder Questionnaire.

though the rate of other tic disorders was not reported. Pitman et al. (26) reported that of 16 OCD subjects, 6 (5 men and 1 woman) had a tic disorder, specifically 3 chronic motor, 2 transient, and 1 (6%) with TS. In two pediatric studies, in which TS was exclusionary, the rate of tics was reported to be 20% by Swedo et al. (5) and 24% by Riddle et al. (27). These studies suggest that there is an increased rate of tics in OCD probands.

OCD IN TS

Conversely, early reports of patients with tic disorders noted significant obsessionality. As early as 1907, Meige and Feindel (28) in their textbook on tics, reported that "the frequency with which obsessions, or at least a proclivity for them and tics are associated, cannot be a simple coincidence" (29). This association was one rea-

son that TS was originally classified as a functional illness (29), but by 1935, Creak and Guttman (30) had noted the neurological findings in TS patients and concluded that the illness was of an organic origin, although the debate over its classification has continued. Fernando's 1967 (31) review of the literature reported that less than 30% of 85 TS were "obsessional." In the four detailed case reports presented, one "spinster" with TS was "excessively religious," which suggests a diagnosis of scrupulosity. Morphew and Sim in their 1969 (29) report of six TS cases listed two cases as having obsessional personality, one of which had "sadistic fantasies involving knife attacks on his children" and "folie du doute," again suggesting an OCD and not an obsessive–compulsive personality (OCP) diagnosis.

In the 1980s, with the increased interest in TS, larger studies examined the associated features of the illness, although often the distinction between compulsive rituals and tics was not made. These studies are summarized in Table 2. Nee et al. (32) found that 68% (34 of 50) of TS patients had "DSM-III obsessive compulsive behavior," concluding that it was one of the most commonly associated behaviors. In a later report (33), they noted a high comorbidity with OCD, finding that 90% of 30 patients (not stated if these patients are presented in the 1980 report) had "obsessive compulsive behavior . . . , most commonly touching". Yarvura-Tobias et al. (34) reported that 89% (49 of 55) of TS patients had "OC symptoms," but the high percentage in this study may be due to the inclusion of nonspecific symptoms, such as the "urge to tic." Jagger et al. (35) reported that two-thirds of their patients had "compulsive actions," but they included tics, such as touching, tapping, kicking, and self-destructive actions of biting and head banging in the count. Montgomery et al. (36) distinguished rituals from vocal and motor tics, and, using a structured interview, reported that 67% (10 of 15) of TS patients had "OC illness," although *Diagnostic and Statistical Manual*, 3rd ed. (DSM-III) (37) criteria were not applied. Stefl (38) using a mailed questionnaire of behavioral difficulties, found that 32% of TS respondents had undefined obsessive–compulsive behavior. Comings and Comings (39), in their large sample of 250 TS patients, found that 32% had OC behaviors, although it was not clear that "compulsive tics" were excluded. In their later report (40), 45% had a significant "obsessive compulsive score," however, compulsive echolalia, palilalia, touching, and self-mutilating behavior were included. The blurred distinctions between compulsive rituals and repetitive tics in most of these reports make it difficult to determine the true comorbidity of OCD with TS.

Subsequent studies continued to report an increase in obsessive–compulsive symptomatology, although these too were limited by the lack of standardized DSM-III (37) diagnostic criteria for OCD. Kurlan et al.'s (41) report of 29 TS patients from a large pedigree found that 48% (14 of 29) had obsessions or compulsions, although the actual diagnosis of OCD was not made. Jankovic and Rohaidy (42) reported that 32% of 112 TS patients had OCD traits, but these were not defined. Erenberg et al. (43) found that 32% of 58 TS patients in a mail questionnaire acknowledged obsessive–compulsive behaviors. Robertson et al. (44) reported that 37% (33 of 90) of TS probands had OC behaviors, although DSM-III or ICD-9 criteria were not mentioned. Singer and Rosenberg (45), using the OC subscale on the Child Behavior Checklist, filled out by parents of TS probands found that 43% of the younger children and 40% of the older children had OC symptoms.

Recent studies have attempted to study more systematically the prevalence of OCD in TS probands. Pauls et al. (15), in one of the first studies that systematically evaluated the TS adult proband in person using structured interviews based on DSM-III criteria, reported that 50% (16 of 32) met criteria for OCD. Grad et al. (46), using structured interviews based on DSM-III criteria and rating scales, distinguished compulsive rituals from repetitive tics, and found that 28% (7 of 25) of the TS patients met criteria for OCD in comparison with 8% (2 of 25) of the control group. Frankel et al. (47), using the Leyton Obsessional Inventory, found that 52% (33 of 64) of TS patients had a score greater than 70 (defined as elevated) in comparison to 12% (5 of 41) of normal controls. Pitman et al. (26) reported that 62% of 16 TS probands had OCD in comparison to none of the control subjects. In summary, those studies evaluating TS probands for OCD meeting DSM-III criteria using structured interviews have reported a comorbidity ranging from 28% to 62%.

FAMILY STUDIES OF TS PROBANDS

Additional evidence supporting a relationship between OCD and TS comes from family studies demonstrating an increased rate of OCD in first-degree relatives of TS probands. As seen in Table 3, this association was initially reported in several family history studies; for example, Nee et al. (33) found that 13 of 30 (43%) probands had a family member with OC behavior but did not state the actual number of relatives affected. In a study by Jankovic and Rohaidy (42), 10% of 112 TS probands reported that they had a relative (unspecified if first-degree) with marked (unspecified) OC behaviors. Pitman et al. (26) studied 16 TS patients (of whom 10 had OCD), using the family history method (confirmed by phone interview with a family member when available) and found that 7% of their relatives had OCD, which was equivalent to the rate of relatives of OCD probands and was greater than that in those of controls. Montgomery et al. (36) attempted to interview all first-degree relatives and found that 13% (4 of 30) of first-degree relatives evaluated met criteria for OC illness; however, information about 43% of the relatives was not available.

Two other family studies reported on (different) single large pedigrees. Kurlan (41) identified 29 TS/chronic motor tics (CMT) probands in 69 relatives in one large pedigree with several generations; although he reported a "significant incidence of obsessions and compulsions" in family members unaffected by tics (N = 40), a rate of OCD was not calculated. Robertson and Gourdee's (48) report on 122 members of one family, 85 of whom were evaluated in person, diagnosed 29 cases of TS, 17 cases of CMT, and 4 cases of OCD, although rates of illness were not computed and several generations were used.

Pauls et al. (15), in the first systematic family study wherein all first-degree relatives were evaluated with direct personal structured interviews, found an increased rate of OCD in the first-degree relatives of TS probands over those of the control sample of adoptee relatives, regardless of the OCD status of the TS proband. They hypothesized that some forms of OCD may represent alternative expressions of the underlying cause of TS. In a subsequent study, Pauls et al. (49) blindly interviewed in person the 338 first-degree relatives of 86 TS probands and found that the rates of TS, CMT, and OCD are higher in the biological relatives of TS probands than in the relatives of controls. Sex of the proband did not effect the relatives' diagnosis; however, male relatives were more likely to have TS, and female relatives were more likely to have OCD. There was no significant difference in the rate of OCD between relatives of TS probands with and without OCD, again suggesting that OCD and TS may be etiologically related.

TIC DISORDERS IN 54 OCD CHILD PROBANDS

Fifty-four consecutive children and adolescents (36 boys and 18 girls aged 6–18 years) with severe primary OCD were enrolled in controlled clomipramine treatment trials (50,51) at the National Institute of Mental Health (NIMH). TS was an initial exclusionary criteria; however, chronic and transient tic disorders were not. At initial evaluation, 16 (30%) had a current chronic or transient tic disorder and 31 (57%) had a lifetime (including current) diagnosis of a chronic or transient tic disorder. At baseline, those with a lifetime history of tics could not be distinguished from those without tics on the basis of gender, IQ, comorbid diagnoses, baseline OCD severity age of onset of OCD, rate of OCD in first-degree family members, or response to 5 weeks of clomipramine treatment. Although 23 boys and 8 girls had a positive lifetime history of tics at baseline and 13 boys and 10 girls did not, this gender difference was not significant. Although we had hypothesized that the group with a disorder might have a preponderance of touching and tapping rituals, there was no difference between presenting OC symptoms; washing, checking, hoarding, repeating, and counting predominated in that order of frequency.

TABLE 2. *Studies of TS patients*

Authors	TS subjects	Structured interview/rating scales for OCD	DSM-III-R/ICD-9 diagnosis for OCD	OCD OCP OCB PCS	Tics distinguished from rituals?	Results (OC in TS)
Nee, et al., 1980	N = 50	Clinical interview	Yes	OCD (for OCD)	No	34/50 (68%) OCB
Yaryura-Tobias et al., 1981 (34)	N = 55 $\overline{X}$ = 23 yo (6–62)	Clinical interview	No	OCS	No	49/55 (89%) included are urged to tic Nonspecific OCS
Nee et al. 1982 (33)	N = 30 8 F, 22 M aged 21–71 yr	Clinical interview	Yes	OCB	No	90% had OCB (actual no. patients not stated)
Jagger, et al., 1982 (35)	N = 75 57 M, 18 F aged 8–57 yr	Unspecified self-report questionnaire	No	Compulsive actions	No	Two-thirds of the patients had compulsive actions (including touching and tapping, tics, self-destructive behaviors)
Montgomery et al. 1982 (36)	13 M, 16.7 yo 2 F 12 and 28 yo	RDR	No Feighner criteria	OC illness OCS	Yes	10/15 (67%), 6/10 moderate to severe, 4 mild
Stefl 1984 (38)	N = 425 330 M, 95F	Mail questionnaire of behavioral problems	No	OCB	?	32% often, 41% sometimes, 26% never had OCB (actual no. patients not stated)
Comings and Comings, 1985 (39)	N = 250 201 M, 17 ± 10 yr 49 F, 26.3 ± 17.1 yr	Nonspecific structured standard questionnaire	No	OCB	?	32% had OCB (actual no. patients not stated)
Grad et al., 1987 (46)	25 TS 11.10 ± 1.68 (8–13 yr) 25 controls 10.78 ± 1.72 (8–13) yr	DICA LOI CBCL	Yes	OCD	Yes	More children (7/25) (28%) had OCD than in the control group (2/25) (8%)
Frankel, et al., 1986 (48)	N = 63 <18 yo = 13 >18 yo = 50 41 n.c.	LOI Questionnaire derived from LOI (70 was the cut-off score for OCD)	No	OCD symptoms	No	33/64 (52%) TS pts had LOI of >70; 5/41 (12%) controls had LOI of >70 (note discrepancy of N = 63 vs 64 TS pts not explained)

Study	Sample	Method		Classification		Findings
Kurlan et al., 1986 (41)	N = 29 $\overline{X}$ = 33.4 yo (5–72), all from one pedigree	Clinical interview Standard questionnaire	No	Obsessions Compulsions	Yes	14/29 (48%) had obsessions or compulsions
Pauls, et al., 1986 (49)	N = 32 mean = 20.75 yrs	Clinical and semistructured interview	Yes	OCD	Yes	50% (16/32) had OCD
Pitman, et al., 1987 (26)	16 TS, 90 M, 7 F 31 ± 7.8 yo 16 normal, 8 men, 8 women, 39 ± 9.2 yr	Yale Schedule DIS Maudsley	Yes	OCD	Yes	62% (10/16) had OCD 0 of controls had OCD
Jankovic and Rohaidy, 1987 (42)	N = 112, age unspecific M:F 3.8:1	Clinical interview, unspecific psychological evaluations	No	OCP OCB Undefined	Yes	32% OCP traits
Erenberg et al., 1987 (43)	N = 58, sex unknown 15–25 (± 2.6 yr)	Mail questionnaire sent with unspecific OCB questions	No	OCB	No	32% OCB
Robertson et al., 1988 (44)	N = 90 Dx = 21.5 yr ± 12.7	Clinical interview Leyton OCEI	No	OCB	Unspecified	33/90 (37%) OCB and/or rituals
Singer and Rosenberg, 1989 (45)	78 M, 6–16 yr (48 aged 6–11, 30 aged 12–16)	CBCL OC subscale filled out by parent	No	OCS	No	43% aged 6–11 OCS 40% aged 12–16 OCS

CBCL, Children's Behavioral Checklist; OCEI, Crown Crisp Experimental Index; DICA, Diagnostic Interview for Children; DIS, Diagnostic Interview Schedule; DSM-III, *Diagnostic and Statistical Manual*, 3rd ed.; DSM-III-R, *Diagnostic and Statistical Manual*, 3rd ed. revised; ICD-9, International Classification of Diseases, 9th ed.; LOI, Leyton Obsessional Inventory; Maudsley, Maudsley Obsessive Compulsive Inventory; OCB, obsessive–compulsive behavior; OCD, obsessive–compulsive disorder; OCP, obsessive–compulsive personality; OCS, obsessive–compulsive symptoms; RDR, Renard Diagnostic Review; TS, Tourette syndrome; Yale, Yale Schedule for Tourette and other Behavioral Syndromes; yo, years old.

TABLE 3. *Family studies of TS probands*

Author	Subjects: TS probands and their OCD status	Total no. first-degree relatives evaluated	Structured interview rating scales	DSM-III-(R)/ICD-9 diagnosis for OCD	OCD OCP OCB OCS	Tics distinguished from rituals?	Results: OCD in first-degree relatives
Nee et al., 1982 (33)	N = 30 8 women, 22 men aged 21–71 yr, 90% (34/50) reported OC behavior, "most commonly touching"	Family history on 1,117 patients and relatives, including third and fourth generation, unknown total no.	Family history method — no —	Stated as "yes" but included touching	OCB	No	13/30 (43%) probands had OC behavior in family members but actual no. of relatives with OCD not stated
Montgomery et al., 1982 (36)	N = 15 13 men 16.7 yr, 2 women 12 and 18 yr, 10/15 had OC illness	30 of 53 (57%) first-degree relatives interviewed	RDR	Yes	OCB	Yes	4 relatives (13%) interviewed met criteria for OC illness
Kurlan et al., 1986 (41)	N = 29 X̄ = 33.4 yr all from one pedigree; 14/29 (48%) had obsessions or compulsions	69 relatives evaluated including second-, third-, fourth-degree relatives, unknown total no. relatives	Standardized questionnaire, 47/69 videotaped	No	Obs., comp.	Yes	5/40 (13%) unaffected (tic) relatives had obsessions and 5/40 (13%) had compulsions (not mutual exclusion); unable to calculate rate in relatives
Pauls et al., 1986 (15)	N = 32 X̄ = 20.7 yr, 14/32 probands had OCD	Information on all 122 first-degree relatives obtained, 117/122 (96%) by direct interview	Blind clinical and semistructured interview	DSM-III	OCD	Yes	11/58 (19%) relatives had OCD in TS with OCD probands 12/45 (27%) relatives had OCD in TS without OCD probands; adoptive families 0 cases of OCD

Study	Subjects	Relatives	Method		Disorder		Results
Jankovic and Rohaidy, 1987 (42)	N = 112, 32% OCP traits	Unclear if relatives were first degree, no. evaluated unspecified	Family history method, direct interview if available	No	OCP OCB Undefined	Yes	10% of proband had relative with marked OCD
Pitman et al., 1987	N = 16 TS; N = 16 OCD; N = 16 NC; 10/16 TS pts had OCD	Family members not seen in person	Family history method confirmed by phone interview with a family member when available	Yes	OCD	Yes	5/74 (7%) of relatives of TS probands had OCD; 6/75 (8%) of relatives of OCD proband had OCD; 1/86 (1%) of controls had relative with OCD
Robertson and Gourdie, 1990	122 members of one pedigree: 29 TS, 17 CMT, 4 OCD; 2/29 TS had OCB, 4/17 CMT had OCB	85 of 122 members interviewed of one family; multigenerational	Semistructured interview, LOI Crown Crisp, SADS	No	OCB	No	10/85 members had OCB; 4/85 had OCB without tics
Pauls et al., 1991 (49)	N = 86 TS, 64 M, 22 F, 55 TS only, 31 TS and OCD; N = 21 adopted TS; N = 22 normal	338 biological first-degree relatives of 86 TS probands; 21 biologically unrelated relatives of adopted TS probands; 22 relatives of normal subjects; 297/381 (78%) first-degree relatives interviewed directly	Raters blind to proband diagnosis DIS KSADS-E Structured interview for TS and OCP	DSM-III	OCD	Yes	49/338 (14%) biologic relatives had OCD; 1/43 (2%) relatives of controls had OCD; no significant difference between relatives of TS probands with and without OCD

comp., compulsions; DIS, Diagnostic Interview Schedule; DSM-III, *Diagnostic and Statistical Manual*, 3rd ed.; ICD-9, International Classification, 9th ed.; KSADS-E, Schedule for Affective Disorders and Schizophrenia for School Age Children; LOI, Leyton Obsessional Inventory; obs, obsessions; OCB, obsessive compulsive behavior; OCD, obsessive compulsive disorder; OCP, obsessive compulsive personality; OCS, obsessive compulsive symptoms; RDR, Renard Diagnostic Review; SADS, Schedule for Affective Disorders and Schizophrenia; TS, Tourette syndrome.

At the 2–4 year follow-up, eight (15%) boys met DSM-III-R (1) criteria for a lifetime diagnosis of TS, despite it having been an initial exclusionary criteria (52). The presentation and clinical course of their OCD was indistinguishable from that of OCD patients without TS. Family history of tics, TS, and OCD in first-degree relatives also did not differ between groups. Two of the eight boys might arguably have just met or just missed diagnostic criteria for TS at presentation, but the "development" of TS in even 6 (12%) of 54 children and adolescents with severe primary OCD is higher than expected. This increased incidence of tics and TS in our OCD probands is consistent with the hypothesis that some cases of OCD and TS may be etiologically related.

It is clear from the increased rates of OCD in TS patients, the increased prevalence of tics and TS in OCD patients, and the increased familial rates of OCD and TS in first-degree relatives of both TS and OCD probands, that there is a close association between the two disorders. The nature of that relationship remains unclear. Whether OCD and TS might represent different phenotypic expressions of the same aberrant genotype or merely overlapping disorders must be determined by further systematic investigations.

REFERENCES

1. American Psychiatric Association, Committee on Nomenclature and Statistics. *Diagnostic and Statistical Manual of Mental Disorders*, 3rd ed., revised. Washington, DC: American Psychiatric Association, 1987.
2. Karno M, Golding JM, Sorenson SB, et al. Epidemiology of obsessive compulsive disorder in five U.S. communities. *Arch Gen Psychiatry* 1988; 45:1094–9.
3. Flament MF, Whitaker A, Rapoport JL. Obsessive compulsive disorder in adolescence: an epidemiological study. *J Am Acad Child Adolesc Psychiatry* 1988;27:764–71.
4. Black A. The natural history of obsessional neurosis. In: Beech HR, ed. *Obsessional States*. London: Methuen, 1978.
5. Swedo SE, Rapoport JL, Leonard HL, Lenane M, Cheslow D. Obsessive compulsive disorder in children and adolescents: clinical phenomenology of 70 consecutive cases. *Arch Gen Psychiatry* 1989; 46:335–43.
6. Rasmussen SA, Eisen JL. Epidemiology and clinical features of obsessive–compulsive disorder. In: Jenike MA, Baer L, Minichiello WE, (eds). *Obsessive-compulsive disorders: theory and management*. Chicago: Year Book Medical Publishers, 1990;10–27.
7. Insel TR, Mueller EA, Alterman I, et al: Obsessive compulsive disorder and serotonin: is there a connection? *Biol Psychiatry* 1985;20:1174–88.
8. Pigott TA, Pato MT, Bernstein SE, et al. Controlled comparisons of clomipramine and fluoxetine in the treatment of obsessive-compulsive disorder. *Arch Gen Psychiatry* 1990;47:926–32.
9. Goodman WK, Price LH, Rasmussen SA, Delgado PL. Heninger GR, Charney DS. Efficacy of fluvoxamine in obsessive-compulsive disorder. *Arch Gen Psychiatry* 1989;46:36–44.
10. Luxenberg JS, Swedo SE, Flament MF, Friedland RP, Rapoport JL, Rapoport SI. Neuroanatomic abnormalities in obsessive-compulsive disorder detected with quantitative x-ray computed tomography. *Am J Psychiatry* 1988;145:1089–94.
11. Baxter LR, Phelps ME, Mazziotta JC, Guze BH, Schwartz JM, Selin CE. Local cerebral glucose metabolic rates in obsessive-compulsive disorder. *Arch Gen Psychiatry* 1987;44:211–8.
12. Baxter LR, Schwartz JM, Mazziotta JC, Phelps ME, Pahl JJ, Guze BH. Cerebral glucose metabolic rates in non-depressed obsessive-compulsives. *Am J Psychiatry* 1989;145:1560–3.
13. Nordahl TE, Benkelfat C, Semple WE, Gross M, King AC, Cohen RM. Cerebral glucose metabolic rates in obsessive compulsive disorder. *Neuropsychopharmacology* 1989;2:23–8.
14. Swedo SE, Schapiro ME, Grady CL, et al. Cerebral glucose metabolism in childhood-onset obsessive compulsive disorder. *Arch Gen Psychiatry* 1989;46:518–23.
15. Pauls DL, Towbin KE, Leckman JF, Zahner GEP, Cohen DJ. Gilles de la Tourette's syndrome and obsessive-compulsive disorder. *Arch Gen Psychiatry* 1986;43:1180–2.
16. Von Economo C (trans., ed.). *Encephalitis Lethargic, its Sequellae and Treatment*. New York: Oxford University Press, 1931.
17. Laplane D, Baulac M, Widlocher D, Dubois B. Pure psychic akinesia with bilateral lesions of basal ganglia. *J Neurol Neurosurg Psychiatry* 1984; 47:377–85.
18. Swedo SE, Rapoport JL, Cheslow DL, et al. Increased incidence of obsessive compulsive symptoms in patients with Sydenham's chorea. *Am J Psychiatry* 1989;146:246–9.
19. Singer HS, Walkup JT. Tourette syndrome and other tic disorders: diagnosis, pathophysiology and treatment. *Medicine* 1991;70:15–32.
20. Lenane M, Swedo S, Leonard H, et al. Psychiatric disorders in first degree relatives of children and adolescents with obsessive compulsive disorder. *J Am Acad Child Adolesc Psychiatry* 1990; 29:407–12.
21. Pitman RK. Pierre Janet on obsessive-compulsive

disorder (1903). *Arch Gen Psychiatry* 1987; 44:226–32.

22. Schilder P. The organic background of obsessions and compulsions. Presented at the ninety-third annual meeting of The American Psychiatric Association, Pittsburg, PA, May 10–14, 1937.

23. Grimshaw L. Obsessional disorder and neurological illness. *J Neruol Neurosurg Psychiatry* 1964; 27:229–31.

24. Robinson JF, Vitale LJ. Children with circumscribed interest patterns. *Am J Orthopsychiatry* 1959;27:755–66.

25. Rasmussen SA, Tsuang MT. Clinical characteristics and family history in DSM-III obsessive-compulsive disorder. *Am J Psychiatry* 1986; 143:317–22.

26. Pitman RK, Green RC, Jenike MA, Mesulam MM. Clinical comparison of Tourette's disorder and obsessive-compulsive disorder. *Am J Psychiatry* 1987;144:1166–71.

27. Riddle MA, Scahill L, King R, et al. Obsessive compulsive disorder in children and adolescents: phenomenology and family history. 1990; 29:766–72.

28. Meige H, Feindel E. *Tics and their treatment.* London: Sidney Appleton, 1907.

29. Morphew JA, Sim M. Gilles de la Tourette's syndrome: a clinical and psychopathological study. *Br J Psychol* 1969;42:293–301.

30. Creak M, Guttman E. Chorea, tics, and compulsive utterances. *J Ment Sci* 1935;82:834–9.

31. Fernando SJM. Gilles de la Tourette's syndrome. *Br J Psychiatry* 1967;113:607–17.

32. Nee LE, Caine ED, Polinsky RJ, Eldridge R, Ebert MH. Gilles de la Tourette syndrome: clinical and family study of 50 cases. *Ann Neurol* 1980;7:41–9.

33. Nee LE, Polinsky RJ, Ebert MH. Tourette syndrome: clinical and family studies. In: Friedhoff AJ, Chase TM, ed. *Gilles de la Tourette syndrome.* New York: Raven Press, 1982;1291–4.

34. Yaryura-Tobias JA, Neziroglu F, Howard S, Fuller B. Clinical aspects of Gilles de la Tourette syndrome. *J Orthomolecular Psychiatry* 1981; 10:263–8.

35. Jagger J, Prusoff BA, Cohen DJ, Kidd KK, Carbonari CM, John K. The epidemiology of Tourette's syndrome: a pilot study. *Schizophr Bull* 1982; 8:267–78.

36. Montgomery MA, Clayton PJ, Friedhoff AJ. Psychiatric illness in Tourette syndrome patients and first-degree relatives. In: Friedhoff AJ, Chase TN (eds.). *Gilles de la Tourette syndrome.* New York: Raven Press, 1982;335–9.

37. American Psychiatric Association: *Diagnostic and Statistical Manual of Mental Disorders*, 3rd ed.

Washington, DC: American Psychiatric Association, 1980.

38. Stefl ME. Mental health needs associated with Tourette syndrome. *Am J Public Health* 1984; 74:1310–3.

39. Comings DE, Comings BG. Tourette syndrome: clinical and psychological aspects of 250 cases. *Am J Hum Genet* 1985;37:435–50.

40. Comings DE, Comings BG. A controlled study of Tourette syndrome. IV. Obsessions, compulsions, and schizoid behavior. *Am J Hum Genet* 1987; 41:782–803.

41. Kurlan R, Behr J, Medved L, et al. Familial Tourette's syndrome: report of a large pedigree and potential for linkage analysis. *Neurology* 1986; 36:772–6.

42. Jankovic J, Rohaidy H. Motor, behavioral and pharmacologic findings in Tourette's syndrome. *Can J Neurol Sci* 1987;14:541–6.

43. Erenberg G, Cruse RP, Rothner AD. The natural history of Tourette syndrome: a follow-up study. *Ann Neurol* 1987;22:383–5.

44. Robertson MM, Trimble MR, Lees AJ. The psychopathology of the Gilles de la Tourette syndrome. A phenomenological analysis. *Br J Psychiatry* 1988;152:383–90.

45. Singer HS, Rosenberg LA. Development of behavioral and emotional problems of Tourette syndrome. *Pediatr Neurol* 1989;5:41–4.

46. Grad LR, Pelcovitz D, Olson M, Matthews M, Grad GJ. Obsessive-compulsive symptomatology in children with Tourette's syndrome. *J Am Acad Child Adolesc Psychiatry* 1987;26,1:69–73.

47. Frankel M, Cummings JL, Robertson MM, Trimble MR, Hill MA, Benson DF. Obsessions and compulsions in Gilles de la Tourette syndrome. *Neurology* 1986;36:378–82.

48. Robertson MM, Gourdie A. Familial Tourette's syndrome in a large British pedigree. Associated psychopathology, severity, and potential for linkage analysis. *Br J Psychiatry* 1990;156:515–21.

49. Pauls DL, Raymond CL, Stevenson JM, Leckman JF. A family study of Gilles de la Tourette syndrome. *Hum Genet* 1991;48:154–63.

50. Flament MF, Rapoport JL, Berg CJ, et al. Clomipramine treatment of childhood compulsive disorder. *Arch Gen Psychiatry* 1985;42:977–83.

51. Leonard HL, Swedo S, Rapoport JL. Treatment of obsessive compulsive disorder with clomipramine and desipramine in children and adolescents: a double-blind crossover comparison. *Arch Gen Psychiatry* 1989b;46:1088–92.

52. Leonard HL, Lenane MC, Swedo SE, Rettew DC, Gershon ES, Rapoport JL. Tics and Tourette's syndrome: a two to seven year follow-up of 54 obsessive-compulsive children. *Am J Psychol* (in press).

Advances in Neurology, Vol. 58, edited
by T. N. Chase, A. J. Friedhoff, and
D. J. Cohen. Raven Press, Ltd.,
New York © 1992.

12

Comorbidity, Tourette Syndrome, and Anxiety Disorders

Barbara Coffey, Jean Frazier, and Stephen Chen

Tufts New England Medical Center, Boston, Massachusetts 02111

The relationship between tics, Tourette syndrome (TS), and anxiety is not well understood. Although authors often refer to the presence of "anxiety" in TS and an association between "tics and nervous tension," there has been a paucity of well-designed studies of these phenomena. The scientific literature on anxiety and tics is particularly limited. The one association that has been carefully explored in the past 5 years is the relationship between TS and obsessive–compulsive disorder (OCD). Evidence has accumulated that there is a genetic link between these disorders (1). The relationship between TS and other psychopathology in general, and non-OCD anxiety disorders in particular, continues to be intriguing but controversial.

The scientific literature contributes a historical perspective to the relationship between tics and anxiety. In Freud's *Studies in Hysteria* (1895) (2), Frau Emmy von N. had anxiety and multiple motor tics and verbal utterances, although she was not diagnosed at the time as having TS.

Zausmer (1954) (3) studied a group of 96 children with tics and anxiety; 53 were evaluated before 1952 (Group I) and 43 afterward (Group II). Of the two groups, results of 41 patients in Group I and 34 in Group II were analyzed following treatment. Anxiety symptoms of four types (sleep disturbance, tension habits, motor unrest, phobias/worries/poor concentration) were noted in over 80% of the patients. Severity of the anxiety symptoms did not always correlate with severity of tics, and the anxiety symptoms tended to persist longer than tics following therapy. Patients with mild anxiety improved with brief therapy, while those with severe anxiety responded better to longer term therapy.

Corbett et al. (4) studied 171 children and 9 adults with tics through retrospective chart review (1948–1965). One-half, or 89, had presented with tics as the primary complaint. Seventy-three (82%) of these 89 patients were available for follow-up through mail, hospital records, or interview 1–18 years after initial assessment. Thirty were available through interview, 16 were assessed through hospital records, 16 through mailed questionnaires, and 11 through other sources. Of the 30 patients assessed for psychiatric symptoms during interview at follow-up, anxiety was described as the most commonly reported symptom. Clinical observation and direct questioning yielded 17 patients with anxiety symptoms including 5 with phobias and 3 with obsessive compulsive symptoms.

The Comings team (5) studied anxiety disorders in 246 TS patients and 47 controls. In this study 16% of TS patients and none of the controls had more than three panic attacks a week. Nineteen percent of TS patients and none of the controls had phobias that interfered with their life; 26% of TS patients had more than three phobias while only 8.5% of controls had more than three. Fourteen percent of TS patients and 4.2% of controls had both panic attacks and phobias.

Robertson et al. (1988) (6) reported on 90 adults with TS who were assessed for the presence of psychopathology. Mean anxiety levels in TS patients as measured by the Mood Adjective Checklist and Crown Crisp Experiential Index were noted to be higher than those noted for normals.

The Tufts New England Medical Center Hospital Tourette's and Movement Disorder Clinic, jointly sponsored by the Departments of Pediatrics and Psychiatry, is a multidisciplinary setting for the evaluation and treatment of movement disorders in patients of all ages. Of 134 patients evaluated over the first 3 years, 84 had TS, 18 had chronic motor tics (CMT), and 22 had non-TS/CMT movement disorders. An additional ten patients had other disorders. Seventy-six percent were younger than 18 years and 24% were 18 or older. The average age was 15.3 years and the ratio of males to females was approximately 4/1 (Table 1).

Of the first 84 TS patients, 45 (53.6%) had attention deficit hyperactivity disorder (ADHD) by *Diagnostic and Statistical Manual*, 3rd ed., revised (DSM-III-R) criteria. Eleven (13.1%) had obsessive–compul-

TABLE 2. *Tourette syndrome and comorbidity*

Group/subgroup	No. (%)
TS	84
TS with ADHD	45 (54)
TS with OCD	11 (13)
TS with anxiety disorder (non-OCD)	16 (19)

For abbreviations, see footnote to Table 5.

sive disorder (OCD) or symptoms and 16 (19%) had non-OCD anxiety disorders. The subgroup of patients with non-OCD anxiety disorders included separation anxiety disorder, panic attacks/disorder, phobias, and overanxious or generalized anxiety disorder. One patient had posttraumatic stress disorder. The majority of these patients had TS of mild to moderate severity (Table 2).

Global adjustment to peers, school or work, and family was assessed. Interestingly, severity of tics, particularly motor and vocal, did not parallel severity of maladjustment or adaptation. Patients did not necessarily view their motor and vocal tics as the primary problem. Frequently, these patients were most distressed by the associated features such as the severe attention deficits, obsessions, compulsions, phobias, and separation anxiety. These symptoms were as much a target of treatment intervention as were the motor and vocal tics.

BENZODIAZEPINE TREATMENT

A pilot study of benzodiazepine treatment was conducted in 9 of the first 84 patients with anxiety disorder and Tourette syndrome. Criteria for entry included the following: (a) age above 6 years, (b) DSM-III criteria for TS, (c) IQ above 80, and (d) absence of other neurological disorders, seizures, or major medical illness. Patients were allowed to continue on a neuroleptic or other TS medication such as clonidine if they were already receiving it and showing a positive response in terms of at least some control of tics.

TABLE 1. *Demographic data on patients with movement disorders evaluated at NEMCH Tourette Syndrome (TS)/Movement Disorder Clinic*

	No. (%)
Total patients	124
TS	84
CMT (chronic motor tic)	18
Non-TS, non-CMT	22
No movement disorder	10
Age: total patients	
<18 yr	102 (76)
≥18 yr	22 (24)
Average age: 15.3	
Ratio male to female: 3.9/1	

Assessment procedures included the following:

1. A general physical and neurological exam conducted by a child neurologist
2. A psychiatric screening exam by a child psychiatrist and/or psychiatric nurse clinical specialist
3. Completion of the Tufts NEMC TS and Movement Disorder History Form, for history of tics, associated problems, and family and medical history
4. Family history obtained by direct interview of the parents or patient if adult and completion of a three-generation genogram with a particular reference to presence of tics, TS, and associated behavioral problems in close (first- or second-degree) relatives

Entry into the pilot study was possible if the patient met DSM-III or -III-R criteria for TS and one or more of the following anxiety disorders: (a) separation anxiety disorder, (b) overanxious disorder (for patients <18 years), (c) generalized anxiety disorder (for patients ≥18 years), (d) panic disorder, and (e) phobic disorder. The anxiety had to be disabling to the patient and interfere with key aspects of development such as school, family, or peer relations. Two patients also met criteria for OCD.

Patients were treated in an open, nonblind fashion by one of the two physicians involved in the study. Dosage of the benzodiazepine was individualized, and corresponded to dosages for non-TS patients with anxiety disorders. Four adults (18 years or over) and five children/adolescents were treated in this study. The children ranged in age from 8 to 13 years. Patients were assessed at baseline and 6–8 weeks after the benzodiazepine was started. Overall response was assessed through the clinician's global assessment. In addition, tics and anxiety symptoms were evaluated separately for response.

Table 3 illustrates the results of the study. Alprazolam was used in three adults and lorazepam in one; three had generalized anxiety disorders with panic attacks and/or phobias and one had panic disorder. Two of the adults were on no other TS medications. All four adults showed at least some improvement overall; one showed marked improvement in both tics and anxiety on no other medication, and the other three showed at least some improvement in tics and anxiety.

Children and adolescents were treated with lorazepam. In contrast to the adult patients, all of the children and adolescents were on other TS medications. Three of the five improved at least somewhat; all of these patients were peripubescent or postpubertal. Interestingly, one child, with severe TS and OCD, worsened on lorazepam due to disinhibition. Although his anxiety decreased, he became irritable and explosive. This was the youngest child in the study.

In general, side effects were infrequent. Four patients, including two adults and two children, had no side effects whatsoever. Mild fatigue was the most common problem; it was seen in three patients, including one adult and two children. One adult had decreased appetite and lost 10 pounds, which he attributed to improved mood. Cognitive effects were not systematically assessed; however, no decrements in school performance were spontaneously reported. Of note is the fact that five of nine patients remain on benzodiazepines at the present time.

Results of this early work suggested there may be a subgroup of TS patients with non-OCD anxiety disorders that may be responsive to anxiolytic treatment.

Thus, a series of questions arose:

1. Does *non-OCD anxiety* disorder occur in TS?
2. If so, *how frequently* does non-OCD anxiety disorder occur in TS?
3. What *kinds* of non-OCD anxiety occur in TS? Can this be specifically empirically described?
4. Are there *differences* between non-OCD anxiety in children and adults with TS?

TABLE 3. *Pilot study: benzodiazepine treatment in TS patients with anxiety disorders*

Patient	Age (yr)/sex	TS/plus	Benzodiazepine/max. dose (mg)		Other dose (mg)	
1	Adult/M	GAD/PA/PH	Alprazolam	6	None	
2	Adult/M	GAD/PA	Alprazolam	4	None	
3	Adult/M	PD	Alprazolam	2	Haloperidol	4
4	Adult/M	GAD	Lorazepam	2	Amoxapine	100
5	(13)/M	OD/OCD	Lorazepam	0.75	Clonidine	0.25
6	(8)/M	SAD/OCD	Lorazepam	3	Amoxapine	250
7	(12)/F	SAD/OD	Lorazepam	3	Pimozide	3
8	(13)/M	OD	Lorazepam	2.5	Pimozide	3
9	(13)/M	OD	Lorazepam	1	Clonidine	0.4

PA, panic attacks; PD, panic disorder; GAD, generalized anxiety disorder; OD, overanxious disorder; SAD, separation anxiety disorder; OCD, obsessive compulsive disorder; PH, phobias; AG, agoraphobia; ADAM, adjustment disorder with anxious mood; TS, Tourette syndrome.

TABLE 4. *Clinician ratings[a]*

Patient	Baseline			After benzodiazepine treatment			
	CGI[b]	Tics	Anxiety	CGI[b]	Tics	Anxiety	Side effects
1	3	3	2	2	2	1	None
2	3	2	3	1	1	0	Decreased weight
3	2	2	3	1	1	1	Mild fatigue
4	2	2	1	1	1	.5	None
5	2	2	1	2	2	.5	Fatigue
6	3	3	3	3	3	2	Disinhibition
7	2	2	2	.5	.5	1	None
8	3	3	3	0	1	0	None
9	2	2	2	1	1	1	Fatigue

[a] 0, no symptoms; .5, minimal symptoms; 1, mild symptoms; 2, moderate symptoms; 3, severe symptoms.
[b] CGI, Clinical Global Impression.

5. Can *subjective and objective ratings* of anxiety in standardized instruments assess/quantify this?

6. Do standardized rating scales *correlate* with clinical diagnosis obtained in semistructured interview using DSM-III-R criteria? Could clinical diagnosis be predicted by standardized instruments and vice versa?

7. Is there a correlation between *two standardized rating scales* that measure anxiety?

8. Does the presence of *OCD anxiety* correlate with or predict non-*OCD anxiety*? What is the pattern of coexistence or comorbidity?

COMORBIDITY OF TS AND ANXIETY

An expanded data base was developed for all new TS patients referred for evaluation and for those currently in active treatment. This included the following assessment tools (see Table 5):

1. *Tufts New England Medical Center Tourette's and Movement Disorder History Form* for detailed history and course of TS and three-generation family genogram for family history

2. *TSGS (Global Severity Scale)* with quantitative clinician's assessment of motor and vocal tic severity and index of work, school and behavior dysfunction. Global Scale Scores of 0–24 are considered mild; 25–39 are moderate; and scores over 40 are considered severe (7)

3. *OCD Inventory.* A 40-question self-report inventory adopted by Frankel from the Leyton Obsessional Inventory. Each question has a range of scores

TABLE 5. *Rating instruments*

Name	Population	Range/description	Positive score	
Hamilton Anxiety Scale	Adults	0–56	>10	
Obsessive Compulsive Inventory	Adults and children/ adolescents 40 questions; screening (Frankel/Leyton)	0–200	>70	
Revised Children's Manifest Anxiety Scale (RCMAS)	Children and adolescents 6–19 years old	37 items, 9 lie scale, 3 subscales	T > 60 (1 SD from norm)	
Spielberger State-Trait Anxiety Inventory				
Y_1–Y_2	Adults (high school →)	20–80 raw score	T > 60 or 80%	
C_1–C_2	Children/adolescents trait scale	20–60 raw score		
Tourette Syndrome Global Scale (TSGS)	Children/adolescents and adults	0–100	Mild	0–24
			Moderate	25–39
			Severe	40–59
			Extreme	60–100

from 0 to 5; total score greater than 70 is considered positive (8).

4. *Hamilton Anxiety Scale* for assessment of anxiety in adults. Clinician administered, scores range from 0 to 56 with scores greater than 10 considered positive (9)

5. *Conners Parent and Teacher Abbreviated Forms.* Quantitative assessments of signs of ADHD as rated independently by parents and teacher. Forms are administered by parents and teacher simultaneously for 5 consecutive days and averaged. Scores for each of ten individual items range from 0 to 3; average scores of 1.5 or greater are considered positive (10)

6. *Spielberger State-Trait Inventory* for adults and children. A standardized subjective rating scale that differentiates situational (state) from ongoing (trait) anxiety. It is standardized for children, adolescents, and adults (11)

7. *Revised Children's Manifest Anxiety Scale.* A 37-item subjective report in which three subscales of anxiety are reported, and a lie scale to document reliability. T scores of greater than sixty are considered positive (12)

A mailing of these rating scales and other forms was sent out in March, 1991 to patients who had not already completed them as part of their initial evaluation; this included approximately 150 patients evaluated in the TS Clinic. Approximately 75 of these patients were considered active cases. Of those active cases (75), about one-third were adults (38%) and 25% were female. Clinical diagnoses had been made at the time of initial evaluation in the clinic, and updated in charts at the time of the mailing. For most patients, the length of time between clinical diagnosis and completion of scales was within 3 months.

The active patient group is thus currently slightly older and more female than the first 84 patients described. The study was con-

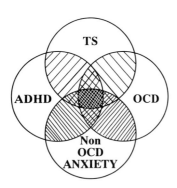

FIG. 1. Possible comorbidity in TS.

TABLE 6. *First data set, children and adolescents*

Pt.	Age (years)	Sex	TS/plus	Medications
1	5	M	OCD/ADHD	Haloperidol
2	13	M	PDD/SDD	Pimozide/cogentin
3	9	F	OCsx.	Fluphenazine
4	11	M	ADHD/SAD	Clonidine
5	13	F	—	—
6	13	F	GAD	Clonidine
7	9	F	ADHD/SAD	Haldol/DMI/clonazepam/clonidine
8	13	M	ADHD/SDD	Clonidine
9	17	F	OAD	Pimozide/lorazepam
10	17	M	CD/OCD/DYS	Pimozide/clonidine
11	5	F	OCsx./ADHD	Clonidine
12	8	M	—	
13	13	M	SDD	Clonidine
14	15	M	ADHD/ODD/SDD	Clonidine
15	14	F	ADHD/OCD/OAD	—
16	11	M	OCD	Fluphenazine
17	13	M	SDD/ADHD	Haloperidol

OCD, obsessive–compulsive disorder; SDD, specific developmental disorder; GAD, generalized anxiety disorder; PDD, pervasive developmental disorder; ADHD, Attention deficit hyperactivity disorder; SAD, separation anxiety disorder; DYS, dysthymia; CD, conduct disorder; TS, Tourette syndrome; OCsx., obsessive compulsive symptoms; ODD, oppositional defiant disorder; OAD, overanxious disorder; blank = none.

ducted on a subgroup of this currently active population of TS patients.

Twenty-five data sets are currently complete, including 17 children ranging in age from 5 to 17 years, and 8 adults; thus 68% of the sample was under 18 and 32% was 18 or over. Mean age of the children was 11.7 and the adults 27.9. Mean age of the total sample was 19.8. Fourteen (56%) were male and eleven (44%) were female.

Tables 6 and 7 illustrate the patient composition of each group.

Clinical diagnoses were established by semistructured interview using DSM-III-R criteria. Of the children and adolescents, 6 of 17 had OCD or symptoms (35%); 8 of 17 met criteria for ADHD (47%), and 5 of 17 met criteria for non-OCD anxiety disorders (29%).

Of the adults, four of eight met DSM-III-R criteria for OCD (50%); and six of eight met criteria for non-OCD anxiety (75%).

Children and Adolescents

Non-OCD Anxiety

Results of the anxiety assessment for children and adolescents are summarized in

TABLE 7. *First data set, adults*

Pt.	>18 yr	Sex	TS/plus	Medications
1	23	F	PD/DYS/AG	Haloperidol/clonazepam
2	30	M	PD/OCD/SDD	Fluoxetine
3	23	M	PA/OCD/Ph	Fluoxetine
4	27	M	PA/GAD	Alprazolam/pimozide
5	26	F	GAD/OCD/DYS	Haloperidol
6	20	F	—	—
7	39	M	—	—
8	35	F	OCD/GAD	Lorazepam

OCD, obsessive compulsive disorder; SDD, specific developmental disorder; GAD, generalized anxiety disorder; AG, agoraphobia; PD, panic disorder; DYS, dysthymia; Ph, phobia; PA, panic attack.

TABLE 8. *Non-OCD anxiety rating scale scores. First data set, children/adolescents*

Pt.	Age (years)	Sex	TS plus	RCMAS			Spielberger			
				R	%	T	C_1	C_2	%	T
1	5	M	ADHD/OCsx.	28	99	90*	58	52	75	99*
2	13	M	PDD/SDD	18	91	63*	37	41	57	75*
3	9	F	OCsx.	10	36	46	39	37	41	50
4	11	M	ADHD/SAD	18	89	62*	40	38	50	49
5	13	F	—	6	10	37	32	31	41	19
6	13	F	OAD	11	60	53	27	33	55	28
7	9	F	ADHD/SAD/OAD	16	69	55	34	35	45	38
8	13	M	ADHD/SDD	8	40	47	24	30	39	13
9	17	F	OAD/SAD	25	99	74*	46	45	70	92*
10	17	M	OCD/CD/DYS	7	49	50	41	29	37	10
11	5	F	ADHD/OCsx.	7	10	37	33	—	—	—
12	9	M	OCsx.	3	9	36	28	24	33	5
13	13	M	SDD	17	86	61*	34	43	57	77*
14	15	M	ADHD/ODD/SDD	4	20	42	32	28	9	36
15	14	F	OCsx./ADHD/OAD	21	94	66*	45	51	73	99*
16	11	M	OCD	5	24	43	26	33	31	45
17	13	M	SDD/ADHD	4	21	42	26	24	1	27

For abbreviations, see Table 6 footnote.
* = positive score.

Table 8. Five patients (nos. 4, 6, 7, 9, 15) met DSM-III-R criteria for non-OCD anxiety disorder. Six patients (nos. 1, 2, 4, 9, 13, 15) met criteria for anxiety disorder based on Revised Children's Manifest Anxiety Scale (RCMAS) scores; five (nos. 1, 2, 9, 13, 15) of those six patients had concordant positive scores for anxiety by the Spielberger Trait Scale. The one patient (no. 4) who was discordant just met DSM-III-R clinical criteria for separation anxiety disorder; the intensity would vary from interview to interview over several months.

Of the six patients with positive anxiety ratings as measured by RCMAS, four (1, 4, 9, 15) had anxiety disorders by DSM-III-R clinical criteria (OCD and non-OCD). Of these six with positive anxiety scales, three had non-OCD anxiety (nos. 4, 9, 15).

For the two patients with concordant-positive rating scales but without clinically apparent anxiety, one (no. 2) had TS plus pervasive developmental disorder and was frequently silly and socially inappropriate and acted up. He was prone to deny his anxiety on direct interview. The other patient (no. 13) had TS plus specific developmental disorder and tended to be rather quiet and inhibited in direct interview. Patients 6 and 7 met clinical criteria for non-OCD anxiety but did not achieve positive scores in the rating scales; for both patients a greater than usual interval (6 months) had elapsed between initial clinical diagnosis and time of rating, and both had been treated during this interval.

Obsessive–Compulsive Disorder

Six of 17 patients met DSM-III-R criteria for OCD or symptoms. Those who had symptoms that did not significantly interfere with daily life were classified as symptoms and not disorder. Results of the OCD Inventory are summarized in Table 9. Five of 17 patients (nos. 1, 4, 5, 15, 16) had positive OCD inventories. Three patients (nos. 1, 15, 16) of five with positive OCD inventories correlated with clinical diagnostic criteria. Only one patient (no. 10) with clinical OCD didn't score positively on the OCD Inventory. This patient showed a close to positive score (no. 60). In addition, three of the five patients with positive OCD Inventories (nos. 1, 4, 15) also had positive RCMAS scores. Two of those patients (nos. 4, 15) met DSM-III-R criteria for non-OCD anxiety disorder.

TABLE 9. *OCD anxiety rating scale scores, children/adolescents*

Pt.	Age (years)	Sex	TS plus	OCD
1	5	M	ADHD/OCsx.	126*
2	13	M	PDD/SDD	21
3	9	F	OCsx.	21
4	11	M	ADHD/SAD	71*
5	13	F	—	102*
6	13	F	OAD	30
7	9	F	ADHD/SAD/OAD	3
8	13	M	ADHD/SDD	46
9	17	F	OAD/SAD	62
10	17	M	OCD/CD/DYS	60
11	5	F	ADHD/OCsx.	(50)
12	9	M	OCsx.	35
13	13	M	SDD	37
14	15	M	ADHD/ODD/SDD	32
15	14	F	OCsx./ADHD/OAD	94*
16	11	M	OCD	81*
17	13	M	SDD/ADHD	31

For abbreviations, see footnote to Table 6.
* = positive score.

TABLE 11. *Rating scale scores, adults*

Pt.	Sex	Age (years)	TS plus	OCD
1	F	23	PD/DYS/AG	68
2	M	30	PD/OCD/SDD	135*
3	M	23	PA/OCD/Ph	100*
4	M	27	PA/GAD	45
5	F	26	GAD/OCD/DYS	120*
6	F	20	—	12
7	M	39	—	26
8	F	35	OCD/GAD	89*

For abbreviations, see Table 6 footnote.
* = positive score.

Adults

Non-OCD Anxiety

Results of the anxiety assessments of the adults are summarized in Table 10. Six patients had non-OCD anxiety by DSM-III-R clinical criteria; four of six also had OCD. Six of eight patients (nos. 1, 2, 3, 4, 5, 8) had positive Spielberger Trait Scores and four of seven Hamilton Scales were positive (nos. 1, 2, 5, 8).

Four of seven adult patients with completed data bases were concordant for anxiety as measured by Spielberger and Hamil-ton (nos. 1, 2, 5, 8). Of the six patients with positive Spielbergers, all had anxiety disorders by clinical criteria. Of the six with positive Spielbergers, all had identifiable non-OCD anxiety disorders, but four of six (nos. 2, 3, 5, 8) also had OCD. In the one patient with discordant Spielberger and Hamilton scores, the Hamilton was 8.

Obsessive–Compulsive Disorder

Table 11 summarizes results of the obsessive–compulsive inventory ratings for adults. Four patients (nos. 2, 3, 5, 8) met DSM-III-R criteria for OCD. Four of eight patients (nos. 2, 3, 5, 8) had positive OCD Inventories. All of the four positive OCD Inventories correlated with DSM-III-R clinical criteria. Of the four positive OCD Inventories, all also had positive Spielbergers. All of these patients (nos. 2, 3, 5, 8) had comorbid non-OCD anxiety.

TABLE 10. *Anxiety rating scale scores, adults*

Pt.	Sex	Age (years)	TS plus	Spielberger				Hamilton
				Y₁	Y₂	%	T	
1	F	23	PD/DYS/AG	81	65	100	80*	31*
2	M	30	PD/OCD/SDD	73	70	100	85*	26*
3	M	23	PA/OCD/Ph	53	51	94	66*	—
4	M	27	PA/GAD	34	53	95	68*	8
5	F	26	GAD/OCD/DYS	52	62	100	77*	22*
6	F	20	—	24	34	50	40	7
7	M	39	—	53	39	69	54	8
8	F	35	OCD/GAD	54	62	100	77*	16*

For abbreviations, see Table 6 footnote.
* = positive score.

TABLE 12. *Family history (1⁰ and 2⁰). first data set (N = 25)[a]*

	TS	Tics	OCD/sx	Anx	ADHD	Affective	EtoH[b]
Child/Adol.	1	9	5	5	1	2	8
Adult	1	5	2	3	1	3	1
Total (%)	2 (9)	14 (63)	7 (32)	8 (36)	2 (9)	5 (23)	9 (41)

[a] 17 (children/adolescents) − 3 (adopted) = 14 biological (including 1 DZ twin); 8 adults (including 1 DZ twin).
[b] EtoH, alcohol abuse. For other abbreviations, see Table 6 footnote.

Family History

Family history data was obtained by direct interview of the parent when the patient was a child, or the adult patient during the initial evaluation. Direct interviews of family members other than adult patients and parents of patients were not conducted.

Results are summarized on Table 12. This sample of 17 children and adolescents included 3 adopted children; thus, biological family histories were available on 14 children and adolescents including 1 dizygotic twin. Family histories were obtainable on eight adults, including one dizygotic twin. Parents and adults patients were specifically asked about the presence of TS, tics, OCD symptoms, anxiety disorders, ADHD, affective illness, and alcohol abuse in their family histories, as well as other medical or psychiatric illness.

Tics were reported as present in 63% of first- and second-degree relatives and TS in 9%. OCD or symptoms were reported in 32% and non-OCD anxiety in 36% of relatives. ADHD was reported in 9% of relatives, affective illness in 23%, and alcohol abuse in 41%.

ROLE OF ANXIETY IN TS

Preliminary responses can be made to some of the questions about the relationship between non-OCD anxiety and TS that led to this study. Potential sources of bias are the small number of patients, and the absence of controls. It is also possible that, since the proportion of females in this data set is larger than the percentage of females in the current active case group, this may bias the data toward greater proportions of anxiety. In addition, it is possible that the more anxious patients are likely to complete their forms earlier rather than later. Completion of the remaining data sets of the 75 active cases will clarify any observed trends. Another potential source of bias occurs in one of the instruments. The OCD Inventory, while used in Frankel's study with patients less than 18 years old, is not yet, to our knowledge, standardized in terms of language and items for children and adolescents. This may bias our data toward more frequent reports of obsessive–compulsive symptoms in the adults.

An additional confounding variable is the use of medication in most of the patients at the time of the study. None of these patients, to our knowledge, had developed anxiety symptoms as a *result* of their current TS medications (neuroleptics and clonidine); however, patient 1 had developed haldol-induced separation anxiety prior to his clonidine trial, and was switched off haloperidol. Some of the patients were on anxiolytics at the time of the study and, without medications, may have had even more symptoms of anxiety.

Non-OCD anxiety disorders appear to co-exist with TS in a subgroup of patients. These non-OCD anxiety disorders include overanxious disorder, generalized anxiety disorder, phobias, separation anxiety disorder, and panic disorder. There appears to be overlap or comorbidity of OCD and non-OCD anxiety disorders in this subgroup of TS patients (see Fig. 1).

In this preliminary study, non-OCD anxiety appears to occur in this subset of TS patients at a rate more frequent than that reported in the literature for normal populations; however, a comparison group of psychiatric patients or normal controls has not been studied yet. Non-OCD anxiety and OCD may be detected by standardized reliable and valid rating instruments. In the first subset of TS patients to complete standardized rating instruments of anxiety, there is a trend for both OCD and non-OCD anxiety to be reported in a greater proportion of adults than children. Preliminary data indicate that standardized measures of anxiety correspond more directly with clinical diagnosis in adults than children. Specific correlations of scales and subscale items is needed. Rates of sensitivity and specificity of these instruments must be clarified in future studies, particularly the OCD Inventory, which is not yet standardized for children. A study of anxiety in TS patients at baseline prior to medication treatment and compared to a control population is planned.

These preliminary findings, and the results of the open study of benzodiazepine treatment of anxious TS patients, point to anxiolytic treatment as a potential therapeutic avenue for some patients with TS in the future.

REFERENCES

1. Pauls DL, Raymond CL, Stevenson JM, Leckman JF. A family study of Gilles de la Tourette syndrome. *Am J Hum Genet* 1991;48:154–63.
2. Freud S. Frau Emmy Von N. In: *Studies in Hysteria. Standard Edition of Complete Psychological Works*, vol 2 (1893–96). London: Hogarth Press, 1955;48–105.
3. Zausmer DM. The treatment of tics in childhood. *Arch Dis Child* 1954;29:537–42.
4. Corbett JA, Matthews AM, Connell PH, Shapiro DA. Tics and Gilles de la Tourette's syndrome: a follow-up study. *Ann Neurol* 1969;22:383–5.
5. Comings DE, Comings BG. A controlled study of Tourette syndrome: III. Phobias and panic attacks. *Am J Hum Genet* 1987d;41:761–81.
6. Robertson MM, Trimble MR, Lees AJ. The psychopathology of the Gilles de la Tourette syndrome. *Br J Psychiatry* 1988;152:383–90.
7. Harcherik DJ, Leckman JD, Detlor J, Cohen DJ. A new instrument of clinical studies of Tourette's syndrome. *J Am Acad Child Psychiatry* 1984;23:153–60.
8. Frankel M, Cummings J, Robertson M, Trimble M, Hill MA, Benson DF. Obsessions and compulsions in Gilles de la Tourette's syndrome. *Neurology* 1986;36:378–82.
9. Hamilton M. The assessment of anxiety states by rating. *Br J Med Psychol* 1959;32:50–5.
10. Conners CK. Ratings scales for use in drug studies with children. In: *Assessment Manual (Early Clinical Drug Evaluation Unit)*. Rockville, MD: National Institute of Mental Health, 1976.
11. Spielberger CP, Gorsuch RL, Lushene RE. *Manual for the State-Trait Anxiety Inventory (Self Evaluation Questionnaire)*. Palo Alto: Consulting Psychologists Press, 1970.
12. Reynolds CR, Richard BO. What I think and feel: a revised measure of children's manifest anxiety. *J Abnorm Child Psychol* 1978;6:271–180.

Advances in Neurology, Vol. 58, edited by T. N. Chase, A. J. Friedhoff, and D. J. Cohen. Raven Press, Ltd., New York © 1992.

13

Self-Injurious Behavior and Tourette Syndrome

Mary M. Robertson

Institute of Neurology and Department of Psychiatry, The National Hospital for Neurology and Neurosurgery and Academic Department of Psychiatry, University College and Middlesex Schools of Medicine, Middlesex Hospital, London, England W1N 8AA

Self-injurious behaviour (SIB) is a dramatic but poorly studied phenomenon, and successful treatments of it remain elusive (1). SIB, which may be categorized by both the type of patient and clinical context in which it occurs, is being recognized in more and more disorders and as a result may lead to further understanding of these disorders and their pathophysiology.

In *Diagnostic and Statistical Manual*, 3rd ed., revised (DSM-III-R) impulsive SIB among nonpsychotic intellectually normal individuals is acknowledged as an impulse disorder in its own right (2); several authors have documented their patients' symptoms and suggested there is a specific and impulsive SIB syndrome (3,4). SIB is self-inflicted, nonaccidental injurious behavior, variously referred to as self-mutilation, self-injury, self-destructive behavior, and deliberate self-harm. It is seen in patients with a variety of disorders including the Tourette syndrome (TS).

In his original paper published in 1885, Georges Gilles de la Tourette (5) described two patients with TS who injured themselves. The first, a 24-year-old man, bit his tongue, and the second, a 14-year-old boy, bit his lower lip. It has also been suggested that Dr. Samuel Johnson was afflicted with TS (6); he also exhibited mild SIB.

A number of case reports of SIB in TS patients have subsequently appeared, including accounts of picking at sores (7), punching the abdomen (8), lip biting, filing of teeth (9), head banging (10), tongue or cheek biting (11), pummelling of the head and chest (12), repeated digging of the forefinger into the hollow of the cheek (13), eye damage (14,15), and tooth extraction (16). In one large study of 145 patients, hitting of self or others was the second most frequent complex movement, making up 35% of a total of 252 complex movements found in 106 patients (17).

Several studies have specifically investigated SIB in the context of TS. Moldofsky and colleagues (18) examined 15 patients with TS and found that 8 had SIB, with the patients biting their lips, cheeks, or tongues or striking themselves. Van Woert and colleagues (19) described a patient who had typical symptoms of TS, but who also had lip and tongue biting. This resulted in a questionnaire study of SIB in TS, involving members of the US Tourette's Syndrome Association (TSA). One hundred and eleven questionnaires were completed by patients or their parents, and 43% reported SIB, of which the most common were head banging, biting of the tongue, cheeks, lips and extremities, and self-hitting.

Nee and colleagues (20) investigated 50 patients with TS. Forty-eight percent had SIB; examples included repeatedly and forcefully pushing a sharpened pencil into the ear canal; pressing vigorously on the eyeball; persistent biting of the lips to the point of drawing blood and causing difficulty with healing, and placing fingers on a hot stove, resulting in painful, serious burning. Stefl (21) mailed a questionnaire to 555 members of the TSA of Ohio, and 431 questionnaires were returned completed: 34% admitted to SIB.

In an epidemiological study Caine et al. (22) found 41 TS subjects among over 142,000 pupils enrolled in the public and private schools of Monroe County, New York. Seventeen percent had SIB, including hitting themselves, touching hot objects, repetitive lip biting, scab pulling, or repetitively sticking pins under the skin.

Robertson et al. (23) studied 90 patients fulfilling DSM-III criteria (24) for TS (the first Queen Square cohort). Thirty-three percent admitted to SIB. Twenty-three types of SIB were reported and included head banging, body punching or slapping, head or face punching or slapping, body to hard object banging, poking sharp objects into body, scratching parts of body, and putting hands through window. Several other single types of SIB including putting the head through a window, pinching the face, dislodging teeth due to excess grinding, knees hitting the chin, scraping a leg against hard or rough surfaces, poking the umbilicus with the forefinger, violent head shaking, attempting to dislocate joints, purposely walking into obstacles with the intention of injury, reckless driving with the specific aim of being injured, and finally two eye injuries including pressing hard on the eyeballs and sticking a fork into the eye. Fourteen of the patients showed more than one type of SIB. Thirteen of 14 head bangers had computed tomography (CT) brain scans, and two showed cavum septum pellucidum cavities. Only these 2 scans of the total of 73 scans performed were abnormal, which is statistically significant.

Of the total group of 90 TS patients, 54 adults completed psychiatric rating scales including the Hostility and Direction of Hostility Questionnaire (HDHQ), and the Leyton Obsessional Inventory (LOI). Results indicated that TS patients had much higher scores than those of normal control populations and that SIB was significantly related to all aspects of hostility and obsessionality in that the SIB patients obtained significantly higher scores on the rating scales than did those subjects without such behavior. In addition, patients with SIB were more anxious and neurotic and had more general psychopathology. In the total group, SIB was significantly related to the cumulative number of motor tics and tics of the legs (that is, the severity of TS motor symptoms), as well as a past psychiatric history. No relationships with other demographic or motor or other aspects of TS emerged.

Patients who had a history of head banging gave a history of having had to attend a special school, being aggressive towards other people, and experiencing a greater number of motor tics than those without head banging. There were no other differences between those with or without head banging with regard to demographic data or TS symptoms. Patients who had exhibited head banging rated themselves as significantly more psychiatrically disturbed, with depression, criticism of others, and neurosis (23).

Robertson et al. (23) also reported four TS patients who had severe SIB resulting in serious eye injuries. They were all refractory to treatment, and one died as a result of severe head shaking, while a second required psychosurgery. Investigators interested in eye mutilation (25,26) conclude that it is invariably associated with psychosis such as schizophrenia. None of the TS patients were psychotic, but the last two mentioned were disturbed, aggressive, and maladjusted individuals.

In the second Queen Square cohort (Robertson et al., in preparation) there are now over 150 patients. Preliminary results on the first 50 of the second cohort indicate that 44% exhibit SIB. Examples of SIB in the second cohort were similar to those in the first cohort, and, once again, head banging was the most common. Hitting themselves and lacerating were followed by various biting maneuvers.

Robertson and Gourdie (27) studied a British pedigree spanning six generations and multiply affected by TS. Of 122 members identified, 85 were individually examined and 50 diagnosed as cases; 48 of these were mild. Cases could be distinguished from noncases on the basis of various behaviors including obsessive–compulsive features and SIB. Although severity of TS symptomatology was related to SIB in one large cohort (23), the finding of SIB in both pedigree (27) and epidemiological (22) settings suggests that SIB may be found in TS of all severities.

How frequent is SIB? In psychiatric populations, several studies have addressed the question of the frequency of SIB. In inpatients of a large psychiatric hospital screened for SIB, between 1 and 4% were found to have such behavior (28,29). On the other hand, SIB among mentally retarded people occurs in between 7 and 9% of such individuals, increasing to 14–19% of institutionalized retarded children, and occurring in as many as 40% of institutionalized psychotic children (30). The incidence of SIB in the TS cohorts is therefore much more than in psychiatric populations, being found in 17% (22), 33% (23), 34% (21), 44% (Robertson et al., in preparation), 48% (20), and 53% (18) of TS individuals.

In which other conditions is SIB found, and what are the links, if any, between those disorders and TS? It is worth noting that some types of SIB are found in normal children and may be accepted as ritual in some cultures (see ref. 23), but in most cases SIB is associated with psychopathology.

SIB resulting in mutilative lesions has been described in a variety of conditions, but perhaps the paradigm is the Lesch-Nyhan syndrome (LNS). LNS is an X-linked recessive disorder of purine metabolism, with increased excretion of urinary uric acid; it is characterized by hypotonia, spasticity, chorea, athetosis, dystonia, dysarthria, dysphagia, mental and growth retardation, aggression, and SIB (31–33). Decreased homovanillic acid (34) and 3-methoxy-4-hydroxy phenylethylene (35) in the cerebrospinal fluid (CSF), indicating reduced dopamine and norepinephrine turnover, and high 5-hydroxyindoleacetic acid (35) in the CSF, suggesting increased serotonin turnover in LNS, have been reported, providing support for the theory of abnormal central monoamine metabolism in LNS. Since the early descriptions many authors have reported on SIB in the syndrome; most authors note the lip and finger biting, tongue biting, poking of the eyes and nose, and head banging (36–38).

An early report of raised serum uric acid in three patients with TS (39), a suggestion of similarities between the SIB encountered in LNS and that in TS (40), and the control by L-5-hydroxytryptophan of SIB in LNS (41) and in one patient with TS (42) set the stage for studies into purine and serotonin metabolism in TS. Then Moldofsky et al. (18) found normal serum uric acid and adenine and hypoxanthine guanine phosphoribosyl transferase (HPGT) in a group of 15 TS patients, of whom over half had SIB. Van Woert et al. (42) confirmed normal activity of HPGT in fresh erythrocytes in TS patients compared with controls, but reported less stable HGPT from the hemolysates of patients compared with controls; in addition, the hemolysates of TS patients that had the most abnormal patterns were from cases exhibiting severe SIB. The authors therefore suggested that TS was a disorder of purine metabolism. Robertson et al. (23) measured serum uric acid in a few TS patients, and in all, the values were normal.

What about the relationship between SIB and intelligence? In the only study of TS patients with SIB that addressed this issue, there was no association with intelligence. The mean full-scale IQ of that cohort of patients on the Wechsler Intelligence Scales was 99.7 (23). However, the type of SIB seen in that cohort was similar to the type seen in mentally retarded populations, which can include face rubbing resulting in broken facial skin and bleeding, head-to-object banging, hand-to-hand punching and slapping, face scratching, skin picking, hand biting, lip chewing, and eye gouging (43).

de Lange syndrome is characterized by retarded mental and physical development and distinctive clinical features (44). SIB in the syndrome takes the form of self-scratching, biting the fingers, lips, shoulders, and knees (45), and head and face slapping (44) and occurs in approximately half of the population with the condition (43). None of the patients in the Robertson et al. (23) cohort had this diagnosis.

An important diagnosis to consider when SIB occurs in the setting of a movement disorder is neuroacanthocytosis. The disorder usually presents in the third or fourth decade with orofacial dyskinesias, jerking of limbs, (46–48), vocalizations (48), and echolalia (49). SIB including tongue, lip, and cheek biting are characteristic (47,48). Approximately 5–15% of the erythrocytes are acanthocytes (46), and the diagnosis is confirmed by the characteristic blood picture. None of the TS patients in one large cohort received a diagnosis of neuroacanthocytosis (23).

The type of SIB seen in psychotic disorders such as schizophrenia may be violent and severe, including cutting the radial artery or jugular vein (50), although wrist cutting is more common (51,52). Other examples of SIB committed by schizophrenic patients include autocastration (53), severe eye injuries (25), limb amputation (54,55), glossectomy (56), and gun shot wounds (57). These injuries are bizarre and relatively uncommon. It is of particular interest therefore that four patients in one TS cohort with severe SIB injured their eyes seriously (23).

The majority of injuries in schizophrenia seem to be in response to psychotic experiences (25,58,59). Others have suggested that a severe disturbance in body image seen in some 15% of these patients accounts for such destructive acts (60). A previous act of SIB is also a significant risk factor (57). Psychosis in TS patients is rare (23); more specifically, no patients were psychotic in one large TS cohort in which SIB was common (23).

Some patients with depressive illness also exhibit SIB; examples are wrist cutting (61), head banging (62), dermatitis artefacta (63), lacerations of the body (29), and eye injuries (25). Of importance is that all adult patients in one cohort filled in the Beck Depression Inventory (64) and the depression subscale of the Crown Crisp Experimental Index (CCEI) (65), and no associations were found between depression scores on either rating scale and the presence of SIB (23).

SIB, regarded as "secondary self-stimulation," such as head banging, self-biting, and self-scratching, is common in children with autism (66). Studies indicate that SIB occurs in 37–40% of such children, with biting of the wrist or back of hand and head banging being the most common forms (67,68). No patients in one study had a diagnosis of autism (23).

SIB can also occur in people with personality disorders; this is most commonly manifest as wrist slashing (51) or cutting of various parts of the body including forearms, antecubital fossi, abdomen, and thighs (69). One review of the literature (59) found that 7% of male genital self-mutilators had character or personality disorders. Of the patients with personality disorders who slash their wrists, it has been suggested that those with the "borderline personality" are particularly liable to this form of behavior (70,71). Self-inflected eye injuries are rare outside the setting of psychosis, but there has been one case report of a young man who repeatedly injured his left eye and who was diagnosed as suffering from borderline personality disorder (72). Of importance is that adult patients in one study completed the Borderline Syndrome Index (BSI) (73), a rating scale measuring aspects of the Borderline Personality but also reflecting general psychopathology, and those with SIB had significantly higher scores on this particular rating scale (23). However, wrist cutting was not typical of the patients' SIB.

Some sensory neuropathies may lead to unintentional oral SIB, including trigeminal sensory loss from any cause (and, for example, syringobulbia and anesthesia dolorosa) and the congenital sensory neuropathy associated with anhidrosis (74). None of the patients in the Robertson et al. (23) cohort had any evidence of a sensory neuropathy.

Are any types of personality overrepresented in SIB populations, and, more specifically, what is the relationship between SIB and obsessionality? Several studies have assessed aspects of psychopathology in people who injure themselves using standardized rating scales and have found that obsessionality and SIB are significantly associated (75,76). It seems that obsessionality is associated with SIB although it should be noted that scores of obsessionality as measured by rating scales are increased by depression (77). The results of the Robertson et al. (23) study compare favorably with these previous investigations, in that significantly and specifically high obsessionality and BSI scores were found associated with SIB.

Are there any biochemical links between SIB and TS? A biochemical basis for TS has been suggested for some time; an abnormal dopaminergic system has received the most support (78). It is of interest therefore that the dopaminergic system has not only been implicated in LNS (35,79) but, in addition, several studies and reviews have implicated dopaminergic systems in SIB in both animal experiments and human studies (80,81).

Neuropeptides are receiving much attention in the SIB literature. Thus Corbett and Campbell (82), in a review, note possible links between endorphins and the clinical observations in stereotyped SIB. Others (30) have also suggested the role of β-endorphins in SIB. Coid and colleagues (83) found significantly raised mean plasma metenkephalin concentration in patients with diagnosis of borderline personality disorder who habitually mutilated themselves compared with healthy controls. In addition, the raised levels of metenkephalin appeared to depend on the severity of the patients' symptoms and how recently they had mutilated themselves. Recently Sandman et al. (84) showed that patients with SIB and stereotypy have elevated β-endorphin plasma levels when compared with controls. Of interest in this context is that patients with SIB have been successfully treated with naloxone (85) and naltrexone (86–90), suggesting that they play a role in the regulation of the endorphin/enkephalin systems and can alter SIB. It is of special interest therefore that recently both overactivity (91) and underactivity (92) of the endogenous opioid system have been postulated in TS. In addition, a post mortem examination of a patient with TS showed total absence of dynorphin-like (DLI) positive woolly fibers in the dorsal part of the external segment of the globus pallidus; the ventral pallidum exhibited very few DLI-positive fibers (93). This study has been replicated and similar results found in six TS patients (Haber et al., *this volume*). Recently Kurlan et al. (94) reported a significant reduction in TS tic symptomatology in a controlled trial of naloxone and placebo, confirming previous case reports (95,96). Moreover, several recent case reports of exacerbation of TS symptomatology by jogging (97) and withdrawal of chronic opiate have been documented (98–100), giving further support to an involvement with the opioid system in TS. Clearly, further investigations into the role of neuropeptides and the basal ganglia in TS and SIB need to be carried out.

Interestingly, abnormalities of serotonin have been demonstrated in both TS (78) and the LNS (101). In the light of animal data that have tied aggression to serotonergic depletion and the suggestion that SIB represents a form of aggression, Mizuno and Yugari (41) successfully gave 5-hydroxy-tryptophan to four patients with SIB and LNS. Subsequent studies have shown fewer successes. Another basis for consideration of a role for the serotonin system in SIB is the similarity of some of its features to OCD. Three early clinical studies specifically reported severe eye SIB occurring in patients with OCD (76,102,103). In addition, compulsive lip biting in a person of normal intelligence has been reported (104). Yaryura-Tobias and Neziroglu (105) have, moreover, suggested a compulsive mutilatory syndrome that possibly involved the hypothalamus/serotonergic pathways. Finally, two studies have reported successful treatment of OC SIB with specific serotonin re-uptake inhibitors (SSRIs) such as clomipramine (103) and fluoxetine (106).

The term trichotillomania was first used by Hallopeau in 1889 (107) for a form of alopecia resulting from excessive hair pulling. It may represent a form of SIB. In DSM-III-R (2), this is recognized as a disorder of impulse control; in this context there are a few reports of successful treatment with lithium (108). However, recently, Swedo and colleagues (109) suggested that it is related to OCD and there are now several reports of successful treatment with SSRIs such as clomipramine and fluoxetine (109–112). It has also been documented that there is an increase of OCD individuals in the families of trichotillomania patients (113). With respect to SIB there have been reports of comorbidity of trichotillomania and SIB (114).

Onychophagia or severe nail biting has recently been shown in a single case study by Lipinski (115) and a double-blind study by Leonard and colleagues (116) to respond to clomipramine in a manner that was significantly superior to desipramine. It is suggested that onychophagia may well be related to the OCD spectrum of disorders, which in some cases may include SIB.

What about head banging? CT scans were performed on 73 of 90 TS patients, and the only two abnormalities encountered were cavum septum pellucidum cavities, both in subjects who exhibited repetitive head banging; both abnormal scans, in addition, showed ventricular enlargement (23). Cavum septum pellucidum cavities are normal occurrences during fetal life (117); at autopsy in a large series of premature births, the incidence was found to be 100% (18). The incidence decreases with age, and has been reported to be 12% in children aged 6 months to 16 years (118) and 30% in children of unspecified age (119), but in adults the incidence has been found in only 0.9% of adult autopsies (119) and between 0.1% and 0.4% in pneumoencephalographic (PEG) studies on adult neurological patients (120,121).

Looking at one TS population (23), the incidence is much greater. Considering first the whole cohort of 73 who had CT scans, the incidence was 2.7%, and when only head bangers were taken into account the incidence rose to 15%. This may well be relevant in the light of the literature on the incidence of such cavities in boxers, in whom it has been found to occur in between 56% and 60% in PEG and air-encephalographic studies (122–124); in postmortem studies the incidence was as high as 92% (125). In addition, some 3% of nonboxers in the same investigation had a penetrated cavum, compared with 77% of the boxers, however, in 5 of the 15 nonboxers showing the abnormality, there was firm clinical or neuropathological evidence of past head injury (125). It would appear therefore that the anomaly can be either developmental (a normal occurrence) or acquired (due to head injury); in TS patients the latter mechanism is proposed (23).

In conclusion, SIB is encountered in various clinical syndromes, including that of TS. Taking the review of the literature into account, it would appear that this behavior in TS may well be underreported to date, and those studies addressing the subject specifically have found a substantial proportion of patients exhibiting such behavior. Results suggest that SIB may occur in mild cases, but in general, the clinical correlates of SIB are the severity of TS symptoms and psychopathology. In particular, TS patients with SIB and self-mutilators in other studies scored high on obsessionality and hostility measures. This is particularly interesting in that Robertson et al. (126) have also found links between obsessionality and hostility in TS patients and copro- and echophenomena, core features of TS. Thus, SIB may be part of the TS syndrome in some patients, which would fit in with the suggestion that TS may be a heterogeneous condition (127).

The types of SIB in TS patients were, in general, not typical of those encountered in patients with LNS, neuroanthocytosis, schizophrenia, depression, or personality disorders, but were nonspecific and somewhat similar to that found in mentally retarded populations. Of importance is that the patients were of average intelligence. There are, however, difficulties in comparing the results of studies investigating SIB, as there are many varying definitions of such behavior (43,61,128). In the majority of cases of deliberate SIB the more usual means is ingestion of toxic substances or drugs (129); such cases were not included in most studies.

Some TS patients incur serious injuries, perhaps exemplified by blindness, cavum septum pellucidum cavities, and death. With regard to a biochemical substrate for TS patients with SIB, the most likely areas appear to be the dopaminergic, serotonergic, and endogenous opioid systems.

Another question to be addressed is that of management. As SIB in one cohort (23) was related to both severity of TS symptoms and psychopathology, one possibility is that with treatment of the manifestations of TS or the psychopathology, the SIB may itself disappear and/or reduce as a consequence. Based on biochemical abnormalities that have been suggested in both TS and SIB, it is suggested that the following agents be used alone or in combination; dopamine antagonists, SSRIs, clonidine, naloxone and naltrexone, lithium, and β-blockers (130,131).

Finally, there is a new class of psychoactive compounds with uniquely selective behavioral effects in animals and putative value in the management of pathologically destructive behavior in humans. Eltoprazine is one of the serenics (132), which reduces aggression and may be of use in the SIB of TS. Finally, psychosurgery must be borne in mind as a life-saving treatment in the most severe cases.

REFERENCES

1. Winchel RM, Stanley MS. Self-injurious behavior: a review of the behavior and biology of self-mutilation. *Am J Psychiatry* 1991;148:306–17.
2. American Psychiatric Association *Diagnostic and Statistical Manual of Mental Disorders*, 3rd ed, revised. Washington, DC: American Psychiatric Association, 1984.
3. Siomopoulos V. Repeated self-cutting: an impulse neurosis. *Am J Psychother* 1974;28:85–94.
4. Pattison EM, Kahan J. The deliberate self-harm syndrome. *Am J Psychiatry* 1983;140:867–72.
5. Gilles de la Tourette G. Etude sur une affection nerveuse caracterisée par de l'incoordination motrice accompagnée d'echolalie et de copralalie. *Arch Neurol* 1885;9:19–42, 158–200.
6. Murray TJ. Dr Samuel Johnson's movement disorders. *Br Med J* 1979;1:1610–4.
7. Ascher E. Psychodynamic consideration in Gilles de la Tourette's disease (maladie des tics): with a report of five cases and discussion of the literature. *Am J Psychiatry* 1948;105:267–76.
8. Dunlap JR. A case of Gilles de la Tourette's disease (maladie des tics): a study of the intrafamily dynamics. *J Nerv Ment Dis* 1960;130:340–4.
9. Bruun RD. Gilles de la Tourette's syndrome: an overview of clinical experience. *J Am Acad Child Psychiatry* 1984;23:126–33.
10. Eldridge R, Sweet R, Lake CR, Shapiro AK. Gilles de la Tourette's syndrome: clinical, genetic, psychologic, and biochemical aspects in 21 selected families. *Neurology* 1977;27:115–24.
11. Ericksson B, Persson T. Gilles de la Tourette's syndrome, two cases with an organic brain injury. *Br J Psychiatry* 1969;115:315–53.
12. Morphew JA, Sim M. Gilles de la Tourette's syndrome: a clinical and psychopathological study. *Br J Med Psychol* 1969;42:293–301.
13. Obendorf CP. Simple tic mechanism. *JAMA* 1916;16:99–100.
14. Eisenhauer GL, Woody RC. Self-mutilation and Tourette's disorder. *J Child Neurol* 1987;2:265–7.
15. Stevens JR, Blachly PH. Successful treatment of

the maladie des tics. *Am J Dis Child* 1969; 112:541–5.

16. Woody RC, Eisenhauer G. Tooth extraction as a form of self-mutilation in Tourette's disorder. *South Med J* 1986;79:1466.

17. Shapiro AK, Shapiro E, Bruun RD, Sweet RD. *Gilles de la Tourette syndrome,* New York: Raven Press, 1978.

18. Moldofsky H, Tullis C, Lamon R. Multiple tics syndrome (Gilles de la Tourette's syndrome). *J Nerv Ment Dis* 1974;15:282–92.

19. Van Woert MH, Jutkowitz R, Rosenbaum D, Bowers MB. Gilles de la Tourette's syndrome: biochemical approaches. In: Yahr MD, ed. *The basal ganglia.* New York: Raven Press, 1976; 459–465.

20. Nee LE, Caine ED, Polinsky RJ, Eldridge R, Ebert MH. Gilles de la Toureete syndrome: clinical and family study of 50 cases. *Ann Neurol* 1980;7:41–9.

21. Stefl ME. Mental health needs associated with Tourette syndrome. *Am J Public Health* 1984; 74:1310–3.

22. Caine ED, McBride MC, Chiverton P, Bamford KA, Rediess S, Shiao J. Tourette syndrome in Monroe County School Children. *Neurology* 1988;38:472–5.

23. Robertson MM, Trimble MR, Lees AJ. Self-injurious behaviour and the Gilles de la Tourette syndrome: a clinical study and review of the literature. *Psychol Med* 1989;19:611–25.

24. American Psychiatric Association. *Diagnostic and Statistical Manual of Mental Disorders,* 3rd ed. Washington, DC: American Psychiatric Association, 1980.

25. Crowder JE, Gross CA, Heiser JF, Crowder AM. Self-mutilation of the eye. *J Clin Psychiatry* 1979; 40:420–3.

26. Rogers T, Pullen I. Self-inflicted eye injuries. *Br J Psychiatry* 1987;151:691–3.

27. Robertson MM, Gourdie A. Familial Tourette's syndrome in a large British pedigree. Associated psychopathology, severity, and potential for linkage analysis. *Br J Psychiatry* 1990;156:515–21.

28. Hassanyeh F. Self-mutilation in psychiatric inpatients. *Br J Clin Soc Psychiatry* 1985;3:27–9.

29. Phillips RH, Alkan M. Recurrent self-mutilation. *Psychiatr Q.* 1961;35:424–31.

30. Barron J, Sandman CA. Relationship of sedative-hypnotic response to self-injurious behaviour and stereotypy by mentally retarded clients. *Am J Ment Def* 1983;88:177–86.

31. Lesch M, Nyhan WL. A familial disorder of uric acid metabolism and central nervous system function. *Am J Med* 1964;36:561–70.

32. Nyhan WL. Introduction—clinical and genetic features. *Fed Proc* 1968;27:1027–33.

33. Nyhan WL. Clinical features of the Lesch-Nyhan syndrome. *Arch Intern Med* 1972;130:186–92.

34. Silverstein F, Smith CB, Johnston MV. Effect of clonidine on platelet alpha 2-adrenoreceptors and plasma norepinephrine of children with Tourette syndrome. *Dev Med Child Neurol* 1985;27:793–9.

35. Jankovic J, Caskey TC, Stout T, Butler IJ. Lesch-Nyhan syndrome: a study of motor behavior and cerebrospinal fluid neurotransmitters. *Ann Neurol* 1988;23:466–9.

36. Gilbert S, Spellacy E, Watts RWE. Problems in the behavioural treatment of self-injury in the Lesch-Nyhan syndrome. *Dev Med Child Neurol* 1979;21:795–800.

37. Scully C. The orofacial manifestations of the Lesch-Nyhan syndrome. *Int J Oral Surg* (Copenh) 1981;10:380–3.

38. Christie R, Bay C, Kaufman IA, Bakay B, Borden M, Nyhan WL. Lesch-Nyhan disease: clinical experience with nineteen patients. *Dev Med Child Neurol* 1982;24:293–306.

39. Pfeiffer CC, Ilie Y, Nichols RE, Sugerman AA. The serum urate level reflects degree of stress. *J Clin Pharmacol* 1969;9:384–92.

40. Seegmiller JE. In discussion, Hoefnagel D (1968). Seminars on Lesch-Nyhan syndrome, summary. *Fed Proc* 1968;27:1046.

41. Mizuno T, Yugari Y. Prophylactic effect of L-5-hydroxytryptophan on self-mutilation in the Lesch-Nyhan syndrome. *Neuropediatrics* 1975; 6:13–23.

42. Van Woert MH, Yip LC, Ballis ME. Purine phosphoribosyltransferases in Gilles de la Tourette syndrome. *N Engl J Med* 1977;297:210–2.

43. Murphy GH. Self-injurious behaviour in the mentally handicapped: an up-date. *Newsletter Assoc Child Psychol Psychiatry* 1985;7:2–11.

44. Singh NN, Pulman RM. Self-injury in the De Lange syndrome. *J Ment Defic Res* 1978; 23:79–81.

45. Fadel KM. Self-Mutilation. *Psychiatry in Practice* 1985;4:19–26.

46. Bird TD, Cederbaum S, Valpey RW, Stahl WL. Familial degeneration of the basal ganglia with acanthocytosis: a clinical, neuropathological, and neurochemical study. *Ann Neurol* 1978;3:253–8.

47. Sakai T, Mawatari S, Twashita H, Goto I, Kuroiwa Y. Choreoacanthocytosis. Clues to clinical diagnosis. *Arch Neurol* 1981;38:335–8.

48. Critchley EMR, Clark DB, Wikler A. Acanthocytosis and neurological disorder without betalipoproteinemia. *Arch Neurol* 1968;18:134–40.

49. Kito S, Itoga E, Hiroshige Y, Matsumoto N, Miwa S. A pedigree of amyotrophic chorea with acanthocytosis. *Arch Neurol* 1980;37:514–17.

50. Pao PN. The syndrome of delicate self-cutting. *Br J Med Psychol* 1969;42:195–206.

51. Graff H, Mallin R. The syndrome of the wrist cutter. *Am J Psychiatry* 1967;124:36–42.

52. Rosenthal RJ, Rinzler C, Wallsh R, Klausner E. Wrist-cutting syndrome: the meaning of a gesture. *Am J Psychiatry* 1972;128:47–52.

53. Blacker KH, Wong N. Four cases of autocastration. *Arch Gen Psychiatry* 1963;8:169–76.

54. Hall DC, Lawson BZ, Wilson LG. Command hallucinations and self-amputation of the penis and hand during a first psychotic break. *J Clin Psychiatry* 1981;42:322–4.

55. Arons BS. Self-mutilation: clinical examples and reflections. *Am J Psychother* 1981;35:550–7.

56. Tenzer JA, Orozco H. Traumatic glossectomy. *Oral Surg* 1970;30:182–4.

57. Sweeny S, Karizamecnik K. Predictors of self-

mutilation in patients with schizophrenia. *Am J Psychiatry*, 1981;138:1086–9.

58. Kushner AW. Two cases of auto-castration due to religious delusions. *Br J Med Psychol* 1967; 40:293–8.

59. Greilsheimer H, Groves JE. Male genital self-mutilation. *Arch Gen Psychiatry* 1979;36:441–6.

60. Lukianowicz N. Body image disturbances in psychiatric disorders. *Br J Psychiatry* 1967; 113:31–47.

61. Bennun I. Depression and hostility in self-mutilation. *Suicide Life Threat Behav* 1983;13:71–84.

62. Yesavage JA. Direct and indirect hostility and self-destructive behaviour by hospitalized depressives. *Acta Psychiatr Scand* 1983;68:345–50.

63. Fabisch W. Psychiatric aspects of dermatitis artefacta. *Br J Dermatol* 1980;102:29–34.

64. Beck AT, Ward CH, Mendelson M, Mock J, Erbaugh J. An inventory for measuring depression. *Arch Gen Psychiatry* 1961;4:561–71.

65. Crown S, Crisp AH. A short clinical diagnostic self-rating scale for psychoneurotic patients: the Middlesex Hospital Questionnaire (MHQ). *Br J Psychiatry* 1966;122:917–23.

66. Zealley AK. Mental handicap. In: Kendell RE, Zealley AK eds. *Companion to psychiatric studies*, 3rd ed. Edinburgh: Churchill Livingstone, 1983.

67. Green AH. Self-mutilation in schizophrenic children. *Arch Gen Psychiatry* 1967;17:234–44.

68. Rutter M, Lockyer I. A five to fifteen year follow-up study of infantile psychosis. Description of sample. *Br J Psychiatry* 1967;113:1169–82.

69. Bach-Y-Rita G. Habitual violence and self-mutilation. *Am J Psychiatry* 1974;131:1018–20.

70. Rinzler C, Shapiro DA. Wrist-cutting and suicide. *J Mt Sinai Hospital* 1968;25:485–88.

71. Schaffer CB, Carroll J, Abramowitz SI. Self-mutilation and the borderline personality. *J Nerv Ment Dis* 1982;170:468–73.

72. Griffin N, Webb MGT, Parker RR. A case of self-inflicted eye injuries. *J Nerv Ment Dis* 1982; 170:53–6.

73. Conte HR, Plutchik R, Karsau TB, Jerrett IL. A self-report borderline scale: discriminative validity and preliminary norms. *J Nerv Ment Dis* 1980; 168:428–35.

74. Vassella F, Emrich HM, Krause-Ruppert R, Aufdermaur F, Tonz O. Congenital sensory neuropathy with anhidrosis. *Arch Dis Child* 1968; 43:124–130.

75. McKerracher DW, Loughnane T, Watson RA. Self-mutilation in female psychopaths. *Br J Psychiatry* 1968;114:829–32.

76. Gardner AR, Gardner AJ. Self-mutilation, obsessionality and narcissism. *Br J Psychiatry* 1975; 127:127–32.

77. Kendell RE, Discipio WJ. Eysenck personality scores of patients with depressive illness. *Br J Psychiatry* 1968;114:767–70.

78. Caine ED. Gilles de la Tourette's syndrome: a review of clinical and research studies and consideration of future directions for investigation. *Arch Neurol* 1985;42:393–7.

79. Casas-Bruge M, Almenar C, Grau IM, Jane J,

Herrerea-Marschitz M, Ungerstedt V. Dopaminergic receptor supersensitivity in self-mutilatory behaviour of Lesch-Nyhlan disease. *Lancet* 1985; i:991.

80. Jones IH, Barraclough BM. Auto-mutilation in animals and its relevance to self-injury in man. *Acta Psychiatr Scand* 1978;58:40–7.

81. Breese GR, Criswell HE, Duncan GE, Mueller RA. Deopamine deficiency in self-injurious behavior. *Psychopharmacol Bull* 1989;25:353–7.

82. Corbett JA, Campbell HJ. Causes of severe self-injurious behaviour. In: Mittler P, De Jong JM eds. *Mental retardation new horizons, vol II, Biomedical aspects*. Baltimore: University Park Press, 1980;285–92.

83. Coid JM, Allolio B, Rees LH. Raised plasma met-enkephalin in patients who habitually mutilate themselves. *Lancet* 1983;ii:545–6.

84. Sandman CA, Barron JL, Chicz-DeMet A, DeMet EM. Plasma β-endorphin levels in patients with self-injurious behavior and stereotypy. *Am J Ment Retard* 1990;95:84–92.

85. Richardson HS, Zaleski WA. Naloxone and self-mutilation. *Biol Psychiatry* 1983;18:99–101.

86. Herman BH, Hammock MK, Arthur-Smith A, Egan J, Chatoor I, Werner A, Zelnik N. Naltrexone decreases self-injurious behaviour. *Ann Neurol* 1987;22:550–2.

87. Herman BH, Hammock MK, Egan J, Arthur-Smith A, Chatoor I, Werner A. Role for opioid peptides in self-injurious behavior: dissociation from autonomic nervous system functioning. *Dev Pharmacol Ther* 1989;12:81–9.

88. Barrett RP, Feinstein C, Hole WT. Effects of nalonone and naltrexone on self-injury: a double-blind, placebo-controlled analysis. *Am J Ment Retard* 1989;93:644–51.

89. Smith KC, Pittelkow MR. Naltrexone for neurotic excoriations. *J Am Acad Dermatol* 1989; 20:860–1.

90. Sandman CA, Barron JL, Colman H. An orally administered opiate blocker, naltrexone, attenuates self-injurious behavior. *Am J Ment Retard* 1990;95:93–102.

91. Sandyk R. The effects of naloxone in Tourette's syndrome. *Ann Neurol* 1985;18:367–8.

92. Gillman MA, Sandyk R. Opiatergic and dopaminergic function and Lesch-Nyhan syndrome. *Am J Psychiatry* 1985;142:1226.

93. Haber SN, Kowall NW, Vonsattel JP, et al. Gilles de la Tourette's syndrome: a postmortem neuropathological and immunohistochemical study. *J Neurol Sci* 1986;75:225–41.

94. Kurlan R, Majumdar L, Deeley C, Mudholkar GS, Plumb S, Como PG. A controlled trial of propoxyphene and naltrexone in Tourette's syndrome. *Ann Neurol* 1991 (in press).

95. Sandyk R, Iacono RP, Allender J. Naloxone ameliorates compulsive touching behavior and tics in Tourette's syndrome. *Ann Neurol* 1986;20:437.

96. Gadoth N, Gordon CR, Streifler J. Naloxone in Gilles de la Tourette's syndrome. *Ann Neurol* 1987;21:415.

97. Jacome DE. Jogging and Tourette's disorder. *Am J Psychiatry* 1987;144:1100–1.

98. Lichter D, Manjumdar L, Kurlan R. Opiate withdrawal un-masks Tourette's syndrome. *Clin Neuropharmacol* 1988;11:559–64.

99. Walters AS, Hening W, Chokroverty S. Letter to the editor. *Move Dis* 1990;5:89–91.

100. Bruun R, Kurlan R. Opiate therapy and self-harming behavior in Tourette's syndrome. *Move Dis* 1991;6:184–5.

101. Lloyd KG, Hornykiewics O, Davidson L, et al. Biochemical evidence of dysfunction of brain neurotransmitters in the Lesch-Nyhan Syndrome. *N Engl J Med* 1981;305:1106–11.

102. Stinnett JL, Hollender MH. Compulsive self-mutilation. *J Nerv Ment Dis* 1970;150:371–5.

103. Primeau F, Fontaine R. Obsessive disorder with self-mutilation: a subgroup responsive to pharmacotherapy. *Can J Psychiatry* 1987;32:699–701.

104. Lyon LS. A behavioural treatment of compulsive lip-biting. *J Behav Ther Exp Psychiatry* 1982; 14:275–6.

105. Yaryur-Tobias JA, Neziroglu F. Compulsions, aggression, and self-mutilation: a hypothalamic disorder? *Orthomolec Psychiatry* 1978;7:114–7.

106. Hollander E, Fay M, Cohen B, Campeas R, Gorman JM, Liebowitz MR. Serotonergic and noradrenergic sensitivity in obsessive-compulsive disorder: behavioral findings. *Am J Psychiatry* 1988; 148:1015–7.

107. Hallopeau M. Alopecie par grattage (trichomanie ou trichotillomanie) *Ann Dermatol Venereol* 1889;10:440–1.

108. Christenson GA, Popkin MK, Mackenzie TB, Realmuto GM. Lithium treatment of chronic hair pulling. *J Clin Psychiatry* 1991;52:116–20.

109. Swedo SE, Leonard HL, Rapoport JL, Lenane MC, Goldberger EL, Cheslow DL. A double-blind comparison of clomipramine and desipramine in the treatment of trichotillomania (hair pulling). *N Engl J Med* 1989;321:497–501.

110. George MA, Brewerton TD, Cochrane C. Trichotillomania (hair pulling). *N Engl J Med* 1990; 322:470–1.

111. Dech B, Budow L. The use of fluoxetine in an adolescent with Prader-Willi syndrome. *J Am Acad Child Adolesc Psychiatry* 1991;30:298–302.

112. Pollard CA, Ibe O, Krojanker DN, Kitchen AD, Bronson SS, Flynn TM. Clomipramine treatment of trichotillomania: a follow-up report on four cases. *J Clin Psychiatry* 1991;52:128–30.

113. Swedo SE, Rapoport JL. Annotation: trichotillomania. *J Child Psychol Psychiatry* 1991;32:401–9.

114. Adam BS, Kashani JH. Trichotillomania in children and adolescents: review of literature and case report. *Child Psychiatry Hum Dev* 1990; 20:159–68.

115. Lipinski JF. Clomipramine in the treatment of self-mutilating behaviors. *N Engl J Med* 1991; 324:1441.

116. Leonard HL, Lenane MC, Swedo SE, Rettew DC, Rapoport JL. A double-blind comparison of clomipramine and desipramine treatment of severe onychophagia (nail biting). *Arch Gen Psychiatry* 1991;(in press).

117. Bruyn GW. Agenesis septi pellucidi, cavum septi pellucidi, cavum vergae and cavum veli interpositi. In: Vinken PJ, Bruyn GW eds. *Handbook of clinical neurology,* vol 30. Amsterdam; Elsevier/North Holland, 1977;299–336.

118. Shaw CM, Alvord EC. Cava septi pellucidi et vergae: their normal and pathological states. *Brain* 1969;92:213–24.

119. Swenson O. Nature and occurrence of the cavum septi pellucidi. *Arch Pathol* 1944;37:119–23.

120. Bonitz G. Sur klinische-diagnostischen Bedeutung des Erweiterten und Kommunizierenden cavum septi pellucidi. *Nervenarzt* 1969;40:121–8.

121. Sonntag I, Nadjmi M, Lajosi F, Fuchs G. Anlage-bedingte Gehirnanomalien der Mittellinie. *Nervenarzt* 1971;42:531–9.

122. Isherwood I, Mawdsley C, Ferguson FR. Pneumoencephalographic changes in boxers. *Acta Radiol* 1966;5:654–61.

123. Johnson J. Organic psychosyndromes due to boxing. *Br J Psychiatry* 1969;115:45–53.

124. Spillane JD. Five boxers. *Br Med J* 1962; ii:1205–10.

125. Corsellis JAN, Bruton CJ, Freeman-Browne D. The aftermath of boxing. *Psychol Med* 1973; 3:270–303.

126. Robertson MM, Trimble MR, Lees AJ. The psychopathology of the Gilles de la Tourette syndrome: a phenomenological analysis. *Br J Psychiatry* 1988;152:383–90.

127. Lees AJ, Robertson MM, Trimble MR, Murray NMF. A clinical study of Gilles de la Tourette syndrome in the United Kingdom. *J Neurol Neurosurg Psychiatry* 1984;47:1–8.

128. Corbett J. Aversion for the treatment of self-injurious behaviour. *J Ment Defic Res* 1975;19:79–95.

129. Odejide AO, Williams AO, Ohaeri JU, Ikusean BA. The epidemiology of deliberate self-harm. The Ibadan experience. *Br J Psychiatry* 1986; 149:734–7.

130. Luchins DJ, Dojka D. Lithium and propranolol in aggression and self-injurious behaviour in the mentally retarded. *Psychopharmacol Bull* 1989; 25:372–5.

131. Ruedrich SL, Grush L, Wilson J. Beta adrenergic blocking medications for aggressive or self-injurious mentally retarded persons. *Am J Ment Retard* 1990;95:110–9.

132. Olivier B, Mos J, Hartog J, Rasmussen D. Serenics. *DN P* 1990;3:261–71.

Advances in Neurology, Vol. 58, edited by T. N. Chase, A. J. Friedhoff, and D. J. Cohen. Raven Press, Ltd., New York © 1992.

14

Immunohistochemical Study of the Basal Ganglia in Normal and Parkinsonian Monkeys

Brigitte Lavoie, Pierre-Yves Côté, and André Parent

Centre de Recherche en Neurobiologie, Université Laval et Hôpital de l'Enfant-Jésus, Québec, Canada G1J 1Z4

Tourette syndrome (TS) is a neuropsychiatric disorder characterized by multiform motor and phonic tics and complex behavioral symptoms. The neurochemical mechanisms and anatomical substrates involved in this syndrome have not been clearly identified (1). The dopaminergic system is believed to be involved in the genesis of tic disorders. Indeed, dopamine blocking agents, such as haloperidol, can improve the clinical symptoms in numerous TS patients. Furthermore, serotonin (5-hydroxytryptamine) has been implicated in obsessive–compulsive disorder (OCD), which is a clinical entity closely associated with TS in a large proportion of patients (2). In recent studies abnormal interactions between neurochemical systems such as dopaminergic–noradrenergic systems and dopaminergic–cholinergic systems have been proposed (1). In addition to classical neurotransmitters, opiate peptides have also been involved in TS. For example, dynorphin was shown to be significantly reduced in the pallidum of patients with severe forms of TS (3).

The basal ganglia are a possible neuroanatomical substrate for TS. Indeed, this set of structures integrates information from most cortical areas and some subcortical structures and plays an important role in the control of psychomotor behaviors. Although very little information is presently available on the neurotransmitters involved in TS, there exists a wealth of information on neurotransmitter alterations at the basal ganglia level in other diseases, such as parkinsonism, which also involves motor as well as cognitive deficits (4). Furthermore, an excellent animal model of Parkinson's disease was recently developed in primates (5–7). Valuable information on the interactions between various chemospecific systems in the basal ganglia can be derived from studies of this animal model, and these data may help our understanding of the possible involvement of the basal ganglia in the pathophysiology of TS. In the present study the organization and integrity of some chemospecific systems implicated in basal ganglia function in primates will be analyzed in both normal and parkinsonian monkeys. Each system will be studied with a particular attention to the functional territories imposed upon the basal ganglia by the massive cortical input.

The results of the present immunohistochemical study were obtained from brains of normal squirrel monkeys (*Saimiri sciureus*) and cynomolgus monkeys (*Macaca fascicularis*). Tyrosine hydroxylase-, substance P-, enkephalin-, serotonin- and the calcium-binding protein calbindin D-28k-immunoreactive neuronal profiles were revealed according to the standard immunohistochemical procedures of Sternberger (8) and/or Hsu et al. (9), as described in detail elsewhere (10). The antibodies were purchased from Immunonuclear Corp. Inc. (Stillwater, MN), except the monoclonal calbindin antibody, which was generously donated by Dr. M.R. Celio (11). No significant species differences between *Saimiri* and *Macaca* were noted in regard to the distribution of the various neuromediators mentioned above. In addition to normal monkeys, eight cynomolgus monkeys were rendered parkinsonian following the systemic administration of 1-methyl-4-phenyl-1,2,3,6-tetrahydropyridin (MPTP) (total dose: 4–8 mg/kg), a neurotoxin that selectively affects the mesostriatal dopaminergic pathway. All MPTP-treated monkeys were severely bradykinetic at the moment of sacrifice.

NORMAL MONKEYS

The striatum is the major receptive component of the basal ganglia. This structure receives its major inputs from the cerebral cortex, the thalamus, and the brainstem. The cortex gives rise to the most massive striatal afferent, and almost all cortical areas contribute to this projection. These areas topographically project to the striatum and impose on this structure a functional organization that is maintained throughout the basal ganglia. The cortical inputs define three distinct striatal territories: the sensorimotor (SM), the associative (AS), and the limbic (LI) territories (Fig. 1A–C) (12). The SM striatal territory includes most of the postcommissural putamen, the lateral border of the body of the caudate nucleus and of the precommissural putamen, and the dorsolateral rim of the head of the caudate nucleus (Fig. 1A–C).

The SM striatal territory receives its inputs from neurons of both sensory and motor cortical areas. The AS striatal territory comprises most of the head of the caudate nucleus, the precommissural putamen, except its lateral border, and the medial border of the body of the caudate nucleus and of the postcommissural putamen (Fig. 1A–C). The AS striatal territory is afferented by neurons of the associative areas of the prefrontal, temporal, parietal, and anterior cingulate cortices. The LI striatal territory, which includes the ventral region of both caudate nucleus and putamen, the nucleus accumbens, and the deep layers of the olfactory tubercle, receives its afferents from limbic and paralimbic cortical areas and from the amygdala and hippocampus (Fig. 1A–C). These three functional territories are not sharply defined and form a continuum in the striatum, as exemplified by the significant degree of overlap that exists between the territories.

In addition to this topographical organization, studies of the distribution of the neuromediators and receptors reveal another level of organization in the striatum. For instance, small acetylcholinesterase-poor zones, termed striosomes, are found embedded in a large and homogeneous acetylcholinesterase-rich matrix (13). Several chemospecific systems, including neurons containing calbindin, as well as afferent and efferent striatal projections, are known to respect this compartmental organization (14). In both macaques and squirrel monkeys, the striosomal organization is particularly obvious in the AS striatal territory (10, 15,16).

The thalamostriatal projection is the second most prominent afferent to the striatum. The posterior intralaminar nuclei, the centromedian and parafascicular nuclei, give rise to a dense striatal projection that is topographically organized. Neurons of the centromedian nucleus mainly project to the SM striatal territory, whereas those of the parafascicular nucleus arborize in both AS and LI striatal territories (17).

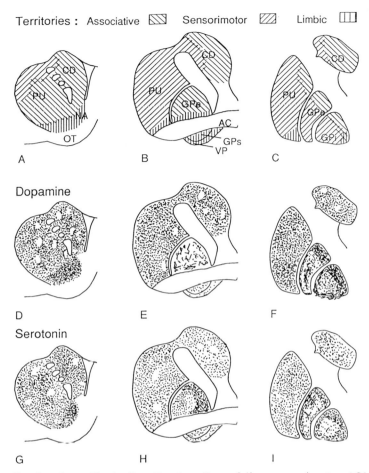

FIG. 1. Schematic drawings illustrating the location of the sensorimotor (*SM*), associative (*AS*), and limbic (*LI*) territories **(A–C)** and the distribution of dopaminergic **(D–F)** and serotoninergic **(G–I)** fibers and axon terminals at three rostrocaudal levels of the basal ganglia in normal monkeys. The dopamine innervation was revealed by using an antibody raised against the enzyme tyrosine hydroxylase, whereas serotonin was visualized with an antibody raised directly against 5-hydroxytryptamine. *AC*, anterior commissure; *CD*, caudate nucleus; *GPe*, external pallidal segment; *GPi*, internal pallidal segment; *GPs*, subcommissural pallidum; *VP*, ventral pallidum; *NA*, nucleus accumbens; *OT*, olfactory tubercle; *PU*, putamen.

The striatum also receives an important input from the dopaminergic neurons of the ventral mesencephalon. These neurons are mainly located in the substantia nigra pars compacta (SNc) and the ventral tegmental area (VTA) (see Fig. 3B). In the SNc, the dopaminergic cells, as revealed by tyrosine hydroxylase immunohistochemistry, are particularly abundant in the ventral tier of the structure, where they form several columns impinging deeply in the underlying substantia nigra pars reticulata (SNr). The dopaminergic neurons lying in the dorsal tier of SNc form a thin layer scattered along the rostrocaudal extent of the structure. The neurons of this cellular layer merge imperceptibly with the neurons of the VTA. The dopaminergic fibers reaching the striatum are thin and varicose and arborize extensively in the entire structure, with an increasing dorsoventral gradient. They form dense terminal fields composed of a multitude of isolated varicosities (Fig. 1D–F) (16). In regard to the functional territories, the densest dopaminergic innervation is found in the LI striatal territory. The AS and SM striatal territories receive a dense dopaminergic innervation, and fibers are more heterogeneously distributed in the AS than in the SM striatal territories. In the AS striatal territory, some dopamine-poor zones are observed (Fig. 1D) (16) that closely correspond to the striosomal compartment as revealed by acetylcholinesterase staining on adjacent sections (18).

Another striatal monoaminergic afferent arises from the serotoninergic neurons of the dorsal raphe nucleus. It is mainly composed of varicose fibers, among which are scattered numerous isolated varicosities. The topographic distribution of the serotoninergic profiles is comparable, although less abundant, to that of the dopaminergic profiles (Fig. 1G–I) (15). Analysis of the distinct striatal territories shows that the serotoninergic fibers are more numerous in the LI striatal territory than in the AS and SM striatal territories. The serotoninergic innervation is uniform in the SM striatal territory and heterogeneous in the AS striatal territory. In the latter territory, some zones of poor serotonin immunostaining are observed (Fig. 1G). These serotonin-poor zones, which are in register with the dopamine-poor zones, could correspond to the striosomes (15).

The striatum mainly projects to the pallidum and the SNr (12). The present study focuses on the pallidum, where the striatopallidal projections remain segregated according to the striatal territories defined above. In the substantia nigra, the striatal afferents appear less well segregated than in the pallidum (Haber, *this volume*). The striatopallidal fibers originating in the AS territory arborize in the rostral external pallidal segment and more caudally in the dorsal third of both the internal and the external pallidal segment. Those arising from the SM striatal territory terminate in the ventral two-thirds of the postcommissural pallidum

(Fig. 1B,C) (12). Neurons located in the LI striatal territory innervate the medial tip of the internal pallidal segment and the ventral pallidal complex (19), comprising the ventral pallidum proper and subcommissural pallidum as defined by Russchen et al. (20). Results obtained from anatomical and immunohistochemical studies suggest that distinct neuronal subpopulations of striatal neurons project to each pallidal segment (12,21–23). Virtually all striatopallidal neurons use γ-aminobutyric acid (GABA) as a neurotransmitter (22). However, most striatopallidal neurons projecting to the external pallidal segment coexpress enkephalin, whereas those arborizing in the internal pallidal segment contain substance P (Fig. 2C,D). The enkephalin-containing fibers are more abundant in the small dorsal AS pallidal territory than in the larger ventral SM pallidal territory of the external pallidum (Fig. 2C). The substance P-containing fibers arborize uniformly in both SM and AS pallidal territories of the internal pallidum

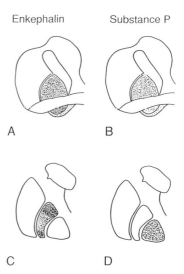

Enkephalin   Substance P

A   B

C   D

FIG. 2. Schematic drawings illustrating the terminal arborization of enkephalin- **(A,C)** and substance P- **(B,D)** immunoreactive striatopallidal fibers at rostral **(A,B)** and caudal **(C,D)** levels of the pallidal complex in normal monkeys. For the localization of structures, see abbreviations in Figure 1B,C.

(Fig. 2D). In the LI pallidal territory, enkephalin-containing fibers arborize profusely in the subcommissural pallidum, whereas substance P-containing fibers terminate particularly in the ventral pallidum (Fig. 2A,B) (20). Also worth noting is the presence of both enkephalin- and substance P-containing fibers in the rostral region of the external pallidal segment, which is considered an AS pallidal territory (Fig. 2A,B).

The pallidum also receives extrastriatal inputs from the dopaminergic and serotoninergic neurons of the brainstem (15,16,24). These two afferents arborize more profusely in the internal pallidal segment than in the external pallidal segment (Fig. 1F,I). The dopaminergic pallidal innervation consists of thin varicose fibers and a few isolated varicosities, whereas the serotoninergic pallidal innervation is characterized by numerous isolated varicosities. The dopaminergic fibers are abundant in the entire medial part of the internal pallidal segment, particularly its medial tip. In the lateral part of internal pallidal segment and in the entire external pallidal segment, dopaminergic fibers are more abundant dorsally (Fig. 1F). The serotoninergic innervation is dense in the medial tip of the internal pallidal segment and along the internal medullary lamina. In both the internal and the external pallidal segment, isolated serotoninergic varicosities are more abundant dorsally (Fig. 1I). In respect to pallidal territories, both dopaminergic and serotoninergic innervations are more abundant in the AS pallidal territory than in the SM pallidal territory. In the LI pallidal territory, the serotoninergic innervation is homogeneously dense compared with the dopaminergic innervation, which is light in the ventral pallidal complex and dense in the medial tip of the internal pallidal segment.

PARKINSONIAN MONKEYS

In parkinsonian monkeys, a massive dopaminergic cell loss is observed at midbrain levels. The neurons located in the ventral tier of SNc are more severely affected than those in the dorsal tier of the SNc and in the VTA. Most of the spared dopaminergic neurons in both SNc and VTA contain calbindin (25). At striatal levels, the dopaminergic innervation is severely reduced, the dorsolateral part of the striatum being more affected than the ventromedial part (Fig. 3A). In regard to the striatal territories, the most severe loss of the dopaminergic innervation is observed in the SM striatal territory, whereas the LI striatal territory is the least affected. The dopaminergic denervation of the AS striatal territory is generally moderate but varies greatly from one animal to the other (25). The dopaminergic deple-

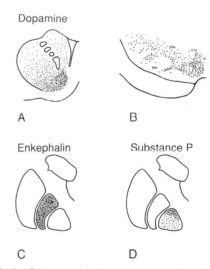

FIG. 3. Schematic drawings showing the decrease of dopaminergic innervation at striatal level in a parkinsonian monkey **(A)**. The distribution of dopaminergic neurons within the middle third of the substantia nigra—ventral tegmental area (*SN-VTA*) complex is illustrated in **B**. The neurons of the ventral tier of the SN pars compacta (*SNc*) are those that degenerate massively in parkinsonian monkeys, whereas the neurons of the dorsal tier are spared and contain calbindin (see ref. 25 for a detailed description). The increase of enkephalin immunoreactivity and decrease of substance P immunoreactivity in the SM pallidal territory of parkinsonian monkeys are shown in **C** and **D**, respectively. *SNr*, SN pars reticulata; *III*, oculomotor nerve root fibers.

tion affects the intensity of peptide immuno-staining in the striatopallidal neurons differentially according to the various striatal territories. The striatopallidal neurons containing enkephalin, and whose cell bodies are located in the SM striatal territory, show an increase of immunostaining, which is particularly obvious in the SM pallidal territory of the external pallidal segment (Fig. 3C). In contrast, striatopallidal neurons containing substance P, and whose cell bodies are located in the SM striatal territory, display a decrease of immunostaining, which is particularly evident in the SM pallidal territory of the internal pallidal segment (Fig. 3D). At variance with findings in the SM territory, enkephalin immunostaining is decreased and substance P immunostaining is increased in the LI territory; these changes are particularly evident in the ventral striatum (25). In the AS territory, enkephalin and substance P immunostaining is highly heterogeneous and varies from one animal to the other. For example, cell patches displaying intense enkephalin or substance P immunostaining are noted in the AS striatal territory of some animals. In other animals, zones containing cells weakly stained for substance P and corresponding to striosomes, as visualized on adjacent sections stained for calbindin, are rimmed by a dense substance P-immunostained neuropil in the AS striatal territory (25). These results reveal that in parkinsonian monkeys dopamine depletion has differential effects on the expression of peptides according to the various functional territories.

The analysis of the monoaminergic innervation of the basal ganglia in normal monkeys, in the light of the three major functional territories defined by the cortical input, has revealed that both dopaminergic and serotoninergic innervations are denser in the LI striatal territory than in the SM and AS striatal territories. The monoaminergic innervation is uniform in the SM striatal territory, whereas it is particularly heterogeneous in the AS striatal territory, where some zones of poor immunostaining are observed.

In regard to peptide immunostaining, the present findings reveal that enkephalin and substance P are not uniformly distributed at pallidal levels. The enkephalin-positive fibers arborize in the external pallidal segment where they are more abundant in the AS pallidal territory than in the SM pallidal territory. The substance P-positive fibers are distributed homogeneously in the internal pallidal segment. In the LI pallidal territory, enkephalin-positive fibers arborize mostly in the subcommissural pallidum, whereas substance P-positive fibers are mainly confined to the ventral pallidum.

Our results in parkinsonian monkeys confirm that midbrain dopaminergic neurons do not form a homogeneous population. The neurons of the ventral tier of the SNc degenerate massively, whereas those of the dorsal tier of the SNc and of the VTA are much less affected. Most of the spared neurons were found to contain calbindin, a finding suggesting that this calcium-binding protein may protect the dopaminergic neurons from the neurotoxic effect of MPTP. Our data also show that dopamine inhibits the expression of enkephalin and stimulates that of substance P in striatopallidal neurons located in the SM territory, whereas the inverse situation occurs in the LI territory. This finding indicates that the influence of dopamine on peptide expression may be different in the three major functional territories of the basal ganglia.

The results of the present immunohistochemical study reveal that the monoaminergic innervation of the basal ganglia in primates is highly heterogeneous. The distribution of the monoaminergic fibers varies according to the three functional territories imposed upon the basal ganglia by the massive cortical input. Data obtained in parkinsonian monkeys suggest that dopamine differentially influences the expression of peptides in these three territories. Therefore, the existence of the three major functional territories in the basal ganglia should be taken into account when interpreting the results of neuromediator changes encountered in various neuropathologies, including TS.

REFERENCES

1. Leckman JF, Walkup JT, Riddle MA, Towbin KE, Cohen DJ. Tic disorders. In: Meltzer HY, ed. *Psychopharmacology: the third generation of progress*. New York: Raven Press, 1987;1239–46.
2. Goodman WK, McDougle CJ, Price LH, Riddle MA, Pauls DL, Leckman JF. Beyond the serotonin hypothesis: a role for dopamine in some forms of obsessive compulsive disorders? *J Clin Psychiatry* 1990;51:36–58.
3. Haber SN, Kowall NW, Vonsattel JP, Bird ED, Richardson Jr EP. Gilles de la Tourette's syndrome. A postmortem neuropathological and immunohistochemical study. *J Neurol Sci* 1986; 75:225–41.
4. Agid Y, Javoy-Agid F, Ruberg M. Biochemistry of neurotransmitters in Parkinson's disease. In: Marsden CD, Fahn S, eds. *Movement disorders*, vol 2. London: Butterworths, 1987;166–230.
5. German DC, Dubach M, Askari S, Speciale SG, Bowden DM. 1-methyl-4-phenyl-1,2,3,6-tetrahydropyridine-induced parkinsonian syndrome in *Macaca fascicularis*: which midbrain dopaminergic neurons are lost? *Neuroscience* 1988; 24:161–74.
6. Langston JW, Forno LS, Rebert CS, Irwin I. Selective nigral toxicity after systemic administration of 1-methyl-4-phenyl-1,2,5,6-tetrahydropyridine (MPTP) in the squirrel monkey. *Brain Res* 1984; 292:390–4.
7. Schneider JS, Yuwiler A, Markham CH. A selective loss of subpopulations of the ventral mesencephalic dopaminergic neurons in the monkey following exposure to MPTP. *Brain Res* 1987; 411:144–50.
8. Sternberger LA. *Immunocytochemistry*. New York: John Wiley & Sons, 1986.
9. Hsu SM, Raine L, Fanger H. Use of avidin-biotin-peroxidase complex (ABC) in immunoperoxidase techniques: a comparison between ABC and unlabelled antibody (PAP) procedures. *J Histochem Cytochem* 1981;21:557–80.
10. Côté PY, Sadikot AF, Parent A. Complementary distribution of calbindin D-28k and parvalbumin in the basal forebrain and midbrain of the squirrel monkey. *Eur J Neurosci* 1991; 3:1316–29.
11. Celio MR. Calbindin D-28k and parvalbumin in the rat nervous system. *Neuroscience* 1990;35: 375–475.
12. Parent A. Extrinsic connections of the basal ganglia. *Trends in Neurosci* 1990;13:254–8.
13. Graybiel AM, Ragsdale Jr CW. Histochemically distinct compartments in the striatum of human, monkey, and cat demonstrated by acetylcholinesterase staining. *Proc Natl Acad Sci USA* 1978; 75:5723–6.
14. Graybiel AM. Neurotransmitters and neuromodulators in the basal ganglia. *Trends Neurosci* 1990; 13:244–54.
15. Lavoie B, Parent A. Immunohistochemical study of the serotoninergic innervation of the basal ganglia in the squirrel monkey. *J Comp Neurol* 1990; 299:1–16.
16. Lavoie B, Smith Y, Parent A. Dopaminergic innervation of the basal ganglia in the squirrel monkey as revealed by tyrosine hydroxylase immunohistochemistry. *J Comp Neurol* 1989;288:36–52.
17. Sadikot AF, Parent A, François C. The centremédian and parafascicular nucleus project respectively to the sensorimotor and associative-limbic striatal territories in the squirrel monkey. *Brain Res* 1990;510:161–5.
18. Graybiel AM, Hirsch EC, Agid Y. Differences in tyrosine hydroxylase-like immunoreactivity characterize the mesostriatal innervation of the striosomes and extrastriosomal matrix at maturity. *Proc Natl Acad Sci USA* 1987;84:303–7.
19. Haber SN, Lynd E, Klein C, Groenewegen HJ. Topographic organization of the ventral striatal efferents projections in the rhesus monkey: an anterograde tracing study. *J Comp Neurol* 1990; 293:282–8.
20. Russchen FT, Amaral DG, Price JL. The afferent connections of the substantia innominata in the monkey, *Macaca fascicularis*. J Comp Neurol 1985; 242:1–27.
21. Haber SN, Elde R. Correlation between met-enkephalin and substance P immunoreactivity in the primate globus pallidus. *Neuroscience* 1981; 6:1291 7.
22. Parent A. *Comparative neurobiology of the basal ganglia*. New York: John Wiley & Sons, 1986.
23. Parent A, Smith Y, Filion M, Dumas J. Distinct afferents to internal and external pallidal segments in the squirrel monkey. *Neurosci Lett* 1989; 96:140–4.
24. Parent A, Lavoie B, Smith Y, Bédard PJ. The dopaminergic nigropallidal projection in primates: distinct cellular origin and relative sparing in MPTP-treated monkeys. In: Streifler MB, Korczyn AD, Melamed E, Youdim MBH, eds. *Advances in neurology*, vol 53. New York: Raven Press, 1990;111–6.
25. Lavoie B, Parent A, Bédard PJ. Effects of dopamine denervation on striatal peptide expression in parkinsonian monkeys. *Can J Neurol Sci* 1991; 18:373–5.
26. Smith Y, Parent A. Differential connections of caudate nucleus and putamen in the squirrel monkey (*Saimiri sciureus*). *Neuroscience* 1986;18: 347–71.

Advances in Neurology, Vol. 58, edited by T. N. Chase, A. J. Friedhoff, and D. J. Cohen. Raven Press, Ltd., New York © 1992.

15

Postmortem Analysis of Subcortical Monoamines and Amino Acids in Tourette Syndrome

George M. Anderson, Eleanor S. Pollak, Diptendu Chatterjee, James F. Leckman, Mark A. Riddle, and Donald J. Cohen

Child Study Center, Yale University School of Medicine, New Haven, Connecticut 06510

Tourette's syndrome (TS), a childhood-onset, familial neuropsychiatric disorder, has been well described for over a century. In typical cases, tics first emerge in the early school age years and the natural history is characterized by many years or a lifetime of multiple, ever-changing motor and phonic tics that wax and wane in severity (1–7). The neuroanatomical substrate for TS is not known. Based on the nature of symptoms, hypotheses have been offered about the possible role of the basal ganglia (8–12) and the cortex (12,13) and midbrain (14) regions. There is a relative paucity of neuroanatomical studies (15–26). These have included neuropathological examinations (15), histochemical study of neuropeptides in basal ganglia regions (16), positron emission tomography (PET) scan studies using [^{18}F]fluorodeoxyglucose (17,18) and dopaminergic ligands (19–21), a study of regional cerebral blood flow (22), x-ray tomographic (23,24) and magnetic resonance imaging studies (25), and a study of receptors and enzymes in cortical tissues (26).

Various neurochemical systems have been implicated in the pathogenesis of TS, base primarily on drug response and studies of cerebrospinal fluid (CSF) and other fluids

in patients with TS. However, no specific neurochemical defect has been identified. A role for dopamine is suggested by the amelioration of tics by neuroleptics such as haloperidol and pimozide (27,28), exacerbation of symptomatology by stimulant medications such as amphetamine and methylphenidate (29,30), the findings of reduced group mean concentrations of the dopamine metabolite (homovanillic acid) in the cerebrospinal fluid of patients (31), and the importance of dopamine pathways in mediating motor behavior (32). The noradrenergic system has been suggested to play a modifying role in symptom expression because of the therapeutic effects of clonidine (33,34), an agent that reduces noradrenergic activity, and the role of noradrenergic pathways in the modulation of arousal (35). Serotonin (5-HT) has been implicated on the basis of reduced levels of the major 5-HT metabolite, 5-hydroxyindoleacetic acid (5-HIAA), in the CSF of TS patients (31,36), as well as the neurophysiological role of 5-HT in the modulation of arousal and sensory gating (37). The finding of reduced dynorphin in the lateral globus pallidus in one postmortem brain specimen (16), the observation of elevated CSF dynorphin in a small group of

TS patients (36), and neuroendocrine studies (38,39) have suggested a role for opioids. Acetylcholine (40) and γ-aminobutyric acid (GABA) (41,42) have been discussed due to their importance in basal ganglia functioning and because of pharmacological response. A lack of neuroanatomic resolution and problems of peripheral contamination have limited most previous neurochemical studies.

In this report, we present analyses of monoamines, monoamine metabolites, amino acids, and related compounds in subcortical regions of postmortem brains of four individuals with the diagnosis of TS. Because of the limited number of brains and other methodological issues, this report must be considered preliminary. However, this study represents a detailed examination of subcortical neurotransmitters in TS and provides hypotheses that can guide future research.

Brains of four patients, diagnosed before death as having TS, were obtained at autopsy. One-half of each brain was frozen and stored at −70°C to 80°C. Information regarding age, sex, behavior, medication history, cause of death, and postmortem interval is given below. A total of 22 control brains were used to assemble the two to six age-, sex-, and postmortem interval-matched control specimens for each region of interest.

CASE REPORTS

Patient 1 was a 57-year-old man with eye blinking, facial tics, phonic tics and coprolalia, self-injurious behavior, self-inflicted blindness, and obsessive–compulsive disorder (OCD). The age of onset was 5 years and there was no family history of TS, tics, or OCD. The patient was heavily medicated (haloperidol 10 mg three times daily, cogentin 1 mg each day, lasix 40 mg intravenously three times daily, depo/provera 1g intramuscularly once a month) and died of complications of renal cell carcinoma after long-term hospitalization. The postmortem interval was 6 hours.

Patient 2 was a 38-year-old man with vocalizations, eye blinking, and tics of the head, face, neck, shoulders, legs, and arms. The age of onset was 7 years, there was a history of drug abuse (alcohol and diazepam) and depression, and the family history was unknown. Medications included haloperidol (5 mg daily) and clozapine (9 mg twice daily). The cause of death was suicide by carbon monoxide inhalation, and the postmortem interval was 5.5 hours.

Patient 3 was an 86-year-old man with vocalizations, lip smacking, and facial and head tics. The age of onset was unknown. There was a family history of tics in a sister and in grandchildren. There was no history of medication being administered for tics or related problems. Death was caused by a stroke (brainstem). The postmortem interval was 9.0 hours.

Patient 4 was 57-year-old woman who had been diagnosed as having TS; however, behavioral and medication history were unavailable. There was a family history of OCD in the patient's daughter and of motor and phonic tics in grandsons. Death resulted from complications of carcinoma of the bowel. The postmortem interval was 9.0 hours.

Brain dissections were carried out at the Brain Tissue Resource Center in Belmont, MA. Partially thawed half-brains were sliced coronally (1-cm slabs) and areas dissected on a −10°C cold plate (43,44). Individual areas were then cut into small pieces weighing approximately 10–50 mg each. After thorough mixing, aliquots of 100–250 mg each were separated and stored at −70°C. TS and control aliquots were coded to ensure blinded sample preparation and analyses. Regions dissected included the caudate (CAU), accumbens (ACC), globus pallidus (medial, MGP; lateral, LGP), substantia nigra (reticulata, SNR; compacta, SNC), subthalamus (STN), thalamus (ventral-lateral, TVL; anteriomedial, TAM; anteriolateral, TAL; dorsal-medial, TDM), olfactory tubercle (OLF), and amygdala (AMY).

Tissue was homogenized by sonication in 10/1 v/w of homogenation solution consisting of pH 6.5, 0.1 M MOPS buffer, 0.1% disodium EDTA, 0.1% ascorbic acid, and the internal standards 3,4-dihydrobenzylamine (DHBA, 200 ng/ml), α-methylnorepinephrine (MNE, 200 ng/ml), N-methylserotonin (NMS, 200 ng/ml), homoserine (HS, 50 μg/ml), and δ-aminovaleric acid (DAVA, 50 μg/ml). After sonication on ice (setting 3, model 185 Sonifier, Branson Sonic Power, Bridgeport, CT, three cycles of 10 seconds on/10 seconds off; occasionally additional cycles were required to completely disrupt tissue), the homogenate was split. One portion was immediately frozen ($-70°C$) as homogenate while the other was first deproteinated by adding 10% by volume of 3.2 M $HClO_4$ and centrifuging (5 minutes, 12,000 xg).

Tryptophan (TRP), 5-HT, 5-HIAA, and homovanillic acid (HVA) were determined, after direct injection of centrifuged supernate, by high-performance liquid chromatography (HPLC) with serial fluorometric and electrochemical detection (45,46). Norepinephrine (NE), dopamine (DA), and 3,4-dihydroxyphenylacetic acid (DOPAC) were determined, after alumina extraction, by HPLC with electrochemical detection (47,48). The amino acids glutamate (GLU), glycine (GLY), aspartate (ASP), γ-aminobutyric acid (GABA), serine (SER), glutamine (GLN), and taurine (TAU) were analyzed by HPLC-fluorometry following precolumn derivatization with orthophthaldehyde (OPT) (49). Tyrosine hydroxylase (TH) was determined by measuring ^3H_2O released from [3,5-^{3}H]tyrosine (50). Choline acetyltransferase activity was assayed by extracting and measuring labeled acetylcholine produced from ^{14}C-labeled acetyl CoA (51). Protein was determined by the method of Bradford (52). All analyses within a particular area were performed on the same day. Results were expressed as weight of analyte per gram wet weight of tissue or per milligram of protein. Statistical analyses were performed using two-tailed Student's t tests and Wilcoxon Sum Rank (WSR) tests.

In both the TS and control groups coefficients of variation were typically about 50%. In most cases, the distribution of values observed in the two groups were highly overlapping. In several areas, suggestive group mean differences were seen for particular analytes.

SEROTONIN AND RELATED COMPOUNDS

In general, the group means and within-group distributions observed for 5-HT, its precursor TRP, and its major metabolite 5-HIAA, were fairly similar in the two groups (Table 1). However, when the group means for the three compounds are inspected across all the subcortical areas, one sees a distinct trend to lower values in the TS group. Lower TS group means were observed for 5-HT in 11 of the 13 areas, and for TRP and 5-HIAA in 12 of 13 areas examined. On the average, group means ($\pm$ SD) for 5-HT, TRP, and 5-HIAA in the TS patients were 79.5 $\pm$ 22.8%, 72 $\pm$ 16%, and 74 $\pm$ 13%, respectively, of those seen for control subjects. An ANOVA of concentration by group showed significant main effects of group for TRP and 5-HIAA (p = 0.17, 0.002, and 0.015 for 5-HT, TRP, and 5-HIAA, respectively). When individual patient values were examined, it was observed that patient 2, who had committed suicide, had the lowest 5-HIAA level in most (9/13) of the regions. Levels of TRP and 5-HT seen for this patient were similar to the TS group mean in nearly all areas. When patient 2 was deleted, TS group means for 5-HIAA were still lower than the control mean in 12/13 areas; however, the TS group means for 5-HIAA then averaged 86 $\pm$ 13% of the control means.

The tendency for serotonin and related compounds to be lower in the subcortical regions examined prompted us to measure

TABLE 1. *Brain TRP, 5-HT, 5-HIAA, and [³H]citalopram binding in Tourette syndrome (expressed as a % of control means)*

Region	No. (C/TS)	TRP	5-HT	5-HIAA	[³H]citalopram binding
CAU	4/4	55 ± 14**	63 ± 25	89 ± 42	102 ± 20
ACC	4/3	60 ± 23	77 ± 12	104 ± 33	110 ± 25
SNC	4/4	71 ± 15	127 ± 17	85 ± 26	98 ± 22
SNR	2/4	44 ± 7***	72 ± 20	88 ± 39	55 ± 50
STN	3/4	68 ± 66	119 ± 17	48 ± 31	—
LGP	5/4	85 ± 35	92 ± 38	78 ± 21	120 ± 24
MGP	6/4	69 ± 19**	92 ± 33	76 ± 18	126 ± 19
TVL	2/3	74 ± 21**	58 ± 32	36 ± 3	77 ± 29
TAM	2/4	94 ± 22	67 ± 25	61 ± 8	79 ± 10
TAL	2/4	104 ± 24	79 ± 29	87 ± 4	83 ± 18
TDM	2/3	68 ± 22	48 ± 24	43 ± 19	52 ± 19
AMY	5/4	63 ± 23	71 ± 30	69 ± 15	83 ± 15
OLF	4/3	88 ± 29	70 ± 44	74 ± 57	68 ± 14

** $p < 0.05$.
*** $p < 0.01$, Wilcoxon Sum Rank test.
ACC, accumbens; AMY, amygdala; C, control; CAV, caudate; 5-HIAA, 5-hydroxyindoleacetic acid; 5-HT, serotonin; LGP, lateral globus pallidus; MGP, medial globus pallidus; OLF, olfactory tubercle; SNC, substantia nigra compacta; SNR, substantia nigra reticulata; STN, subthalamus; TAL, thalamus, anterolateral; TAM, thalamus, anteromedial; TDM, thalamus, dorsal-medial; TRP, tryptophan; TS, Tourette syndrome.

levels of [³H]citalopram binding. [³H]citalopram binds to the presynaptic 5-HT uptake site, and binding site density can be considered to be an index or marker for serotonergic neurons. As seen in Table 1, the density of [³H]citalopram binding sites was *not* consistently lower in the TS group.

There has been considerable speculation concerning serotonergic functioning in TS (2,3,31,36,53–57). This has been based on neurochemical and neuropharmacologic observations as well as neuroanatomic, neurophysiological, and behavioral considerations. In essence, the rich serotonergic innervation of basal ganglia areas (58), the predominantly inhibitory role for 5-HT in DA neurotransmission and functioning (59), the reports of lowered CSF 5-HIAA in TS mentioned above (31,37), and the beneficial effects of serotonergic agents on related obsessive–compulsive symptoms (60) can be taken to suggest that central 5-HT functioning might be reduced in TS. The relatively pervasive reductions seen for TRP, 5-HIAA, and 5-HT in the face of apparently normal levels of [³H]citalopram binding suggest that, while serotonergic innervation is

normal, serotonergic neurotransmission may be reduced in TS. The widespread nature of the reductions in subcortical levels of the precursor, TRP, suggests the possibility of an alteration in TRP metabolism or transport, which in turn affects 5-HT metabolism. The postmortem data indicate that these issues, and the general area of 5-HT functioning in TS, deserve further study.

CATECHOLAMINES

For most areas, little difference in mean NE concentration was seen between the TS and control groups, with distributions greatly overlapping. Although a lower TS group mean was observed for NE in the ventral-lateral thalamus (TVL: TS vs. control, 154 ± 1 vs. 60.1 ± 16.8 µg/g, $p = 0.02$) the small size of the groups (two subjects each) gives this little weight.

The results for DA are less clear. Although nonsignificantly lower TS group means were observed in all areas examined except the olfactory bulb (OLF), the ranges of values were quite high. Less variation was seen for levels of the major DA metabolite, HVA, and little difference was seen for HVA between the groups. Likewise, group mean values observed for activities of the rate-limiting synthetic enzyme tyrosine hydroxylase (TH) were usually similar in the TS and control groups. The ranges of TH activities observed in each area were relatively small. In the one area (anterio-lateral thalamus, TAL) in which a low p value ($p < 0.01$, WSR) was seen, the groups were small, and means for TH activity differed by less than 20%. Taken together, the HVA and TH data suggest that DA metabolism in the subcortical regions of TS subjects is not greatly altered. However, the high variability in DA and NE levels, and the use of haloperidol by at least two of the TS subjects, require any statements concerning the catecholamines to be extremely tentative.

AMINO ACIDS

To a large extent, the amino acid concentrations were found to have similar means and distributions in the TS and control groups (Table 2). The data for taurine,

aspartate, and glutamine (not shown) were quite unremarkable, with no t test p values less than 0.06. Although lower mean levels were seen for serine in the substantia nigra reticulata (SNR, $p = < 0.01$) and the anterio-lateral thalamus (TAL, $p < 0.01$), and for glycine in the SNR ($p = < 0.05$), in each case the control group was composed of only two subjects.

One of the very few instances in which there was no overlap in the TS and control values occurred for glutamate in the medial globus pallidus. Mean values of $1,120 \pm 201$ µg/g and 796 ± 95 µg/g were observed in the control and TS groups, respectively ($p = < 0.01$, WSR). As shown in Figure 1, the difference was also seen when glutamate concentrations were expressed as µg/mg protein (15.4 ± 2.4 versus 10.4 ± 1.1, $p = < 0.01$, WSR). Although the p values are not significant given the number of tests carried out, and the TS group means are reduced by only about 30%, the lack of overlap is striking. The MGP glutamate levels in patient 2, who had committed suicide by carbon monoxide inhalation, were 795 µg/g and 9.94 µg/mg protein. The closeness of these values to the group mean was reassur-

TABLE 2. *Brain GLU, ASP, GLY, and GABA in Tourette syndrome (expressed as % of control mean)*[a]

Region	No. (C/TS)	GLU	ASP	GLY	GABA
CAU	4/4	109 ± 25	88 ± 60	101 ± 23	117 ± 36
ACC	4/3	113 ± 30	76 ± 21	86 ± 41	104 ± 11
SNC	4/4	87 ± 6	79 ± 30	61 ± 9	122 ± 51
SNR	2/4	72 ± 6*	65 ± 34	49 ± 6***	106 ± 40
STN	3/4	111 ± 27	103 ± 29	106 ± 25	77 ± 25
LGP	5/4	70 ± 19**	80 ± 51	80 ± 21	160 ± 51
MGP	6/4	70 ± 9***	99 ± 62	70 ± 28	143 ± 44
TVL	2/3	113 ± 24	190 ± 116	127 ± 54	99 ± 34
TAM	2/4	119 ± 6	215 ± 86	173 ± 40	113 ± 30
TAL	2/4	134 ± 40	251 ± 141	235 ± 101	104 ± 33
TDM	2/3	120 ± 38	195 ± 131	170 ± 97	222 ± 250
AMY	5/4	91 ± 12	78 ± 20	80 ± 11	105 ± 16
OLF	4/3	117 ± 9	139 ± 72	154 ± 60	150 ± 102

[a] Mean GLU concentrations in the control group ranged from 733 ± 275 µg/g (STN) to $1,420 \pm 266$ µg/g (CAU)
* $p < 0.1$.
** $p < 0.05$.
*** $p < 0.01$, Wilcoxon Sum Rank test.
For abbreviations, see footnote to Table 1.

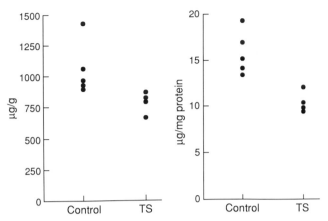

FIG. 1. Concentrations of glutamate measured in the medial globus pallidus (*MGP*) of control (*C*) and Tourette syndrome (*TS*) subjects.

ing, given the suggestion that the globus pallidus might be especially sensitive to carbon monoxide intoxication (61).

The suggestive decreases seen for glutamate in the MGP of TS subjects (Fig. 1) are quite consistent with the models developed for hyperkinetic disorders (9,62–64). The decreased excitatory input to the MGP would be expected to decrease activity in the inhibitory, pallidal projection to the thalamus, leading to increased thalamocortical activation (Fig. 2b).

It is interesting to note the levels seen for glutamate and GABA in related basal ganglia areas of the TS subjects. Glutamate also shows a trend to lower levels in the SNR and LGP, while levels in the STN appear normal (Table 2). GABA levels in the caudate, SNR, STN, and all areas of the thalamus were similar in TS and control subjects; however, somewhat elevated levels were seen in the medial and lateral pallidum (MGP and LGP) in the TS subjects. The lower glutamate levels in the SNR and MGP are consistent with both areas receiving their main glutamatergic afferents from the subthalamic nucleus (STN). The lowered LGP glutamate further tends to implicate decreased STN output, as it too receives glutamatergic fibers from the STN (64,65). The suggestive changes in glutamate, all potentially traceable to the STN, are similar to

those expected in hemiballismus after STN lesion and in Huntington's disease.

According to the models, one possibility for decreased glutamatergic output of the STN is increased GABAergic inhibition by the LGP. However, the relatively normal levels of GABA in the STN would indicate that changes in MGP glutamate are not a result of increased inhibition of the STN. This contrasts with the situation in Huntington's disease, in which a reduction in GABAergic projections from the striatum to the LGP (66,67) apparently results in disinhibition of the LGP, leading in turn to excessive inhibition of the STN. So, unlike Huntington's disease, in which presumed changes in the output nuclei (MGP and SNR) can be traced back to the degeneration of particular GABAergic striatal neurons, in TS the alteration does not appear to extend back past the STN. If anything, the MGP and LGP levels of GABA, both presumably arising from striatal projections, appear somewhat higher in TS subjects (Table 2). The report of normal saccadic eye movements in TS also suggests that strionigral projections are intact in TS (68). This again stands in contrast to Huntington's disease, in which loss of inhibitory striatal projections to the SNR leads to abnormal saccades.

The speculation concerning lowered subthalamic glutamatergic output in TS is in

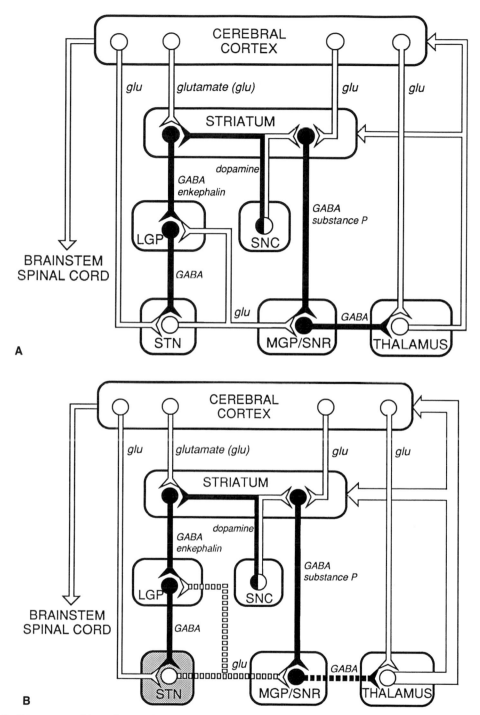

FIG. 2. Diagrams of basal ganglia circuitry. *Filled* and *open lines* represent inhibitory or excitatory projections, respectively. Increased activity is indicated by increased line width; decreased activity is shown by dotted lines. Normal circuitry is shown **(A),** along with a diagram illustrating the possible changes occurring in hemiballismus following STN lesions **(B).** *LGP,* lateral globus pallidus; *MGP,* medial globus pallidus; *SNR,* substantia nigra reticulata; *SNC,* substantia nigra compacta; *STN,* subthalamic nucleus; *GLU,* glutamate; *GABA,* γ-aminobutyric acid. Adapted from Alexander and Crutcher (64) and DeLong (63).

line with a previous suggestion that hemiballismus, choreoathetosis, and tics all result from decreased STN activity (9). One can speculate that, neurochemically, TS is more like hemiballismus, and several clinical similarities can be noted. In both disorders, it has been reported that movements can be exacerbated by stress, can be suppressed for brief periods, and are responsive to haloperidol and tetrabenazine (4,27, 28,69,70). There is a case report of the sudden simultaneous appearance of hemiballismus and coprolalia, both of which responded to tetrabenazine (71). In addition, TS and hemiballismus both often involve involuntary facial movements (69,72). On the other hand, TS is usually clearly distinguished from hemiballismus in terms of the nature and magnitude of the movements observed. The flinging movements of hemiballismus are characterized by their coarseness and irregularity, while the tics of TS are, by contrast, usually coordinated, more elaborate, stereotypical, and accompanied by a predisposing urge. Also, the oculomotor disturbances frequently seen in TS (73) have not been reported in hemiballismus.

Assuming that STN output is reduced in TS, the nature of the circuitry suggests that simply changing overall glutaminergic or GABAergic functioning would probably not have beneficial effects in TS. However, it might be possible to increase selectively the function of the subthalamic glutamatergic projections to the MGP/SNR depending upon the specific types of pre- and postsynaptic receptors present. Recent demonstration of anti-parkinsonian effects of NMDA antagonists, apparently mediated through the MGP (74,75), suggests that NMDA agonists might possibly be used to advantage in hyperkinetic disorders. The localization of substance P to striatal-MGP/SNR projections and of enkephalin to striatal-LGP projections (9,62,65) might also offer an opportunity to modulate selectively the activities of these pathways using peptidergic agents.

In conclusion, it is apparent, given the in-

herent limitations of postmortem analyses, the problems specific to these groups of samples, and issues of statistical power, that speculation and conclusions based on this study must be highly qualified. However, it can be noted that the suggestive differences seen occur against a background of general normality in that, for most regions, concentrations or activities of the analytes were highly overlapping in the TS and control groups. Also, the trends observed for 5-HT and related compounds, and for glutamate, were self-consistent. In the case of 5-HT, TRP and 5-HIAA were decreased along with 5-HT in most areas examined. As for glutamate, decreases were seen in the three major projection areas (LGP, MGP, and SNR) of the subthalamus (STN). While the nature of the trends tends to lend them more weight, it is difficult to choose between the two (5-HT vs. glutamate) as to which might be more likely to be involved in the pathobiology or etiology of TS. Certainly it would be of interest to try to relate or connect the two possible alterations. Finally, the glutamate findings draw attention to the STN and globus pallidus, raise issues regarding the relationship of TS and hemiballismus, and might guide the development of animal models for TS.

REFERENCES

1. American Psychiatric Association: *Diagnostic and Statistical Manual of Mental Disorders,* 3rd ed. Washington, DC: American Psychiatric Association, 1980.
2. Shapiro AK, Shapiro ES, Young JG, Feinberg TE (eds.), *Gilles de la Tourette Syndrome,* 2nd ed. New York: Raven Press, 1988.
3. Cohen DJ, Riddle MA, Leckman JF, Ort SI, Shaywitz BA: Tourette's syndrome. In: Jeste DV, Wyatt RJ, eds. *Neuropsychiatric movement disorders.* New York: American Psychiatric Press, 1984;20–52.
4. Jankovic J: The neurology of tics. In: Marsden C, Fahn S, eds. *Movement disorders,* 2nd ed. Cornwall: Butterworth & Co., 1987;383–405.
5. Chappell PB, Leckman JF, Pauls DL, Cohen DJ: Biochemical and genetic studies of Tourette's syndrome: implications for treatment and future research. In: Deutsch SI, Weizman A, Weizman R,

eds. *Application of basic neuroscience to child psychiatry.* New York: Plenum, 1990;241–60.

6. Leckman JF, Riddle MA, Cohen DJ: Pathobiology of Tourette syndrome. In: Cohen DJ, Bruun RD, Leckman JF, eds. *Tourette's syndrome and tic disorders: clinical understanding and treatment.* New York: John Wiley & Sons, 1988;95–116.

7. Kurlan R: Tourette's syndrome: current concepts. *Neurology* 1989;39:1625–30.

8. Hassler R, Dieckmann G: Stereotaxic treatment of tics and inarticulate cries or coprolalia considered as motor obsessional phenomena in Gilles de la Tourette's disease. (English translation.) *Rev Neurol (Paris),* 1970;123:89–100.

9. Albin RL, Young AB, Penney JB: The functional anatomy of basal ganglia disorders. *Trends Neurosci* 1989;12:366–75.

10. Baxter LR, Schwartz JM, Guse BH, Bergman K, Szuba MP: PET imaging in obsessive compulsive disorder with and without depression. *J Clin Psychiatry* 1990;51(Suppl):61–9.

11. Leckman JF, Knorr AM, Rasmusson AM, Cohen DJ. Basal ganglia research and Tourette's syndrome. *Trends Neurosci* 1991;14:94.

12. Pitman RK: Animal models of compulsive behavior. *Biol Psychiatry,* 1989;26:189–98.

13. Sutherland RJ, Kolb B, Schoel WM, Whishaw IQ, Davies D: Neuropsychological assessment of children and adults with Tourette syndrome: a comparison with learning disabilities and schizophrenia. In: Friedhoff AJ, Chase TN, eds. *Gilles de la Tourette syndrome.* 1982;311–22.

14. Devinsky O: Neuroanatomy of Gilles de la Tourette syndrome: possible midbrain involvement. *Arch Neurol* 1983;40:508–14.

15. Richardson EP: Neuropathological studies of Tourette syndrome. In: Friedhoff AJ, Chase TN, eds. *Advances in neurology: Gilles de la Tourette syndrome,* vol 35. New York: Raven Press, 1982; 83–7.

16. Haber SN, Kowall NW, Vonsattel JP, Bird ED, Richardson EP: Gilles de la Tourette's syndrome: a postmortem and neurohistochemical study. *J Neurol Sci* 1986;75:225–41.

17. Chase TM, Foster NL, Fedro P, et al. Gilles de la Tourette syndrome: studies with the fluorine-18-labelled fluorodeoxyglucose positron emission topographic method. *Ann Neurol* 1984;15:S175.

18. Chase TN, Geoffrey V, Gillespie M, Burrows GH: Structural and functional studies of Gilles de la Tourette syndrome. *Rev Neurol (Paris)* 1986; 142:851–5.

19. Singer HS, Wong DF, Tiemeyer M, et al. Pathophysiology of Tourette syndrome: a positron emission tomographic and postmortem analysis. *Ann Neurol* 1985;18:416.

20. Wong DF, Singer H, Pearlson G, et al. D2 dopamine receptors in Tourette's syndrome and manic depressive illness. *J Nucl Med* 1989;29:820–1.

21. Wong DF, Young LT, Pearlson G, et al. D2 dopamine receptor densities measured by PET are elevated in several neuropsychiatric disorders. *J Nucl Med* 1989;30:731.

22. Hall M, Costa DC, Shields J, Heavens J, Robertson M, Ell PJ: Brain perfusion patterns with Tc-

99m-HMPAO/SPECT in patients with Gilles de la Tourette syndrome. *Eur J Nucl Med,* 1990; 16:WP18.

23. Harcherik DF, Cohen DJ, Ort S, et al. Computed tomographic brain scanning in four neuropsychiatric disorders of childhood. *Am J Psychiatry* 1985; 142:731–4.

24. Caparulo BK, Cohen DJ, Rothman SL, et al. Computed tomographic brain scanning in children with developmental neuropsychiatric disorders. *J Am Acad Child Psychiatry* 1981;20:338–47.

25. Riddle MA, Lidov M, Abrahams J, Leckman JF: Magnetic resonance imaging in Tourette's syndrome. *Am Cong Neuropsychopharmacol Abstr* 1989;187.

26. Singer HS, Hahn I-H, Krowiak E, Nelson E, Moran T: Tourette's syndrome: a neurochemical analysis of postmortem cortical brain tissue. *Ann Neurol* 1990;27:443–6.

27. Shapiro AK, Shapiro E: Treatment of tic disorders with haloperidol. In: Cohen DJ, Bruun RD, Leckman JF, eds. *Tourette's syndrome and tic disorders: clinical understanding and treatment.* New York: John Wiley & Sons, 1988;267–81.

28. Ross MA, Moldofsky H: A comparison of pimozide and haloperidol in the treatment of Gilles de la Tourette syndrome. *Am J Psychiatry* 1978; 135:585–7.

29. Golden GS: Gilles de la Tourette syndrome following methylphenidate administration. *Dev Med Child Neurol* 1974;16:76–8.

30. Price A, Leckman JF, Pauls DL, Cohen DJ, Kidd KK: Gilles de la Tourette's syndrome: tics and central nervous system stimulants in twins and nontwins. *Neurology* 1986;36:232–7.

31. Cohen DJ, Shaywitz BA, Caparulo B, Young JG, Bowers MB: Chronic, multiple tics of Gilles de la Tourette's disease: CSF acid monoamine metabolites after probenecid administration. *Arch Gen Psychiatry* 1978;35:245–50.

32. Iversen SD, Alpert JE: Functional organization of the dopamine system in normal and abnormal behavior. In Friedhoff AJ, Chase TN, eds. *Gilles de la Tourette syndrome.* New York: Raven Press, 1982;69–76.

33. Cohen DJ, Detlor JG, Lowe T: Clonidine ameliorates Gilles de la Tourette syndrome. *Arch Gen Psychiatry* 1980;37:1350–7.

34. Leckman JF, Detlor JG, Harcherik DF, Ort SI, Shaywitz BA, Cohen DJ: Short and long term treatment of Tourette's syndrome with clonidine: a clinical perspective. *Neurology* 1985;35:343–51.

35. Amaral DG, Sinnamon HM: The locus coerulus: neurobiology of a central noradrenergic nucleus. *Prog Neurobiol* 1977;9:147–96.

36. Leckman JF, Riddle MA, Berrettini WH, et al. Elevated CSF dynorphin A[1–8] in Tourette's syndrome. *Life Sci* 1988;43:2015–23.

37. Singer HS, Pepple JM, Ramage AL, Butler IS: Gilles de la Tourette syndrome: further studies and thoughts. *Ann Neurol* 1978;4:21–5.

38. Sandyk R, Bamford CR, Crinnin CT: Abnormal growth hormone response to naloxone challenge in Tourette syndrome. *Int J Neurosci* 1987;37:191–2.

39. Chappell PB, Leckman JF, Riddle MA, et al. The

neuroendocrine and behavioral aspects of naloxone in Tourette's syndrome. In: Chase TN, Friedhoff AJ, Cohen DJ. Tourette syndrome: Genetics, neurobioloigy, and treatment. Chapter 31, this volume.

40. Stahl SM: Neuropharmacology of movement disorders: comparison of spontaneous and drug-induced movement disorders. In: Shah NS, Donald AG, eds. *Movement disorders.* New York: Plenum, 1986;1–36.

41. Gonce M, Barbeau A: Seven cases of Gilles de la Tourette syndrome: partial relief with clonazepam: a pilot study. *Can J Neurol Sci* 1977;4:279–83.

42. Mondrup K, Dupont E, Braendgaard H: Progabide in the treatment of hyperkinetic extrapyramidal movement disorders. *Acta Neurol Scand* 1985; 72:341–3.

43. Stevens TJ, Bird ED: Microdissections of nuclear areas from human brain slices. In: Cuello AC, ed. *IBRO handbook series: methods in the neurosciences: brain microdissection techniques,* vol 2. New York: John Wiley & Sons, 1983;171–83.

44. Bird ED, Iversen LL: Huntington's chorea: postmortem measurement of glutamic acid decarbonxylase, choline acetyltransferase and dopamine in basal ganglia. *Brain* 1974;97:457–72.

45. Anderson GM, Young JG, Batter DK, Young SN, Cohen DJ, Shaywitz BA: Determination of indoles and catechols in rat brain and pineal using liquid chromatography with fluorometric and amperometric detection. *J Chromatogr* 1981;223:315–20.

46. Anderson GM, Feibal FC, Cohen DJ: Determination of serotonin in whole blood, PRP, PPP and plasma ultrafiltrate. *Life Sci* 1987;40:1063–70.

47. Anderson GM, Riddle MA, Hoder EL, Fiebel FC, Shaywitz BA: The ontogeny of 3,4-dihydroxyphenylacetic acid in human cerebrospinal fluid. *J Neurol Neurosurg Psychiatry* 1988;51:1100–2.

48. Felice LJ, Felice JD, Kissinger PT: Determination of catecholamines in rat brain parts by reverse-phase ion-pair liquid chromatography. *J Neurochem* 1978;31:1461–5.

49. Durkin TA, Anderson GM, Cohen DJ: High performance liquid chromatographic analysis of neurotransmitter amino acids in the brain. *J Chromatogr* 1988;428:9–15.

50. Reinhard JF, Smith GK, Nichol CA: A rapid and sensitive assay for tyrosine-3-monooxygenase based upon the release of ^3H_2O and adsorption of [^{3}H]-tyrosine by charcoal. *Life Sci* 1986; 39:2185–9.

51. Fonnum F: A rapid radiochemical method for the determination of choline acetyltransferase. *J Neurochem* 1988;24:407–9.

52. Bradford MM: A rapid and sensitive method for the quantitation of microgram quantities of protein utilizing the principle of protein-dye binding. *Anal Biochem* 1976;72:248–54.

53. Comings DE: Blood serotonin and tryptophan in Tourette syndrome. *Am J Med Genet* 1990; 36:418–30.

54. Knott PJ, Hutson PH: Stress-induced stereotypy in the rat: neuropharacological similarities to Tourette syndrome. In: Friedhoff AJ, Chase TN, eds. *Gilles de la Tourette syndrome: advances in neurology,* vol 35. New York: Raven Press, 1982; 233–8.

55. Jacobs BL, Trulson ME, Heym J, Steinfels GF: On the role of CNS serotonin in the motor abnormalities of Tourette syndrome: behavioral and single-unit studies. In: Friedhoff AJ, Chase TN, eds. *Gilles de la Tourette syndrome: advances in neurology,* vol 35. New York: Raven Press, 1982; 93–8.

56. Crosley CJ: Decreased serotoninergic activity in Tourette syndrome. *Ann Neurology* 1979;5:596–7.

57. Comings DE: *Tourette syndrome and human behavior.* Duarte, CA: Hope Printing, 1990.

58. Parent A: Extrinsic connections of the basal ganglia. *Trends Neurosc* 1990;13:254–8.

59. Korsgaard S, Gerlach J, Christensson E: Behavioral aspects of serotonin-dopamine interaction in the monkey. *Eur J Pharmacol* 1985;118:245–52.

60. Riddle MA, Hardin MT, King RA, Scahill L, Woolston JF: Fluoxetine treatment of children and adolescents with Tourette's and obsessive compulsive disorders: preliminary clinical experience. *J Am Acad Child Adolesc Psychiatry* 1990;29:45–8.

61. Brierly JB: Cerebral hypoxia. In: Arnold E, Blackwood W, Corsellis JAN, eds. *Greenfields neuropathology,* 3rd ed. London: E. Arnold, 1976; 68–71.

62. Crossman AR: Neural mechanisms in disorders of movement. *Comp Biochem Physiol* 1989; 93A:141–9.

63. DeLong MR: Primate models of movement disorders of basal ganglia origin. *Trends Neurosci* 1990; 13:281–5.

64. Alexander GE, Crutcher MD: Functional architecture of basal ganglia circuits: neural substrates of parallel processing. *Trends Neurosci* 1990; 13:266–71.

65. Graybiel AM: Neurotransmitters and neuromodulators in the basal ganglia. *Trends Neurosci* 1990; 13:245–53.

66. Reynolds GP, Pearson SJ: Brain GABA levels in asymptomatic Huntington's disease. *N Engl J Med* 1990;323:682.

67. Reynolds GP, Pearson SJ: Decreased glutamic acid and increased 5-hydroxytryptamine in Huntington's disease brain. *Neurosci Lett* 1987; 78:233–8.

68. Bollen EL, Roos RAC, Cohen AP, et al. Oculomotor control in Gilles de la Tourette syndrome. *J Neurol Neurosurg Psychiatry* 1988;51:1081–3.

69. Shannon KM: Hemiballismus (review). *Clin Neuropharmacol* 1990;13:413–25.

70. Wolfson L, Brown LL, Makman M, Warner C, Dvorkin B, Katzman R: Dopamine mechanisms in the subthalamic nucleus and possible relationship to hemiballismus and other movement disorders. In: Friedhoff AJ, Chase TN, eds. in: *Gilles de la Tourette syndrome: advances in neurology,* vol 35. New York: Raven Press, 1982;203–11.

71. Marti-Masso JF, Obeso JA: Coprolalia associated with hemiballismus: response to tetrabenazine. *Clin Neuropharmacol* 1985;8:189–90.

72. Dewey RB, Jankovic J: Hemiballism-hemichorea: clinical and phaurmacologic findings in 21 patients. *Arch Neurol* 1989;46:862–7.

73. Frankel M, Cummings JL: Neuro-ophalamic abnormalities in Tourette's syndrome: functional and anatomical implications. *Neurology* 1984; 34:359–61.

74. Graham WC, Robertson RG, Sambrook MA, Crossman AR: Injection of excitatory amino acid antagonists into the medial pallidal segment of a 1-methyl-4-phenyl-1, 2, 3, 6-tetrahydropyridine (MPTP) treated primate reverses motor symptoms of parkinsonism. *Life Sci* 1990;47:PL91–P197.

75. Klockgether T, Turski L. NMDA antagonists potentiate antiparkinsonian actions of L-dopa in monoamine-depleted rats. *Ann Neurol* 1990; 28:539–46.

Advances in Neurology, Vol. 58, edited
by T. N. Chase, A. J. Friedhoff, and
D. J. Cohen. Raven Press, Ltd.,
New York © 1992.

16

Neurochemical Analysis of Postmortem Cortical and Striatal Brain Tissue in Patients with Tourette Syndrome

Harvey S. Singer

*Departments of Neurology and Pediatrics, Johns Hopkins University School of
Medicine, Baltimore, Maryland 21205*

Tourette syndrome (TS) is a chronic neurological disorder characterized by the presence of involuntary motor and phonic tics. Despite an estimated frequency of 150,000 affected persons in the United States, little is known about the neuroanatomic localization or underlying pathophysiological abnormality in this disorder. Computer tomography and magnetic resonance imaging in living patients have demonstrated only isolated or minor structural alterations (1–3). Similarly, routine postmortem studies in patients who had classical TS during their lifetime have shown no specific focus of disease (4). Despite the lack of a clear neuroanatomic localization, neurochemical abnormalities have been proposed as the potential underlying mechanism.

Dysfunction of central neurotransmitter systems has been suggested as an underlying cause of TS, based primarily on the responsiveness of symptoms to specific medications, on studies of neurotransmitter metabolites in blood and cerebrospinal fluid, and on limited analyses of postmortem brain samples. To date, the dopaminergic, serotoninergic, noradrenergic, cholinergic, γ-aminobutyric acid (GABA)ergic, and opiate systems have had their proponents. Since many synaptic transmitter systems are integrated in the production of complex neurologic actions, it has been speculated that imbalances within different transmitter systems might lead to similar groups of symptoms (5). It is also possible that an abnormality involving a second messenger system could unify findings of alterations within multiple transmitter systems. In an attempt to clarify a potential neurotransmitter abnormality in patients with TS, my laboratory has examined synaptic neurochemical characteristics in postmortem cortical and striatal samples (6,7).

OVERVIEW OF SYNAPTIC NEUROTRANSMISSION

Neurons in the brain are distinct cells primarily interconnected via axonal processes. It has long been known that neurons transfer signals predominantly by the release of neurotransmitters from knob-like branches on axonal terminals that approximate, but do not touch, the cell body and dendrites of other neurons. An individual neuron receives multiple inputs, about 30,000 for large neurons within the human cortex. The list of putative neurotransmitters is long and includes the widely recognized amines dopamine, norepinephrine, serotonin, and acetylcholine; the amino acids GABA and glutamate; and the peptides enkephalin, substance P, and somatostatin as well as many others. Neurotransmitters are often synthesized within the axon terminal and then stored in vesicles. Some neurons contain both a classical neurotransmitter (e.g., dopamine, acetylcholine) and a neuropeptide.

With the arrival of an axon potential, the terminal membrane is depolarized, calcium enters the axon terminal, vesicles containing neurotransmitters fuse with the presynaptic membrane, and their contents are released into the synaptic cleft (Fig. 1). The released transmitter diffuses across the synaptic cleft, where it binds to a postsynaptic receptor. The concentration of transmitter within the cleft can be lowered very efficiently by rapid re-uptake into the axon terminal via an energy-dependent pump, or degradation by specific enzymes. Receptors are complex proteins, within synaptic membranes, that possess a transmitter recognition site (binding site) closely linked to action-related subunits (e.g., ion channels or second messenger systems). Specific recep-

tors exist for each transmitter and its structural analogs. In addition to postsynaptic membrane receptors, most transmitter systems have presynaptic receptors on their own or other presynaptic terminals. Some of these receptors monitor the amount of transmitter within the cleft and regulate further release via a negative feedback control mechanism.

Contact between a neurotransmitter and its specific postsynaptic receptor initiates a series of reactions within its action-related subunit. In its simplest form the transmitter-receptor complex brings about opening of ion channels leading to depolarization or hyperpolarization of the resting membrane potential. A second type of action subunit results in the synthesis of second messengers such as adenosine 3′,5′-monophosphate (cyclic AMP). Cyclic AMP, in turn, influences the activity of various cytoplasmic and membrane enzymes.

Several steps in synaptic transmission can be assayed biochemically. Presynaptic function can be evaluated by measuring the activity of synthesizing enzymes, levels of a particular neurotransmitter and its metabolism and turnover, and neurotransmitter re-uptake. Postsynaptic events can be investigated by evaluating membrane receptors for the neurotransmitter, ionic fluxes, or the synthesis of second messengers.

Frozen postmortem brain samples from four adults with a lifetime diagnosis of TS and control subjects were made available by the Brain Tissue Resource Center in Belmont, MA and the John Hopkins Brain Bank. Small blocks of tissues were available from frontal superior cortex (A7), supplemental motor cortex (A6), occipital lobe (A17), temporal lobe (A38), caudate, and putamen. Ages of the TS patients ranged from 38 to 86 years, at least two had a childhood onset, two a positive family history, and two had received neuroleptics. The age range for controls was 23 to 96 years. The postmortem interval (the time interval between death and autopsy) was less than 9 hours in TS samples and less than 15 hours

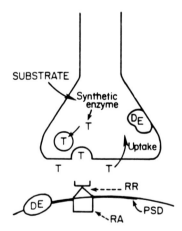

FIG. 1. Schematic diagram of chemical synapse. *T*, endogenous transmitter; *DE*, degradative enzymes; *RR*, receptor recognition site; *RA*, receptor action subunit (e.g., ion channels or second messenger systems); *PSD*, postsynaptic density. From Johnston and Singer (44).

in control tissues. These tissues were further characterized and used for a series of studies. The presynaptic marker for GABAergic interneurons was glutamate decarboxylase (GAD), a highly specific synthesizing enzyme (8). The cholinergic system was assessed presynaptically with the acetylcholine-producing enzyme choline acetyltransferase (ChAT) and postsynaptically by the specific binding of 0.3 μM [³H]quinuclidinyl benzilate (QNB) to muscarinic cholinergic receptors (9,10). Concentrations of dopamine and its metabolites homovanillic acid (HVA) and 3,4-dihydroxyphenylacetic acid (DOPAC), norepinephrine, and the serotonin metabolite 5-hydroxyindoleacetic acid (5-HIAA) were measured by high-pressure liquid chromatography (HPLC) and electrochemical detection (11). Postsynaptic binding to β-adrenergic receptors was determined with 65 pM iodinated iodocyanopindolol ([¹²⁵I]ICYP) as the ligand (12). Cortical membrane preparations from frozen caudate and putamen were assayed for both pre- and postsynaptic receptor binding. Binding to the dopamine uptake carrier (transporter) site was measured by use of 4.0 nM [³H]mazindol (13); to the D1 receptor by a modification of the method of Billard et al. (14) with 1 nM [³H]SCH 23390; and to the D2 receptor with 0.3 nM [³H]spiperone (15). Cyclic AMP was measured as described by Brown et al. (16).

In this study we evaluated synaptic markers in several regions of the cortex and striatum. In the cortex we examined markers for local GABAergic neurons, cholinergic terminals from the basal forebrain, and neurons that have long projections to the cortex: dopaminergic mesocortical projections, ascending noradrenergic tracts from the locus coeruleus, and serotonergic fibers from the median raphe. In the striatum we focused primarily on the dopaminergic system.

Cortex

In the cortical regions studied there was no significant difference between the mean activity of choline acetyltransferase or glutamate decarboxylase from patients with TS and control subjects (Fig. 2). Levels of the neurotransmitters dopamine, norepinephrine, and the serotonin metabolite 5-HIAA showed a broad range, but were not clearly abnormal. Similarly, postsynaptic receptor binding to two different receptor types, muscarinic cholinergic receptors and β receptors, was essentially normal (Fig. 3). In area A38, the mean binding with ICYP from three TS brain samples was reduced when compared with average binding in two available control tissues. No specific dopamine (D2) receptor binding was detected in any TS or control cortical region with [³H]spiperone as the ligand.

In contrast to the above lack of findings,

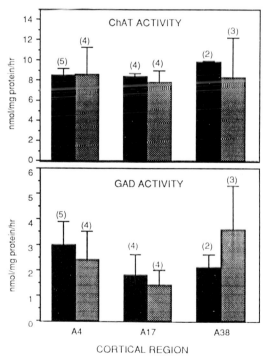

FIG. 2. Neurotransmitter synthesizing enzyme activity in cortical regions from patients with TS and control subjects. *ChAT,* choline acetyltransferase; *GAD,* glutamate decarboxylase. Values are plotted as the mean ± SEM (error bars); controls, *solid bars;* TS, *hatched bars.* Numbers of subjects are shown in parentheses.

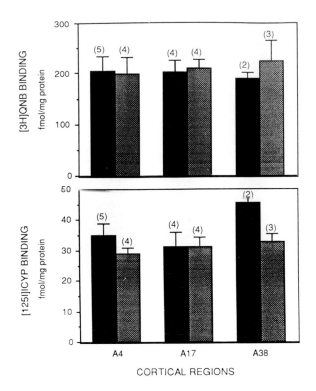

FIG. 3. Postsynaptic receptor binding in cortical regions from patients with TS and control subjects. Values are plotted as the mean ± SEM (error bars); controls, *solid bars;* TS, *hatched bars.* Numbers of subjects are shown in parentheses.

the mean concentrations of cyclic AMP in TS samples were reduced in all four cortical regions available for study (Table 1). As shown in Figure 4, in three of four patients with TS, values were below the mean for control samples in all cortical regions studied. Normal cyclic AMP values were obtained only from samples from a single patient with TS. Adenylate cyclase activity, determined as both basal levels and after forskolin stimulation, did not significantly differ in patients with TS compared with control samples (7).

Striatum

Pre- and postsynaptic markers of dopamine metabolism were analyzed in postmortem striatum (caudate and putamen) from three adults with the diagnosis of TS. Binding of [^{3}H]mazindol, which is associated with the striatal dopamine uptake carrier site, was significantly increased in the striatum of patients with TS compared with controls (Fig. 5). Binding was increased by 37% in the caudate and by 50% in the putamen. After evaluating an abnormality on single-point analyses, saturation isotherms were obtained on a putamen membrane preparation from a single TS sample. Values showed a K_D of 7.0 with a B_{max} of 3,650 fmol/mg protein compared with a control K_D of 6.1 nM with a B_{max} of 2,052 fmol/mg protein. These data suggested that the

TABLE 1. *Concentrations of cyclic AMP in different regions*[a]

Region	Controls	TS
A4	59 ± 9 (5)	39 ± 7 (4)
A6	48 ± 9 (5)	26 ± 9 (2)
A17	64 ± 6 (4)	28 ± 5 (4)
A38	58 ± 4 (2)	28 ± 12 (3)
Putamen	54 ± 18 (8)	70 ± 15 (3)

Values (mean ± SEM) are expressed as femtomoles per milligram of tissue. The numbers of samples are shown in parentheses. TS, Tourette syndrome.

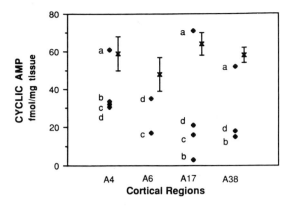

FIG. 4. The concentration of cyclic AMP in cortical regions of control subjects and patients with TS. Control values (*x*) are plotted as the mean ± SEM (for areas A4 and A6, n = 5; area A17, n = 4; area A38, n = 2). Individual values from TS patients are plotted separately. From Singer et al. (7).

differences in TS samples represent an increase in the number of binding sites and not a change in affinity.

The mean concentrations of dopamine and its major metabolites HVA and DOPAC were not significantly different from control values (Fig. 6). Because dopamine interacts with at least two pharmacologically distinct receptor recognition sites, D1 and D2, binding to each was evaluated. Results of single-point studies were not statistically different for binding to the D1 receptor (Fig. 7), whereas mean values for D2 receptors were slightly increased in both caudate and putamen (Fig. 7). This slight upregulation of [³H]spiperone binding in the TS patients

probably represents an increase in D2 receptors associated with chronic haloperidol therapy in two of the three subjects.

NEUROANATOMICAL LOCALIZATION

This study focused on a neurochemical evaluation of the cortex and the striatum because both have been prominently considered as putative sites of pathology. Although the precise neuroanatomic localization of the dysfunction in TS remains unknown, circumstantial evidence suggests involvement of the "motor" circuit within the basal ganglia (17). At the

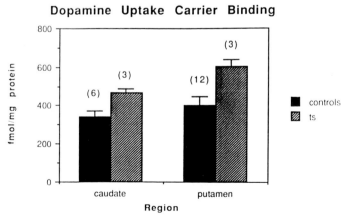

FIG. 5. Receptor binding to dopamine carrier sites ([³H]mazindol) in caudate and putamen from control subjects and TS syndrome patients. Values are shown as the mean ± SEM (error bars) with the number of samples given in parentheses. Control *solid bars;* TS, *hatched bars.* From Singer et al. (6).

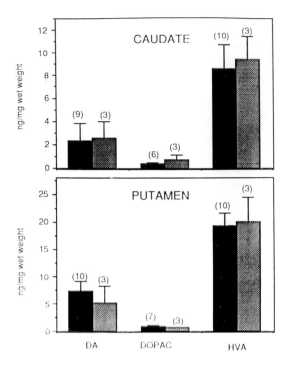

FIG. 6. Concentrations of dopamine and its major metabolites homovanillic acid (*HVA*) and 3,4-dihydroxyphenylacetic acid (*DOPAC*) in caudate and putamen from control subjects and patients with TS. Values are means ± SEM (error bars) with the number of samples given in parentheses. Control, *solid bars;* TS, *hatched bars.*

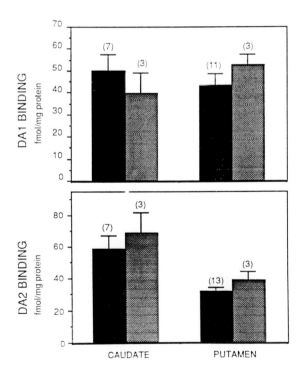

FIG. 7. Receptor binding to dopamine-1 and -2 receptors in caudate and putamen from control subjects and patients with TS. Values are means ± SEM (error bars) with the number of subjects given in parentheses. Control, *solid bars;* TS, *hatched bars.*

level of the striatum this circuit is largely based in the putamen, which receives substantial somatotypically organized projections from the motor and somatosensory cortices. The putamen sends organized projections to both the internal and external segments of the globus pallidus and caudolateral portions of the substantia nigra. These structures, in turn, project to the ventrolateral, ventroanterior, and centromedian nuclei of the thalamus, from which projections proceed to their cortical terminus, the supplementary motor area.

Supporting evidence for an abnormality in the "motor" circuit in TS includes its established role in other movement disorders (18–20); its postulated function in obsessive–compulsive disorder and attention deficit hyperactivity disorder (21–23); and an abnormality of glucose utilization in the basal ganglia of TS patients (24).

NEUROCHEMICAL FINDINGS IN THE CORTEX

In the present study, the majority of indicators evaluated in postmortem tissue were normal. These results suggest the presence of intact extrathalamic pathways to the cortex, including the dopaminergic, noradrenergic, and serotonergic systems. Similarly, pre- and postsynaptic markers for the cholinergic system (ChAT activity and QNB binding) and glutamate decarboxylase, the specific presynaptic marker for GABAergic interneurons, were unaffected.

The striking finding in the cortex was the reduction of cyclic AMP in most individuals with TS. Indeed, the mean level of cyclic AMP was reduced in measurements from frontal, temporal, and occipital cortices and in the putamen. Cyclic AMP is generated via receptor-regulated activation of a stimulatory guanine nucleotide protein (Gs) associated with adenylate cyclase and is degraded by phosphodiesterase. The association between cyclic AMP and TS symptoms, if any, is unknown. It is intriguing, however, to note that in a variety of neurotransmitter systems there is an interaction between the receptor-recognition site and cyclic AMP (Fig. 8). For example, the D1 subpopulation of dopamine receptors and β-adrenergic receptors activates adenylate cyclase activity (25,26). In contrast,

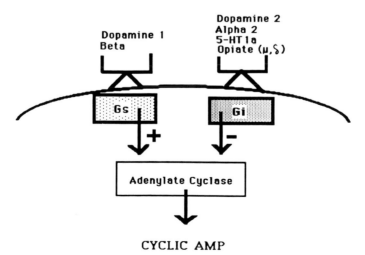

CYCLIC AMP

FIG. 8. Diagramatic representation of receptor recognition sites and linkage to the adenylate cyclase system. D1 and β-adrenergic receptors are associated with the stimulatory guanine nucleotide protein (*Gs*) whereas opiate (μ and δ), α 2, D2, serotonergic (*5-HT1a*), and muscarinic M2 receptors are associated with the inhibitory guanine nucleotide protein (*Gi*).

opiate (μ and δ), α 2-adrenergic, D2 dopaminergic, serotonergic (5-HT1a), and muscarinic (M2) receptors inhibit cyclase activity (26–30). Hence, it is possible that an abnormality involving a second messenger could explain why alterations are found in multiple transmitter systems. Additional studies are planned to clarify potential interactions between cyclic AMP metabolism and TS symptoms. For example, studies of the D2 receptor-linked inhibitory G-protein (Gi)-adenylate cyclase system and of the degradative enzyme phosphodiesterase could provide further information on the mechanism underlying the reduction of cyclic AMP.

NEUROCHEMICAL FINDINGS IN THE STRIATUM

A defect in the dopaminergic system, either an excessive amount of dopamine or an increased sensitivity of dopamine receptors, has previously been hypothesized as the pathophysiologic mechanism in TS (31,32). Several lines of evidence are usually cited to support this contention: the therapeutic effectiveness of dopamine D2 receptor antagonists such as haloperidol, fluphenazine, and pimozide (33,34); the reduction of tics by agents that block dopamine synthesis or accumulation (35,36); the appearance of tics after withdrawal from neuroleptic drugs (37); the exacerbation of tics by agents that increase central monoaminergic activity (38); and the reduction of basal and turnover levels of cerebrospinal fluid HVA, a major metabolite of brain dopamine (31,32,39).

Dopaminergic fibers originate from the substantia nigra pars compacta and provide a major input into the striatum. In our biochemical evaluation of striatal tissue, the most impressive finding was the significant increase in the number of striatal presynaptic dopamine carrier sites. We believe that this change is potentially important in TS. We think that it is unlikely to be due to sampling errors, since changes in mazindol binding were not accompanied by alterations of either dopamine, D1, or D2 receptors. Moreover, changes are not readily explained as an effect of medication, since patients were not receiving drugs such as cocaine or L-deprenyl, which have been shown to increase striatal uptake carrier binding. Lastly, neuroleptic medications used by TS subjects in this study have not been shown to affect the density of dopamine uptake carrier sites (40,41)

The neuroanatomical correlate of increased dopamine transporter sites remains speculative. We postulate that the increased [3H]mazindol binding in TS patients is associated with hyperinnervation of the dopaminergic system. We recognize, however, that this increase in binding may be associated with an increase in the concentration of uptake sites on normal numbers of dopamine terminals. Furthermore, it may also be associated with an excessive release of dopamine from the axon terminal. The latter, however, appears inconsistent with findings of reduced levels of the dopamine metabolite HVA in CSF of patients with TS (31,32,39). In contrast, increased dopamine uptake might explain the lower levels of CSF HVA via a mechanism of increased clearance of dopamine from the synaptic cleft. Although the presence of excess terminals might be expected to be accompanied by increased levels of dopamine, discrepancies between innervation and levels of neurotransmitter have been previously reported in other diseases affecting the basal ganglia (42). In the future, a dopamine hyperinnervation hypothesis can be confirmed through a parallel investigation of anatomic markers for cellular components of the dopaminergic system. For example, in adjacent postmortem striatal sections, staining for the synthesizing enzyme tyrosine hydroxylase could be correlated with dopamine transporter sites, and D2 receptors. Nevertheless, it is intriguing to speculate that increased innervation of dopamine terminals, projecting to motor and/or limbic areas in the striatum, may be associated with TS symptoms.

Our preliminary data do not support previous speculations that there are abnormal supersensitive dopamine D2 receptors in TS. Single-point analyses of D1 and D2 binding showed no significant changes from controls. A slight upregulation of [^{3}H]spiperone binding in the TS patients is probably associated with the use of haloperidol in at least two of the three subjects. No similar alteration in the D1 system is noted, presumably because of its relative resistance to up regulation (43).

In conclusion, two abnormalities in postmortem brain tissue from patients with TS have been identified: a reduction in the second messenger cyclic AMP, and an increased number of dopamine uptake carrier sites in the striatum. Both require additional studies to clarify whether these represent epiphenomena or potential pathogenetic associations with Tourette symptoms.

REFERENCES

1. Robertson M, Trimble MR, Lees AJ. The psychopathology of the Gilles de la Tourette syndrome: a phenomenological analysis. *Br J Psychiatry* 1988; 152:383–90.
2. Chase TN, Geoffrey V, Gillespie M, Burrows GH. Structural and functional studies of Gilles de la Tourette syndrome. *Rev Neurol (Paris)* 1986; 142:851–5.
3. Harcherik DF, Cohen DJ, Ort S, et al. Computed tomographic brain scanning in four neuropsychiatric disorders of childhood. *Am J Psychiatry* 1985; 142:731–4.
4. Richardson EP. Neuropathological studies of Tourette syndrome. In: Friedhoff AJ, Chase TN, eds. *Gilles de la Tourette syndrome.* New York: Raven Press, 1982;83–7.
5. Singer HS, Pepple JM, Ramage AL, Butler IJ. Gilles de la Tourette syndrome. Further studies and thoughts. *Ann Neurol* 1978;4:21–5.
6. Singer HS, Hahn I-H, Moran TH. Abnormal dopamine uptake sites in postmortem striatum from patients with Tourette syndrome. *Ann Neurol* 1991; 30:558–62.
7. Singer HS, Hahn IH, Krowiak E, Nelson BA, Moran T. Tourette's syndrome: a neurochemical analysis of postmortem cortical grain tissue. *Ann Neurol* 1990;27:443–6.
8. Wilson SH, Schrier RK, Farber JL, et al. Markers for gene expression in cultured cells from the nervous system. *J Biol Chem* 1972;247:3159–69.
9. Bull G, Oderfeld-Nowak B. Standardization of a radio chemical assay of choline acetyltransferase and a study of the activation of the enzyme in rabbit brain. *J Neurochem* 1971;18:935–41.
10. Yamamura H, Snyder S. Muscarinic cholinergic binding in rat brain. *Proc Natl Acad Sci USA* 1977; 71:1725–9.
11. Zaczek R, Coyle JT. Rapid and simple method for measuring biogenic amines and metabolites in brain homogenates by HPLC-electrochemical detection. *J Neurol Transm* 1982;53:1–5.
12. Engel ED, Hoyer D, Berthold R, Wagner H. ($\pm$)[^{125}Iodo]-cyanopindolol, a new ligand for β-adrenoceptors: identification and quantification of subclasses of β-adrenoceptors in guinea pigs. *Naunyn Schmiedebergs Arch Pharmacol* 1981; 317:277–85.
13. Javitch JA, Blaustein RO, Snyder SH. [^{3}H]mazindol binding associated with neuronal dopamine and norepinephrine uptake series. *Mol Pharmacol* 1984;26:35–44.
14. Billard WV, Ruperto V, Crosby G, et al. Characterization of the binding of [^{3}H]SCH 23390, a selective D-1 receptor antagonist ligand, in rat striatum. *Life Sci* 1984;35:1885–93.
15. Briley M, Langer SZ. Two binding sites for [^{3}H]spiroperidol on rat striatal membranes. *Eur J Pharmacol* 1978;50:283–4.
16. Brown BL, Albano JDM, Ekins RP, Sgherzi AM. A simple and sensitive saturation assay method for the measurement of adenosine $3',5'$-cyclic monophosphate. *Biochem J* 1971;121:561–2.
17. Alexander GE, DeLong MR, Strick PL. Parallel organization of functionally segregated circuits linking basal ganglia and cortex. *Annu Rev Neurosci* 1986;9:357–81.
18. Albin RL, Young AB, Penny JB. The functional anatomy of basal ganglia disorders. *Trends Neurosci* 1989;12:366–75.
19. DeLong MR. Primate models of movement disorders of basal ganglia origin. *Trends Neurosci* 1990; 13:281–5.
20. Sacks OW. Acquired tourettism in adult life. In: Friedhoff AJ, Chase TN, eds. *Gilles de la Tourette syndrome.* New York: Raven Press, 1982;89–92.
21. Baxter LR, Jr, Phelps ME, Mazziotta JC, Guze NH, Schwartz JM, Selin CE. Local cerebral glucose metabolic rates in obsessive-compulsive disorder: a comparison with rates in unipolar depression and normal control. *Arch Gen Psychiatry* 1987;44:211–8.
22. Lou HC, Henriksen L, Bruhn P, Borner H, Nielsen JB. Striatal dysfunction in attention deficit and hyperactivity disorder. *Arch Neurol* 1989; 46:48–52.
23. Luxenberg JS, Swedo SE, Flament MF, Friedland RP, Rapoport J, Rapoport SI. Neuroanatomical abnormalities in obsessive compulsive disorder detected with quantitative x-ray computed tomography. *Am J Psychiatry* 1988;145:1089–93.
24. Chase TN, Foster NL, Fedro P, et al. Gilles de la Tourette syndrome. Studies with the fluorine-18-labeled fluorodeoxyglucose positron emission tomographic method. *Ann Neurol* 1984;15:S175.
25. Cassel D, Selinger Z. Mechanism of adenylate cy-

clase activation through the β-adrenergic receptor: catecholamine-induced displacement of bound GDP by GTP. *Proc Natl Acad Sci USA* 1978; 75:4155–59.

26. Kaiser C, Jain T. Dopamine receptors: functions, subtypes and emerging concepts. *Med Res Rev* 1985;5:145–229.

27. Cooper DMF, Londos C, Gill DL, Rodbell M. Opiate receptor-mediated inhibition of adenylate cyclase in rat striatal plasma membrane. *J Neurochem* 1982;38:1164–7.

28. Schoffelmeer ANM, Hansen HA, Stoff JC, Mulder AH. Blockade of D-2 dopamine receptors strongly enhances the potency of enkephalins to inhibit dopamine-sensitive adenylate cyclase in rat neostriatum: involvement of σ- and μ-opioid receptors. *J Neurosci* 1986;6:2235–9.

29. Peroutka SJ. 5-Hydroxytryptamine receptor subtypes. *Annu Rev Neurosci* 1988;11:45–60.

30. Olianas MC, Onabi P, Neff HN, Costa E. Adenylate cyclase activity of synaptic membranes from rat straitum. Inhibition by muscarinic receptor agonists. *Mol Pharmacol* 1983;23:393–8.

31. Butler IJ, Koslow SH, Seifert WE, Caprioli RM, Singer HS. Biogenic amine metabolism in Tourette syndrome. *Ann Neurol* 1979;6:37–9.

32. Singer HS, Butler IJ, Tune LE, Seifert WE, Coyle JT. Dopaminergic dysfunction in Tourette syndrome. *Ann Neurol* 1982;12:361–6.

33. Shapiro E, Shapiro AK, Fulop G, et al. Controlled study of haloperidol, pimozide, and placebo for the treatment of Gilles de la Tourette's syndrome. *Arch Gen Psychiatry* 1989;46:722–30.

34. Singer HS, Gammon K, Quaskey S. Haloperidol, fluphenazine and clonidine in Tourette syndrome: controversies in treatment. *Pediatr Neurosci* 1986; 12:71–4.

35. Jankovic J, Glaze DG, Frost JD. Effects of tetrabenazine on tics and sleep of Gilles de la Tourette's syndrome. *Neurology* 1984;34:688–92.

36. Sweet RD, Brunn RD, Shapiro E, Shapiro AK. Presynaptic catecholamine antagonists as treatment for Tourette syndrome: effects of alpha-methyl-paratyrosine and tetrabenazine. *Arch Gen Psychiatry* 1974;31:857–61.

37. Klawans HL, Falk DK, Nausieda PA, Weiner WJ. Gilles de la Tourette syndrome after long-term chlorpromazine therapy. *Neurology* 1978; 28:1064–6.

38. Golden GS. The relationship between stimulant medication and tics. *Pediatr Ann* 1988;17:405–8.

39. Cohen DJ, Shaywitz BA, Caparulo BK, Young JG, Bowers MB, Jr. Chronic multiple tics of Gilles de la Tourette's disease. CSF acid monoamine metabolites after probenecid administration. *Arch Gen Psychiatry* 1978;35:245–50.

40. Pearce RKB, Seeman P, Jellinger K, Tourtellote WW. Dopamine uptake sites and dopamine receptors in Parkinson's disease and schizophrenia. *Eur Neurol* 1990;30(suppl 1):9–14.

41. Czudek C, Reynolds GP. [^{3}H]GBR 12935 binding to dopamine uptake sites in schizophrenia. *Br J Pharmacol* 1988;95:765P.

42. Janowsky A, Vocci F, Berger P, et al. [^{3}H]GBR-12935 binding to the dopamine transporter is decreased in the caudate nucleus in Parkinson's disease. *J Neurochem* 1987;49:617–21.

43. Friedhoff AJ. Insights into the pathophysiology and pathogenesis of Gilles de la Tourette syndrome. *Rev Neurol (Paris)* 1986;142:860–4.

44. Johnston MV, Singer HS. Brain neurotransmitters and neuromodulators in pediatrics. *Pediatrics* 1982;70:57–68.

Advances in Neurology, Vol. 58, edited by T. N. Chase, A. J. Friedhoff, and D. J. Cohen. Raven Press, Ltd., New York © 1992.

17

Basal Ganglia Peptidergic Staining in Tourette Syndrome

A Follow-up Study

*Suzanne N. Haber and †D. Wolfer

*Department of Neurobiology and Anatomy, University of Rochester School of Medicine, Rochester, New York 14642. †Institute of Anatomy, University of Zürich-Irchel, Zürich, Switzerland

We recently reported (1) the distribution of immunoreactivity of three neuropeptides, enkephalin, substance P, and dynorphin, and of acetylcholinesterase in the basal ganglia of a patient showing the typical clinical manifestations of Tourette syndrome (TS), a disease for which no characteristic or consistent neuropathological features have been discerned. In that case, routine neuropathological examination showed no abnormalities to which the patient's illness could be ascribed. Enkephalin-like-immunoreactive (ELI) and substance P-like immunoreactive (SPLI) fibers were densely stained and normally distributed. Dynorphin-like immunoreactivity (DLI) was, however, considerably less dense throughout the basal ganglia. The most striking finding was the total absence of DLI-positive fibers in the rostral part of the external segment of the globus pallidus and in the ventral pallidum.

RECENT FINDINGS

Since our original findings we have had the opportunity to study the basal ganglia of four additional patients diagnosed as having

TS and to compare them with controls. The tissue was provided by the Brain Tissue Resource Center, Belmont, MA (Table 1). Tissue blocks arrived in 10% formalin and were immediately placed in phosphate buffer containing 10% sucrose for several days before immersion in a 20%, and finally a 30%, sucrose-containing phosphate buffer solution. The blocks were frozen and cut on a sliding microtome at 50 μm. The sections were processed for immunohistochemistry using antisera directed against substance P (Cambridge Research Biochemicals, Atlantic Beach, NY), Met-enkephalin, and dynorphin A. The antisera to enkephalin and dynorphin were generously provided by Dr. R. Elde, University of Minnesota, and Dr. S. Watson, University of Michigan, respectively. These antibodies have been characterized in detail elsewhere (2–4). A modified peroxidase–antiperoxidase technique, as described elsewhere for human tissue (5), was used throughout this study. Sequential sections were stained respectively with enkephalin, substance P, and dynorphin antisera as well as with cresyl violet and acetylcholinesterase (AChE) (6). Additional sections were incubated in primary antisera

TABLE 1. *Summary of information on patients with Tourette syndrome and controls[a]*

Case	Age	Sex	PMI (hours)
T1	38	M	5.5
T2	61	F	12.5
T3	60	M	21.8
T4	57	F	9.0
C1	32	F	2.4
C2	73	M	13.9
C3	74	F	109.5
C4	63	M	4.9

[a] Age, sex, and postmortem interval (PMI) of Tourette syndrome (TS) patients and controls (C) included in this study.

TABLE 2. *Summary of opiate peptide staining densities in patients with Tourette syndrome and controls[a]*

Case	DYN	ENK
Previously reported result	1	4
T1	2	3
T2	1	4
T3	2	4
T4	4	4
C1	3	4
C2	4	4
C3	4	4
C4	3	4

[a] Density of staining of dynorphin (DYN) and enkephalin (ENK) in the rostral globus pallidus and ventral pallidum in TS patients and controls. 1 = very light staining; 2 = light staining; 3 = moderate staining; 4 = dense staining.

preabsorbed with the corresponding synthetic peptide. In each of the compartments in which sections were being stained for the substances named, corresponding sections from rat brain were run to ensure that the system was working properly and that the appropriate staining was observed in normal brain regions. With the exception of the primary antisera, the immunohistochemical methods used were identical for all compartments.

Staining density on randomly selected sections was rated by three different observers who did not know the nature of the study. Each section was rated for density of immunoreactivity as follows: 0 = none, 1 = very light, 2 = light, 3 = moderate, and 4 = dense.

Although some variation in rating did occur between levels 3 and 4, interrater reliability was high for all other density levels. Intense staining for all substances in question (enkephalin, substance P, dynorphin, and AChE) was observed in all the appropriate regions of control brains. All three neuropeptides, enkephalin, substance P, and dynorphin, as well as AChE, in the normal controls, appeared dense throughout the extent of the striatum and were distributed in a patch-like manner. In the globus pallidus, ELI, SPLI, and DLI all appeared in a distinct morphological pattern termed woolly fibers, which are composed of an unstained

central core (corresponding to a nonreactive pallidal dendrite) ensheathed in a dense plexus of thin striatal peptide-positive efferent fibers (7). As in the normal situation, AChE staining in the globus pallidus was light. More ventral regions exhibited densely stained cells, which are considered to be part of the basal nucleus of Meynert (8).

The distribution and density of enkephalin and AChE appeared normal in the TS brains. Densely stained enkephalin-positive woolly fibers were noted in the appropriate regions of the globus pallidus (Fig. 1a). Substance P-positive woolly fibers were also normally distributed in the globus pallidus in the TS brains, but in one brain appeared to be less densely stained. Dynorphin-like immunoreactivity was barely detectable in one case (T2) and light in two other TS cases (T1, T3; Table 2) (Fig. 1). In one case (T4) dense staining was found in the globus pallidus.

GENERAL COMMENTS

These results support our previous findings of a trend toward decreased dynorphin-like immunoreactivity in the globus pallidus. Several hypotheses for an underlying

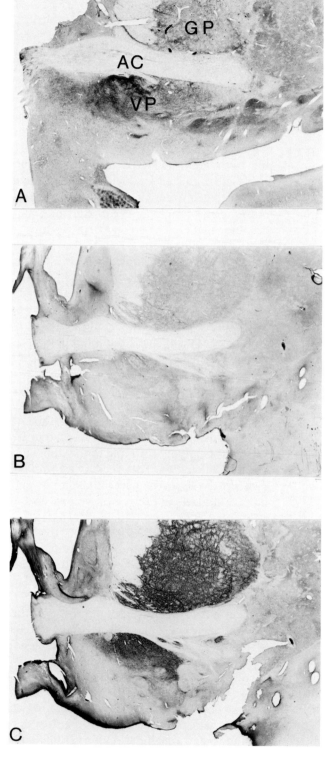

FIG. 1. Peptide immunohistochemistry in the human forebrain. A. Dynorphin-like immunoreactivity in a normal control. B. Dynorphin-like immunoreactivity in a TS brain. C. Enkephalin-like immunoreactivity in a TS brain. AC, anterior commissure; VP, ventral pallidum; GP, globus pallidus.

biochemical etiology for TS have been put forward over the years as various investigators have grappled with the enigmatic nature of this disease. Some are based on neurochemical and pharmacological studies that implicate monoaminergic, cholinergic, and opiate abnormalities (9–17). If a deficiency of dynorphin in the striatopallidal fibers is indeed related to TS, this phenomenon may be the result of one (or a combination) of several factors involving the synthesis, metabolism, or transport of this peptide. For example, the deficiency could be due to faulty processing of precursor molecules, increase of release, abnormally rapid peptide breakdown, or some other mechanism.

The effects on dynorphin may also be secondary to the primary deficit in the disease. Of the various hypotheses that have been suggested concerning the etiology of TS, one of the most viable has been the dopamine hypothesis (9,12–15). This proposes that TS may be the result of an increase in activity in the dopamine pathways. Dynorphin is found in medium spiny neurons of the striatum and is one of the main targets of the midbrain dopaminergic cells. Manipulation of the dopamine system has been shown to affect the regulation of dynorphin directly (18–20). It is of interest to note that striatal fibers containing the other endogenous opiate, enkephalin, maintained high staining density in the TS brains. Both these neuropeptides are found in the medium spiny projection neurons of the striatum. However, they are found in different populations of neurons and are under different regulatory mechanisms. Dynorphin (18–20) and enkephalin (21) are both modulated by the dopamine system but in different ways. A primary deficit of dopamine or of one of the dopamine receptors on a subpopulation of cells may have a selective effect on the regulation of dynorphin. Alternatively, it may affect a number of peptidergic systems differently, not all of which may be detectable immunohistochemically.

Limbic and Motor Interactions in the Basal Ganglia

TS is a chronic movement and behavioral disorder. Symptoms include components of both the motor system and the limbic system. The findings presented here are intriguing but should be considered within the context of basal ganglia pathways. One important question is how the transmitter pathways through the basal ganglia can affect both limbic and motor function. Recent anatomical and physiological studies have shown that different cortical areas project onto the striatum in an organized and topographic manner (22–24) and that this topography is maintained through the pallidal complex and the thalamus, which, in turn, projects topographically back to the cortex (for review, see ref. 25). Thus the cortex and basal ganglia have been considered to be arranged in parallel, functionally segregated circuits, in which each individual circuit has a specific, functionally distinct region of cortex as a nodal point. In addition to the motor circuit, other circuits have been proposed that involve association and limbic cortex (25). The ventral striatum has been associated with the limbic system by virtue of its inputs from the limbic lobe and the amygdala (26). This region in primates projects to the rostral part of the globus pallidus and to the entire region ventral to the anterior commissure and is referred to as the ventral pallidum (27).

We have recently demonstrated that projections arising from different ventral striatal regions in monkeys remain segregated in their projection to the ventral pallidum (27). Projections from different regions of the ventral pallidum to the subthalamic nucleus also remain segregated (28). This is consistent with the idea of segregated pathways through the pallidum described for the dorsal striatum. However, interestingly, there is an extensive overlap between terminating fibers arising from the different ventral striatal and ventral pallidal regions in the substantia nigra. Thus, unlike the striatopallidal and pallidosubthalamic/thalamic pathways, the striatonigral and pallidonigral pathways do not terminate in specific regions of the SN, but rather throughout the dorsal part of the nucleus.

The distribution of terminals over a wide mediolateral range of dopamine neurons suggests an influence of these fibers on dopamine neurons that project not only to the ventral striatum, but also to the dorsolateral portions of the striatum. The fact that the ventral striatum and ventral pallidum project to the entire mediolateral range of dorsally located dopamine cells indicates that the limbic-related ventral basal ganglia influences a greater proportion of the striatum via the dopamine neurons than it receives input from. This may provide a mechanism by which the ventral striatum and ventral pallidum output can influence dorsal portions of the striatum. Thus a deficit in the function of dopamine in the substantia nigra or receptors in the striatum, even if limited to a small region, is likely to affect wide areas of the striatum and several of the cortical loops. In this way specific regions of the substantia nigra or striatum can modulate and integrate both limbic and motor circuits.

REFERENCES

1. Haber SN, Kowall NW, Vonsattel JP, Bird ED, Richardson EP, Jr. Gilles de la Tourette's syndrome. A postmortem neuropathological and immunohistochemical study. *J Neurol Sci* 1986; 75:225–41.
2. Ho RH, DePalatis LR. Substance P immunoreactivity in the median eminence of the North American apossum and domestic fowl. *Brain Res* 189:565–9.
3. Haber S, Elde R. The distribution of enkephalin immunoreactive fibers and terminals in the monkey central nervous system—an immunohistochemical study. *Neuroscience* 1982;7:1049–95.
4. Haber SN, Watson SJ. The comparative distribution of enkephalin, dynorphin and substance P in the human globus pallidus and basal forebrain. *Neuroscience* 1985;14:1011–24.
5. Haber SN, Groenewegen HJ. Interrelationship of the distribution of neuropeptides and tyrosine hydroxylase immunoreactivity in the human substantia nigra. *J Comp Neurol* 1989;290:53–68.
6. Geneser-Jensen FA, Blackstad JW. Distribution of acetylcholinesterase in the hippocampal region of the guinea pig. I. Entorhinal area, para subiculum, and presubiculum. *Z Zellforsch Mikrosk Anat* 1971;114:460–81.
7. Haber SN, Nauta WJH. Ramifications of the globus pallidus in the rat as indicated by patterns of immunohistochemistry. *Neuroscience* 1983;9: 245–60.
8. Saper CB, Chelimsky TC. A cytoarchitectonic and histochemical study of nucleus basalis and associated cell groups in the normal human brain. *Neuroscience* 1984;13:1023–39.
9. Sweet RD, Solomon GE, Wayne H, Shapiro E, Shapiro AK. Neurological features of Gilles de la Tourette's syndrome. *J Neurol (Paris)* 1973; 9:19–42, 158–200.
10. Stahl SM, Berger PA. Physostigmine in Tourette syndrome—evidence for cholinergic underactivity. *Am J Psychiatr* 1981;138:240–1.
11. Leckman JR, Anderson GM, Cohen DJ, et al. Whole blood serotonin and tryptophan levels in Tourette's disorder—effects of acute and chronic clonidine treatment. *Life Sci* 1984;35:2497–503.
12. Sverd J, Kupietz S. Effects of high dose propranodol in Tourette syndrome. *J Clin Psychopharmacol* 1984;4:359–61.
13. Uhr SB, Berger PA, Pruitt B, Stahl SM. Treatment of Tourette's syndrome with R022-1319, a D-2 receptor antagonist (Letter). *N Engl J Med* 1984; 311(15):989.
14. Singer HS, Butler IJ, Tune LE, Seifert WE, Coyle JT. Dopaminergic dysfunction in Tourette syndrome. *Ann Neurol* 1982;12:361–6.
15. Singer HS, Hahn IH, Krowiak E, Nelson E, Moran TH. Tourette syndrome: a neurochemical analysis of postmortem cortical brain tissue. *Ann Neurol* 1990;27:443–6.
16. Sandyk R. The opioid system in Gilles de la Tourette's syndrome. *Neurology* 1985;35:449.
17. Leckman JF, Riddle MA, Berrettini WH, et al. Elevated CSF dynorphin A [1–8] in Tourette's syndrome. *Life Sci* 1988;43:2015–23.
18. Jiang HK, McGinty JF, Hong JS. Differential modulation of striatonigral dynorphin and enkephalin by dopamine receptor subtypes. *Brain Res* 1989; 507:57–64.
19. Li S, Sivam SP, Hong JS. Regulation of the concentration of dynorphin A1–8 in the striatonigral pathway by the dopaminergic system. *Brain Res* 1986;398:390–2.
20. deleted in proof.
21. Normand E, Popovici T, Onteniente B, et al. Dopaminergic neurons of the substantia nigra modulate preproenkephalin A gene expression in rat striatal neurons. 1988.
22. Goldman-Rakic PS, Selemon LD. Topography of corticostriatal projections in nonhuman primates and implications for functional parcellation of the neostriatum. In: Jones EG, Peters A, eds. *Cerebral cortex,* vol 5. New York: Plenum, 1986;447–66.
23. Kunzle H. An autoradiographic analysis of the efferent connections from premotor and adjacent prefrontal regions (areas 6 and 9) in *Macaca fascicularis. Brain Behav Evol* 1978;15:135–234.

24. Yeterian EH, Van Hoesen GW. Cortico-striate projections in the rhesus monkey: the organization of certain cortico-caudate connections. *Brain Res* 1978;139:43–63.
25. Alexander GE, DeLong MR, Strick PL. Parallel organization of functionally segregated circuits linking basal ganglia and cortex. *Annu Rev Neurosci* 1986;9:357–81.
26. Heimer L. The olfactory cortex and the ventral striatum. In: Livingston KE, Hornykiewicz O, eds. *Limbic mechanisms.* New York: Plenum, 1978;95–187.
27. Haber SN, Lynd E, Klein C, Groenewegen HJ. Topographic organization of the ventral striatal efferent projections in the rhesus monkey: an anterograde tracing study. *J Comp Neurol* 1990;293:282–98.
28. Haber SN, Lynd-Balta E, Mitchell SJ. The ventral pallidal link in the limbic circuit through the monkey basal ganglia. 1991 (Submitted).

Advances in Neurology, Vol. 58, edited by T. N. Chase, A. J. Friedhoff, and D. J. Cohen. Raven Press, Ltd., New York © 1992.

18

Issues in Genetic Linkage Studies of Tourette Syndrome

Phenotypic Spectrum and Genetic Model Parameters

David L. Pauls

Department of Genetics, Child Study Center, Yale University School of Medicine, New Haven, Connecticut 05610

Understanding of the inheritance of Tourette syndrome (TS) has advanced considerably over the last decade. At the time of the first International Tourette Syndrome Symposium in 1981, the first family history studies were being completed and hypotheses regarding genetic factors were being proposed. Now, at the time of the second International Tourette Syndrome Symposium, a consortium of researchers from the Untied States and several countries throughout the world is engaged in genetic linkage studies designed to localize a gene or genes for TS.

Genetic linkage studies were undertaken because all published reports of genetic analyses suggested that the TS spectrum is inherited as a single gene (1–7). Genetic linkage studies provide a powerful method for confirming the conclusions of segregation analysis studies, since linkage results can demonstrate the existence of a major locus and help clarify the pattern of inheritance.

The localization of a gene or genes responsible for the expression of TS will be a major step forward in our understanding of the genetic/biological risk factors important for the expression of this syndrome. In addi-

tion, this work will allow the potential identification of nongenetic factors associated with the manifestation or the amelioration of the symptoms of the disorder (8,9). On the one hand, the identification of a linked marker will permit the design of much more incisive studies to illuminate the physiological/biochemical etiology of TS by examination of the gene product and its impact on the manifestation of the syndrome. On the other hand, by controlling for genetic factors it will be possible to document more carefully the environmental/nongenetic factors important for the expression of the TS spectrum.

For these linkage studies to be successful, there are a number of issues that need to be resolved. This paper will focus on two: (a) characterization of the phenotype; and (b) estimation of the parameters of the genetic model that best describes the mode of inheritance of the phenotype. With regard to the phenotype, it is necessary to understand what range of behaviors constitutes the full spectrum of TS. For example, it is important to know to what extent chronic tics and/or obsessive–compulsive symptoms are variant expressions of TS. Inclusion of individuals as affected, when in fact they are not, can be ruinous to genetic linkage studies. With regard to the genetic model, it is necessary to obtain reliable estimates of the parameters of the model that best describes the mode of transmission of this phenotype within families. Including the wrong genetic model in the linkage analyses can lead to spurious results (10). For example, if an inappropriate model is used, it could be falsely concluded that there is no linkage (11).

CHARACTERIZATION OF THE PHENOTYPE

All of the early studies examining the familiality of TS combined individuals with chronic tics (CT) or TS into a single affected category because it was assumed that chronic tics represented a milder manifestation of the syndrome. Based on this assumption, several studies were published that were consistent with the hypothesis that TS was familial. Two studies demonstrated an increased frequency of a positive family history of tics in the families of TS patients (12,13). Since these studies did not estimate rates of illness among relatives, it was not possible to determine if the increase in positive family history of tics actually represented a significant increase in the rate of TS and CT among the relatives of TS probands (14). The first study to estimate rates of TS and CT was reported by Kidd and coworkers (15). These investigators also combined TS and CT into a single category and demonstrated that the rate of tics among the first-degree relatives was significantly elevated over what would be expected by chance.

Pauls and colleagues (16) examined empirically this hypothesis of relationship between TS and CT. Their results suggested that: (a) CT appeared to represent a variant expression of TS; (b) the rate of both TS and CT was elevated in families of TS probands; and (c) the patterns of occurrence of TS and CT were consistent with hypotheses of vertical transmission. Several additional studies have replicated these early results regarding TS and CT (17–19).

As will be discussed below, it may be necessary to reconsider the relationship between TS and CT in the light of findings from segregation analyses. Given the frequency of tics in the general population, it is possible that many of the relatives in TS families have tics that are not genetically related to TS. Inclusion of these individuals in genetic linkage analyses could be problematic.

In addition to CT, other disorders have been hypothesized to be part of the spectrum of behaviors associated with TS (17,20–24). These include obsessive–compulsive disorder (OCD), attention deficit hyperactivity disorder, and learning disorders, among others. There is considerable controversy regarding this hypothesis (25), with one exception; the majority of investigators who have studied TS agree that obsessive–compulsive-like symptoms are related to the syndrome (26).

The hypothesis that OCD is a variant manifestation of the syndrome grew out of a number of studies documenting the increased frequency of obsessive–compulsive symptomatology among TS patients (27–38). Preliminary results from the Yale Family Study of Gilles de la Tourette's syndrome suggested that OCD alone (no current or past history of tics) could represent a variant expression of TS (39). Several recent studies have supported these findings (19,40–42).

The most convincing support for the hypothesis that OCD is a variant expression of the syndrome comes from family data showing that the rate of OCD is increased significantly regardless of whether the TS proband has a concomitant diagnosis of OCD (Table 1), that is, the rate of OCD is equally high in families of probands with both TS and OCD, and families of probands with TS only.

It is particularly noteworthy that the

TABLE 1. *Age-corrected rates of TS, CT, and OCD among first-degree relatives of TS probands with and without OCD*

Diagnosis of relative	Diagnosis of proband	
	TS − OCD	TS + OCD
TS	0.090 ± 0.020	0.081 ± 0.026
CT	0.176 ± 0.027	0.170 ± 0.036
OCD	0.104 ± 0.023	0.136 ± 0.036

CT, chronic tics; OCD, obsessive–compulsive disorder; TS, Tourette syndrome.

expression of OCD appears to be sex-related. It is a common observation that more males than females exhibit TS. Initial studies suggested that the transmission of the syndrome was related to this sex difference, since relatives of females with TS were at greater risk for TS and CT than relatives of TS males (15,16). Recent data do not support this early finding (43). Nevertheless, there appears to be a sex-related expression of the syndrome. OCD by itself occurs more frequently in female relatives of TS probands (19). Data in Table 2 illustrate this pattern; males are more likely to express TS and females are more likely to express OCD in the absence of any tics. The rate of CT is slightly elevated among males but the difference is not significant. This pattern of relationship has been replicated in several studies (37,41).

There is debate as to whether the individuals in TS families who manifest obsessive compulsive–compulsive-like symptoms actually meet diagnostic criteria for obses-

TABLE 2. *Age-corrected rates of TS, CT, and OCD among first-degree relatives of TS probands*

Diagnosis	Sex of Relative	
	Male (n = 158)	Female (n = 180)
TS	0.150 ± 0.030	0.034 ± 0.014
CT	0.215 ± 0.034	0.138 ± 0.024
OCD	0.072 ± 0.023	0.152 ± 0.030
Total	0.430 ± 0.042	0.318 ± 0.037

For abbreviations, see footnote to Table 1.

sive–compulsive disorder (see Leonard, *this volume*). However, there is general agreement that these individuals have obsessive-like symptoms and that in many of them, these symptoms do interfere with daily functioning. Thus, it is important to assess all relatives carefully for obsessive–compulsive symptomatology in families being studied for genetic linkage so that they may be included in the analyses.

ESTIMATION OF THE GENETIC MODEL PARAMETERS

Most linkage analyses require that the parameters of the genetic model for the mode of inheritance be specified. Misspecification of the genetic model results in reduced power (10) and could lead to false-negative results when included in multipoint linkage analyses (11). Thus, it is important to obtain valid and reliable estimates of the genetic model parameters before linkage analyses are undertaken.

A number of studies designed to test specific hypotheses regarding the mode of transmission of TS and related conditions have been completed over the last decade. Five studies (1–5) analyzed family history data and two used family study data (6,7).

Of the five studies using family history data, all reported that the pattern of inheritance within families was consistent with a genetic hypothesis that postulated the existence of a single gene of major effect that conferred susceptibility to TS and/or CT. However, this was not the only hypothesis supported. Kidd and Pauls (2) were unable to reject an hypothesis of multifactorial-polygenic transmission. (This hypothesis posits that there are many genes, each with equal and additive effect, which contribute to the expression of the disorder.) Although the single-locus hypothesis provided the best fit to the data, the multifactorial-polygenic hypothesis could not be rejected statistically. Comings and colleagues (3) also could not reject the multifactorial-polygenic hypothesis unless extended relatives were included and the population prevalence for TS and CT was restricted to be less than 0.0075. Nevertheless, the consistent conclusion in all studies was that a two-allele single major-locus genetic model best explained the observed data.

A single locus with two alleles results in three possible genotypes. Let *TS* represent the susceptibility allele for the Tourette syndrome spectrum of behaviors and *TSTS*, *TSts* and *tsts* represent the three possible genotypes. The probability that a specific genotype will result in a particular phenotype (e.g., TS or CT) is defined as the penetrance. By convention f_2 is the penetrance for the genotype with two susceptibility alleles (*TSTS*); f_1 is the penetrance for the heterozygous genotype (*TSts*); and f_0 is the penetrance for the genotype with no susceptibility alleles (*tsts*). For classical autosomal dominant mendelian inheritance $f_2 = f_1 = 1.0$ and $f_0 = 0.0$. For recessive inheritance $f_2 = 1.0$ and $f_1 = f_0 = 0.0$. When f_2 is less than 1.0, the disorder is said to be incompletely penetrant, and is referred to as a complex disorder because the pattern of inheritance is not strictly mendelian. If $f_2 > f_1 > f_0$ then the disorder does not follow either a dominant or recessive pattern and, each genotype has a unique probability of expressing the phenotype.

The maximum likelihood solutions for the best single-locus models obtained in each of the five studies are presented in Table 3. The estimates of penetrance (f_2, f_1, f_0) var-

ied considerably from study to study. Thus, while the results from all studies were consistent with a single-locus hypothesis, not all studies supported an identical model of inheritance. Results from three of the studies (1,3,5) were consistent with an autosomal dominant hypothesis. The remaining two studies reported unequal f_2 and f_1 values that were not consistent with dominant inheritance. Using any of these parameter sets in genetic linkage analyses could lead to spurious evidence regarding the location of a gene for TS.

Comings et al. (44) have recently hypothesized that the mode of inheritance for TS is not strictly dominant or recessive. They suggest that the inheritance of TS may be best described as "semi-dominant, semi-recessive." This hypothesis is based on the assumption that a wide range of other behaviors are also manifestations of the TS gene. Family history data are presented that suggest that obsessive–compulsive behavior, panic attacks, attention deficit hyperactivity disorder, alcohol and/or drug abuse, eating disorders (including obesity), and other psychiatric conditions are elevated among first-, second- and third-degree relatives of TS probands. Since many of their families have relatives with these disorders on both maternal and paternal sides of the family, these authors propose that a single dose of the TS gene will be likely to result in these variant expressions and a double dose (i.e., homozygosity) will be more likely to result in TS. No formal segregation

TABLE 3. *Results of genetic analyses including TS and CT as affected Sex-specific penetrance[a]*

Study	f_2		f_1		f_0	
	Male	Female	Male	Female	Male	Female
Baron et al. (1)	0.953	0.875	0.812	0.640	0.018	0.004
Kidd and Pauls (2)	0.933	0.774	0.309	0.106	0.000	0.000
Comings et al. (3)	0.987	0.893	0.677	0.297	0.006	0.000
Devor (4)	0.999	0.999	0.125	0.015	0.001	0.000
Price et al. (5)	0.789	0.763	0.789	0.763	0.004	0.003
Pauls and Leckman (6)	0.999	0.560	0.999	0.560	0.009	0.000
Pauls et al. (7)	0.999	0.600	0.999	0.600	0.010	0.000

For abbreviations, see footnote to Table 1.

analyses are presented to support their hypothesis, and no genetic model parameters are provided for inclusion in linkage analyses.

As indicated, all of these studies relied on family history data, that is, the diagnosis of the relatives was based on information obtained from one or two informants within a family; not all of the relatives were personally interviewed. It has been demonstrated that family history data underestimate the "true" rates of neuropsychiatric disorders (including TS and CT) obtained with direct interviews (18,45,46). Thus, segregation analyses using family history data could give inaccurate genetic model parameters. To address the potential problem of underestimation of rates in family history studies, the Yale Family Study of Tourette's Syndrome was undertaken in 1981. In this study, all available first-degree relatives were personally assessed using a structured psychiatric interview. These interview data were then used to assign a wide range of diagnoses, including TS and CT. All diagnoses were made independently by two raters who were blind to the diagnosis of the proband.

Segregation analyses of these family study data suggested that the most likely mode of transmission for TS and related conditions was autosomal dominant inheritance and provided estimates of the genetic model parameters that were based on direct interview data (6). Of note is that the autosomal dominant hypothesis was supported with three different diagnostic schemes: (a) when only relatives with TS were considered to be affected; (b) when relatives with TS or CT were considered to be affected; and (c) when relatives with TS, CT, or OCD were included as affected. Furthermore, these results were replicated with data collected for a linkage study of TS (7) (see Table 3). While some nuclear families within the large extended Canadian family are consistent with the hypothesis proposed by Comings and colleagues (44), the segregation analysis findings suggest that when

the entire multigenerational data set is used, the most likely mode of inheritance is autosomal dominant. These results are observed even when very high population prevalences for TS and CT are used in the analyses. Segregation analyses of additional families have also provided results consistent with autosomal dominant inheritance (Pauls, unpublished data).

While the segregation analyses suggest an autosomal dominant mode of transmission, goodness-of-fit tests using the parameters obtained from segregation analyses suggest that including just TS and CT may be inappropriate. Price et al. (5) reported that, even though segregation analyses suggested that inheritance was autosomal dominant, the comparison between observed rates in the families and those predicted from the best genetic model obtained with segregation analyses were significantly different from one another when CT was assumed to be part of the spectrum of the syndrome. Pauls and Leckman (6) also reported that the goodness-of-fit comparison of the observed and expected rates for the solution, including only individuals with TS and CT, resulted in a significant chi square. Thus, it appears that not all individuals with CT in the families of TS probands have a form of the syndrome.

It would be helpful to have some observable characteristic that would allow the identification of those individuals who have the tics that are related to the syndrome. One such possible characteristic could be the co-occurrence of obsessive–compulsive symptoms and tics (CT + OCD). To determine if that subset would be likely to represent a form related to the TS spectrum, the rates of TS, CT + OCD, and OCD alone were tabulated in the families included in the Yale Family Study. The results are presented in Table 4. There is a remarkable symmetry observed in males and females, suggesting that these individuals may represent an etiologically related subset of tics. What remains to be done is to include these individuals in formal segregation analyses

TABLE 4. *Age-corrected rates of TS, CT, and OCD among first-degree relatives of TS probands*

Diagnosis	Sex of relative	
	Male (n = 158)	Female (n = 180)
TS	0.150 ± 0.030	0.034 ± 0.014
CT + OCD	0.016 ± 0.012	0.038 ± 0.015
OCD	0.072 ± 0.023	0.152 ± 0.030
Total	0.231 ± 0.036	0.215 ± 0.033

For abbreviations, see footnote to Table 1.

to determine if the results are consistent with a simple genetic model and whether the parameters of that model accurately predict the rates observed in the relatives of TS probands.

Determining the range of expression of the TS spectrum is critical for linkage studies. If there are individuals with tics that are not genetically related to TS in these families, including them in the linkage analyses will result in reduced power and the possibility of missing a linkage relationship altogether. False-positive diagnoses can be fatal to any genetic linkage studies. The most conservative approach would be to include only individuals in the linkage analysis who have a definite diagnosis of TS. At the present time, however, the number of relatives with TS is too small in any given family to allow definitive analyses for that family. Thus it is necessary to include relatives with a variant form of the illness most likely to be due to the same underlying genes as TS itself. Given the replication of the OCD findings and the pattern when relatives with CT + OCD are included, it seems reasonable to reanalyze the existing data including relatives with these diagnoses.

REFERENCES

1. Baron M, Shapiro E, Shapiro A, Ranier JD. Genetic analysis of Tourette syndrome suggesting a major gene. *Am J Hum Genet* 1981;33:767–75.
2. Kidd KK, Pauls DL. Genetic hypotheses from Tourette syndrome. In: Friedhoff AJ, Chase TN, eds. *Gilles de la Tourette syndrome.* New York: Raven Press, 1982;243–9.
3. Comings DE, Comings BG, Devor EJ, Cloninger CR. Detection of a major gene for Gilles de la Tourette syndrome. *Am J Hum Genet* 1984; 36:586–600.
4. Devor EJ. Complex segregation analysis of Gilles de la Tourette syndrome: further evidence for a major locus mode of transmission. *Am J Hum Genet* 1984;36:704–9.
5. Price RA, Pauls DL, Kruger SD, Caine ED. Family data support a dominant major gene for Tourette syndrome. *Psychiatr Res* 1988;24:251–61.
6. Pauls DL, Leckman JF. The inheritance of Gilles de la Tourette's syndrome and associated behaviors: evidence for autosomal dominant transmission. *N Engl J Med* 1986;315:993–7.
7. Pauls DL, Pakstis AJ, Kurlan R, et al. Segregation and linkage analyses of Gilles de la Tourette's syndrome and related disorders. *J Am Acad Child Adolesc Psychiatry* 1990;29:195–203.
8. Pauls DL. Emerging genetic markers and their role in potential preventive intervention strategies. In: Muehrer P, ed. *Conceptual research models for preventing mental disorders.* Rockville, MD: NIMH, 1990;184–95.
9. Leckman JF, Dolnansky ES, Hardin M, et al. The perinatal factors in the expression of Tourette's syndrome. *J Am Acad Child Adolesc Psychiatry* 1990;29:220–6.
10. Clerget-Darpoux F, Bonaiti-Pellie C, Hochez J. Effects of misspecifying genetic parameters in lod score analysis. *Biometrics* 1986;42:393–400.
11. Guiffra LA. *Genetic analysis of complex traits.* PhD Thesis, Yale University 1991.
12. Eldridge R, Sweet R, Lake CR, Ziegler M, Shapiro AK. Gilles de la Tourette's syndrome: clinical, genetic, psychological and biochemical aspects in 21 selected families. *Neurology* 1977;27:115–24.
13. Shapiro AK, Shapiro ES, Bruun RD, Sweet RD. *Gilles de la Tourette's syndrome.* New York: Raven Press, 1978.
14. Wilson RS, Garron DC, Klawans HL. Significance of genetic factors in Gilles de la Tourette syndrome: a review. *Behav Genet* 1978;8:503–10.
15. Kidd KK, Prusoff BA, Cohen DJ. The familial pattern of Tourette syndrome. *Arch Gen Psychiatry* 1980;37:1336–9.
16. Pauls DL, Cohen DJ, Heimbuch R, Detlor J, Kidd KK. Familial pattern and transmission of Gilles de la Tourette syndrome and multiple tics. *Arch Gen Psychiatry* 1981;38:1091–3.
17. Comings DE, Comings BG. A controlled study of Tourette syndrome. I. Attention deficit disorder, learning disorders and school problems. *Am J Hum Genet* 1987;41:701–41.
18. Pauls DL, Kruger SD, Leckman JF, Cohen DJ, Kidd KK. The risk of Tourette syndrome (TS) and chronic multiple tics (CMT) among relatives of TS patients: obtained by direct interview. *J Am Acad Child Psychiatry* 1984;23:134–7.
19. Pauls DL, Raymond CL, Leckman JF, Stevenson JM. A family study of Tourette's syndrome. *Am J Hum Genet* 1991;48:154–63.
20. Comings DE, Comings BG. A controlled study of

Tourette syndrome. II. Conduct. *Am J Hum Genet* 1987;41:742–60.

21. Comings DE, Comings BG. A controlled study of Tourette syndrome. III. Phobias and panic attacks. *Am J Hum Genet* 1987;41:761–81.

22. Comings DE, Comings BG. A controlled study of Tourette syndrome. IV. Obesessions, compulsions and schizoid behaviors. *Am J Hum Genet* 1987;41:782–803.

23. Comings DE, Comings BG. A controlled study of Tourette syndrome. V. Depression and mania. *Am J Hum Genet* 1987;41:804–21.

24. Comings DE, Comings BG. A controlled study of Tourette syndrome. VI. Early development, sleep problems, allergies and handedness. *Am J Hum Genet* 1987;41:823–38.

25. Pauls DL, Cohen DJ, Kidd KK, Leckman JF. Tourette's syndrome and neuropsychiatric disorders: is there a genetic relationship? *Am J Hum Genet* 1988;43:206–9.

26. Towbin KE. Obsessive-compulsive symptoms in Tourette's syndrome. In: Cohen DJ, Bruun R, Leckman JF, eds. *Tourette syndrome and tic disorders: clinical understanding and treatment.* New York: John Wiley & Sons, 1988;138–49.

27. Kelman DH. Gilles de la Tourette's disease in children: a review of the literature. *J Child Psychol Psychiatry* 1965;6:219–26.

28. Fernando SJM. Gilles de la Tourette's syndrome. *Br J Psychiatry* 1967;113:115–24.

29. Morphew JA, Sim M. Gilles de la Tourette's syndrome: a clinical and psychopathological study. *Br J Med Psychol* 1969;42:293–301.

30. Nee LE, Caine ED, Polinsky RJ, Eldridge R, Ebert MH. Gilles de la Tourette syndrome: clinical and family study of 50 cases. *Ann Neurol* 1980;7:41–9.

31. Yaryura-Tobias JA, Neziroglu F, Howard S, Fuller B. Clinical aspects of Gilles de la Tourette syndrome. *Orthomolec Psychiatry* 1981;10:263–8.

32. Jagger J, Prusoff BA, Cohen DJ, Kidd KK, Carbonari CM, John K. The epidemiology of Tourette's syndrome: a pilot study. *Schizophr Bull* 1982; 8:267–78.

33. Montgomery MA, Clayton PJ, Friedhoff AJ. Psychiatric illness in Tourette syndrome patients and first-degree relatives. In: Friedhoff AJ, Chase TN, eds. *Gilles de la Tourette syndrome.* New York: Raven Press, 1982;335–9.

34. Nee LE, Polinsky RJ, Ebert MH. Tourette syndrome: clinical and family studies. In: Friedhoff

AJ, Chase TN, eds. *Gilles de la Tourette syndrome.* New York: Raven Press, 1982;291–5.

35. Stefl ME. Mental health needs associated with Tourette syndrome. *Am J Public Health* 1984; 74:1310–3.

36. Cummings JL, Frankel M. Gilles de la Tourette syndrome and the neurological basis of obsessions and compulsions. *Biol Psychiatry* 1985;20: 1117–26.

37. Robertson MM, Trimble MR, Lees AJ. The psychopathology of the Gilles de la Tourette syndrome: a phenomenological analysis. *Br J Psychiatry* 1988;152:383–90.

38. Robertson MM. The Gilles de la Tourette syndrome: the current status. *Br J Psychiatry* 1989; 154:147–69.

39. Pauls DL, Towbin KE, Leckman JF, Zahner GEP, Cohen DJ. Gilles de la Tourette syndrome and obsessive compulsive disorder: evidence supporting an etiological relationship. *Arch Gen Psychiatry* 1986;43:1180–2.

40. Frankel M, Cummings JL, Robertson MM, Trimble MR, Hill MA, Benson DF. Obsessions and compulsions in the Gilles de la Tourette syndrome. *Neurology* 1986;36:379–82.

41. Pitman RK, Green RC, Jenike MA, Mesulam MM. Clinical comparison of Tourette's disorder and obsessive-compulsive disorder. *Am J Psychiatry* 1987;144:1166–71.

42. Walkup JT, Leckman JF, Price RA, Harden MT, Ort S, Cohen DJ. The relationship between Tourette syndrome and obsessive compulsive disorder: a twin study. *Psychopharmacol Bull* 1988;24: 375–9.

43. Pauls DL, Leckman JF. The genetics of Gilles de la Tourette's syndrome. In: Cohen DJ, Bruun R, Leckman JF, eds. *Tourette syndrome and tic disorders: clinical understanding and treatment.* New York: John Wiley & Sons, 1988;91–102.

44. Comings DE, Comings BG, Knell E. Hypothesis: homozygosity in Tourette syndrome. *Am J Med Genet* 1989;34:413–21.

45. Andreason NC, Endicott J, Spitzer RL, Winokur G. The family history method using diagnostic criteria: reliability and validity. *Arch Gen Psychiatry* 1977;34:1229–35.

46. Orvaschel H, Thompson WD, Belanger A, Prusoff BA, Kidd KK. Comparison of the family history method to direct interview: factors affecting the diagnosis of depression. *J Affective Disord* 1982; 4:49–59.

Advances in Neurology, Vol. 58, edited by T. N. Chase, A. J. Friedhoff, and D. J. Cohen. Raven Press, Ltd., New York © 1992.

19

Tourette Symptoms in 161 Related Family Members

*William M. McMahon, †Mark Leppert, ‡Francis Filloux, §Ben J.M. van de Wetering, and ‖Sandra Hasstedt

Department of Psychiatry and Primary Children's Hospital, University of Utah Health Sciences Center, Salt Lake City, Utah 84132, †Department of Human Genetics and Howard Hughes Medical Institute, University of Utah Health Sciences Center, Salt Lake City, Utah 84132, ‡Departments of Neurology and Pediatrics, University of Utah Health Sciences Center, Salt Lake City, Utah 84132, ‖ Department of Human Genetics, University of Utah Health Sciences Center, Salt Lake City, Utah 84132, §University Hospital Rotterdam, Rotterdam, The Netherlands

This report summarizes our preliminary clinical and genetic research on a family that provides unusual potential for genetic study. This remarkable pedigree descended from one man, deceased in 1954, who manifested a history of Tourette syndrome (TS) and who produced 43 offspring and over 500 living descendants.

In the autumn of 1988, a 10-year-old boy came with his mother seeking consultation at the Learning Problems Clinic of Primary Children's Hospital in Salt Lake City. He exhibited chronic multiple motor and vocal tics with the characteristic waxing and waning course. More importantly, he was 1 of 15 living sibs, of which 4 others presented a similar history of tics. The mother listened attentively as we discussed the genetics of TS, and responded with the belief that her family could be of help. She described the size of the family and its historical and religious doctrine encouraging large families. She left the clinic with the promise that she would discuss TS with family members, and would call if family members were interested. That call came 4 months later, initiating our project.

Our proband's grandfather, born in 1894, had a history of multiple vocal and motor tics, as reported by a number of family members. During the course of his lifetime, he had married ten women and produced 43 children. Four of his wives were still living, although advanced in age. Extensive pedigree information was available, tracing family lineage back in time to the 1600s. Counting our proband as a member of Generation III, and his grandfather as Generation I, we could identify four living generations in the five family branches thought to exhibit TS. Many large sibships (16 siblings) adorned the family tree. Counting married-in spouses, 523 living members filled in the five branches (Table 1).

All diagnoses are based on direct assessment of each subject by at least one research physician expert in diagnosis of TS and associated conditions. For children, parent interview supplemented direct interview of the child. For diagnostic interviewing, we adapted the Tourette's Syndrome Association (TSA) Unified Tic Rating Scale by adding the Shapiro Checklist (1). We in-

TABLE 1. *Kindred 1591, all branches*

Branch number	Living members	Interviewed	No TS-OCD	TS CMT	History TS-CMT	Tics (≥5)	OCD	TIC	#	STUT
8	127	71	21	34	5	36	4	2	12	18
6	37	7	0	7	0	5	0	0	2	3
5	105	22	11	6	0	4	0	1	2	6
4	177	39	13	9	7	12	1	2	6	9
3	77	22	5	3	3	7	0	1	1	7
Total	523	161	50	59	15	64	5	6	23	43

CMT, chronic multiple tics; OCD, obsessive–compulsive disorder; STUT, stuttering; TS, Tourette syndrome, habitual counting.

cluded educational and medical history with specific items for obsessive–compulsive disorder (OCD) and attention deficit hyperactivity disorder (ADHD). We have also begun collecting Yale-Brown Obsessive Compulsive Scales (2). Diagnostic criteria are those specified in the *Diagnostic and Statistical Manual* of the American Psychiatric Association, 3rd ed, revised (DSM-III-R) (3).

CLINICAL FINDINGS

Our findings should be regarded as preliminary since we have interviewed only 161 family members, 31% of the 523 living members in the five Tourette branches we have studied (Table 1). Our initial efforts have probably biased this sample toward increased incidence, since we began with those family members who expressed interest. Presumably those interested are more likely to have recognized symptoms in themselves and close relatives. However, no family member had previously ever been clinically diagnosed or treated for TS or OCD. Both affected and unaffected individuals showed unusual tolerance for what they referred to as "the family twitch." As Table 1 shows, the five branches range in size from 37 to 177 members. We have interviewed more members of Branch 8 than any other, 71 of 127, or 56%. Of those interviewed, we define "No TS-OCD" to mean no history or manifestations of any tic disorder, or OCD. We found 50 of 161 interviewed subjects (31%) to be "No TS-OCD."

We have combined the categories of TS and chronic multiple tic (TS-CMT) but separated those who manifested definite tics during an interview from those who gave a history for TS or CMT but did not show tics during the interview (History TS-CMT in Table 1.). Thus 37%, 59 of 161, presented signs of at least CMT; another 9% (15 of 161) gave only a history of TS or CMT. Using number of simple and complex tics reported as a measure of severity, 64 of 74 subjects (86%) who remembered past tics recalled at least five tics. Several members reported having up to 25 separate tics during their lifetime. Adults typically reported that tic number, frequency, intensity, and interference peaked in late childhood and early adolescence with subsequent decrease in adulthood. OCD was diagnosed in five individuals. Finally, six members presented with only a single tic. Because of our uncertainty about the boundaries of the TS phenotype, we were particularly interested in complex repetitive phenomena. Habitual counting (arithromania) was present in 23 family members. Stuttering occurred in 43.

TABLE 2. *Diagnosis by sex*

	Definite TS	Definite CMT	OCD	Total
Male	25	9	0	34
Female	22	3	5	30

For abbreviations, see footnote to Table 1.

TABLE 3. *Complex symptoms in 47 individuals with definite Tourette syndrome*

	Coprolalia	Mental coprolalia	Palilalia	Echolalia	Echopraxia	Stutter
Male (no.)	0	2	5	12	6	10
Female (no.)	2	0	6	9	5	7
Percent	4	4	23	45	23	36

The sex ratio in this pedigree for individuals with definite TS was surprisingly near equal: 25 males and 22 females, or 1.1:1. For definite CMT, the ratio was 3:1, with 9 males and 3 females. OCD was found only in five females (Table 2).

To examine the phenotype further using the most clearly affected, we examined the history of complex symptomatology in the 47 members with definite TS (Table 3). Near equal gender rates were evident for echophenomena, with echolalia the most common, found in 21 subjects (45%). Coprolalia was quite rare, reported by only 2 of this 47 (4%). Mental coprolalia was also present in two members. No copropraxia was ascertained. We found stuttering in 17 (36%) of definite TS subjects.

Focusing more narrowly on the incidence of stuttering in different diagnostic categories, we noted that the presence of TS or CMT coincided with a twofold increase in stuttering over cases without chronic tics or OCD (Table 4). In subjects without tics or OCD, stuttering occurred in 17%, or 8 of 48. For 58 individuals with definite TS or CMT, 21 (36%) had a history of stuttering. Likewise, a history of TS or CMT but no tics on current exam showed a similar increase: 40%, or 6 of 15, such tic cases were also stutterers. Contrary to this finding in tic categories, no stutterers were found among the five individuals with OCD.

Because we were concerned about the possibility of inbreeding within this relatively isolated population, we examined mating relationships for potential consanguinity. We were able to trace the relatives of Generation I spouses back to 1831 in two wives, to 1793 in one, and to 1777 in another (Fig. 1). No inbreeding loops were identified, although records were incomplete in four of the five branches. In Branch 8, records were more complete: five of eight married-in spouses could be traced back to 1869 or earlier. Again, inbreeding loops could be ruled out for all married-in subjects traced in this branch.

On the other hand, assortative mating occurred in Generations II and III. Surprisingly, a total of six married-in spouses (three men and three women) were diagnosed with TS, CMT, or OCD. All men had definite TS, while one woman each had TS, CMT, and OCD. Only 11 spouses of the existing 90 have been interviewed.

SEGREGATION ANALYSIS

The unusually large size of Kindred 1591 allowed us to utilize segregation analysis on

TABLE 4. *Stuttering by diagnosis[a]*

	Definite TS-CMT	History TS-CMT	OCD	No TS-OCD	Total
Stutter	21 (36)	6 (37.5)	0 (0)	8 (17)	34 (27)
Nonstutter	37 (64)	10 (62.5)	5 (100)	40 (83)	91 (73)
Total	58	16	5	48	125

[a] Percent in parentheses.
For abbreviations, see footnote to Table 1.

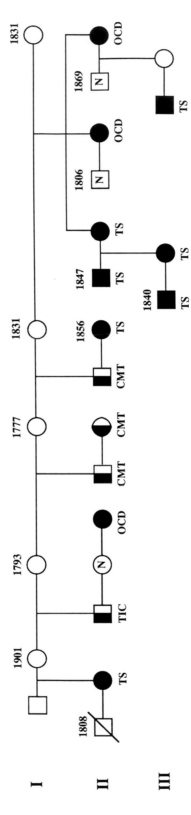

FIG. 1. Affection status of spouses in Kindred 1591. Dates refer to historical records ruling out inbreeding. For abbreviations, see footnote to Table 1.

this single family. We applied segregation analysis (4) to test for major locus inheritance of TS in the family. The genetic model specified each phenotype as the sum of independent effects attributed to segregation of two alleles at one locus, polygenic inheritance, and individual-specific random effects. We computed likelihoods of the genetic models (5) using the Pedigree Analysis Package (PAP) (6) and obtained the maxima using NPSOL (7). Table 5 presents chi-square statistics computed as the natural logarithm of the ratio of the likelihood of a submodel relative to the likelihood of a general model multiplied by negative two; the degrees of freedom equal the number of parameters restricted when specifying the submodel from the general model. The chi-square statistics support major locus inheritance of TS in this family. However, significant polygenic inheritance partially accounts for incomplete penetrance of the TS disease allele.

Unfortunately, the transmission of the TS allele within the pedigree deviates from mendelian ratios. One possible explanation of the nonmendelian transmission, that penetrance differs with age, proved nonsignificant when tested. We are still pursuing other explanations of the nonmendelian transmission, such as assortative mating. Nevertheless, assuming mendelian transmission, the most likely genetic model specified that 60% of individuals with at least one copy of the TS allele and 0.07% of individuals lacking the disease allele are affected. In this model, 49% of the variance within major locus genotypes was attributed to polygenic heritability.

TABLE 5. *Segregation analysis*

Null hypothesis	Chi-square	df	Significance (p value)
No major locus	34.74	3	<0.001
No polygenic effect	18.42	1	<0.001
Mendelian transmission	10.68	3	<0.05
No age effect	4.30	3	>0.5

Again, results should be considered preliminary because of incomplete sampling. Our results best support a major gene model, but cannot rule out a polygenic component.

LINKAGE ANALYSIS

Scoring of subjects as affected, unaffected, or unknown was first carried out using the categories developed under the auspices of the TSA (8). We included as affected three diagnostic groups: (a) definite Tourette on exam; (b) Tourette by history; (c) definite chronic multiple motor tic when tics were unambiguous and complex; and (d) positive diagnosis of OCD. Subjects with no tics and no OCD were considered unaffected. Finally, we scored as unknown those individuals with chronic single tic, transient tic, or chronic multiple tics when equivocal or absent on exam.

As segregation analysis in Kindred 1591 supported a single major gene mode of inheritance, we attempted to find a polymorphic DNA marker that cosegregated with the TS/CMT/OCD phenotype. We adopted both candidate and general linkage search approaches. Candidate genes tested for linkage in the entire Kindred 1591 included the dopamine D1 receptor on chromosome 5 and the dopamine D2 receptor on chromosome 11. Two regions of the genome in which cytogenetic anomalies were uncovered in sporadic TS patients were also tested with polymorphic markers for evidence of linkage: the chromosome 3p21-14 region (9) and the chromosome 9p23-pter region (10). Neither the candidate genes (D1 and D2 receptors) nor the probes in the candidate regions (c-raf and E41 on chromosome 3p, and ovc 2.2 on chromosome 9p) supported linkage. The LOD scores for all candidate markers were heavily negative, with the exception of the D1 locus, which yielded a small positive LOD score of 0.47 at a recombination distance of 0.001. Fifty-eight additional markers were typed in

Kindred 1591 and analyzed for linkage assuming for the disease allele a penetrance of 0.8 and a frequency of 0.001. The two-point LOD scores for all markers at a recombination fraction of 0.001 in Kindred 1591 are listed in Table 6. None of the markers gave evidence of genetic linkage to the TS phenotype.

While much of Kindred 1591 remains to be examined, our results nevertheless support some conclusions about the phenotypic expression of the putative TS gene(s) in this family. First, TS need not be a crippling disorder. No member of this pedigree had ever been diagnosed or treated for TS or OCD. This lack of interference with life may reflect both a mild intensity of tics and a remarkable tolerance for "the family twitch." Further quantification of both biological and psychosocial stressors and protectors in this family may provide a model for understanding the TS phenotype in others. Second, severity of tics decreases in most cases with age, particularly after early adolescence. Third, compared with the 30–40% rate of coprolalia reported in 11 published studies, coprolalia is quite uncommon (4%) in this family (11). On the other hand, echophenomena are common, with echolalia in 45% of those with definite TS. Fourth, the near equal male–female sex ratio for definite TS in this sample is discrepant with the ratios of 3:1 for adults and 9:1 for children found in the North Dakota epidemiologic study (12). Fifth, repetitive counting phenomenon occurs commonly and may be an alternative expression of the TS gene(s). Finally, stuttering as determined from personal history was observed in both TS/CMT individuals (36%) and in family members without TS, CMT, or tics (17%). The significance of these preliminary findings concerning stuttering is unclear. However, when a genetic marker is discovered for the TS locus, this family may elucidate the role of stuttering within the TS phenotype.

Assortative mating in this TS family deserves special mention. We have evidence that "like marries like." A total of six unre-

TABLE 6. *Linkage analysis in kindred 1591*

Chromosome	Probe	LOD score (0.001)
1	MCT58	−3.61
	MCT118	−4.05
2	YNH24	−14.0
	MCOE32	−6.08
3	c-RAF	−9.63
	30-1-60	−6.25
	E41	−3.15
	EFD145.1	−3.45
	YNZ86.1	−9.71
	MCOB29	+0.46
	CI3-340	−2.50
	HCP-1	−0.63
	MCT32.1	−5.90
	HHH129	−6.70
	Mfd2	−3.56
	Mfd4	−4.02
	Mfd17	−2.47
	Mfd30	−1.99
5	213-205-ED	−11.6
	JO157E-A	−6.73
	HF12-65	+0.20
	D1	+0.47
	L1200	+0.22
6	YNB3.6	−8.05
	YNZ132	−6.64
	MCOB12	−6.63
7	JCZ76	−15.0
8	HNFL	−0.38
	PLAT	−5.71
	YNM3	−5.95
	MCT128	−3.42
9	OVC2.2	−2.31
	THH22	−0.46
	MCOA112	−3.29
	EKZ19.3	−1.44
	MHZ13	−5.28
10	TBQ7	−1.64
	EFD75	−12.07
11	HGTH 4	−2.76
	TBB2	−5.89
	3C7	−4.27
	D2	−1.72
13	IE8	−3.52
14	HHH160	−9.19
	CMM101	−7.73
15	CMW-1	−2.07
	MS1-14	−10.9
	DP151	−3.15
	EFD52.1	−8.59
	EKZ104	−7.36
	THH55	−5.71
	EFD85.7	−10.89
16	CJ52.94	−8.28
	KKA22	−11.8
	CJ52.161	+0.17
17	KKA35	−5.85
20	MS1-27	−1.51
	RMR6	−1.73
21	D21S72	−3.60
	E8	+0.45
	EFD70.3	−2.40
	MCT15	−3.98
	G21RK	−3.62

lated spouses were found to have TS, CMT, or OCD. Since only 11 of 90 marry-in spouses have been interviewed, this number is a minimal estimate. Prevalence for adult TS reported by Burd et al. (12) is 1 in 13,000 in males. The three TS husbands that married into this family occurred in 7% of matings (3 of 45). Thus, husbands coming into the family have a rate of TS at least 1,000 times higher than the rate in the general population. Similar figures can be calculated for the three affected incoming wives. Furthermore, these rates may increase as the other 79 marry-in spouses are examined. Whether this represents a cultural phenomenon specific to this kindred or a more generalized attachment behavior remains to be seen.

REFERENCES

1. Shapiro AK, Shapiro ES, Brown RD, Sweet D. 1978; Gilles de la Tourette Syndrome. Raven Press: New York.
2. Goodman WL, Delgado P, Heninger GR, Charney DS. The Yale-Brown Obsessive Compulsive Scale. I. Development, use, reliability. *Arch Gen Psychiatry* 1989;46:1006–11.
3. American Psychiatric Association. *Diagnostic and statistical manual of mental disorders,* 3rd ed., revised. Washington, DC: American Psychiatric Association, 1987.
4. Lalouel JM, Rao DC, Morton NE, Elston RC. A unified model for complex segregation analysis. *Am J Hum Genet* 1983;35:816–26.
5. Elston RC, Stewart J. A general model for the genetic analysis of pedigree data. *Hum Hered* 1971; 21:523–42.
6. Hasstedt SJ. *PAP: pedigree analysis package,* rev 3. Salt Lake City: Department of Human Genetics, University of Utah, 1989.
7. Gill PE, Murray W, Saunders MA, Wright MH. *NPSOL: A fortran package for nonlinear programming.* Tech rep SOL 86-2, Department of Operations Research, Stanford University, 1986.
8. Kurlan R. Tourette's syndrome: current concepts. *Neurology* 1989;39:1625–30.
9. Brett P, Curtis D, Gourdie A, et al. Possible linkage of Tourette syndrome to markers on short arm of chromosome 3 (C3p21–14). Lancet 1990; 336:1076.
10. Krizman D. Report of the seventh genetic workshop on Tourette syndrome, June 15, 1991. Bayside, New York: Tourette Syndrome Association, 1991.
11. Brunn RD. The natural history of Tourette's syndrome. In: Cohen DJ, Bruun RD, Leckman JF, eds. *Tourette's syndrome and tic disorders.* New York: John Wiley & Sons, 1988;22–39.
12. Burd L, Kerbeshian J, Wikenheiser M, Fisher W. Prevalence of Gilles de la Tourette's syndrome in North Dakota adults. *Am J Psychiatry* 1986; 143:787–8.

Advances in Neurology, Vol. 58, edited by T. N. Chase, A. J. Friedhoff, and D. J. Cohen. Raven Press, Ltd., New York © 1992.

20

Genetic Study on Tourette Syndrome in The Netherlands

*Peter Heutink, †B.J.M. van de Wetering, *G.J. Breedveld, and ‡B.A. Oostra

Department of Clinical Genetics, Erasmus University and University Hospital Dijkzigt, 3000 DR Rotterdam, The Netherlands, †Department of Psychiatry, University Hospital Dijkzigt, 3015 GD Rotterdam, The Netherlands, ‡Department of Cell Biology, Erasmus University, 3000 DR Rotterdam, The Netherlands

When the biochemical cause of a genetic disease is known, it is possible to characterize the genetic defect by isolating and purifying the protein. With antibodies raised against this protein it is possible to isolate complementary DNA (cDNA) clones from an expression library. The messenger RNA (mRNA) sequence resulting from these cDNA clones can be used to localize and isolate the complete gene on genomic DNA. For Tourette syndrome (TS) the biochemical cause is not known. There have been reports on the involvement of the dopaminergic system, but the precise localization of the defect in the brain and the nature of the defect itself is still not clear. For disorders in which no biochemical defect is known, use of polymorphic DNA markers provide a way to isolate a gene. This method is called "positional cloning" (1). By correlating the inheritance of a distinct well-localized polymorphic marker with the inheritance of a disease, it is possible to determine the localization of the disorder on the human genome. With the use of more polymorphic markers in this region it may be possible to focus on the region in which the defective gene must be localized. When the region is small enough, genomic DNA li-

braries can be used to close the gap to the gene, and finally cDNAs from this region can be isolated that are candidate genes for the disorder. Either by carrying out expression studies with mRNA or by mutation analysis of these genes in patients, the defective gene can be isolated and the biochemical causes of the disorder studied (Fig. 1).

To find the gene(s) that is (are) involved in the development of TS, several research groups are performing "reverse genetics" studies on TS. At the Department of Clinical Genetics, Erasmus University, Rotterdam, an ongoing genetic study is making use of several strategies to localize the defective gene responsible for TS. Table 1.

SEARCH FOR CHROMOSOMAL ABNORMALITIES

Generally the karyotypes of patients with TS do not demonstrate chromosomal abnormalities (2). In our study we have examined the karyotypes of 18 sporadic cases of TS. All karyotypes were found to be normal. However, some TS patients have been described to have a chromosomal aberration. Comings et al. (3) presented evidence for

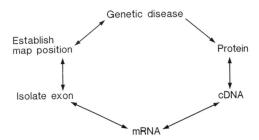

FIG. 1. Schematic presentation of the use of "positional cloning."

TABLE 2. *Candidate genes tested for linkage with TS*

Gene	Chromosomal localization
Dopamine receptor D1	5q
Dopamine receptor D2	11q22
Gastrin-releasing peptide	18
Tyrosine hydroxylase	11p15
Dopamine β-hydroxylase	9q34

the localization of the TS gene. They reported a 46,t,(7;18) (q22;q22.1) reciprocal translocation in six relatives suffering from TS. Their evidence suggested a localization of the TS gene near the 18q22.1 breakpoint. Donnai (4) reported a TS patient with a deletion of the long arm of chromosome at 18q22.1. These findings led to the tentative assignment of the TS gene to chromosome 18q22.1. In our family material, however, strong evidence for nonlinkage of TS with this localization was found (5), as described below.

SEARCH FOR OTHER DISEASES INHERITED WITH THE DISEASE

For a complex disorder like TS, linkage analysis could be simplified if the disorder would cosegregate, in one of the families that are studied, with a disorder that is already localized or segregates in an mendelian way. In all our families that are sampled for linkage analyses on TS there are no known diseases cosegregating with TS, pro-

TABLE 1. *Strategies to localize/isolate the TS gene*

Search for chromosomal abnormalities associated with the disease
Search for other diseases cosegregating with the disease
Candidate gene approach
Screening for restriction fragment length polymorphism (RFLP) markers linked to the disease locus

viding no clue about the possible localization of TS.

CANDIDATE GENE APPROACH

For TS a number of candidate genes have been proposed and tested, especially genes related to the dopaminergic system. None of the candidate genes tested in the Dutch and Norwegian families showed linkage with TS (5–7, unpublished results) (Table 2). Other candidate genes for TS are the dopamine receptors D3–D5 that have recently been cloned but remain to be tested. Also, one could regard several other neurotransmitter receptor genes or neurotransmitter genes as candidate genes.

The candidate gene approach appears to be an attractive approach to linkage analysis. The hypothesis of the involvement of a certain gene in the etiology of the disorder of interest can be directly tested. A number of candidate genes are proposed without a very strong indication that they are involved in causing TS. Those candidate genes that have been cloned, localized, and are polymorphic, however, can easily be included in a systematic screening of the human genome.

LINKAGE ANALYSIS IN THE DUTCH FAMILIES

The focus of the genetic studies carried out in Rotterdam is on a systematic screening of the human genome with polymorphic markers. In order to perform such a study it is necessary to obtain DNA from families in which TS segregates.

Ten extended families, comprising 321 subjects, participated in the study. The size of the available families varied from 6 to 60 subjects. All families were Dutch Caucasian, except for one Norwegian family of 32 subjects. All subjects were interviewed with a semistructured interview (D.L. Pauls, Yale University, New Haven, CT). This schedule includes an extensive questionnaire about tics in addition to a standardized psychiatric interview. Furthermore, a Dutch version of the Leyton Obsessional Inventory (LOI) was filled in by all Dutch subjects over the age of 15 years. TS and other tic syndromes were diagnosed using information from observation and the structured interview. Obsessive–compulsive symptoms (OCS) were assessed in two ways: (a) the method of structured interview; and (b) the Dutch version of the LOI.

There were four probands (all male, mean age 11 ± 2.6 years) without any OCS and six probands (three males, three females, mean age 21 ± 10.8 years) with OCS. Of 241 biologic relatives, 27 suffered from TS. The number of biologic relatives (36) with chronic multiple tics (CMT) was scarcely higher. Just above 60% of these subjects had no characteristics of the tic syndromes. Fifty-seven biologic relatives (23%) were affected by one or more OCSs. Of 70 nonbiologic relatives, none had TS, and two showed chronic tics.

Genetic analysis of family data of TS families has been extensive. Most studies have been consistent with the hypothesis that susceptibility to the disorder is most likely due to a single genetic locus with an autosomal dominant mode of inheritance and reduced penetrance, although other models cannot always be excluded (8). There is general agreement that in families affected by TS the CMT syndrome is a variant, milder phenotype of the disorder (9,10). Whether OCSs are etiologically related is still a matter of discussion.

By defining the phenotypes in this way there are four possible models to perform linkage analysis. The four models will show a broadening of the diagnostic criteria (Table 3). For each model the penetrance values, phenocopy rates, and gene frequencies must be determined.

The first goal for our study was to find evidence for the tentative assignment of the TS gene to chromosome 18q22.1. We selected polymorphic markers distributed over the whole length of chromosome 18. The selection was based on information from the Chromosome 18 Committee at Human Gene Mapping 9 (11). No evidence for linkage was found. Instead, strong evidence for nonlinkage was found. Combining the marker data in multipoint analyses enabled us to exclude the complete chromosome 18 as being the site of the TS gene in the Dutch families and the Norwegian family (5). The approach we used for chromosome 18 is the same as we employ for the rest of the human genome. We select polymorphic markers with a known localization and with the combination of two-point and multipoint analyses we try to find evidence for linkage. When no evidence can be found we calculate which area of the genome can be excluded for linkage with TS (7).

At present, 175 markers have been tested in the Dutch families. No strong and definite evidence for linkage was obtained. Although several markers produce positive LOD scores in a subset of families, these LOD scores have not yet reached a significant level and need further work in order to obtain more conclusive results. Approxi-

TABLE 3. *Genetic model used in linkage analysis*

Mode of inheritance: Autosomal dominant with reduced penetrance and variable expression
Diagnostic categories:
   Tourette syndrome (TS)
   TS and chronic multiple tics (CMT)
   TS, CMT, and obsessive–compulsive symptoms (OCS)
   TS, CMT, OCD, and other psychiatric symptoms

mately 45% of the human genome can be excluded as a site for the TS gene in the Dutch and Norwegian families. An estimation of those regions of the human genome that have been excluded in the Dutch study is depicted in Figure 2.

LINKAGE RESULTS OF THE COLLABORATING GROUPS

All the results obtained from linkage analyses were shared with the other groups in the consortium in order to work as efficiently as possible. Not all the groups work with the same family material. Under the assumption of homogeneity the data obtained in different families can be combined if the genetic parameters that are used in the linkage analysis are the same. The collaborating groups agreed to use the outcome of two segregation analyses (12,13) as the basis for the genetic parameters used in the linkage analyses. The most likely genetic model was used to combine the data (Table 4). The results of the linkage analyses from the collaborating groups are combined in exclusion maps as an extension of the data published by Pakstis et al. (7). An exact calculation of

the proportion of the human genome that has been excluded under homogeneity cannot be carried out. First, the exact length of the human autosomal map is not known; second, a number of markers are not exactly localized and therefore it is unknown whether their exclusion zones overlap with those of well-localized markers. If we make a conservative estimate based only the well-localized loci in the largest sex-specific maps, at least 80% of the human autosomes has been excluded. The remaining gaps in the map are mainly located on chromosomes 3, 4, 6, 9, 14, and 16. The number of well-localized polymorphic markers on these chromosomes is limited, and more markers have to be generated in order to gain conclusive results on these chromosomes.

Now that approximately 80% of the human genome has been excluded under the assumption of genetic homogeneity, several questions arise. Is there genetic heterogeneity? If there is genetic heterogeneity, the family material in Rotterdam is sufficient to detect a linkage with a subset of the families that are tested. Simulation analysis on the Dutch families makes clear that at least four families can detect a linkage by themselves. All the statistical analyses on the Dutch families are carried out on separate families prior to pooling the data for an overall outcome. Another important question is: Which phenotype should be regarded as an expression of the gene causing TS? Absolute certainty can only be given after the gene has been cloned. Until then we have to use the best estimate, and we will be testing the four different genetic models with broadening diagnostic criteria as described above. The collaborating groups have

TABLE 4. *Genetic model parameters*

Parameter	
Tourette syndrome including chronic multiple tic syndromes[a]	
Gene frequency	0.003–0.005
Penetrance	
Male	0.900
Female	0.600
Phenocopies	
Male	0.0002–0.005
Female	0.0000–0.0001

[a] Single autosomal dominant gene.

→

FIG. 2. Estimation of the chromosomal regions that can be excluded as a site for the TS gene in the Dutch and Norwegian families. Human autosomes are presented in chronological order from left to right. On the right side of each chromosome a *black bar* represents that part of the chromosome that can be excluded as the site for the TS gene when chronic multiple tics are included as a milder phenotype of the disorder.

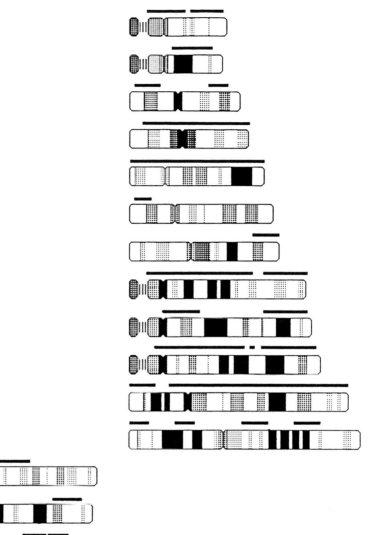
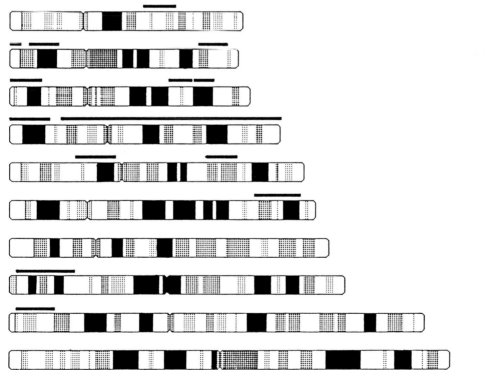

agreed to share more of their family material in order to screen the human genome more efficiently. Working this way is not only more efficient but allows independent replication of results, and it will certainly shorten the time until a positive linkage will be found.

Linkage will open the search for the isolation of the gene that is causing TS and will make it possible to define the genetic model in more detail. It will be the first step towards the unraveling of the defect in this gene.

REFERENCES

1. Orkin SH. Reverse genetics and human disease. *Cell* 1986;47:845–50.
2. Shapiro AK, Shapiro E, Bruun RD, Sweet RD. *Gilles de la Tourette syndrome*. New York: Raven Press, 1978.
3. Comings DE, Coming BG, Dietz G, et al. Evidence the Tourette syndrome gene is at 18q22.1. *Am J Hum Genet* 1986;39:447.
4. Donnai D. Gene location in Tourette syndrome. *Lancet* 1987;i:627.
5. Heutink P, van de Wetering BJM, Breedveld GJ, et al. No evidence for genetic linkage of Gilles de la Tourette syndrome on chromosome 7 and 18. *J Med Genet* 1990;27:433–6.
6. Devor EJ, Grandy DK, Civelli O, et al. Genetic linkage is excluded for the D2-dopamine receptor HD2G1 and flanking loci on chromosome 11q22-q23 in Tourette syndrome. *Hum Hered* 1990; 40:105–8.
7. Pakstis AJ, Heutink P, Pauls DL, et al. Progress in the search for genetic linkage with Tourette syndrome: an exclusion map covering more than 50% of the autosomal genome. *Am J Hum Genet* 1991; 48:281–94.
8. Shapiro AK, Shapiro ES, Young JG, Feinberg TE. *Gilles de la Tourette syndrome*, 2nd ed. New York: Raven Press, 1988.
9. Kurlan R, Behr J, Medved L, Shoulson I, Pauls D, Kidd KK. Severity of Tourette's syndrome in one large kindred: implication for determination of disease prevalence rate. *Arch Neurol* 1987;44:268–9.
10. Kurlan R. Tourette's syndrome: current concepts. *Neurology* 1989;39:1625–30.
11. Shaw D, Eiberg H. Report of the committee for chromosomes 17, 18, and 19. *Cytogenet Cell Genet* 1987;46:242–56.
12. Pauls DL, Leckman JF. The inheritance of Gilles de la Tourette syndrome and associated behaviours: evidence for autosomal dominant transmission. *N Engl J Med* 1986;315:993–7.
13. Pauls DL, Pakstis AJ, Kurlan R, et al. Segregation and linkage analyses of TS. *Am Acad Child Adolesc Psychiatry* 1990;29:195–203.

Advances in Neurology, Vol. 58, edited by T. N. Chase, A. J. Friedhoff, and D. J. Cohen. Raven Press, Ltd., New York © 1992.

21

Application of Microsatellite DNA Polymorphisms to Linkage Mapping of Tourette Syndrome Gene(s)

Patricia J. Wilkie, Peter A. Ahmann, Jeff Hardacre, Robert J. LaPlant, Bradley C. Hiner, and James L. Weber

Marshfield Medical Research Foundation, Marshfield, Wisconsin 54449

Mutations are one of the most powerful tools available to biologists. The study of chemotaxis in bacteria, protein secretion in yeast, development in flies, and many other systems has been greatly enhanced through analysis of mutations. In humans, the many thousands of available mutations in the form of genetic diseases represent a gold mine of new biological information. Genetic diseases like cystic fibrosis or Tourette syndrome (TS) warrant study simply because of the large numbers of individuals affected. However, even rare genetic diseases, which may affect <1/100,000 individuals, merit study because of the important biological information that can be extracted.

For the vast majority of genetic diseases, the affected proteins remain unknown. In these cases investigators must take a difficult and circuitous route to reach the disease gene and mutation. First, families that are afflicted by the disorder must be identified and family members examined. The mode of inheritance and inheritance parameters must also be established. Second, the disease gene must be assigned to an approximate chromosomal location through linkage mapping. This step often requires that hundreds of different DNA polymorphisms distributed throughout the genome be tested. Third, the initial, crude map position for the disease gene must be refined, and the correct gene within this interval identified. This last step has been accomplished to date only for a handful of genes. We have concentrated on the second step in this process, the initial linkage mapping of disease genes. A new class of human DNA polymorphisms, microsatellite DNA polymorphisms, have been used to improve the efficiency of this step significantly.

MICROSATELLITE DNA POLYMORPHISMS

Microsatellites are defined as relatively short runs of simple sequence tandem repeats. Repeat lengths for the microsatellites typically range from one up to five or six bases, and the total length of the run of repeats is usually <40 nucleotides; in virtually all cases it is <60 nucleotides. Examples of microsatellites with mononucleotide, dinucleotide, and tetranucleotide repeats are shown in Table 1.

In 1988, we found that microsatellites based on CA/GT dinucleotide repeats were polymorphic in length (1). In Europe, Bé Wieringa (2) and Diethard Tautz (3) inde-

TABLE 1. *Examples of human microsatellite DNA sequences*

AACCCCGCCA CCTTCCTTTT TTTTTTTTTT TTTTGAGATG GAGTTTCACT CTTATTGCCC ATGCTAGAGT
CCCCCACCCA ACACACACAC ACACACACAC ACACACACAC ACACACACAC CCTGCAATTA
CTAATTTTGT GTGTGTGTGT ATTGTTTGTG TGTGTGTGTG TGTGCGTGTG TGTGTGTGTG TATTT
CATGACTGTG TGTGTGTGTG TGTGTGTGTG TGTGTGTGTG TGTGTGTGTG TGAGAGAGAG
  AGAGAGGGAG ATGGAG
GTTTAATTGT AGATTTATTT ATTTATTTAT TTATTTATTT ATTTATTTAT TTATTTATAT GGAGTCTCTT

pendently and at about the same time also reached the same conclusion. Since then, several groups have demonstrated that microsatellites with other repeat sequences such as $(A)_n$, $(AAT)_n$, and $(AAAG)_n$ are also polymorphic in length (4–6). Microsatellite polymorphisms are analyzed by amplifying a short fragment of genomic DNA that contains a run of repeats. The polymerase chain reaction (PCR) primers for this amplification anneal to unique DNA that flanks the block of repeats on either side. The relatively short amplified DNA fragments are sized by electrophoresis through denaturing polyacrylamide gels. An example of the results obtained with this procedure are shown in Figure 1. All of the individuals represented in Figure 1 are heterozygous for the dinucleotide repeat polymorphism at the D19S49 locus, with the exception of the individual represented in lane H. Note that alleles differ in size by multiples of two nucleotides.

Microsatellite DNA polymorphisms have two particularly important advantages over polymorphisms detected by restriction enzyme digestion, blotting, and hybridization (RFLPs). One is that the microsatellite polymorphisms are, in general, about twice as informative as RFLPs. Average heterozygosities for microsatellite polymorphisms are about 70% (7). This improvement in informativeness means that many more individuals within genetic disease families will provide information that can allow the detection or the exclusion of linkage. The second major advantage is that microsatellites can be typed much more rapidly than RFLPs. Routine microsatellite genotyping rates of 1,000 genotypes/week/person have been achieved by us. In comparison, the average rate for RFLP typing from several labs is only about 350 genotypes/week person (8). Peak genotyping rates for microsatellites achieved in our center have been 1,600 genotypes/week/person; through au-

D19S49

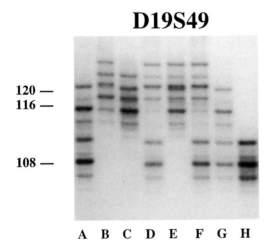

120 —
116 —

108 —

A B C D E F G H

FIG. 1. Analysis of microsatellite DNA polymorphisms. Shown is an autoradiograph of a polyacrylamide gel loaded with amplified DNA fragments from a dinucleotide repeat polymorphism at the D19S49 locus. Sizes of the DNA fragments in nucleotides are shown at the left. **Lanes A–H** each contained samples amplified using as template genomic DNA from a single individual. Genotypes of these individuals were **A**: 116,108; **B**: 120,118; **C**: 118,116; **D**: 120,108; **E**: 120,116; **F**: 120,108; **G**: 116,108; and **H**: 108,108.

TABLE 2. *Disease genes mapped using microsatellites*

Situs inversus viscerum (murine)
Facioscapulohumeral muscular dystrophy
Limb–girdle muscular dystrophy (dominant)
Non-insulin-dependent diabetes
Progressive degenerative myeloencephalopathy
  (bovine)

tomation of various portions of the genotyping process using pipetting robots, image analysis, and other technologies, it is expected that microsatellite genotyping rates will continue to climb. Together, the superior informativeness of the microsatellites and the increase in genotyping rate translate into a sixfold improvement in the rate at which disease genes can be mapped. At least five genetic disease genes have now been mapped using microsatellite polymorphisms (Table 2) (9–11, and unpublished results), and this list is expected to grow rapidly.

About 200 microsatellite DNA polymorphisms, nearly all based on CA/GT dinucleotide repeats, have now been developed in our laboratory. At least 100 additional microsatellite polymorphisms have been developed in other laboratories, and many more will be coming in the near future. Nearly all of our markers have been assigned to a specific chromosome. The distribution of the markers by chromosome is displayed in Figure 4. Note that the distribution of the microsatellite markers closely parallels the relative size of the chromosomes, indicating that the CA/GT repeat sequences are, at least to a first approximation, uniformly distributed throughout the genome. Both DNA from panels of somatic cell hybrids containing rearranged human chromosomes and linkage analysis using the reference CEPH families have been used to localize the new markers regionally. In Figure 3, maps for four different human chromosomes showing the approximate positions of microsatellite DNA polymorphisms are presented. Similar maps for the other chromosomes are under construction. The

regional mapping information, particularly linkage mapping data, will make the process of initial linkage mapping of disease genes more efficient. Markers that are very close together need not all be tested, and it will be possible to construct exclusion maps.

TOURETTE SYNDROME GENE MAPPING

For about the past 2 years we have attempted to map TS genes using microsatellite DNA polymorphisms. Families available for study include the Wisconsin A pedigree shown in Figure 2. Wisconsin A contains living affected individuals in four generations. At least three different neurologists have independently diagnosed TS in different members of this family. A number of the individuals in the most recent generation in Wisconsin A have shown amelioration of tics during the teenage years. Relatively few of the adult members of the kindred still exhibit multiple tics. Also available are nine families from the Netherlands, generously provided by Ben Oostra, Peter Heutink, and Ben Van de Wetering and also Branch C of the large Canadian Mennonite Tourette kindred (12) provided by Ken Kidd.

To date, approximately 125 microsatellite DNA polymorphisms have been tested with the available Tourette families. Almost all of the markers have been typed through at least Wisconsin Family A and Dutch Family 7; a few markers have been typed through all available families. The numbers of markers tested on each chromosome are shown in Table 3. For calculation of LOD scores only individuals with either tics or full-blown Tourette syndrome were considered affected. Autosomal dominant inheritance was assumed, with penetrance values of 90% in males and 56% in females along with phenocopy rates of 0.005 and a gene frequency of 0.003. No LOD scores greater than 3.0 have yet been obtained. Moderately positive LOD scores for individual

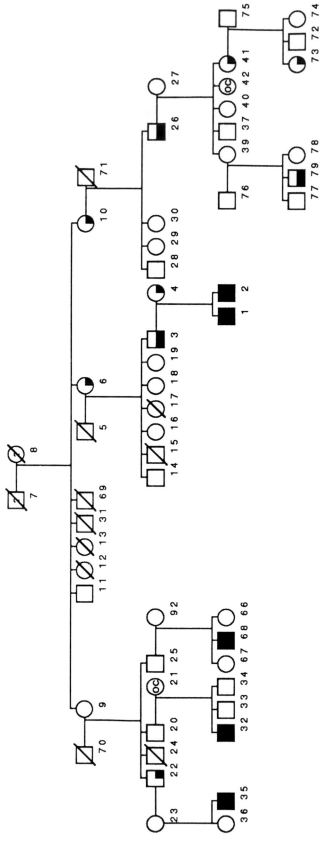

FIG. 2. Pedigree drawing of Tourette family Wisconsin A. *Completely filled symbols* represent individuals with full-blown Tourette syndrome, *half-filled symbols* individuals with multiple motor tics, and *quarter-filled symbols* individuals with single motor tics. *OC,* significant obsessive–compulsive behavior based on neuropsychological testing. Diagnosis of the Wisconsin A family members was purposely conservative so as to try to avoid false positives.

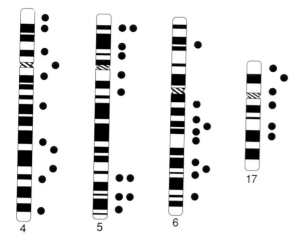

FIG. 3. Regional assignment of microsatellite polymorphisms located on chromosomes 4, 5, 6, and 17. Mapping was accomplished using both linkage analysis and panels of somatic cell hybrids containing rearranged chromosomes. The *black circles* represent markers developed at Marshfield, while the *gray circles* represent markers developed by Mihael Polymeropoulos at the National Institute of Mental Health.

families have been obtained with markers located on chromosomes 3, 8, and 9. Assuming locus homogeneity for the major Tourette syndrome gene, roughly two-thirds of the genome have now been excluded using the microsatellite polymorphisms.

Selected regions of the genome have been examined in greater detail. In particular, because of a report of a Tourette syndrome patient with a de novo deletion at 9pter (Taylor et al., submitted), the short arm of chromosome 9 has received special attention. The terminal portion of the short arm of chromosome 9 is a particularly poorly mapped region. Fortunately, however, one microsatellite marker was found, D9S54 (Mfd141), with moderate informativeness (heterozygosity 0.54) that mapped to this region. Evidence for the assignment of D9S54 to the 9pter region included the facts that this marker could be amplified with DNA from a hybrid (provided by David Krizman) that contained only the region 9pter to 9p22, and that this marker when typed in the

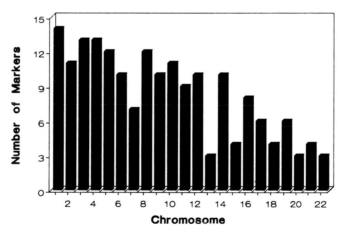

FIG. 4. Chromosome distribution of human microsatellite polymorphisms developed at Marshfield.

TABLE 3. *Numbers of microsatellite polymorphisms typed with Tourette families*

Chromosome	No. of markers	Chromosome	No. of markers
1	6	12	7
2	6	13	2
3	12	14	2
4	11	15	4
5	11	16	4
6	6	17	1
7	3	18	2
8	7	19	10
9	10	20	3
10	5	21	2
11	7	22	2

CEPH reference families was found to be tightly linked to D9S25 (CRI-L1022), which was previously placed on the distal portion of 9p (13). None of the other eleven chromosome 9 polymorphisms tested could be amplified from the 9pter-9p22 hybrid, and none of these markers could be linked to D9S54 or D9S25 by CEPH family typing. The new 9p microsatellite was analyzed using DNA from all of the available Tourette families, with the results shown in Table 4. Most of the families gave strongly negative LOD scores. The sum of the LOD scores clearly excluded the region about this marker under the assumption of locus homogeneity. Three families, however, gave weakly positive LOD scores. Also, since D9S54 is currently unlinked to other chromosome 9 microsatellite polymorphisms, the entire terminal portion of 9p has not yet been excluded.

The tryptophan oxygenase gene has been proposed as a candidate for mutation in TS patients (14). This gene has been mapped to 4q31 close to the MNS blood group gene(s) (15). We have tested in Tourette families two microsatellite markers that map to the region 4q25-q34.3, including one (D4S175) located approximately 7 cM from MNS. All resulting LOD scores were negative. Intervals of 40 cM for each marker could be excluded for the location of a Tourette gene in the families tested.

WHY ARE TOURETTE GENES PROVING SO DIFFICULT TO MAP?

Over 500 DNA polymorphisms, both RFLPs and microsatellite markers, have now been tested in various Tourette families by members of the Tourette genetics con-

TABLE 4. *LOD scores for Tourette syndrome plus tics vs. D9S54*

Family	Recombination frequency						
	0.001	0.05	0.10	0.15	0.20	0.25	0.30
Wisconsin A	−9.21	−5.91	−4.21	−3.06	−2.22	−1.60	−1.12
Canadian C	−3.71	−1.68	−1.14	−0.91	−0.79	−0.73	−0.64
Dutch 1	0.34	0.32	0.29	0.25	0.20	0.14	0.09
Dutch 2	−3.68	−1.70	−1.04	−0.64	−0.38	−0.21	−0.11
Dutch 5	0.24	0.20	0.16	0.13	0.10	0.07	0.05
Dutch 6	−3.72	−2.29	−1.65	−1.22	−0.91	−0.66	−0.47
Dutch 7	−3.29	−1.23	−0.51	−0.13	0.09	0.20	0.23
Dutch 9	0.55	0.54	0.49	0.42	0.34	0.26	0.17
Dutch 10	−1.74	−0.54	−0.27	−0.14	−0.06	−0.02	−0.00
Dutch 15	−2.56	−1.23	−0.85	−0.61	−0.44	−0.31	−0.21
Totals	−26.8	−13.5	−8.7	−5.9	−4.1	−2.9	−2.0

sortium (16 and unpublished results). No convincing evidence for linkage has been found. Why is the TS gene so difficult to map compared with other genetic disease genes?

The possibility that the critical region of the genome still has not been tested always remains. Five hundred markers are more than usually required to detect linkage to a disease gene, but at the present stage of development of the human linkage map, it cannot be concluded that every last bit of the genome has been covered. Still, with so many markers tested, it is possible, maybe even probable, that the relevant region(s) of the genome have already been excluded.

A number of factors contribute to the difficulty of linkage mapping of Tourette syndrome gene(s); one of these is the possibility of locus heterogeneity. Although locus heterogeneity has a reputation of being used as a crutch to explain the inability to reproduce linkage findings, the distinct possibility of heterogeneity in Tourette syndrome cannot be ignored. If several loci are involved in different Tourette families, then our gene mapping task becomes much more difficult. The LOD scores shown in Table 4 for D9S54, for example, clearly do not exclude linkage in every family tested. Tens of thousands of additional genotypes would probably need to be collected for Tourette families under the assumption of heterogeneity.

Another complication involves difficulties in diagnosis. While it is relatively simple to diagnose an individual with full-blown Tourette syndrome, those family members with subtle tics are virtually impossible to diagnose. Carefully defined rules for classification of family members can be devised, but the relationship of the actual genetics to the classification schemes is very difficult to determine. It is unlikely that any of the large Tourette kindreds currently under study for linkage analysis are completely free of diagnostic errors, including Wisconsin A. As has been demonstrated for bipolar affective disorder (17), diagnostic changes can strongly affect the resulting LOD scores.

The mode of inheritance of Tourette syndrome and the parameters of the inheritance model are another cause for concern. Although autosomal dominant inheritance as a result of a major Tourette gene has been concluded to be the most likely mode of inheritance for TS, other models, particularly multigenetic models, have not been firmly excluded (18–20). Similarly, sex-specific penetrance values and correction factors for age of onset have not been accurately specified. The incomplete penetrance observed for TS means that LOD scores even for tightly linked and highly informative markers will be reduced. Sib pair and affected pedigree member methods of analysis may become useful in TS since these methods do not require assumption of a particular mode of inheritance.

Another uncertainty is whether to score individuals as affected within the Tourette families who exhibit only obsessive–compulsive behaviors or attention deficit disorders. Since the diagnosis of these behavioral disorders is even more difficult than the detection of tics, inclusion of these traits will be problematic. It has also proved difficult to determine whether these trials are alternative manifestations of Tourette gene(s) (21).

Although application of highly informative microsatellite DNA polymorphisms to the initial linkage mapping of genetic disease genes represents a substantial improvement in this process, mapping of a disorder as complicated as TS remains extremely challenging. If a single, major Tourette gene existed, then given the large effort that has already been devoted to linkage mapping, it is likely that a location for the gene would have been found by now. Successful mapping of Tourette gene(s) may well require accumulation of significant amounts of new genotyping data, and, in addition, pooling of data from different laboratories for joint (and creative) analysis. On a more positive note, the continued progress of the human genome initiative, particularly the effort now under way to sequence and map all genes expressed in the central nervous system, will undoubtedly make the task of identifying Tourette genes easier. Also, because it is inherently simpler to diagnose tics as opposed to behavioral or psychiatric disorders, Tourette syndrome gene mapping may be intermediate in difficulty between mapping of single gene disorders and mapping of disorders such as schizophrenia and alcoholism. Success with Tourette syndrome may indicate the correct path to follow for mapping many common, heritable human traits.

REFERENCES

1. Weber JL, May PM. Abundant class of human DNA polymorphisms which can be typed using the polymerase chain reaction. *Am J Hum Genet* 1989; 44:388–96.
2. Smeets HJM, Brunner HG, Ropers HH, Wieringa B. Use of variable simple sequence motifs as genetic markers: application to study of myotonic dystrophy. *Hum Genet* 1989;83:245–51.
3. Tautz D. Hypervariability of simple sequences as a general source for polymorphic DNA markers. *Nucleic Acids Res* 1989;17:6463–71.
4. Economou EP, Bergen AW, Warren AC, Antonarakis SE. The polydeoxyadenylate tract of Alu repetitive elements in polymorphic in the human genome. *Proc Natl Acad Sci USA* 1990; 87:2941–54.
5. Zuliani G, Hobbs HH. A high frequency of length polymorphisms in repeated sequences adjacent to Alu sequences. *Am J Hum Genet* 1990;46:963–9.
6. Polymeropoulos MH, Rath DS, Xiao H, Merril CR. Trinucleotide repeat polymorphism at the human intestinal fatty acid binding protein gene (FABP2). *Nucleic Acids Res* 1990;18:7198.
7. Weber JL. Human DNA polymorphisms based on length variations in simple sequence tandem repeats. In: Tilghman S, Davies K, eds. *Genome analysis series: genetic and physical mapping*, vol 1. Cold Spring Harbor, NY: Cold Spring Harbor Laboratory Press, 1990;159–81.
8. Weber JL, Human DNA polymorphisms and methods of analysis. *Curr Opin Biotechnol* 1990; 1:166–71.
9. Hanzlik AJ, Binder M, Layton WM, et al. The murine situs inversus viscerum (iv) gene responsible for visceral asymmetry is linked tightly to the Igh-C cluster on chromosome 12. *Genomics* 1990; 7:389–93.
10. Wijmenga C, Frants RR, Brouwer OF, Moerer P, Weber JL, Padberg GW. Location of the fascioscapulohumeral muscular dystrophy gene on chromosome 4. *Lancet* 1990;336:651–3.
11. Bell GI, Xiang KS, Newman MV, et al. Gene for non-insulin-dependent diabetes mellitus (maturity-onset diabetes of the young subtype) is linked to DNA polymorphisms on human chromosome 20q. *Proc Natl Acad Sci USA* 1991;88:1484–8.
12. Kurlan R, Behr J, Medved L, et al. Familial Tourette's syndrome: report of a large pedigree and potential for linkage analysis. *Neurology* 1986; 36:772–6.
13. Donis-Keller D, Green P, Helms C, et al. A genetic linkage map of the human genome. *Cell* 1987; 51:319–37.
14. Comings DE. Blood serotonin and tryptophan in Tourette syndrome. *Am J Med Genet* 1990; 36:418–30.
15. Comings DE, Muhleman D, Dietz GW Jr, Donlon T. Human tryptophan oxygenase localized to 4q31: possible implications for alcoholism and other behavioral disorders. *Genomics* 1991; 9:301–8.
16. Pakstis AJ, Heutink P, Pauls DL, et al. Progress in the search for genetic linkage with Tourette syndrome: an exclusion map covering more than 50% of the autosomal genome. *Am J Hum Genet* 1991; 48:281–94.
17. Kelsoe JR, Ginns EI, Egeland JA, et al. Re-evaluation of the linkage relationship between chromosome 11p loci and the gene for bipolar affective disorder in the Old Order Amish. *Nature* 1989; 342:238–43.
18. Pauls DL, Leckman JE. The inheritance of Gilles de la Tourette's syndrome and associated behaviors. Evidence for autosomal dominant transmission. *N Engl J Med* 1986;315:993–7.
19. Price RA, Pauls DL, Kruger SD, Cainc ED. Family data support a dominant major gene for Tourette syndrome. *Psychiatr Res* 1988;24:251–61.
20. Comings DE, Comings BG, Devor EJ, Cloninger CR. Detection of major genes for Gilles de la Tourette syndrome. *Am J Hum Genet* 1984; 36:586–600.
21. Pauls DL, Hurst CR, Kruger SD, Leckman JF, Kidd KK, Cohen DJ. Gille de la Tourette's syndrome and attention deficit disorder with hyperactivity, evidence against a genetic relationship. *Arch Gen Psychiatry* 1986;43:1177–9.

Advances in Neurology, Vol. 58, edited by T. N. Chase, A. J. Friedhoff, and D. J. Cohen. Raven Press, Ltd., New York © 1992.

22

Linkage Studies in 16 St. Louis Families

Present Status and Pursuit of an Adjunct Strategy

Eric J. Devor

Department of Psychiatry, Washington University School of Medicine, St. Louis, Missouri 63110

More than 100 years have passed since Gilles de la Tourette first described the syndrome that bears his name (1). During this time Tourette syndrome (TS) has run the etiological gamut from hereditary disorder to psychogenic malady and back again (2). Today, armed with an arsenal of sophisticated and robust quantitative tools, geneticists appear to have won the day for the hereditary position (3–6). Thus, even though details of the exact genetic model of transmission of TS are being debated, that the disorder is hereditary is unquestioned (2,7–8).

With the issue of hereditary transmission all but in hand, the focus of research among geneticists has shifted toward attempting to map the gene(s) responsible (9). In this chapter I will briefly review the contribution made to the gene mapping effort by Washington University in St. Louis and then outline a new, adjunct strategy currently being developed in my laboratory. This strategy utilizes TS families themselves to generate DNA probes for mapping.

THE ST. LOUIS LINKAGE STUDY

As is evident from other contributions to this volume, the TS gene mapping effort encompasses several different groups, each having a role to play. Some laboratories, like those in New Haven and Rotterdam, have made major contributions to the linkage exclusion map. Other, smaller, laboratories like those in St. Louis and Houston, have taken on smaller, more specific tasks.

My laboratory in St. Louis has been a member of the gene mapping consortium since the third Tourette Syndrome Genetics Workshop held in New York in 1988. By that time we had ascertained 16 multiplex TS families (Fig. 1) and had begun to prepare DNA samples for use in linkage studies. Since then, we have participated in the study of specific gene loci such as red-cell acid phosphatase (ACP1) on chromosome 2p (10) and D2-dopamine receptor on chromosome 11q (11). In addition, we have contributed to the general exclusion maps on chromosomes 3, 9, 11, 15, 18, 20, 21, and 22 (cf, ref. 12). Most recently, we have investigated the human XY psedoautosomal region (13).

Finally, we too shared our family data with the other members of the consortium. Pedigree information was contributed for the joint segregation analyses reported in this volume, and DNA samples from many

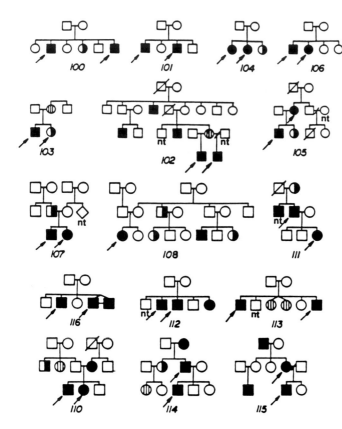

FIG. 1. Pedigrees of the 16 St. Louis Tourette syndrome linkage study families. *Fully shaded symbols* indicate Tourette syndrome while *half-shaded symbols* refer to chronic tics only. *Hatched symbols* indicate obsessive–compulsive behaviors in the absence of other symptoms. Probands are identified with *arrows*.

of the St. Louis families have been sent to Rotterdam, Toronto, and Houston. In turn, we have received DNA samples from both Rotterdam and Houston.

TOURETTE SYNDROME-SPECIFIC PROBES (TSSP): AN ADJUNCT STRATEGY FOR MAPPING THE TS GENE

For all its hard work and good will, the gene mapping consortium has been so far frustrated in its efforts to find the TS gene. Leads, both curious and spurious, have come and gone (10,12,14–16) and still the gene remains elusive. In an editorial in the *Biological Psychiatry*, Dr. Robert Belmaker cautioned (17) that it may be unlikely that a single causal gene with variable penetrance and pleiotropic effects exists for complex hereditary disorders such as TS. Indeed, as Pyeritz has advised,

In all aspects of medical genetics, from clinical service and clinical investigation to molecular analysis of etiology, it is important to remember: *Genetic heterogeneity is the rule, rather than the exception.* (ref. 18:69).

With these caveats in mind, the question of etiologic heterogeneity in TS naturally arises. The answer to this question is, unfortunately, we don't know. Thus, the strategy of searching for the TS gene by systematic genome screening and conventional linkage analysis is the best method at hand. It is not the *only* method, however. Other approaches such as candidate genes and "random mapping" (19) are available. In the former approach specific proteins are proposed as being etiologically relevant and their genes are studied preferentially. To date, however, no viable candidate gene for TS has been proposed (2).

In the absence of a candidate gene, the random mapping approach can be used as an adjunct to systematic genome searches. Random mapping makes use of a unique set of DNA probes termed *minisatellites*, which detect repetitive DNA sequences scattered throughout the human genome (20). These probes produce complex patterns of bands on Southern blots called DNA *fingerprint*. Random mapping involves searching through these patterns in order to find fragments that are cosegregat-ing with the disease in families. Clearly, this is a crude method and it has two significant problems. First, unlike conventional DNA probes, linkage analysis results are not additive between families when using minisatel-lites. Second, many, if not all, minisatellites have a very high mutation rate (21). While these drawbacks do not completely rule out minisatellite probes for use in linkage studies, they do narrow the scope of how they

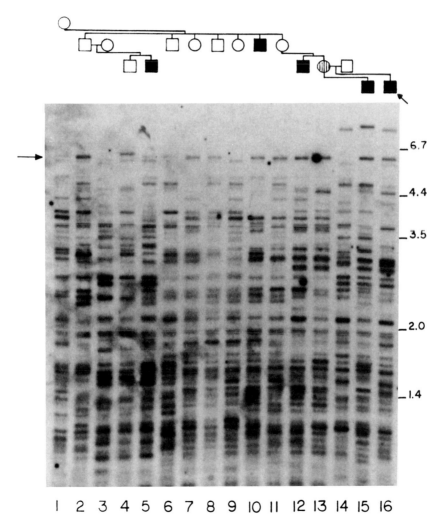

FIG. 2. A DNA "fingerprint" of family TSG102. Genomic DNAs were digested with the restric-tion enzyme *HaeIII* and fragments were size-fractionated by gel electrophoresis. Southern transfer of fragments and hybridization with the M13 minisatellite probe were carried out as described (19). The 6-kb cosegregating fragment is indicated with the *arrow* on the left. Molecu-lar weight markers (λ/*Hind III* + *EcoRI*) are shown on the right. The individual referred to as TSG102-103 is identified by the *hatchings*.

may be applied. The best use of minisatellite probes in a linkage paradigm is restricted to extended families segregating a dominant genetic disorder with high penetrance (21). Fortunately, TS appears to be a dominant genetic disorder with high penetrance and multigenerational, extended families have been identified by all groups studying the disorder.

A Preliminary Example

Vassart and colleagues (22) reported an unusual but useful minisatellite probe in the bacteriophage M13. In a gene that encodes one of the coat proteins of the virus are two blocks of tandem repeats whose 15 base-pair consensus core sequence,

GAGGGTGG(C/T)GG(C/T)TCT, has been found to be present in dozens of sites spread throughout the human genome (22,23). When this DNA sequence is hybridized to genomic DNA digested with the restriction enzyme *HaeIII*, a DNA fingerprint whose fragments are transmitted in a regular mendelian manner is detected.

The M13 minisatellite was used to screen the six multigenerational Tourette families 102, 107, 108, 110, 114, and 115 (Fig. 1). One of these families, 102, showed evidence of a cosegregating fragment among the bands of the DNA fingerprint (Fig. 2). A hybridizing fragment at approximately 6 kilobases (kb) is seen to be shared among the five affecteds and three obligate carriers but does not occur in either married-in persons or

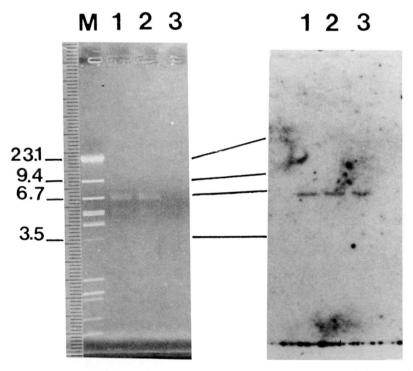

FIG. 3. Preliminary analysis of the 6-kb fragment population. On the left is an ethidium bromide-stained agarose gel. In **lane 1** the DNA is uncut. In **lanes 2 and 3** the DNA was incubated with the restriction enzymes *EcoRI* and *AluI*, respectively. On the right is the autoradiogram resulting from M13 hybridization following Southern transfer of the gel on the left to a nylon membrane. The presence of a strongly hybridizing band in **lane 3** indicates that the repeat-containing fragment is present as an intact piece of DNA. *AluI* digestion of the sample removed the background fragments but did not affect the repeat-containing fragment.

DNA Fingerprint Fragment

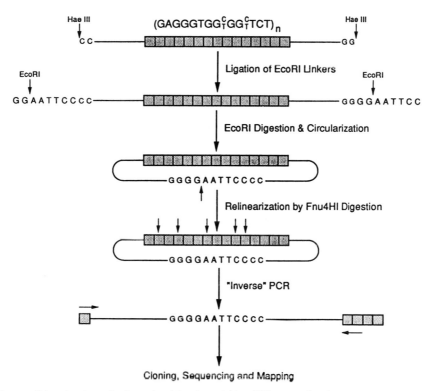

FIG. 4. A possible cloning strategy for blunt-end *HaeIII* fingerprint fragments is presented. The 6-kb fragment will contain an unknown number of copies of the hybridizing core sequence plus nonrepetitive flanking sequences that end in *HaeIII* sites on both sides. Blunt-end ligation of *EcoRI* linkers is carried out in the presence of T4 DNA ligase. Digestion of the linkers with *EcoRI* will create "sticky" ends that will religate and circularize the repeat-containing fragment. Subsequent digestion with the restriction enzyme *Fnu4HI* will "invert" the sequence with the artificial *EcoRI* site inside the fragment. PCR primers specific to the repeat core-sequence can then be used to amplify the two unknown flanking sequences for cloning, sequencing, and mapping. The internal sequence GGGGAATTCCCC created by the linkers will serve as an internal PCR control.

in three of the five remaining unaffecteds. If the individuals carrying the 6-kb fragment are assumed to be heterozygous and those not carrying the fragment are assumed to be homozygous for a presumed alternate allele, then a linkage analysis of the locus in this family can be performed. Using the linkage parameters suggested by Pauls and Leckman (6), the "artificial" locus yields a maximum LOD score of $Z = 1.69$ at $\theta = 0.00$, or zero recombination. Such a high score from a single family suggests that this

DNA fingerprint fragment should be studied further.

The mother of the proband, individual 102-03, is a key member of the family as she has two affected children who are maternal half-sibs. Neither father had symptoms or family history of tics or TS. Thus, the two half-sibs inherited both the TS and the 6-kb DNA fragment from their mother. Therefore, an immortalized lymphoblastoid cell line was established for the mother, 102-03, and sufficient genomic DNA was extracted from cultured cells to permit a detailed study of the potential marker. To begin, fragments in the 6-kb size range were isolated from a *HaeIII* digest of 750 μg of genomic DNA. Aliquots of the purified, size-selected DNA were run out on a minigel following incubation of two of the aliquots with the restriction enzymes *EcoRI* and *AluI* (Fig. 3). The DNA in the gel was then transferred to a charged nylon membrane and hybridized with the M13 minisatellite probe as described (23). The autoradiogram of the hybridization (Fig. 3) clearly indicates that the repeat-containing 6-kb fragment has been isolated in the population of purified DNA fragments.

The final step in the study of this fragment is to clone it out of the background of other fragments. This can be done in several ways. However, these methods all take advantage of the basic strategy shown in Fig. 4 as well as the polymerase chain reaction (24). First, the blunt-ended *HaeIII* fragments are ligated with *EcoRI* linkers. Following *EcoRI* digestion of the linked fragments, circularization is achieved in the presence of DNA ligase (25). The circularized fragments containing the M13 repeat sequence can then be relinearized preferentially in an inverted form by digestion with the restriction enzyme *Fnu4HI*, which cuts the sequence GCGGC. Given the relative rarity of sequences containing the CpG dimer (26), the majority of relinearized fragments should be the repeat-containing target sequence. The polymerase chain reaction (PCR) can then be employed to amplify copies of the flanking sequences using primers specific to the M13 core sequence.

One alternative to the strategy outlined in Fig. 4 is to use PCR primers specific to the M13 core sequence *and* primers that will bind to the linkers. This would allow amplification of the flanking sequences without requiring circularization and inversion. Both methods, however, make assumptions about the human repetitive sequence, such as the fidelity of the core consensus sequence, that have yet to be proved experi-

mentally. If these experiments do work and if the flanking regions can be amplified, cloned, and mapped, then a new and relatively easy means of generating TS linkage probes will be in hand.

REFERENCES

1. Tourette G. Etude sur une affection nerveuse caracteristée par de l'incoordination motrice accompagnée d'echolalie et de coprolalie. *Arch Neurol* 1885;9:19–42.
2. Devor EJ. Untying the Gordian knot: the genetics of Tourette syndrome. *J Nerv Ment Dis* 1990; 178:669–79.
3. Baron M, Shapiro E, Shapiro A, Rainer JD. Genetic analysis of Tourette syndrome suggesting a major gene effect. *Am J Hum Genet* 1981; 33:767–75.
4. Comings DE, Comings BG, Devor EJ, Cloninger CR. Detection of a major gene for Gilles de la Tourette syndrome. *Am J Hum Genet* 1984; 36:586–600.
5. Devor EJ. Complex segregation analysis of Gilles de la Tourette syndrome: further evidence for a major locus mode of transmission. *Am J Hum Genet* 1984;36:704–9.
6. Pauls DL, Leckman JF. The inheritance of Gilles de la Tourette's syndrome and associated behaviors: evidence for autosomal dominant transmission. *N Engl J Med* 1986;315:993–7.
7. Robertson MM. The Gilles de la Tourette syndrome: the current status. *Br J Psychiatry* 1989; 154:147–69.
8. Shapiro AK, Shapiro ES, Young JG, Feinberg TE. *Gilles de la Tourette syndrome*, 2nd ed. New York: Raven Press, 1988.
9. Pakstis AJ, Heutink P, Pauls DL, et al. Progress in the search for genetic linkage with Tourette syndrome: an exclusion map covering more than 50% of the autosomal genome. *Am J Hum Genet* 1991; 48:281–94.
10. Devor EJ, Henderson V, Sparkes RS. Linkage to Tourette syndrome is excluded for red-cell acid phosphatase (ACP1) and flanking markers on chromosome 2pter-2p23. *Hum Biol* 1991;63:221–6.
11. Devor EJ, Grandy DK, Civelli O, et al. Genetic linkage is excluded for the D2-dopamine receptor λHD2G1 and flanking loci on chromosome 11q22-q23 in Tourette syndrome. *Hum Hered* 1990; 40:105–8.
12. Heutink P, van de Wetering BJM, Breeveld GH, et al. No evidence for genetic linkage of Gilles de la Tourette syndrome on chromosomes 7 and 18. *J Med Genet* 1990;27:433–6.
13. Devor EJ, Isenberg KE. A linkage study of the psedoautosomal region in Tourette syndrome. In: *Eighth International Congress of Human Genetics* (abst), 1991.
14. Brett P, Curtis D, Gourdie A, et al. Possible linkage of Tourette syndrome to markers on short

arm of chromosome 3(C3p21-14). *Lancet* 1990; 336:1076.

15. Heutink P, Sandkuyl L, van de Wetering BJM, et al. Unjustified claim for linkage of Gilles de la Tourette syndrome. *Lancet* 1991;337:122–3.

16. Comings DE, Comings BG, Diez G, et al. Evidence the Tourette Syndrome gene is at 18q22.1. In: *Seventh International Congress of Human Genetics* (abst), 1986.

17. Belmaker RH. One gene per psychosis? *Biol Psychiatry* 1991;29:415–7.

18. Pyeritz RE. Formal genetics in humans: mendelian and nonmendelian inheritance. In: McHugh PR, McKusick VA, eds. *Genes, brain, and behavior.* New York: Raven Press, 1991;47–73.

19. Devor EJ, Reich T, Cloninger CR. The genetics of alcoholism and related end-organ damage. *Semin Liver Dis* 1988;8:1–11.

20. Jeffreys AJ, Wilson V, Thein SL, et al. DNA "fingerprints" and segregation analysis of multiple markers in human pedigrees. *Am J Hum Genet* 1986;39:11–24.

21. Jeffreys AJ, Royle NJ, Wilson V, Wong Z. Spontaneous mutation rates to new length alleles at tandem-repetitive hypervariable loci in human DNA. *Nature* 1988;332:278–81.

22. Vassart G, Georges M, Monsieur R, et al. A sequence in M13 phage detects hypervariable minisatellites in human and animal DNA. *Science* 1987; 235:683–4.

23. Devor EJ, Ivanovich AK, Hickok JM, Todd RD. A rapid method for confirming cell line identity: DNA "fingerprinting" with a minisatellite probe from M13 bacteriophage. *Biotechniques* 1988; 6:200–2.

24. Saiki RK, Gelfand DH, Stoffel S, et al. Primer-directed enzymatic amplification of DNA with a thermostable DNA polymerase. *Science* 1988; 239:487–91.

25. Ochman H, Gerber AS, Hartl DL. Genetic applications of an inverse polymerase chain reaction. *Genetics* 1988;120:621–3.

26. Bishop DT, Williamson JA, Skolnick MH. A model for restriction fragment length distributions. *Am J Hum Genet* 1983;35:795–815.

27. Weber JL, May PE. Abundant class of human DNA polymorphisms which can be typed using the polymerase chain reaction. *Am J Hum Genet* 1989; 44:388–96.

Advances in Neurology, Vol. 58, edited by T. N. Chase, A. J. Friedhoff, and D. J. Cohen. Raven Press, Ltd., New York © 1992.

23

Alternative Hypotheses on the Inheritance of Tourette Syndrome

*David E. Comings and †Brenda G. Comings

Department of Medical Genetics, City of Hope National Medical Center, Duarte, California 91010 and †Private Practice, Duarte, California 91010

Other chapters on linkage studies in Tourette syndrome (TS) in this volume have demonstrated that despite a massive effort involving the examination of some 550 different markers and exclusion of over 80% of the genome, the chromosomal location of the TS gene has yet to be determined. Similar difficulties have been experienced in linkage studies of other psychiatric and neuropsychiatric disorders including manic–depressive disorder, schizophrenia, autism, panic attacks, dyslexia, and obsessive–compulsive disorder (OCD). Various theories have been put forward to explain these difficulties. We propose that the major reason for these failures is that the genetic models being used are wrong. We believe there are a number of common assumptions about TS that may not be true. Since they all directly relate to the question of the mechanism of inheritance, we have chosen to list them all. These include statements that we have read in recent reviews or statements we have heard presented at TS conferences.

ASSUMPTION: OTHER THAN OCD NO OTHER BEHAVIORAL DISORDERS ARE PRESENT IN TS PROBANDS

Since the question of how to score family members is critical to linkage studies, the question of what symptoms the *Gts* gene can cause is equally critical. Should only tics be included, or only tics and obsessive–compulsive behaviors (OCB), or other behaviors as well?

In 1987 we presented a series of seven papers reporting a large, controlled study of 247 consecutive, unselected TS probands, most of whom were self-referred (1–7). This showed that TS was actually a neuropsychiatric spectrum disorder. The frequencies of attention deficit hyperactivity disorder (ADHD), learning disorders, OCB, conduct disorder, oppositional disorder, depression and mania, anxiety disorders (including panic attacks, phobias, agoraphobia, separation anxiety and school phobia), sleep disorders, speech problems (including stuttering, dysfluency, and talking too fast or too loud), inappropriate sexual behaviors, addictive behaviors, paranoid tendencies, and hearing voices were 5–20 times more common in TS patients than in the controls. Some (8–11) have objected to the breadth of this spectrum. However, Leckman and Cohen (12) described the associated behavioral traits in TS as including "developmentally inappropriate inattention and impulsivity, disinhibition of thoughts and actions, motoric hyperactivity and restlessness, learning disabilities, emotional lability, increased irritability, maniclike behavior, obsessive-compulsive behaviors, heightened anxiety, phobias, separation anxiety, and depressive reactions," and others (13) who have also used structured instruments found that the frequency of other neuropsychiatric disorders in their proband samples were comparable to those that we reported.

In a recent study of using the Achenback Child Behavioral Checklist, Singer and Rosenberg (14) observed that for a wide range of different psychopatholgies, 19–57% of TS children and adults scored above the 98th percentile. Many of these frequencies were even higher than those we described in 1987.

Many of the papers in this symposium now verify the concept that TS is a broad, neuropsychiatric spectrum disorder. This concept is critically relevant to the correct scoring of affected or unaffected family members in linkage studies. The related concept of whether this spectrum of disorders is present only in probands, or in other family members carrying the Gts gene is discussed below.

ASSUMPTION: THERE IS NOTHING IN THE LITERATURE TO SUGGEST THE CONCEPT OF SPECTRUM DISORDERS

Winokur and colleagues (15,16) were the earliest proponents of the concept that some psychiatric disorders present as a spectrum of disorders. They termed this *depression spectrum disorder*. Van Praag has often championed a similar concept and suggested that nomenclature in psychiatry might make more sense if it was based on pathophysiologic mechanisms that are shared by aggressive, depressive, anxious, and impulsive behavior, rather than obsessing about pigeonholing patients into specific *Diagnostic and Statistical Manual*, 3rd ed., revised (DSM-III-R) diagnostic categories (17–19).

More recently, on the basis of improvement of symptoms with tricyclic and serotonergic antidepressants, Hudson and Pope (20) have suggested that ADHD, OCB, af-

fective disorders, and some types of anxiety, eating, sleep, and somatiform disorders share a common pathogenetic mechanism that constitutes one of the most common disorders affecting humans. They termed this *affective spectrum disorder* and recently added kleptomania to the list (21). This spectrum is identical to our TS spectrum disorder (1,22–26).

Biederman and colleagues (27,28) have reviewed studies showing that ADHD is also a spectrum disorder consisting of comorbidity with depression, learning disorders, anxiety, and conduct and oppositional disorder (27,28). As these children get older, addictive behaviors may also become a problem (22).

Finally, Maser and Cloninger (29) have recently edited a book entitled *Comorbidity of Mood and Anxiety Disorders*, in which 40 contributors explore the evidence that there are common genetic and pathophysiologic factors underlying depression, anxiety, panic attacks, phobias, and related disorders.

In summary, viewing TS as a spectrum disorder (7,22,25,26,30) in which a number of different psychiatric disorders are linked together by a common gene or genes should not be considered a radical idea (8,13).

ASSUMPTION: THE "FAMILY STUDY" TECHNIQUE HAS SHOWN THAT TS AND ADHD SEGREGATE INDEPENDENTLY

In 1984, based on a study of 250 TS probands and families, we proposed that there was an intimate genetic interrelatedness between TS and many cases of ADHD (31). We pointed out that (a) most cases of TS started with symptoms of ADHD, (b) the Gts gene could be expressed as ADHD only, and (c) up to half of ADHD cases might be due to the presence of a Gts gene (1,31–33).

In 1986 Pauls et al. (34) reported a study of 27 TS probands. For the 17 probands who had ADHD, 25% of the 16 affected family members had ADHD. For the 10 probands who did not have ADHD, none of the 14 affected family members had ADHD. From this the authors concluded that TS and ADHD segregated independently and that the presence of ADHD in TS probands was due to ascertainment bias, i.e., the tendency for individuals with two disorders to seek medical help more often than individuals with a single disorder. They predicted that if the TS probands did not have ADHD, the frequency of ADHD in the affected relatives would be no greater than in the general population. However, earlier in that year two of the authors published another paper studying a large TS pedigree in which the proband did not have ADHD (35). Here 9 of 29 or 31% of affected relatives had ADHD. Combining these two studies produced a frequency of ADHD in affected relatives, when the proband did not have ADHD in 9 of 43 or 21%. This was identical to the figure we found for affected relatives of TS probands who did not have ADHD, namely 21% (1,23).

A large number of families have now been studied to examine this issue (24). These show that 50–85% of TS probands have attention deficit disorder (with or without hyperactivity) (ADD). If the proband has ADHD, 25–46% of the affected relatives have ADD. If the proband does not have ADHD, 20–31% of the affected relatives have ADD. These figures are significantly higher than the 3–9% prevalence of ADHD in the general population.

We find the clinical picture of TS to be so identical to that of ADHD that in an interview situation we often do not know which diagnosis we are working with until we have asked the question, "Has there ever been a period of a year or more when your child had almost daily motor or vocal tics?" There was a time when we thought the following equation was valid: TS = (ADHD)^2 meaning TS and ADHD were clinically and genetically related, but TS was more severe and TS patients carried two *Gts-ADHD* genes while ADHD patients carried only one. However, in the process of taking detailed pedigrees we very often see behavioral problems in both the mother or her

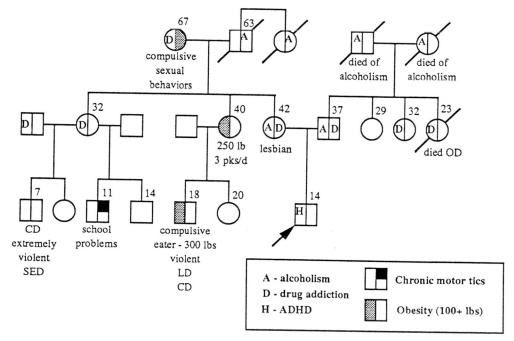

FIG. 1.

family *and* the father or his family, similar to what we see in TS (see below). This is illustrated by the pedigree from an ADHD child shown in Fig. 1. We have seen so many of these pedigrees that we suspect many ADHD patients are also homozygous for the *Gts-ADHD* gene and feel that a more valid equation is: TS = ADHD with tics.

ASSUMPTION: IF THE FREQUENCY OF A COMORBID CONDITION IS LESS IN AFFECTED RELATIVES THAN IN THE PROBAND, THIS MEANS ITS PRESENCE IN THE PROBAND WAS DUE TO ASCERTAINMENT BIAS

We are assuming here that ascertainment bias is defined as the tendency for patients with two independent entities to seek medical care more often than those with a single disorder. Almost universally missed in discussions of this issue is that there is a second major reason why the frequency of a comorbid condition may be much less in affected relatives than in probands. This is that the decrease may simply be due to a lesser degree of expression of the gene or genes. It is true of every medical disorder that the most severely symptomatic patients are the first to seek medical care. For genetic disorders this is termed degree of expression. Those with the greater degree of expression are more likely to seek medical care than those who are mildly affected.

To give an example, it would not be surprising to find that 100% of patients with Marfan syndrome (arachnodactyly, dislocation of the lens, and aortic insufficiency) who had dissecting aneurysm would seek medical help. It would also not be surprising to find that none of their relatives who did not seek medical help had a dissecting aneurysm. From these observations, it would not be valid to conclude that arachnodactyly and dissecting aneurysm were independent, unrelated entities. Dissecting aneurysm is simply the most severe form of expression of the Marfan syndrome.

In a similar fashion, we believe that TS probands who also have ADHD or several of the other comorbid conditions are simply expressing their *Gts* genes (and modifying genes) to a greater degree than those who only have tics. Simply because these behaviors occur less often in affected relatives who do not seek medical care does not mean they are unrelated to the *Gts* gene.

ASSUMPTION: THE FAMILY STUDY TECHNIQUE IS THE GOLD STANDARD FOR STUDYING BEHAVIOR IN TS FAMILIES

There are two general techniques for performing genetic studies to determine the frequency of behavioral problems in relatives. These are the family history technique of asking the probands, or parents of the probands, about the behavioral problems in other relatives, and the family study technique, in which the relatives themselves are interviewed. The family history technique has the advantage that it is inexpensive, allows the examination of large numbers of relatives, is sensitive to the more severe problems, and avoids reverse ascertainment bias (see below). In our hands the family history technique is actually a combination of the family history and family study technique in that the first-degree relatives (parents, siblings, and children) are often seen in the clinic together so they can each be personally interviewed.

The family study technique has the advantage that it usually uses a standardized structured interview that has the potential of being given blind to the diagnosis of the proband, and is more sensitive to subtle symptoms known only to the person interviewed. The major disadvantages are that because of the expense, the number of relatives that can be interviewed may be so limited that there are severe dangers of type II errors in the study, e.g., concluding differences are not significant when in fact they are. A second major disadvantage is reverse ascertainment bias. Since the family studies cannot be done if the relatives are not available, there would be a de facto exclusion of families in which the child is adopted or is a foster child. This often occurs because one or both parents of such children are alcoholics, drug addicts, or otherwise severely impaired. We have several hundred such probands: a TS or ADHD patient is the child of two addicts. This important segment of probands would be missed using a pure family study technique. A second type of reverse ascertainment bias that especially occurs when only first-degree relatives are studied is the tendency to obtain families in which both parents are sufficiently high functioning to have responded to adds soliciting participation in the study. This excludes those families in which one or both parents are so impaired they can't, or don't care to, read newsletters or newspapers. All of these individuals are included in the family history technique but tend to be excluded in the family study technique. As a result of a great deal of psychopathology may be missed.

ASSUMPTION: THE FAMILY STUDY TECHNIQUE SHOWS THAT TS IS NOT A SPECTRUM DISORDER

In a study that has still appeared only in abstract form, the family study technique was used to examine the frequency of various DSM-III-R behavioral disorders in 338 first-degree relatives of 86 TS probands and controls (13). The abstracts states that "the rates of those disorders [see above] among first degree relatives are not significantly elevated compared to controls—except for TS, chronic tics and obsessive-compulsive disorder." However, of the 13 different categories of behaviors examined, in 12 the frequency of the behavior was greater in the first-degree relatives of TS probands than in the relatives of controls. In addition, the critical question on the frequency of psychopathology in relatives of TS probands carrying the *Gts* gene, i.e., having TS,

chronic tics, or OCD, has yet to be presented. The only disorder for which TS relatives were less affected than controls was stuttering; see the chapter entitled *Tourette Symptoms in 161 Related Family Members* showing that stuttering is present in a much higher percent of affected TS relatives than unaffected relatives.

By definition a genetic spectrum disorder may manifest as any one of a number of different behaviors. Again using a genetic syndrome as an example, suppose we had a disorder called "the 13 syndrome," meaning there were 13 different symptoms characteristic of the most fully expressed syndrome, but usually patients only had a small subset of all 13. If 180 family members and 180 members of control families were examined for each of the 13 symptoms individually, the power of the study to detect significant differences would be very low. However, if the question asked was, "What percentage of the syndrome versus control relatives have *any* of the 13 symptoms?" the differences may now be highly significant. When we computer-modeled the Pauls et al.(34) report, and collapsed the 13 groups into an "any behavioral disorder" category, the differences between the TS and control relatives were significant.

We carried out our own family history–family study investigation of 1,851 TS relatives and 541 control relatives. This showed significant increase in the frequency of ADHD, learning disorders, and dyslexia, alcoholism and drug abuse; depression and manic–depression, and other behavioral problems in the relatives of TS versus control families, and most important, an even higher frequency among the relatives with tics (24,25,36). Several of the studies reported in this volume have presented similar results.

ASSUMPTION: TOURETTE SYNDROME IS INHERITED AS AN AUTOSOMAL DOMINANT DISORDER

Linkage studies are doomed to failure if the genetic models used are incorrect. On the basis of our first 250 TS pedigrees, we reported in 1984 that if the gene frequency was held at a low level, and chronic motor or vocal tics were included as well as TS, the data suggested an autosomal dominant mode of inheritance with reduced penetrance (37). We concluded the frequency of the *Gts* gene was 0.006. In 1986, adding OCB to the expression of the gene, Pauls and Leckman (38) also concluded TS was inherited as an autosomal dominant disorder with reduced penetrance and a gene frequency of 0.006. All subsequent linkage studies have assumed this mode of inheritance and used a gene frequency of 0.003 to 0.006.

By the time we had taken our 500th to 1,800th TS pedigree, our clinical experience with this disorder indicated it was necessary to ask about a wide range of behaviors in the relatives, not just tics and OCB. When this was done it became apparent that the whole spectrum of behavioral problems, including alcoholism and drug abuse, were often present in *both* the mother or her family *and* the father or his family (22,39). This, plus studies of platelet serotonin and blood tryptophan, showing decreased levels in both parents (22,40,41), and other evidence (22,39), convinced us that in the more severely affected TS patients the *Gts* gene was coming from both parents, i.e., the probands were recessive-like homozygotes for the gene. However, individuals carrying a single *Gts* gene could still have tics or other parts of the spectrum. In this regard the trait was acting as a dominant gene. Thus, we feel the term semidominant semirecessive is the most accurate representation of the mode of inheritance of TS (22,35,39–42).

ASSUMPTION: TS IS A RARE DISORDER

While almost universally considered to be a very rare disorder, when the DSM-III-R criteria (43) are used, instead of the misperceptions based on watching TV shows, TS is a common disorder. Epidemiologic studies in North Dakota (44) and Monroe County, New York (45) showed the prevalence in males ranged from 1 in 1,500 to 1 in 1,000 (22). When we did on-site monitoring of 3,000 school children over a 2-year period, 1 in 95 boys fulfilled rigid research criteria for TS (46). This is consistent with other studies reporting the frequency of chronic motor *and* vocal tics in schoolchildren (47). Of the ten epidemiologically identified TS patients in our study who came to the City of Hope Clinic for care, *all* had ADHD, *all* had one or more of the associated disorders, and most had a positive family history of chronic tics and associated disorders.

ASSUMPTION: THE *Gts* GENE FREQUENCY IS 0.003 TO 0.006

Just as linkage studies are critically dependent upon the correct model of inheritance, they are also critically dependent upon using the correct assumption of gene frequency. The frequency of the *Gts* gene that has been assumed for all of the TS linkage studies is 0.003 to 0.006 (48–51) (also see this volume). However, if our observation of TS in 1 in 95 schoolboys, and our assumption that most significantly symptomatic TS patients are homozygotes, are correct, then simple calculations using the Hardy-Winberg equation indicate a gene frequency of 0.07 to 0.10—11 to 33 times higher than generally assumed (22). We find it of interest that one of the most common associated behaviors we see in relatives of TS patient is early-onset alcoholism. The suggested frequency of the gene for the type II, early-onset, genetic form of alcoholism, is 0.11 (52), similar to our estimate of the frequency of the *Gts* gene.

ASSUMPTION: THE DOPAMINE D$_2$ RECEPTOR GENE IS NOT INVOLVED IN TS

There are many reasons to believe that a defect in dopamine metabolism might be involved in TS (7,53). Since TS responds well to haloperidol, a specific dopamine D_2 receptor antagonist, there has been special interest in the possibility that these receptors might be defective in TS. Thus, it was of considerable interest when Cevilli and coworkers (54) reported the cloning of the D_2 receptor gene and when a Taq I polymorphism of this gene was found for the human gene (55). Several studies have reported an absence of linkage between the D_2 receptor gene and TS, (56,57) suggesting this gene is not involved in the etiology of TS. However, we have found that the prevalence of the 1 allele of the Taq I polymorphism of the D_2 receptor gene is significantly increased (24.5% to 44.9%) in TS probands (58). There was a similar increase in prevalence for patients with ADHD, autism, alcoholism, conduct disorder, and posttraumatic stress disorder (58,59). The prevalence of the 1 allele increased from 39.8% in mild to moderate TS to 59% in severe TS (58). In ADHD the prevalence of the 1 allele was the same in patients without tics or a family history of tics (46.3%) as in those with a family history of tics (45.8%). Studies of autopsy material have shown that the B_{max} of the D_2 receptor is decreased in individuals carrying the 1 allele (60).

We interpret these results as indicating that variants of the 1 allele of the dopamine D_2 receptor gene act as a modifying gene for the expression of TS and related disorders. These studies also support our proposal that there is a fundamental genetic, pathophysiologic interrelatedness between TS, ADHD, alcoholism, autism, conduct disorder, and PTSD (1,7,22,24–26,42,61,62).

ASSUMPTION: THE PRIMARY DEFECT IN TS IS IN DOPAMINE METABOLISM

Defects in serotonin metabolism have been implicated in all of the associated or comorbid disorders in TS (22,63,64). Studies of cerebrospinal fluid (CSF) 5-hydroxy indoleacetic acid (5-HIAA) show reduced levels in patients with TS (65–67). We have observed significantly decreased levels of both platelet serotonin and blood tryptophan in patients with TS, and both their parents (40). In studies of the level of various neurotransmitters in the brains of TS patients (68), the only changes consistent across many areas was a decrease in serotonin and tryptophan. From a genetic point of view, this suggests the *Gts* mutation may be in the tryptophan oxygenase (TDO2) gene, and that the defect results in the constitutive activation of the gene (22,40,41,61,69,70). We have cloned and sequenced the TDO2 gene. It is located on chromosome 4q31 (69). Interestingly, preliminary linkage studies have suggested that the gene for early-onset alcoholism may be on the same band (71,72). To test the hypothesis that the TDO2 gene may be the TS gene, we are in the process of comparing the DNA sequence of the TDO2 exons in TS patients and controls.

ASSUMPTION: LINKAGE STUDIES ARE THE BEST WAY TO IDENTIFY THE *Gts* GENE

If TS is inherited as an autosomal dominant disorder with a high degree of penetrance, then standard linkage analysis of the type described in this volume and elsewhere (48–51) is the method of choice. However, if the mechanism of inheritance is semidominant semirecessive, then both parents would carry the gene whether they had symptoms or not; often one or both parents might actually be homozygotes themselves, and most or all of the siblings would carry at least one *Gts* gene. Under these circumstances the power of the linkage studies collapses to virtually zero. Even the power of sib pair analysis is impaired if one or both parents are homozygotes, a situation that is likely to occur when families are highly selected for the occurrence of multiple affected sibs.

The technique that we have chosen to use is to identify candidate genes that may be involved either perform association studies, as we did to study the role of the dopamine D_2 receptor allele, or actually compare the sequence of the putative gene in TS patients versus controls. The latter is very labor intensive and requires a high degree of confidence that one might have the right candidate gene.

CONCLUSIONS

These data suggest to us a model of the inheritance of TS and its associated comorbid conditions as shown in Fig. 2. Evidence from animal and human studies indicates there is a serotonin–dopamine axis in which defects in serotonin metabolism both cause and complement hyperactivity of dopamine or dopamine receptors (22,73). We propose that the primary genetic defect in TS, possibly in the TDO2 gene, results in defective serotonin metabolism and that a number of other loci affecting dopamine metabolism, such as the dopamine D_2 receptor allele, can act as modifying genes. This suggests a mechanism we term *CM&M* inheritance, meaning common major genes, common modifying genes (74), i.e., both the primary *Gts* gene, and the genes that modify its action are common, with carrier frequencies in the range of 10–30%. Environmental factors plus a healthy dose of random chaos (22) interact with the genetic substrate to produce an entire spectrum of interrelated behavioral disorders.

There are two aspects of this model that carry with it some degree of urgency. The first is that if the TDO2 model of TS is correct, then hyperinduction of the TDO2 gene carries with it the risk that in addition to an increased breakdown of tryptophan and shunting it away from serotonin, there is also an increased production of quinolinic acid, a neurotoxin that interacts with NMDA receptors (75,76). We wonder how many of the symptoms of TS, especially those involving problems with memory, are

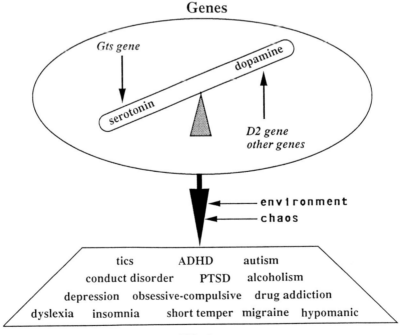

FIG. 2.

secondary to this potentially preventable cause.

The second is a concern one of us had raised before, i.e., the possibility that there may be continuing selection for the *Gts* gene (7,22). Criticism of this concept (8) does not make the possibility go away. If the *Gts* gene causes a spectrum of impulsive–compulsive–aggressive–mood–anxiety and learning disorders, given the problems in our society with addictive, impulsive, compulsive, and violent behaviors, this is not a trivial concern. One could argue that selection for this gene might increase in direct proportion to the increasing technological complexity of society. If for no other reason, this alone suggests that studies of the genetics of TS deserve more national support than they have received to date.

REFERENCES

1. Comings DE, Comings BG. A controlled study of Tourette syndrome. I. Attention-deficit disorder, learning disorders, and school problems. *Am J Hum Genet* 1987;41:701–41.
2. Comings DE, Comings BG. A controlled study of Tourette syndrome. II. Conduct. *Am J Hum Genet* 1987;41:742–60.
3. Comings DE, Comings BG. A controlled study of Tourette syndrome. III. Phobias and panic attacks. *Am J Hum Genet* 1987;41:761–81.
4. Comings DE, Comings BG. A controlled study of Tourette syndrome. IV. Obsessions, compulsions, and schizoid behaviors. *Am J Hum Genet* 1987; 41:782–803.
5. Comings BG, Comings DE. A controlled study of Tourette syndrome. V. Depression and mania. *Am J Hum Genet* 1987;41:804–21.
6. Comings DE, Comings BG. A controlled study of Tourette syndrome. VI. Early development, sleep problems, allergies, and handedness. *Am J Hum Genet* 1987;41:822–38.
7. Comings DE. A controlled study of Tourette syndrome. VII. Summary: a common genetic disorder causing disinhibition of the limbic system. *Am J Hum Genet* 1987;41:839–66.
8. Pauls DL, Cohen DJ, Kidd KK, Leckman JF: Tourette syndrome and neuropsychiatric disorders: is there a genetic relationship? *Am J Hum Genet* 1988;42:206–9.
9. Robertson MM. The Gilles de la Tourette syndrome: the current status. *Br J Psychiatry* 1989; 154:147–69.
10. Devor EJ: Untying the Gordian knot—the genetics of Tourette syndrome. *J Nerv Ment Dis* 1990; 178:669–79.
11. Singer HS, Walkup JT. Tourette syndrome and other tic disorders. Diagnosis, pathophysiology, and treatment. *Medicine* 1991;70:15–32.
12. Leckman JF, Cohen DJ. Descriptive and diagnostic classification of tic disorders. In: Cohen DJ, Bruun RD, Leckman JF (eds). *Tourette's syndrome & tic disorders.* New York: John Wiley & Sons, 1988;4–19.
13. Pauls DL, Leckman JF, Raymond CL, Hurst CR, Stevenson JM. A family study of Tourette's syndrome: evidence against the hypothesis of association with a wide range of psychiatric phenotypes. *Am J Hum Genet* 1988;43:A64.
14. Singer HS, Rosenberg LA. Development of behavioral and emotional problems in Tourette syndrome. *Pediatr Neurol* 1989;5:41–4.
15. Winokur G, Cadoret R, Dorzab J, Baker M. Depressive disease. A genetic study. *Arch Gen Psychiatry* 1971;24:135–44.
16. Winokur G, Tsuang MT, Crowe RR. Affective disorders in relatives of manic and depressed patients. *Am J Psychiatry* 1982;139:209–12.
17. van Praag HM, Kahn RS, Asnis GM, et al. Denosologication of biological psychiatry or the specificity of 5-HT disturbances in psychiatric disorders. *J Affect Disord* 1987;13:1–8.
18. Apter A, van Praag HM, Plutchik R, Sevy S, Korn M, Brown S-L. Interrelationships among anxiety, aggression, impulsivity, and mood: A serotonergically linked cluster? *Psychiatry Res* 1990; 32:191–9.
19. van Praag HM, Asnis GM, Kahn RS, et al. Nosological tunnel vision in biological psychiatry. a plea for a functional psychopathology. *Ann NY Acad Sci* 1990;600:501–9.
20. Hudson JI, Pope HG Jr. Affective spectrum disorder: does antidepressant response identify a family of disorders with a common pathophysiology? *Am J Psychiatry* 1990;147:552–64.
21. McElroy SL, Pope HG Jr, Hudson JI, Keck PE Jr, White KL. Kleptomania: a report of 20 cases. *Am J Psychiatry* 1991;148:652–7.
22. Comings DE. *Tourette syndrome and human behavior.* Duarte, CA: Hope Press, 1990;1.
23. Comings DE, Comings BG. Tourette's syndrome and attention deficit disorder with hyperactivity [Letter]. *Arch Gen Psychiatry* 1987;44:1023–6.
24. Comings DE, Comings BG. A controlled family history study of Tourette syndrome. I. Attention deficit hyperactivity disorder, learning disorders and dyslexia. *J Clin Psychiatry* 1990;51:275–80.
25. Comings DE, Comings BG. A controlled family history study of Tourette syndrome. III. Other psychiatric disorders. *J Clin Psychiatry* 1990; 51:288–91.
26. Sverd J. Clinical presentation of the Tourette's syndrome diathesis. *J Multihandicapped Person* 1989;2:311–26.
27. Biederman J, Newcorn J, Sprich S. Comorbidity of attention deficit hyperactivity disorder with conduct, depressive, anxiety, and other disorders. *Am J Psychiatry* 1991;148:564–77.
28. Faraone SV, Biederman J, Keenan K, Tsuang MT. Separation of DSM-III attention deficit disorder and conduct disorder—evidence from a family-ge-

netic study of American child psychiatric patients. *Psychol Med* 1991;21:109–21.

29. Maser JD, Cloninger CR. *Comorbidity of mood and anxiety disorders.* Washington, DC: American Psychiatric Press, Inc., 1990.

30. Comings DE, Comings BG. A controlled study of Tourette syndrome—revisited. *Am J Hum Genet* 1988;42:209–16.

31. Comings DE, Comings BG. Tourette's syndrome and attention deficit disorder with hyperactivity: are they genetically related? *J Am Acad Child Psychiatry* 1984;23:138–46.

32. Comings DE, Comings BG. Tourette syndrome: clinical and psychological aspects of 250 cases. *Am J Hum Genet* 1985;37:435–50.

33. Comings DE, Comings BG. Tourette's syndrome and attention deficit disorder. In Cohen DJ, Bruun RD, Leckman JF (eds). *Tourette's syndrome and tic disorders: clinical understanding and treatment.* New York: John Wiley & Sons, 1988; 120–35.

34. Pauls DL, Hurst CR, Kruger SD, Leckman JF, Kidd KK, Cohen DJ. Gilles de la Tourette's syndrome and attention deficit disorder with hyperactivity. Evidence against a genetic relationship. *Arch Gen Psychiatry* 1986;43:1177–9.

35. Kurlan R, Behr J, Medved L, et al. Familial Tourette's syndrome: a report of a large pedigree and potential for linkage analysis. *Neurology* 1986; 36:772–6.

36. Comings DE, Comings BG. A controlled family history study of Tourette's syndrome. II. Alcoholism, drug abuse and obesity. *J Clin Psychiatry* 1990;51:281–7.

37. Comings DE, Comings BG, Devor EJ, Cloninger CR. Detection of major gene for Gilles de la Tourette syndrome. *Am J Hum Genet* 1984;36:586–600.

38. Pauls DL, Leckman JF. The inheritance of Gilles de la Tourette's syndrome and associated behaviors. Evidence for autosomal dominant transmission. *N Engl J Med* 1986;315:993–7.

39. Comings DE, Comings BG, Knell E. Hypothesis: homozygosity in Tourette syndrome. *Am J Med Genet* 1989;34:413–21.

40. Comings DE. Blood serotonin and tryptophan in Tourette syndrome. *Am J Med Genet* 1990; 36:418–30.

41. Comings DE, Comings BG. The genetics of Tourette syndrome and its relationship to other psychiatric disorders. In Wetterberg L (ed). *Genetics of neuropsychiatric diseases.* London: MacMillan, 1988:179–89.

42. Comings DE: The genetics of human behavior: lessons for two societies. *Am J Hum Genet* 1989; 44:452–60.

43. American Psychiatric Association. *Diagnostic and statistical manual of mental disorders.* 3rd ed, revised. Washington, DC: American Psychiatric Association, 1987.

44. Burd L, Kerbeshian J, Wikenheiser M, Fisher W. A prevalence study of Gilles de la Tourette syndrome in North Dakota school-age children. *J Am Acad Child Psychiatry* 1986;25:552–3.

45. Caine ED, McBride MC, Chiverton P, Bamford KA, Rediess S, Shiao J. Tourette's syndrome in

Monroe County school children. *Neurology* 1988; 38:472–5.

46. Comings DE, Himes JA, Comings BG. An epidemiological study of Tourette syndrome in a single school district. *J Clin Psychiatry* 1990;51:463–9.

47. Shapiro AK, Shapiro ES, Young JG, Feinberg TE. *Gilles de la Tourette syndrome,* New York: Raven Press, 1988.

48. Heutink P, Sandkuyl LA, van de Wetering BJM, et al. Linkage and Tourette syndrome. *Lancet* 1991; 337:122–3.

49. Pauls DL, Pakstis AJ, Kurlan R, et al. Segregation and linkage analysis of Tourette syndrome and related disorders. *J Am Acad Child Psychiatry* 1990; 29:195–203.

50. Brett P, Curtis D, Gourdie A, et al. Possible linkage of Tourette syndrome to markers on short arm of chromosome-3 (C3p21-14). *Lancet* 1990; 336:1076.

51. Pakstis AJ, Heutink P, Pauls DL, et al. Progress in the search for genetic linkage with Tourette syndrome—an exclusion map covering more than 50 percent of the autosomal genome. *Am J Hum Genet* 1991;48:281–94.

52. Gilligan SB, Reich T, Cloninger CR. Etiologic heterogeneity in alcoholism. *Genet Epidemiol* 1987; 4:395–414.

53. Cohen DJ, Leckman JF. Tourette's syndrome: advances in treatment and research. *J Am Acad Child Psychiatry* 1984;23:123–5.

54. Bunzow JR, Van Tol HHM, Grandy DK, et al. Cloning and expression of a rat D2 dopamine receptor cDNA. *Nature* 1988;336:783–7.

55. Grandy DK, Litt M, Allen L, et al. The human dopamine D2 receptor gene is located on chromosome 11 at q22-q23 and identifies a TaqI RFLP. *Am J Hum Genet* 1989;45:778–85.

56. Devor EJ, Grandy DK, Civelli O, et al. Genetic linkage is excluded for the D2-dopamine receptor lambda-Hd2G1 and flanking loci on chromosome 11Q22-Q23 in Tourette syndrome. *Hum Hered* 1990;40:105–8.

57. Gelernter J, Pakstis AJ, Pauls DL, et al. Gilles-de-La-Tourette syndrome is not linked to D2-dopamine receptor. *Arch Gen Psychiatry* 1990; 47:1073–7.

58. Comings DE, Comings BG, Muhleman D, et al. The dopamine D2 receptor locus as a modifying gene in neuropsychiatric disorders. *JAMA* 1991; 266:1793–800.

59. Comings DE, Muhleman D, Dietz G, Shahbahrami B, Tast D, Kovacs BW. The dopamine D2 receptor gene is a modifier of the expression of the Tourette syndrome (Gts) and ADHD gene. *Am J Hum Genet* 1990;46(abst):A52.

60. Noble EP, Blum K, Ritchie T, Montgomery A, Sheridan PJ. Allelic association of the D2 dopamine receptor gene with receptor-binding characteristics in alcoholism. *Arch Gen Psychiatry* 1991; 48:648–54.

61. Comings DE, Comings BG. Clinical and genetic relationships between autism-PDD and Tourette syndrome: a study of 19 cases. *Am J Med Genet* 1991;39:180–91.

62. Sverd J. Tourette's syndrome and autistic spec-

trum disorders: a significant relationship. *Am J Med Genet* 1991;39:173–9.

63. Brown S-L, van Praag HM. *The role of serotonin in psychiatric disorders*. New York: Brunner/Mazel, 1990.

64. Whitaker-Azmita PM, Peroutka SJ. *The neuropharmacology of serotonin*. New York: Proc. N.Y. Acad. Sci., 1990.

65. Butler IJ, Koslow SH, Seifert WE Jr, Caprioli RM, Singer HS. Biogenic amine metabolism in Tourette syndrome. *Ann Neurol* 1979;6:37–9.

66. Cohen DJ, Shaywitz BA, Young JG, Carbonari CM, Nathanson JA. Central biogenic amine metabolism in children with the syndrome of chronic multiple tics of Gilles de la Tourette: norepinephrine, serotonin, and dopamine. *J Am Acad Child Psychiatry* 1979;18:320–41.

67. Singer HS, Pepple JM, Ramage AL, Butler IJ. Gilles de la Tourette syndrome: further studies and thoughts. *Ann Neurol* 1978;4:21–5.

68. Anderson G. Neuropathology studies on Tourette syndrome brain tissues. In Friedhoff AJ, Chase TN (eds). *2nd International Scientific Symposium on Tourette Syndrome*. New York: Raven Press, 1992; (in press).

69. Comings DE, Muhleman D, Dietz GW, Donlon T. Human tryptophan oxygenase localized to 4q31: possible implications for human behavioral disorders. *Genomics* 1991;9:301–8.

70. Comings DE, Comings BG, Muhleman D, Dietz G. Tourette syndrome, serotonin, tryptophan oxygenase, type II alcoholism and depression. In: *1st World Congress Psychiatric Genetics*. 1989.

71. Hill EM, Wilson AF, Elston RC, Winokur G. Evidence for possible linkage between genetic markers and affective disorders. *Biol Psychiatry* 1988; 24:903–17.

72. Aston CE, Hill SY. Segregation analysis of alcoholism in families ascertained through a pair of male alcoholics. *Am J Hum Genet* 1990;46:879–87.

73. Valzelli L. Animal models of behavioral pathology and violent aggression. *Methods Find Exp Clin Pharmacol* 1985;7:189–93.

74. Comings DE, Comings BG. Common genes for spectrum disorders: implications for psychiatric genetics. *Psychiat Genet* 1991;2:5–6(abst).

75. Stone TW. *Quinolinic acid and the kynurenines*. Boca Raton, FL: CRC Press, 1989.

76. Cotman CW, Bridged RJ, Taube JS, Clakr AS, Geddes JW, Monaghan DT. The role of the NMDA receptor in central nervous system plasticity and pathology. *J NIH Res* 1989;1:65–73.

Advances in Neurology, Vol. 58, edited
by T. N. Chase, A. J. Friedhoff, and
D. J. Cohen. Raven Press, Ltd.,
New York © 1992.

24

Structural Imaging in Tourette Syndrome

Steven Demeter

Department of Neurology, University of Rochester, Rochester, New York, 14642

Since most individuals with Tourette syndrome (TS) lead relatively normal lives, postmortem studies of TS are rare (1). Therefore, morphologic information about the brain in TS has been slow to appear. Fortunately, imaging techniques have made it possible to examine brain structure in living patients. There are a number of reasons why structural abnormalities might be expected in TS. Postmortem studies have not excluded the possibility that there may be abnormalities in TS that could be reflected in gross structural changes (1,2). Although the types of abnormalities that have been reported do not disrupt gross structure as dramatically as do destructive and space-occupying lesions, they could produce more subtle changes that affect certain brain regions in a quantifiable manner. There is precedent for such changes in such disorders as Huntington's disease and schizophrenia. In obsessive–compulsive disorder (OCD), a disorder that may be genetically linked to TS, structural neuroimaging studies have shown abnormalities although subtle (3–5) and not uniformly found (6,7). Functional neuroimaging studies in OCD (8–14) and in TS (15 and *this volume*) have also shown abnormalities, reinforcing the possibility that structural changes might be detectable in TS.

At this point it is useful to ask: why study gross structure at all in TS? On the one hand, both empirical and theoretical considerations suggest that dramatic abnormalities will not be found. On the other hand, functional neuroimaging appears to hold much greater promise for elucidating the pathophysiology of TS and for monitoring its course and response to treatment. There are several reasons why morphologic studies can be useful. Although metabolic and blood-flow studies can be helpful in demonstrating dysfunctional systems, by themselves they are incapable of pinpointing the source of the disturbance. Thus, dysfunction that appears in such studies as widespread may originate from abnormalities that are in fact much more confined. Similarly, receptor imaging studies can point to dysfunctional neural transmission, but even such abnormalities can be due to disturbances elsewhere. Moreover, it is instructive to consider how focal lesions due to unrelated causes might interact with TS and whether they can by themselves cause TS. Are focal lesions affecting particular parts of the brain more likely to have an effect on TS symptomatology than lesions at other locations? Are symptom severity and treatment responsiveness influenced by the concurrent existence of focal lesions? Can cases of "acquired Tourettism" (16) or acquired obsessive compulsiveness provide clues to the localization of abnormalities in TS?

COMPUTED TOMOGRAPHIC AND MAGNETIC RESONANCE IMAGING IN TS

Robertson (17) identified studies or reports of 172 computed tomographic (CT) scans in TS in the published literature. It is appropriate here to provide a precis of this imaging work and add 15 additional cases, some studied with magnetic resonance imaging (MRI). Caparulo et al. (18) reported that 6 of 16 patients with TS had abnormal CT scans. Of these, four had abnormalities that they regarded as severe, including enlarged, symmetric or asymmetric ventricles (either side larger) and (in a single instance) an enlarged right lateral fissure (of Sylvius). The other two patients had mildly enlarged lateral ventricles. The family history was not mentioned. Lees et al. (19) reported that all of their 53 patients who had CT scans had clinically normal studies. Robertson et al. (20) reported that 71 of their 73 cases had normal CT scans. These cases presumably included those reported by Lees et al. (19). Each of the two abnormal CT scans showed a cavum septum pellucidum. Harcherik et al. (21) compared 19 patients with TS with groups of patients with various other kinds of childhood neuropsychiatric disorders and medical controls in a blinded morphometric CT study. No biologically significant differences were found across groups on measures of total ventricular volume, right–left ventricular volume ratio, ventricular asymmetries, ventricle–brain ratio, and brain density. Measurements were not made on specific nuclei.

Regeur et al. (22) reported that 47 of 53 patients with TS had clinically normal CT scans. The abnormalities included two cases of asymmetrical ventricles and one each of a small occipital arachnoid cyst, suprasellar epidermoid, large defect of the right temporoparietal region, and slight cortical atrophy. Since patients were grouped, it is not possible to determine which had relevant family histories. Chase et al. (15) reported that seven of nine patients had normal CT scans and two others had normal MRIs. One of the abnormalities consisted of mild cortical atrophy and the other of ventricular enlargement. The family history was not described. Demeter et al. (in preparation) compared ten adult volunteers with TS with ten medical controls in a blinded morphometric MR study using linear measures. No quantitative differences were found between the TS and control groups on a large number of measures. However, two patients had focal anomalies involving the basal ganglia, one of whom had a family history of tics.

In addition to the foregoing studies, there have been several individual case reports. Yeragani et al. (23) reported a 12-year-old girl without a relevant family history who had had tics since age 10. She was shy, sensitive, timid, and anxious and had a history of enuresis to age 5. CT scan revealed mild increase in the density of the caudate nuclei, thought to be due to calcification. Shaenboen et al. (24) reported a 16-year-old girl with TS, in whom CT revealed enlargement of the occipital horns of the lateral ventricles (colpocephaly). There was a history of cyanosis at 30 hours and of delayed speech development. The family history was not provided. Lakke and Wilmink (25) reported a 27-year-old man with TS who was found to have a pineal tumor on a CT scan performed in the course of his workup for TS. No mention was made of his family history. The CT also revealed calcification in the region of the third ventricle and periaqueductal gray.

Kjaer et al. (26) reported a 28-year-old woman with TS since age 6, who had been born premature by 4 weeks, had a left-sided clonic seizure at 3 weeks of age, convergent strabismus, and hyperactive stretch reflexes on the left. Her CT scan revealed a porencephalic cyst of the right hemisphere measuring $3 \times 5 \times 7$ cm that virtually replaced the temporal lobe and also involved the basal ganglia on the same side. The basal ganglia on the left also showed some contrast enhancement. The family history was not given. Sandyk (27) reported a 7-year-old boy with an unremarkable family history who had TS. MRI revealed asymmetric cerebral peduncles. Vieregge et al. (28) reported twins concordant for TS. There was a family history of TS. CT scan revealed "some" ventricular asymmetry in both, apparently without observable differences. Interestingly, one twin had "soft" neurologic signs. This twin had more lateralized tics. Robertson et al. (29) reported a patient with TS who was a product of a pregnancy complicated by a hemorrhage due to placenta previa. Consequently, the patient spent the first 4 days of her life in an incubator. MRI revealed a high signal lesion in the right globus pallidus.

IMAGING IN
OBSESSIVE–COMPULSIVE DISORDER

Kellner et al. (7) found no differences between groups of 12 OCD patients and 12 normal controls in a morphometric MR study on measures of area of the head of the caudate nucleus, thickness of the cingulate gyrus, intercaudate/frontal horn ratio, and area of the corpus callosum. Luxenberg et al. (5) compared ten patients with OCD with ten normal controls in a morphometric CT study and found that the volume of the caudate nucleus was bilaterally less in OCD patients than in controls. However, they found no differences in the volumes of the lenticular nuclei, third ventricle, and lateral ventricle, and no abnormal asymmetries were noted. Martinot et al. (13) reported 16 patients who had positron emission tomography (PET) and either CT scan or MR neuroimaging. No structural abnormalities were noted on clinical reading.

Garber et al. (4) compared 32 patients with OCD with 14 normals in a nonmorphometric MR study. T_1 was prolonged in patients. Moreover, patients had greater right–left T_1 differences for frontal white matter. Right–left T_1 differences in orbitofrontal cortex were strongly correlated with symptom severity in unmedicated patients and in patients with a family history of OCD. Behar et al. (3) studied 16 adolescents with OCD and 16 matched, normal controls and found that patients had larger ventricle–brain ratios. Insel et al. (6) found no differences in ventricle–brain ratio, asymmetries, or sulcal prominence between ten patients with OCD and ten matched, mixed medical and normal controls.

Weilburg et al. (30) reported a patient with OCD who had history of a birth injury, mild dystonia/hypotonia on the right. A maternal aunt reportedly had a head tic. There was no other family history. MRI revealed an enlarged anterior left lateral ventricle, a smaller left caudate, and a slit-shaped lesion in the left putamen.

ACQUIRED TOURETTISM AND
OBSESSIVE–COMPULSIVENESS

Although there have been numerous reports of lesions and anomalies in cases of TS and OCD, it is usually difficult to ascribe the clinical manifestations to the morphologic abnormalities. It is therefore of interest to consider cases of "Tourettism" and obsessive–compulsiveness that have been clearly related to underlying disorders. Pulst et al. (31) reported a case of carbon monoxide poisoning with features of TS. The patient had been healthy previously. The family history was not provided. CT revealed atrophy with lesions in the basal ganglia, more apparent on the left. Ward (32) observed three patients, who developed transient feelings of compulsion in relation to acquired hemispheric lesions. One was found to have a right frontoparietal glioblastoma, another had a left frontal glioblastoma, and the third had an apparent lacunar infarct in the left basal ganglia.

Laplane et al. (33) reported eight patients with bilateral basal ganglia lesions due to various encephalopathies especially carbon monoxide poisoning. There was no prior history of OCD. The family history was not stated. All patients had obsessive–compulsive symptoms. Turley (34) reported a TS-like disorder after Herpes encephalitis. The family history was not given. CT scan revealed a left temporal lesion. Northam and Singer (35) reported the onset of multiple somatic and vocal tics in relation to presumed Herpes encephalitis that persisted for at least 14 months. CT scan and MR imaging revealed a small hemorrhagic lesion in the right medial temporal region and edema surrounding the affected area and the ipsilateral basal ganglia and thalamus. The family history was not mentioned.

CONCLUSION

Whereas most studies on OCD have revealed abnormalities affecting the circuitry of the caudate nucleus, structural studies on TS have been consistently negative except for uncovering anomalies that may be merely incidental to TS. It is worth noting, however, that only two controlled morphometric studies of TS have been published, and only one of these used more sensitive MR imaging. Moreover, one study exclusively used indirect indices of morphologic abnormalities. The other used linear measurements that do not have the sensitivity of volumetric determinations employed in some studies in OCD. Both used medical controls. The failure to detect structural abnormalities in TS may thus be related to the use of morphometric techniques that are not sufficiently sensitive, use of medical controls that could obscure differences that might otherwise be measurable, and inclusion of subjects at random, thereby diluting effects that might be present only in certain subsets of affected individuals. It is nevertheless possible that there is an intrinsic difference in the extent to which TS and OCD leave structural footprints. Work currently in progress suggests that by selecting patients more carefully and using volumetric techniques, structural abnormalities can in fact be demonstrated. For the present we

can conclude only that structural abnormalities, if they can be demonstrated, will indeed be subtle.

The more interesting observations pertain to case reports of focal lesions that are either coincidental to, contributory to, or causative of TS or OCD. Since TS and OCD are now recognized to be disorders that occur with considerable frequency, it is not surprising that, merely by chance, a variety of underlying lesions and anomalies should be observed in association with these disorders. Of the 177 structural neuroimaging studies of TS published to date, 23 (13%) were abnormal or anomalous. Since abnormal studies are often reported, whereas normal cases are not, the figure of 13% should not be taken as an accurate estimate of the prevalence of structural defects in TS. However, it would be reasonable to regard it as a cap that probably would not be exceeded if the TS population were formally investigated for such abnormalities. The minimum expected rate of abnormalities in TS is the same as that in the general population. If it could be shown that the rate of structural abnormalities in TS indeed exceeded that in the general population, one could conclude that structural defects could in themselves play an etiologic role in genetically unaffected families or a contributory role in genetically susceptible individuals. That structural anomalies can interact with TS could be shown if a higher prevalence of structural anomalies could be demonstrated in certain subgroups such as treatment-resistant cases or cases with severe symptoms. Such information is important for treatment planning, prognosis, and genetic counseling.

Another question relates to the location of abnormalities in TS. A plurality of cases have involved the basal ganglia and a number of others the limbic system with or without basal ganglia involvement. Still others have shown nonspecific findings such as ventricular enlargement or asymmetry without pinpointing the underlying defect, possibly because the techniques used were not sufficiently sensitive to demonstrate them. Cases that involve areas that would not be expected to be affected in light of current thinking show no consistency in pathology or localization. These observations suggest that basal ganglia and possibly the limbic system indeed play important roles in the pathophysiology of TS and that structural lesions in these areas contribute to the occurrence or manifestations of TS.

Cases of acquired Tourettism and obsessive–compulsiveness that have been imaged seem to confirm the localizations suggested by case reports of TS and OCD. Although most such cases have been induced by insults that are less than confined in their localization, they nevertheless seem to point to the basal ganglia and, possibly, to limbic areas as the critical structures responsible for TS.

REFERENCES

1. Richardson EP Jr. Neuropathological studies of Tourette syndrome. In: Friedhoff AJ, Chase TN, eds. *Gilles de la Tourette syndrome*. Advances in neurology, vol 35. New York: Raven Press, 1982; 83–7.

2. Haber SN, Kowall NW, Vonsattel JP, Bird ED, Richardson EP. Gilles de la Tourette's syndrome: a postmortem and neurohistochemical study. *J Neurol Sci* 1986;75:225–41.

3. Behar D, Rapoport JL, Berg CJ, et al. Computerized tomography and neuropsychological test measures in adolescents with obsessive–compulsive disorder. *Am J Psychiatry* 1984;141:363–9.

4. Garber HJ, Ananth JV, Chiu LC, Griswold VJ, Oldendorf WH. Nuclear magnetic resonance study of obsessive–compulsive disorder. *Am J Psychiatry* 1989;146:1001–5.

5. Luxenberg JS, Swedo SE, Flament MF, Friedland RP, Rapoport J, Rapoport SI. Neuroanatomical abnormalities in obsessive–compulsive disorder detected with quantitative X-ray computed tomography. *Am J Psychiatry* 1988;145:1089–93.

6. Insel TR, Donnelly EF, Lalakea ML, Alterman IS, Murphy DL. Neurological and neuropsychological studies of patients with obsessive–compulsive disorder. *Biol Psychiatry* 1983;18:741–51.

7. Kellner CH, Jolley RR, Holgate RC, et al. Brain MRI in obsessive–compulsive disorder. *Psychiatry Res* 1991;36:45–19.

8. Baxter LR Jr, Phelps ME, Mazziotta JC, Guze BH, Schwartz JM, Selin CE. Local cerebral glucose metabolic rates in obsessive–compulsive disorder. A comparison with rates in unipolar depression and in normal controls [published erratum appears in *Arch Gen Psychiatry* 1987;44:800]. *Arch Gen Psychiatry* 1987;44:211–18.

9. Baxter LR Jr, Thompson JM, Schwartz JM, et al. Trazodone treatment response in obsessive–compulsive disorder--correlated with shifts in glucose metabolism in the caudate nuclei. *Psychopathology* 1987;20(Suppl 1):114–22.

10. Baxter LR Jr, Schwartz JM, Mazziotta JC, et al. Cerebral glucose metabolic rates in nondepressed patients with obsessive–compulsive disorder. *Am J Psychiatry* 1988;145:1560–3.

11. Baxter LR Jr, Schwartz JM, Guze BH, Bergman K, Szuba MP. PET imaging in obsessive–compulsive disorder with and without depression. *J Clin Psychiatry* 1990;51(Suppl):61–9; discussion 70.

12. Benkelfat C, Nordahl TE, Semple WE, King AC, Murphy DL, Cohen RM. Local cerebral glucose metabolic rates in obsessive–compulsive disorder. Patients treated with clomipramine. *Arch Gen Psychiatry* 1990;47:840–8.

13. Martinot JL, Allilaire JF, Mazoyer BM, et al. Obsessive–compulsive disorder: a clinical, neuropsychological and positron emission tomography study. *Acta Psychiatry Scand* 1990;82:233–422.

14. Swedo SE, Schapiro MB, Grady CL, et al. Cerebral glucose metabolism in childhood-onset obsessive–compulsive disorder. *Arch Gen Psychiatry* 1989;46:518–23.

15. Chase TN, Geoffrey V, Gillespie M, Burrows GH. Structural and functional studies of Gilles de la Tourette syndrome. *Rev Neurol* 1986; 142:851–5.

16. Sacks OW. Acquired Tourettism in adult life. In: Friedhoff AJ, Chase TN, eds. *Gilles de la Tourette syndrome*. Advances in neurology, vol 35. New York: Raven Press, 1982;89–92.

17. Robertson MM. The Gilles de la Tourette syndrome: the current status. *Br J Psychiatry* 1989; 154:147–69.

18. Caparulo BK, Cohen DJ, Rothman SL, et al. Computed tomographic brain scanning in children with developmental neuropsychiatric disorders. *J Am Acad Child Psychiatry* 1981;20:338–57.

19. Lees AJ, Robertson M, Trimble MR, Murray NMF. A clinical study of Gilles de la Tourette syndrome in the United Kingdom. *J Neurol Neurosurg Psychiatry* 1984;47:1–8.

20. Robertson MM, Trimble MR, Lees AJ. The psychopathology of Gilles de la Tourette syndrome: a phenomenological analysis. *Br J Psychiatry* 1988; 152:383–90.

21. Harcherik DF, Cohen DJ, Ort S, et al. Computed tomographic brain scanning in four neuropsychiatric disorders of childhood. *Am J Psychiatry* 1985; 142:731–4.

22. Regeur L, Pakkenberg B, Fog R, Pakkenberg H. Clinical features and long-term treatment with pimozide in 65 patients with Gilles de la Tourette's syndrome. *J Neurol Neurosurg Psychiatry* 1986; 49:791–5.

23. Yeragani VK, Blackman M, Baker GB. Biological and psychological aspects of a case of Gilles de la Tourette's syndrome. *J Clin Psychiatry* 1983; 44:27–9.

24. Shaenboen MJ, Nigro MA, Martocci RJ. Colpocephaly and Gilles de la Tourette's syndrome. *Arch Neurol* 1984;41:1023.

25. Lakke JP, Wilmink JT. A case of Gilles de la Tourette's syndrome with midbrain involvement. *J Neurol Neurosurg Psychiatry* 1985;48:1293–6.

26. Kjaer M, Boris P, Gadegaard Hansen L. Abnormal CT scan in a patient with Gilles de la Tourette syndrome. *Neuroradiology* 1986;28:362–3.

27. Sandyk R. A case of Tourette's syndrome with midbrain involvement. *Int J Neurosci* 1988; 43:171–5.

28. Vieregge P, Schafer C, Jørg J. Concordant Gilles de la Tourette's syndrome in monozygotic twins: a clinical, neurophysiological and CT study. *J Neurol* 1988;235:366–7.

29. Robertson M, Doran M, Trimble M, Lees AJ. The treatment of Gilles de la Tourette syndrome by limbic leucotomy. *J Neurol Neurosurg Psychiatry* 1990;53:691–4.

30. Weilburg JB, Mesulam M-M, Weintraub S, Buonanno F, Jenike M, Stakes JW. Focal striatal abnormalities in a patient with obsessive–compulsive disorder. *Arch Neurol* 1989;46:233–5.

31. Pulst S-M, Walshe TM, Romero JA. Carbon monoxide poisoning with features of Gilles de la Tourette's syndrome. *Arch Neurol* 1983;40:443–4.

32. Ward CD. Transient feelings of compulsion caused by hemispheric lesions: three cases. *J Neurol Neurosurg Psychiatry* 1988;51:266–8.

33. Laplane D, Levasseur M, Pillon B, et al. Obsessions-compulsions and behavioural changes with bilateral basal ganglia lesions: a neuropsychological, magnetic resonance imaging and positron tomography study. *Brain* 1989;112:699–725.

34. Turley JM (1988) Tourette-like disorder after herpes encephalitis. *Am J Psychiatry* 1988; 145:1604–9.

35. Northam RS, Singer HS. Postencephalitic acquired Tourette-like syndrome in a child. *Neurology* 1991;41:592–3.

Advances in Neurology, Vol. 58, edited by T. N. Chase, A. J. Friedhoff, and D. J. Cohen. Raven Press, Ltd., New York © 1992.

25

SPECT Imaging of Cerebral Blood Flow in Tourette Syndrome

*Mark A. Riddle, †Ann M. Rasmusson, †Scott W. Woods, and ‡Paul B. Hoffer

*Yale Child Study Center, Yale University School of Medicine, New Haven, Connecticut 06510, †Department of Psychiatry, Yale University School of Medicine, New Haven, Connecticut 06510, and ‡Department of Diagnostic Radiology, Yale University School of Medicine, New Haven, Connecticut 06510

Functional brain imaging with single photon emission computed tomography (SPECT) and positron emission tomography (PET) provides a means for direct assessment of blood flow, metabolic activity, and density of neurotransmitter receptors and uptake sites in discrete regions of the brain. Studies using PET to assess regional cerebral metabolic activity and dopamine D-2 receptor densities are presented elsewhere in this volume (see chapters 26, 27, and 28). This chapter focuses on assessment of regional cerebral blood flow (rCBF) using SPECT and presents data from a pilot study of rCBF in adults with Tourette syndrome (TS).

PET AND SPECT

PET and SPECT each have advantages and disadvantages in different situations. Superior resolution can be achieved with PET; in addition, attenuation can be measured directly. The advantages of SPECT include the considerably lower cost and the longer half-life ($t_{1/2}$) of SPECT radionuclides. The longer $t_{1/2}$ of SPECT radionuclides is advantageous for studies requiring that the subject be injected away from the camera site and for receptor displacement studies that require repeated scans in the same patient over a long period of time. The resolution of SPECT devices has significantly improved in recent years. The resolution (measured as full width at half-maximum) of commercially-available SPECT cameras is 7.5–8.0 mm in all three axes, which compares well with that of commercially available PET devices (about 5–6 mm).

UTILITY OF rCBF DETERMINATION

The measurement of rCBF has been shown in a variety of experimental paradigms to reflect dynamic alterations in neuronal activity. For example, discrete physiologic stimuli have been shown in experimental animals to produce increases in cell firing and blood flow in brain regions of nearly identical volume (1,2). The changes in blood flow follow the changes in cell firing by only 1–3 seconds (2,3) or, perhaps, even as little as 250 msec (4). A variety of physiological manipulations believed to alter regional neuronal activity in humans have also been shown to alter rCBF in appropriate brain regions (5–9). Under resting conditions, rCBF and regional glu-

cose or oxygen metabolism are closely correlated across brain regions (5,10). The
mechanism responsible for the tight coupling of neuronal activity and rCBF remains
unknown; potassium release during neuronal depolarization, adenosine, nitric
oxide, or other neuronal factors may play a
role (11).

VALIDITY OF HMPAO DISTRIBUTION AS A REFLECTION OF rCBF

Technetium - 99m - hexamethylpropylene
amine oxime (HMPAO) is a commercially
available radiopharmaceutical that is used
to assess rCBF. There is general agreement
that HMPAO crosses the blood–brain barrier with a high first-pass extraction and that
roughly 4–5% of the intravenously injected
dose is retained in the brain with little redistribution for up to 24 hours postinjection
(12–14). Gray matter and white matter are
distinguishable in the images. Clinical studies have consistently demonstrated regional
decreases in HMPAO uptake in a variety
of clinical conditions under which regional
decreases in rCBF are expected, including
stroke, brain tumors, interictal epilepsy,
and dementia (14–19). HMPAO distribution
has also been reported to show detectable
regional increases in pathological conditions for which rCBF increases are expected, such as luxury perfusion after cerebral infarct (20,21), ictal scans in epileptics
(22,23) and high-flow tumors (24).

Although HMPAO uptake increases in response to increased rCBF, the relationship
between HMPAO uptake and rCBF is not
linear, with HMPAO uptake underestimat-
ing the actual magnitude of increased rCBF
at the highest levels (25–27). The most likely
explanation for this nonlinearity is incomplete cerebral trapping, producing flow-re-
lated back-diffusion of the tracer (25,26), although other possible explanations have
been offered (28–30). Lassen and colleagues (25,26) have developed an algorithm
to correct for this nonlinearity due to back-

diffusion that can be easily applied to the
reconstructed data. Inugami and colleagues
(27) have demonstrated that the Lassen
"linearization" correction is accurate: distribution of HMPAO in the brain as measured by SPECT (with the Lassen correction) revealed an impressive linear
correlation ($r = 0.93$) with CBF as measured by the $C^{15}O_2$ steady-state method and
PET. In a photic stimulation study recently
conducted at Yale, comparison of images
obtained during light-occluded versus
photic stimulation conditions in seven
healthy subjects revealed a significant increase (36.7% ± 6.6%) in distribution of
HMPAO in visual cortex relative to whole
brain [after Lassen correction for back-diffusion (31)].

In summary, HMPAO uptake generally
reflects rCBF, especially under basal conditions. Although HMPAO uptake does not
increase in 1:1 proportion with the actual
rCBF, its increase is generally sufficient to
detect expected rCBF differences, particularly when the Lassen correction is made.

ADVANTAGE OF HMPAO IN PATIENTS WITH TS

Two features of TS render pathophysiological studies, particularly neuroimaging
studies, difficult: head movement caused by
the tics, and the waxing and waning nature
of the symptoms over short periods of time.
Consequently, HMPAO may be uniquely
suited for obtaining scans reflecting rCBF
in patients with TS given the rapid brain uptake and very slow redistribution after uptake of HMPAO (HMPAO uptake is determined by the blood flow during the 1–2
minutes after the injection, not by the blood
flow during the scan acquisition). Rapid
brain uptake is important because tic severity can be observed and rated over the 1–2
minutes during which HMPAO is being
taken up in the brain, so that tic severity can
be compared to rCBF. Slow redistribution
permits a study design in which subjects are

injected while they are having tic symptoms, but are scanned later, when the tics have subsided. If necessary, sedative medication may be administered to diminish or eliminate the tic symptoms during the scanning procedure without changing the pattern of previous HMPAO uptake. This is especially important for studies of children, who may have difficulty holding still, and for provocative studies in which an agent or condition may be invoked to increase tic symptom severity.

LITERATURE REVIEW OF STUDIES OF rCBF USING SPECT

A group of investigators at University College and Middlesex School of Medicine in London are using HMPAO and SPECT to study rCBF in patients with TS. In an ongoing study of 25 subjects with TS and 10 normal control subjects, they reported hypoperfusion in the basal ganglia, thalamus, and frontal and temporal cortical areas (32). The same group of investigators also reported differences in frontal lobe/basal ganglia ratios in "pure TS" versus TS + OCD subjects, although the differences were not significant (33). Unfortunately, the only published data available on these studies are in abstract format.

PRELIMINARY STUDY OF rCBF USING HMPAO

Our group has completed a preliminary study designed to compare rCBF in patients with TS and individually age- and gender-matched controls, and to assess relationships between symptom severity and rCBF in the TS patients. This study was presented in detail elsewhere (34) and is briefly summarized here.

Nine drug-free, right-handed, adults with TS (6 M, 3 F; age, 29.6 ± 6.9 years) and nine individually age- (within 2 years) and gender-matched controls participated. SPECT scans were acquired following IV

injection of 20 mCi HMPAO. Eyes and ears were covered from 2 minutes before until 2 minutes after the injection. The head was positioned using laser lights so that the orbitocanthomeatal (CM) line bilaterally was in the plane of the first slice. Sixteen to 20 transaxial slices, depending on the size of the head, each 6 mm apart, were obtained per study over about 45 minutes [2½ minutes per slice using a Strichman 810X Brain Imager (x–y axis resolution 8 mm at periphery, 10 mm at center; z axis resolution 16 mm)].

Regions of interest (ROIs) were identified by one investigator and outlined using anatomical information from the SPECT scan and an anatomical atlas (35), both cut in slices parallel to the CM line. A series of ROIs were chosen for preliminary analyses, including frontal, parietal, temporal, and occipital cortices, caudate, putamen–globus pallidus, and thalamus, all bilaterally, as well as anterior and posterior cingulate and brainstem. The ROIs were reviewed by a second investigator and any corrections were made by consensus. In each ROI within each slice, the total number of counts, the number of pixels, and the average number of counts per pixel were quantified. ROIs appearing in more than one slice were quantified in each slice in which they appeared. Then a weighted average (counts per pixel), based on relative area, was calculated for each ROI. ROI data were analyzed by calculating ROI-to-whole brain minus cerebellum (WB-CE) ratios. Paired, two-tailed t tests were used for between-group comparisons.

Mean relative HMPAO uptake was reduced in the TS subjects in basal ganglia and frontal cortical areas, reaching statistical significance in the left putamen-globus pallidus, where the relative HMPAO uptake was about 4% lower than in the controls.

Ratings of current tic and obsessive–compulsive symptom severity were also obtained. Pearson correlation coefficients were calculated for these clinical variables versus HMPAO uptake in each of the ROIs. There was a positive correlation between HMPAO uptake in the left thalamus and motor tic severity.

The findings of altered rCBF in frontal cortical and basal ganglia regions are consistent with emerging hypotheses regarding the pathophysiology of TS. Research on the basal ganglia have highlighted the importance of multiple, parallel corticostriatothalamocortical (CSTC) circuits that concurrently subserve a wide variety of motor, oculomotor, sensorimotor, cognitive, and emotive (limbic) processes (36–39).

CONCLUSIONS

Several research groups are beginning to apply PET and SPECT imaging techniques to examine brain function in patients with TS. However, the data that have been presented to date suffer from several methodological limitations including small sample size (in most studies), crude volumetric analytic techniques, and lack of coregistration between magnetic resonance imaging (MRI) and SPECT (or PET) scans for defining anatomically precise ROIs.

Despite these methodological limitations, several provocative findings have emerged including increased relative metabolic activity (41–44) and rCBF in certain frontal cortical areas in OCD and decreased relative metabolic activity (45) and rCBF in basal ganglia in TS. These findings are remarkably consistent with hypotheses concerning the brain regions that are likely to be affected by these disorders.

REFERENCES

1. Leninger-Follert E, Hossmann KA. Simultaneous measurements of microflow and evoked potentials in the somatomotor cortex of the cat brain during specific sensory activation. *Pflugers Arch* 1979; 380:85–9.
2. Lubbers DW, Leniger-Follert E. Capillary flow in the brain cortex during changes in oxygen supply and state of activation. *Ciba Found Symp* 1978; 56:49–67.
3. Silver IA. Cellular microenvironment in relation to local blood flow. *Ciba Found Symp* 1978;56:49–67.
4. Sandman CA, O'Halloran JP, Isenhart R. Is there an evoked vascular response? *Science* 1984; 22:1355–7.
5. Sokoloff L. Relationships among local functional activity, energy metabolism, and blood flow in the central nervous system. *Fed Proc* 1981;2311–6.
6. Fox PT, Raichle ME. Stimulus rate dependence of regional cerebral blood flow in human striate cortex, demonstrated by positron emission tomography. *J Neurophysiol* 1984;51:1109–20.
7. Fox PT, Raichle ME. Focal psychological uncoupling of cerebral blood flow and oxidative metabolism during somatosensory stimulation in human subjects. *Proc Natl Acad Sci USA* 1986; 83:1140–4.
8. Raichle ME, Fox PT, Mintun MA, Dense C. Cerebral blood flow and oxidative blycolysis are uncoupled by neuronal activity. *J Cereb Blood Flow Metab* 1987;7:S300–2.
9. Ginsberg MD, Chang JY, Kelley RE, et al. Increases in both cerebral glucose utilization and blood flow during execution of a somatosensory task. *Ann Neurol* 1988;23:152–60.
10. Raichle ME, Grubb RL Jr., Gado MH, Eighling JO, Ter-Pogossian MM. Correlation between regional cerebral blood flow and oxidative metabolism: in vivo studies in man. *Arch Neurol* 1976; 22:289–97.
11. Lou HC, Edvinsson L, MacKenzie ET. The concept of coupling blood flow to brain function: revision required. *Ann Neurol* 1987;22:289–97.
12. Reichmann K, Biersack HJ, Basso L, et al. A comparative study of brain uptake and early kinetics of ^{99m}Tc-d1 HM-PAO and other PnAO derivatives in baboons. *Nucl Med* 1986;25:134–7.
13. Neirinckz RD, Canning LR, Piper IM, et al. Technetium-99md,1-HM-PAO: a new radiopharmaceutical for SPECT imaging of regional cerebral blood perfusion. *J Nucl Med* 1987;28:191–202.
14. Sharp PF, Smith FW, Gemmell GH, et al. Technetium-99m HM-PAO stereoisomers as potential agents for imaging regional cerebral blood flow: human volunteer studies. *J Nucl Med* 1986; 27:171–7.
15. Podreka I, Suess E, Goldenberg G, et al. Initial experience with technetium-99m HM-PAO brain SPECT. *J Nucl Med* 1987;28:1657–66.
16. Buell U, Stirner H, Braun H, Kreiten K, Ferbert A. SPECT with ^{99}Tc^m-HMPAO with ^{99m}Tc^m-pertechenatate to assess regional cerebral blood flow (rCBF) and blood volume (rCBV): preliminary results in cerebrovascular disease and interictal epilepsy. *Nucl Med Commun* 1987;8:519–24.
17. Stefan H, Pawlik G, Bocher-Schwarz HG, et al. Functional and morphological abnormalities in temporal lobe epilepsy: a comparison of interictal and ictal EEG, CT, MRI, SPECT and PET. *J Neurol* 1987;134:377–84.
18. Gemmell HG, Sharp PF, Besson JAO, et al. Differential diagnosis in dementia using the cerebral blood flow agent ^{99m}Tc HM-PAO: a SPECT study. *J Comput Assist Tomogr* 1987;11:398–402.
19. Neary D, Snowden JS, Shields RA, et al. Single

photon emission tomography using ^{99m}Tc-Hm-PAO in the investigation of dementia. *J Neurol Neurosurg Psychiatry* 1987;50:1101–9.

20. Holmes RA, Gini A, Logan KW. Demonstration of cerebral infarct hyperemia with Tc-99m-HM-PAO. *J Nucl Med* 1987;28:633.

21. Seuss E, Prodreka I, Goldenberg G, et al. Initial experience with ^{99}Tc^m-hexamethyl-propylenea-mineoxine brain SPECT. *Nucl Med Commun* 1986;7:285.

22. Hwang PA, Gilday DL, Ash JM, et al. Perturbations in regional cerebral blood flow detected by SPECT scanning with 99m Tc-HmPAO correlate with EEG abnormalities in children with epilepsy. *J Cereb Blood Flow Metab* 1987;7:S573.

23. Holmes RA, Volkert WA, Gini A, Corlija M. Detection of a high rCBF disorder in patient with Tc-99m-d,1-HMPAO. *J Nucl Med* 1988;977:29.

24. Langen KJ, Herzog H, Kuwert T, et al. Tomographic studies of RCBF with Tc-99m-HM-PAO SPECT in patients with primary brain tumors: comparison with continuous inhalation of Co-15-0 and PET. *J Nucl Med* 1987;28:591.

25. Lassen N, Anderson A, Friberg H. Technetium-99m-HMPAO as a tracer of cerebral blood flow distribution: a kinetic analysis. *J Cereb Blood Flow Metab* 1987a;7:S535(abst).

26. Lassen N, Anderson AR, Neirinckx RD, Ell PJ, Costa DC. Validation of ceretec. In: Ell PJ, Costa DC, Cullum ID, Jarritt PH, Lui D, eds. *rCBF atlas–the clinical application of rCBF imaging by SPECT*. High Wycombe: Brier Press, 1987;14–8.

27. Inugami A, Kanno I, Uemura K, et al. Linearization correction of ^{99m}Tc-labelled hexamethyl-propylene amine oxime (HM-PAO) image in terms of regional CBF distribution: comparison to $C^{15}O_2$ inhalation steady-state method measured by positron emission tomography. *J Cereb Blood Flow Metab* 1988;8:S52–S60.

28. Lear JF. Quantitative local cerebral blood flow measurements with technetium-99m HM-PAO: evaluation using multiple radionuclide digital quantitative autoradiography. *J Nucl Med* 1988;29:1387–92.

29. Lavender J, Peters A, Roddie M. Preliminary clinical experience with Tc-99 HM-PAO for labeling leucocytes and imaging inflammation. *Nucl Med* 1987;26:90(abst).

30. Lui D, Costa D, Jarritt P, et al. Simultaneous, dual radionuclide labeled, white cells: in-111-oxime vs. Tc-99m-HM-PAO. A comprehensive study. *Nucl Med* 1987;26:90.

31. Woods SW, Hegeman IM, Zubal IG, et al. Visual stimulation increases technetium-99m-HMPAO distribution in human visual cortex. *J Nucl Med* 1991;32:210–5.

32. Hall M, Costa DC, Shields J, Heavens J, Robertson M, Ell PJ. Brain perfusion patterns with Tc-99mHMPAO/SPET in patients with Gilles de la Tourette syndrome. *Eur J Nucl Med* 1990;16:56.

33. George MS, Robertson MB, Costa DC, Trimble MR, Eu PJ. HMPAO SPECT scans of comorbid OCD and Tourette's syndrome patients. Abstract NR29. In: *1991 New Research Program and Abstracts*, American Psychiatric Association Annual Meeting, 1991;57.

34. Riddle MA, Rasmusson AM, Woods SW, et al. SPECT imaging of regional cerebral blood flow in Tourette's syndrome. *Psychiatry Res*, (in press).

35. Matusi T, Hirano A. *An atlas of the human brain for computerized tomography*. Tokyo: Igaku-Shoin, 1978.

36. Alexander GE, DeLong MR, Strick PL. Parallel organization of functionally segregation circuits linking basal ganglia and cortex. *Annu Rev Neurosci* 1986;9:357–81.

37. Alexander GE, Crutcher MD. Functional architecture of basal ganglia circuits: neural substrates of parallel processing. *Trends Neurosci* 1990;13:266–71.

38. Alexander GE, Crutcher MD, DeLong MR. Basal ganglia-thalamocortical circuits: parallel substrates for motor, oculomotor, "prefrontal" and "limbic" functions. In: HBM Uylings, CG Van Eden, JPC DeBruin, MA Corner, MGP Feenstra, eds. *Progress in brain research*, vol 85. Amsterdam: Elsevier Science Publishers B.V., 1990; 119–146.

39. Goldman-Rakic PS, Selemon LD. New frontiers in basal ganglia research. *Trends Neurosci* 1990; 13:241–3.

40. Deleted in proof.

41. Baxter LR, Phelps ME, Mazziotta JC, Guze BH, Schwartz JM, Selin CE. Local cerebral glucose metabolic rates in obsessive-compulsive disorder. *Arch Gen Psychiatry* 1987;44:211–8.

42. Baxter LR, Schwartz JM, Mazziotta JC, et al. Cerebral glucose metabolic rates in non-depressed obsessive-compulsives. *Am J Psychiatry* 1988;145:1560–3.

43. Nordahl TE, Benkelfat C, Semple WE, Gross M, King AC, Cohen RM. Cerebral glucose metabolic rates in obsessive compulsive disorder. *Neuropsychopharmacology* 1989;2:23–8.

44. Swedo SE, Shapiro MB, Grady CL, et al. Cerebral glucose metabolism in childhood-onset obsessive-compulsive disorder. *Arch Gen Psychiatry* 1989; 46:518–23.

45. Chase TN, Geoffrey V, Gillespie M, Burrows GH. Structural and functional studies of Gilles de la Tourette syndrome. *Rev Neurol* 1986;142:851–5.

Advances in Neurology, Vol. 58, edited by T. N. Chase, A. J. Friedhoff, and D. J. Cohen. Raven Press, Ltd., New York 1992.

26

Functional Neuroanatomy of Tourette Syndrome

Limbic–Motor Interactions Studied with FDG PET

Brigitte Stoetter, Allen R. Braun, Christopher Randolph, Jeffrey Gernert, Richard E. Carson, Peter Herscovitch, and Thomas N. Chase

Experimental Therapeutics Branch, National Institute of Neurological Diseases and Stroke, National Institutes of Health, Bethesda, Maryland 20892

The pathogenesis of Tourette syndrome (TS) remains nearly as obscure as when the illness was first described more than a century ago (1). TS is clearly a disorder of motor function. The multiple motor and vocal tics that are characteristic of the syndrome must involve brain regions that participate in the organization, initiation, and execution of movement. Yet the tics observed in TS patients differ from abnormal movements typically encountered in other hyperkinetic movement disorders. These are commonly preceded by an experience of motivational tension; their expression is followed by a sense of satisfaction or relief. The urge to tic is consciously experienced by the patients, who may suppress movements for a variable period of time, but will inevitably yield to what they are felt "driven" to do.

For this reason, it appears likely that the pathogenesis of TS is not confined exclusively to the motor domain. Because the disorder is also associated with complex behavior disturbances including obsessions and compulsions (2), attentional difficulties (3), irritability, impulsivity, and self-inju-rious behavior (4), the neuroanatomical substrate underlying symptoms in TS is assumed to include limbic as well as motor mechanisms.

However, the regions of the brain—either limbic or motor—involved in the generation of symptoms have not been identified in studies employing traditional neuro-anatomical or physiological techniques (5–11).

Positron emission tomography (PET), using F-18 fluorodeoxyglucose (FDG), is a well-established method of characterizing functional activity in the living human brain (12), which may be of particular value in illnesses without clear pathophysiological features such as TS. In the present study, we compared regional patterns of glucose metabolism in 18 drug-free individuals with typical TS and 16 age- and sex-matched control subjects in an attempt to characterize the functional neuroanatomy of this illness.

The initial evaluation of these data attempts to identify any changes in metabolic rates for glucose—either global or regional—that distinguish patients with TS from normal volunteers. Brain regions clearly do not operate in isolation, however, but function as elements in a series of neural networks distributed throughout the central nervous system (CNS). Therefore, to identify functional *interactions* between brain regions (13) that might distinguish patients and controls, an analysis of correlations between local metabolic rates for glucose was performed.

Our results suggest that differences in regional metabolic rates can distinguish TS patients and normals and that specific limbic and motor regions of the central nervous system—and altered relationships *between* these regions—may be involved in the pathogenesis of this disorder.

STUDY DESIGN

PET scans were performed in 18 drug-free patients with TS, 16 men and 2 women, aged 33 ± 7 years (mean ± SD; range, 23–49 years), and 16 age- and sex-matched normal volunteer subjects, 11 men and 5 women, aged 34 ± 10 years (mean ± SD; range, 20–50 years).

Scans were performed on the Neuropet (14), a seven-slice positron tomograph with an in-plane resolution of 6–7 mm and an axial resolution of 11–12 mm FWHM. [F-18]-fluoro-2-deoxy-D-glucose (5 m Ci) was injected intravenously over a period of 1 minute, and 10-minute scans were initiated 30–45 minutes after this. Arterialized venous blood was sampled throughout the duration of the study. Local cerebral metabolic rates for glucose were calculated according to the method of Brooks (15).

Results of PET studies are not infrequently inconsistent or difficult to replicate; this can be due to small group numbers, differences in PET instrumentation, or differences in the methods of data analysis. In order to minimize the last source of error, two independent and technically distinct analytic approaches were applied to the PET data by separate investigators, and the results of these analyses were compared.

Eight planes of section were selected for analysis on the basis of recognizable anatomical landmarks; these are illustrated in Figs. 1 and 2.

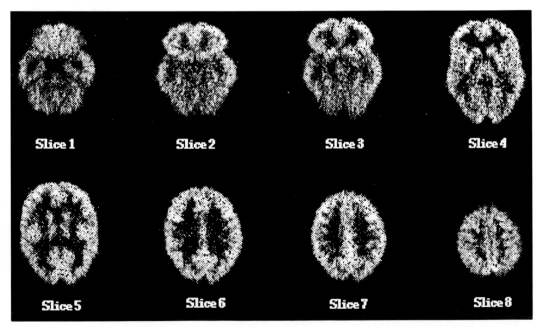

FIG. 1. A typical PET data set, illustrating the eight planes of section chosen for analysis. Inferior regions (cerebellum, temporal pole, and gyrus rectus) are seen at the *upper left* and superior regions (frontal and parietal convexities) *lower right*.

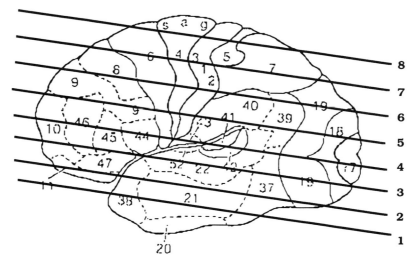

FIG. 2. Approximate location of PET planes of section (see Figs. 1, 4 and 6) illustrated on a lateral representation of the brain in which cytoarchitectonic (Brodman) regions are indicated.

In analysis 1, regional metabolic rates were obtained by placing templates consisting of small circular (7.8 mm in diameter) regions of interest (ROI) on PET planes of section (Fig. 3a). ROIs were independently translated and placed over the local maximum (activity peak). Data reduction was performed by averaging these values.

In analysis 2 irregular regions of interest were applied in the cortex in order to maximize the use of anatomical detail. Cortical–cerebrospinal fluids (CSF) and cortical–white matter boundaries were thresholded interactively and the cortical mantle was divided using a radial template that could be adjusted with reference to the midline and major cortical landmarks (Fig. 3b). Subcortical regions were sampled using circular regions of interest 5.2–7.8 mm in diameter.

For each analysis, templates were designed so that regions could be compared to coded areas in an atlas (16) in which both functional and cytoarchtectonic descriptors are assigned to anatomical areas of interest.

In both analyses 1 and 2, absolute whole-brain glucose metabolic rates (CMRglu) were compared initially, and normalized regional values (regional/whole-brain average

CMRglu) were then analyzed. Repeated measures analyses of variance were performed independently on normalized regional metabolic rates from both data sets. In each case, when overall significance was demonstrated, individual regional metabolic rates were compared by two-tailed t tests in order to identify regions that accounted for significant differences between groups. Regional differences between TS patients and controls that were identified in at least one hemisphere in *both* analyses were considered reliable.

Correlations between metabolic rates were then evaluated in order to identify differences in functional interactions *between* brain regions that might differentiate patients and controls. Pearson product–moment correlation matrices were generated independently for Tourette patients and normal volunteers using normalized metabolic rates estimated for regions of interest in analysis 2. The matrices, in which correlation coefficients serve as an index of functional coupling between brain regions (13,17,18), were calculated utilizing standardized methods (19); their derivation is illustrated schematically in Fig. 4a. TS and control matrices were therefore evaluated

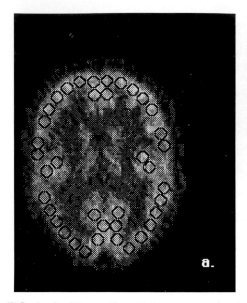 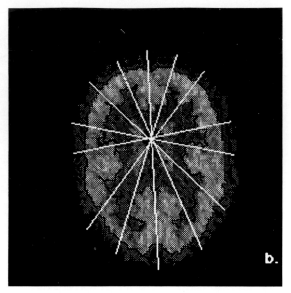

FIG. 3. An illustration of the two methods by which regions of interest were identified in this study. In analysis 1 (**a**), a template consisting of circular regions of interest is placed on the PET image. ROIs are then independently translated and placed over the local maximum (activity peak) in order to minimize the effects of partial volume averaging. In analysis 2 (**b**), irregular regions of interest are applied in the cortex in order to maximize the use of anatomical detail. Cortical–CSF and cortical–white matter boundaries are thresholded interactively. The cortical mantle is then divided using a radial template.

parametrically in a series of steps illustrated schematically in Fig. 4b:

1. A Fisher Z-prime transformation (20) of all the correlation coefficients—necessary to generate a normal distribution of these values—was performed.
2. Interregional correlations in Tourette and control matrices were then compared. Difference scores are calculated by subtracting individual transformed correlation coefficients derived for patients from those derived for controls and weighting these results for the number of subjects in each cohort. Difference scores are themselves Z values for which probability levels can be calculated using a standardized normal distribution table. Z scores greater or less than $\pm$ 1.96 ($p < 0.025$) were retained in the difference matrix and used to identify regional interrelationships that *differed* in patients and controls.

3. Similarities and differences between patients and controls were then represented anatomically by projecting identified correlation coefficients onto brain maps. When significant pairwise differences were identified, the original correlation coefficients themselves were reevaluated. Only instances in which a significant Z score had been obtained *and* one or the other of the correlation coefficients exceeded threshold values (corresponding to a significance level of $p < 0.05$) were used for the purpose of illustrating group differences. Similarities in regional associations were illustrated if correlations between regions in *both* groups exceeded these threshold values.

FINDINGS

Absolute metabolic rates for glucose derived in both analyses were compared ini-

Normalized Regional Metabolic Rates

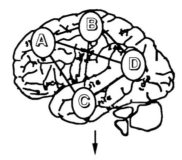

Correlation Matrix

	Reg A	Reg B	Reg C	Reg D
Reg A	1.0	.56	.25	.82
Reg B	.56	1.0	.01	.33
Reg C	.25	.01	1.0	.75
Reg D	.82	.33	.75	1.0

a.

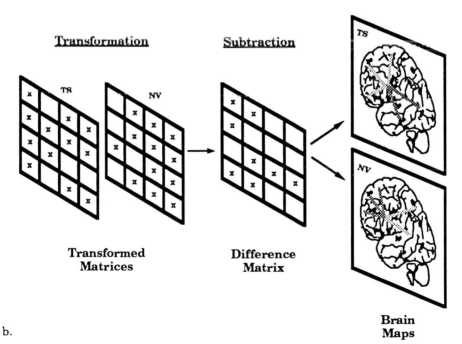

b.

FIG. 4. A schematic illustration of the techniques used to analyze correlations between regional metabolic rates. **a**: Derivation of correlation matrices from regional PET data. **b**: Steps involved in the comparison of Tourette and control matrices. In order to identify differences in regional coupling that distinguish patients from controls, (i) a Z-prime transformation of correlation coefficients is performed; (ii) matrices are subtracted, generating difference scores; and (iii) significant differences are represented by projecting the correlation coefficients back onto brain maps. (These techniques are explained in detail in the Methods section.) *NV*, normal volunteers.

tially. There were no significant differences in overall mean gray matter metabolic rates between Tourette patients and normal volunteers (analysis 1: TS = 8.72 ± 1.24 mg glucose/100 g/min, normals = 8.54 ± 1.32; analysis 2: TS = 8.46 ± 1.28, normals = 8.69 ± 1.44).

When normalized regional metabolic rates in TS and controls were compared by univariate repeated measures analysis of variance, the diagnosis by region interaction was significant in both instances (analysis 1: $F = 2.45$, 111 df, $p < 0.0001$; analysis 2: $F = 1.47$, 163 df, $p < 0.0025$), indicating that TS patients and normals can be distinguished by differences in metabolic rates in distinct brain regions. When the results of analyses 1 and 2 were compared, the distribution of significant differences between normalized metabolic rates identified in post hoc comparison of regional means was markedly congruent. Regional differences identified in at least one hemisphere in *both* analyses were considered the most reliable and are listed in Table 1.

TS patients are characterized by *lower* relative metabolic rates in inferior, limbic regions of the cortex, striatum and subcortical limbic structures, and by *higher* relative metabolic rates in superior, sensorimotor cortices. In the inferior regions, these decreases reached statistical significance, in both analyses, in the orbitofrontal cortices, inferior insular cortex, parahippocampal region, and ventral striatum; normalized metabolic rates were also significantly reduced in the putamen in both data sets, but not to the degree observed in the ventral striatum. In the superior sensorimotor regions, increases reached statistical significance in the supplementary motor area, lateral premotor and Rolandic cortices, and superior parietal lobule.

The foregoing results suggest that altered functional relationships *between* inferior limbic and superior sensorimotor regions might characterize TS patients. In order to examine this possibility more directly, correlations between local metabolic rates for glucose were evaluated. Parametric comparison of correlation matrices permits the evaluation of differences in the magnitude

TABLE 1. *Percent change in normalized regional metabolic rates, Tourette patients vs. normal volunteers*

Regions of interest	Analysis 1 (%)		Analysis 2 (%)	
	Left	Right	Left	Right
Decreases				
Ventral striatum	−10.0****	−7.1**	−7.0***	−5.2*
Anterior putamen	−8.1***	−5.7*	−4.6*	−1.9
Caudal orbital cortex	−8.0*	−8.1*	−3.6	−8.6***
Medial orbital cortex	−8.7*	−4.5	−9.9***	−10.2***
Lateral orbital cortex	−11.6***	−8.7**	−11.6**	−8.1*
Opercular orbital cortex	−13.5****	−6.0*	−7.2***	−2.5
Inferior insula	−12.6****	−6.2*	−9.7****	−3.9*
Parahippocampal region	−4.7*	−3.8	−5.8***	−5.4**
Increases				
Superior lateral premotor cortex	6.0*	8.2***	2.0	3.5*
Anterior SMA[a]	3.8**	7.7**	4.6*	1.2
Posterior SMA	12.0****	11.4***	3.6	5.9*
Inferior rolandic cortex	2.6	5.9**	3.9*	6.1*
Superior rolandic cortex	6.6*	14.4****	4.2*	3.3
Superior parietal lobule	1.4	8.2*	4.7*	5.4**

[a] SMA, supplementary motor cortex.
* $p < 0.05$.
** $p < 0.01$.
*** $p < 0.005$.
**** $p < 0.001$.

of individual pairwise correlation coefficients. Z scores, derived and thresholded as outlined above, identify changes in individual relationships between brain regions that distinguish patients and controls.

When *all* areas of the brain are compared, the region that most consistently distinguishes Tourette patients and normal controls is the ventral striatum. The absolute Z value (Z_{total} = 130.9, sum of absolute values of positive and negative Z scores is markedly higher for this than for any other brain region (the only instance in which this value is greater than three standard deviations above the mean). Changes in the relationships between ventral striatum and other areas also accounted for the highest mean difference score ($Z_{average}$ = 4.85), and the greatest frequency of pairwise differences (34.6% of all possible correlations differed significantly).

In the basal ganglia, therefore, significant differences in regional correlations involve relationships of the ventral striatum more frequently than those of the caudate or putamen. In addition, in the prefrontal cortices, differences between Tourette patients and controls more frequently involve the orbital than dorsolateral or frontal opercular cortices. In limbic regions of interest, differences between patients and controls occur more frequently in the insula and related regions of interest than they do in the cingulate cortex and associated regions (data not illustrated).

Individual relationships of the ventral striatum and other brain regions observed in TS patients and controls are depicted in Fig. 5; these are contrasted with functional relationships the putamen, illustrated in Fig. 6. In general, the most robust differences in the functional relationships of the ventral striatum tend to cluster in sensorimotor regions. In contrast, differences involving the putamen tend to cluster instead in orbital and limbic regions of interest. In each instance, significant differences are found in relationships *between* nuclei of the basal ganglia.

The most striking changes involving the ventral striatum include a *reversal* of functional relationships between this region and sensorimotor cortices—including lateral premotor cortex, supplementary motor area, superior rolandic cortex and parietal cortices—in Tourette patients.

In normal volunteers there is a consistent pattern of *negative* correlations between activity in the ventral striatum and these sensorimotor regions, that is, when the ventral striatum is metabolically active, the sensorimotor areas are relatively silent. In Tourette patients, however, these correlations are uniformly *positive*. Ventral striatum and motor cortices are all active—or activated—concurrently, suggesting that the illness may be characterized, in part, by a distorted relationship between this striatal region and cortical areas involved in motor control.

Metabolic rates in the ventral striatum and putamen are positively coupled in normal volunteers; metabolic rates in these regions of the basal ganglia are uncoupled in TS patients.

In contrast, there is a reversal of functional relationships between the putamen and *ventral limbic* regions in TS patients (Fig. 6). Metabolic rates in the putamen and orbitofrontal cortices, inferior insula, and parahippocampal gyri are in general *negatively* correlated in normal subjects. They are *positively* coupled in patients with Tourette's syndrome.

Although not functionally reversed, relationships between putamen and sensorimotor cortices are altered in TS patients as well. Correlations between metabolic rates in the putamen and rolandic and parietal cortices are positive in normal volunteers. Significant correlations between these regions are absent in TS patients. Metabolic rates in putamen and premotor cortices are *negatively* correlated in TS patients.

Additionally, metabolic rates in putamen, ventral striatum, and caudate nuclei are positively coupled in normal controls. Metabolic rates in nuclei of the basal ganglia are uncoupled in TS patients.

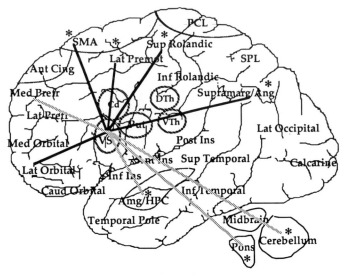

Tourette's Syndrome

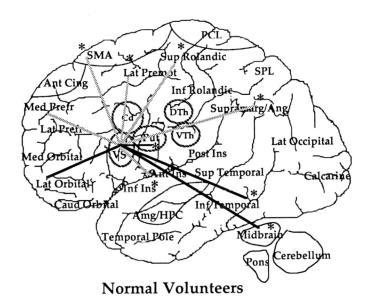

Normal Volunteers

FIGS. 5 and 6. Correlations between regional metabolic rates in Tourette patients (pictured *above*) and normal volunteers (*below*). Functional associations of the ventral striatum (**Fig. 5**) and putamen (**Fig. 6**) are illustrated. *Red* indicates a positive correlation between brain regions, *blue* a negative correlation. Both instances in which functional relationships between brain regions *differentiate* TS patients and controls, or are the *same* in both groups are illustrated. Significant *differences* between TS patients and controls represent instances in which a difference score $\pm$ 1.96 ($p < 0.025$) was obtained *and* one or the other of the correlation coefficients exceeded threshold values ($p < 0.05$); these are indicated with an asterisk. *Similarities* in

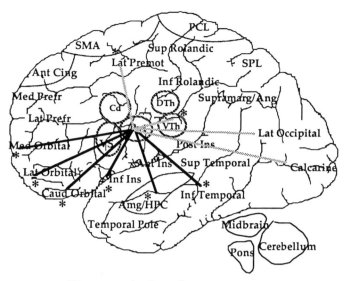

Tourette's Syndrome

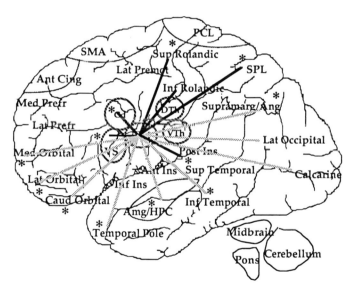

Normal Volunteers

regional associations are illustrated if correlations between regions in *both* groups exceeded threshold values (see Methods section for details). *Prefr*, prefrontal cortices; *cing*, cingulate cortices; *SMA*, supplementary motor area; *Premot*, premotor cortices; *PCL*, paracentral lobule; *SPL*, superior parietal lobule; *Supramarg/Ang*, supramarginal and angular gyri; *Amg/HPC*, amygdala/hippocampus; *Ins*, insula; *Cd*, caudate; *Put*, putamen; *VS*, ventral striatum; *Dth*, dorsal thalamus; *Vth*, ventral thalamus; *Med*, medial; *Lat*, lateral; *Caud*, caudal; *Inf*, inferior; *Sup*, superior; *Ant*, anterior; *Post*, posterior. Each functional/anatomical category depicted in these illustrations may contain several discrete regions of interest.

DISCUSSION

The present results identify altered patterns of cerebral metabolism in patients with TS. The univariate comparison of means pinpoints specific regions of interest in the limbic system, basal ganglia, and sensorimotor cortices in which metabolic rates differ significantly in patients. The analysis of correlations between metabolic rates suggests, furthermore, that altered functional relationships *between* brain regions may distinguish TS patients as well.

The results of both univariate analyses of variance comparing regional means converge in a critical way, suggesting that Tourette patients are characterized by *decreased* metabolic rates in ventral regions of the brain, particularly in the orbitofrontal and inferior insular cortices, striatum, and mesial temporal regions. There are concomitant *increases* in normalized metabolic rates in the superior cortical convexities, including premotor regions [lateral premotor cortex and supplementary motor area (SMA)] and rolandic cortices as well as post-rolandic sensory association areas including the superior parietal lobule.

It is interesting to note that these two general regions of the brain have been implicated in other PET studies as the principal sites of metabolic change in two related illnesses, obsessive–compulsive disorder (OCD) and attention deficit hyperactivity disorder (ADHD). OCD appears to involve metabolic changes in the orbitofrontal cortices and basal ganglia (21, 22), and ADHD changes in superior sensorimotor structures centered in the premotor cortices (23).

The superior regions in which metabolic rates appear to be *increased* in TS patients are clearly involved in the regulation of movement. The rolandic regions, which include primary motor and somatosensory cortices, are directly involved in the execution of somatic motor activity. The medial and lateral premotor cortices as well as the somatosensory association areas of the superior parietal lobule are involved in more complex integrative functions related to the organization and initiation of movement. Their potential relevance to the abnormal movements that characterize TS is relatively straightforward.

With the exception of the putamen, the regions in which glucose utilization is *decreased* in TS also represent elements of an identified brain system. These are limbic structures, but additionally belong to a specific subdivision of the limbic system, a ventral "paleocortical" system centered in the insula (24, 25)—distinct from the dorsal "archicortical" system centered in the cingulate cortices—that may be selectively involved in the pathogenesis of TS.

How might these regions affect motor function in a way that could be relevant to pathogenesis and symptom production in TS? The orbital frontal cortex appears to play a primary role in behavioral inhibition, and regulation of responses to exteroceptive stimuli (26–28). Humans with orbitofrontal lesions are characterized by disinhibition and impulsive behavior. Such patients are stimulus-bound, irritable, emotionally labile, and may exhibit socially inappropriate sexual and aggressive behaviors (29–31). Many of the complex neurobehavioral features of TS—impulsivity, self-injurious behavior, echophenomena, affective and obsessive–compulsive symptoms—may in fact reflect elements of the orbitofrontal syndrome. The parahippocampal region may be involved in integrating sensory and limbic information, and ultimately may also play a significant role in regulating motor responses to exteroceptive stimuli (32). The insula, which has extensive interconnections in virtually *all* regions of the brain including limbic, paralimbic, somatosensory, special sensory, and motor cortices, may perform a complex integrative function that is, at this point, poorly understood (33). The left insular cortex appears to represent an alternative neural relay connecting sensory and motor areas for speech, an association that might be of particular relevence to the generation of complex vocal tics in TS.

Access of orbitofrontal and parahippo-campal cortices to the motor system may occur indirectly, via the projections of these areas to dorsolateral prefrontal cortex or sensory association cortices (26,32). Insular access to the motor system may be more immediate since it projects *directly* to lateral premotor cortex and may project directly to the supplementary motor area as well (33).

On the other hand, orbital and insular cortices as well as mesial temporal structures can influence motor function via their projections to the basal ganglia (34,35), which themselves play a role in regulating inhibitory tone in the premotor cortices (36,37). These areas all project to the ventral region of the striatum, which, in the present study, is also characterized by a relative reduction in metabolic activity in TS patients.

The ventral striatum may ultimately be involved in the regulation of movement by coupling limbic and motor mechanisms (38). The role of dopamine in the pathogenesis of TS might become relevant in this context, for the mesolimbic dopamine system may serve a gating function at the level of the ventral striatum, regulating the flow of information from limbic structures to the pallidum, thereby governing response initiation (39).

It is tempting to speculate that there may exist an altered relationship *between* inferior limbic and superior sensorimotor structures, perhaps mediated by the ventral striatum, which may be significant in the pathophysiology of TS. Such a relationship cannot be directly assessed in an analysis of variance and comparison of regional means. The analysis of *correlations* between regional metabolic rates makes it possible to do so.

These analyses illustrate a reversal in the pattern of correlations between ventral striatum and sensorimotor regions of interest in TS patients (Fig. 5), suggesting that there may be fundamental changes in the functional relationship between these areas, perhaps involving essential shifts in excitatory or inhibitory synaptic tone.

In normal volunteers, metabolic rates in SMA, lateral premotor, rolandic, and superior parietal cortices are by and large *negatively* correlated with those in the ventral striatum, that is, when activity in this limbic region of the striatum increases, activity in the sensorimotor areas is normally depressed. In Tourette patients, however, the situation is reversed. Correlations between limbic and sensorimotor regions are uniformly *positive*. These areas are active—or activated—simultaneously. This may represent a reversal of what is normally an inverse, perhaps inhibitory, relationship between this region of the striatum and cortical areas involved in the initiation of movement.

These results may also be interpreted in another context. DeLong and coworkers (20,34) have suggested that there are neuronal circuits involving cortex, basal ganglia, and thalamus that, in the normal brain, operate in parallel. In this scheme, activity in the premotor regions involved in the initiation of movement is regulated by the putamen and its projections to ventral thalamus via the globus pallidus. The orbitofrontal and insular cortices, on the other hand, are elements of a separate loop, projecting to ventral regions of the striatum, ventral pallidum, and, via the medial thalamus, back to these limbic cortical regions.

In the Tourette brain, the normal relationship between dorsal and ventral striatal regions and motor and limbic cortices appears to be inverted, as if corticostriatal loops had been "short-circuited."

In TS patients, the most striking changes in the relationships of the ventral striatum involve functionally reversed, positive coupling with the sensorimotor cortices—areas related primarily to the putamen. On the other hand, the most robust changes in the relationships of the putamen (Fig. 6) involve reversed, positive coupling with ventral limbic structures—areas normal related primarily to the ventral striatum. In normal volunteers, when the putamen is metabolically active, the limbic cortical areas are relatively silent. In Tourette patients, however, these regions are active—or activated—concurrently. Additionally, positive correlations between putamen and sensorimotor cortices that are observed in normal volunteers are either absent or reversed in TS patients.

Perhaps a functional "cross-wiring" of the basal ganglia-thalamo-cortical circuitry in the Tourette brain results in a more direct connection between the putamen and limbic structures, and between the ventral striatum and cortical regions directly involved in motor control.

Basal ganglia core pathways could subserve such an effect. The putamen projects to external and internal segments of the dorsal globus pallidus and substantia nigra pars reticulata. The ventral striatum projects to the ventral rather than the dorsal pallidum (40). However, the ventral pallidum, while it sends efferents back to limbic structures, sends its densest projections to subthalamic nucleus and substantia nigra pars reticulata (41), where it intersects with the dorsal pallidal system and is in a position to influence activity within premotor and supplementary motor cortices. Indeed Haber and coworkers (42) suggest that the substantia nigra reticulata may be a point of convergence of cortico-striato-thalamocortical loops, and as such represents a site in which functional "short-circuitry" might occur.

Cortical regions involved in the initiation of movement—the supplementary motor area and lateral premotor and rolandic cortices—appear to be associated with what is experienced as intention or will (24). If Tourette patients are characterized by an abnormal, positive coupling between these areas and ventral limbic regions, this might explain certain essential features of the disorder, i.e., that motor and vocal tics, although involuntary, are nevertheless associated with the experience of motivational tension, and that these symptoms (along with obsessions and compulsions) are often experienced as alien or due to the operation of a "second will."

If such dysfunction were located within a network centered upon the striatum and associated with—or predicated upon—an uncoupling of functional relationships within the nuclei of the basal ganglia themselves, this would not be inconsistent with the idea that these nuclei play a cardinal role in the pathophysiology of TS and could account for the salutary effects of dopamine antagonists in this disorder.

Further neuroimaging studies, specifically designed to evaluate motor, behavioral, or cognitive functions in TS patients, and the ways in which these respond to pharmacological intervention, will be needed to extend or modify these hypotheses.

REFERENCES

1. Gilles de la Tourette G. *Etude sur une affection nerveuse caractérisée de l'incoordination motrice accompagnée d'echolalie et de copralalie.* Arch Neurol 1885;9:19–42, 158–200.
2. Towbin KE. Obsessive-compulsive symptoms in Tourette's syndrome. In: Cohen DJ, Bruun RD, Leckman JF, eds. *Tourette's syndrome and tic disorders: clinical understanding and treatment.* New York: John Wiley & Sons, 1988;137–49.
3. Comings DE, Comings BG. Tourette's syndrome and attention deficit disorder. In: Cohen DJ, Bruun RD, Leckman JF, eds. *Tourette's syndrome and tic disorders: clinical understanding and treatment.* New York: John Wiley & Sons, 1988; 119–35.
4. Riddle MA, Hardin MT, Ort SI, Leckman JF, Cohen DJ. Behavioral symptoms in Tourette's syndrome. In: Cohen DJ, Bruun RD, Leckman JF, eds. *Tourette's syndrome and tic disorders: clinical understanding and treatment.* New York: John Wiley & Sons, 1988;151–62.
5. Balthasar K. Uber das anatomishe substrat der generalisierten tic-krankeit (maladie des tics, Gilles de la Tourette): Entwicklungshemmung des corpus striatum. *Arch Psychiatr Nervenkr* 1956; 195:531–49.
6. Haber SN, Kowall NW, Vonsattel JP, Bird ED, Richardson EP. Gille de la Tourette's syndrome: a postmortem neuropathological and immunohistochemical study. *J Neurol Sci* 1986;75:225–41.
7. Harcherik DF, Cohen DJ, Ort S, et al. Computed tomographic brain scanning in four neuropsychiatric disorders of childhood. *Am J Psychiatry* 1985; 23:153–60.
8. Lees AJ, Robertson M, Trimble MR, Marray NMF. A clinical study of Gilles de la Tourette syndrome in the United Kingdom. *J Neurol Neurosurg Psychiatry* 1984;47:1–8.

9. Singer HS, Hahn IH, Krowiak E, Nelson E, Moran T. Tourette's syndrome: a neurochemical analysis of postmortem brain tissue. *Ann Neurol* 1990;27:443–6.

10. Sweet RD, Solomon GE, Wayne JL, Shapiro E, Shapiro AK. Neurological features of Gilles de la Tourette's syndrome. *J Neurol Neurosurg Psychiatry* 1973;36:1–9.

11. Van de Wetering BJM, Martens CMC, Fortgens C, Slaets JPJ, Van Woerkom RCAM. Late components of the auditory evoked potentials in Gilles de la Tourette's syndrome. *Clin Neurol Neurosurg* 1985;87:3181–6.

12. Phelps ME, Huang SC, Hoffman EJ, Selin CE, Sokoloff L, Kuhl DE. Tomographic measurement of local cerebral glucose metabolic rates in humans with (F-18) 2-fluoro-2-deoxyglucose: validation of method. *Ann Neurol* 1979;6:371–88.

13. Horwitz B, Duara R, Rapoport SI. Intercorrelations of glucose metabolic rates between brain regions: application to healthy males in a state of reduced sensory input. *J Cereb Blood Flow Metab* 1984;4:484–99.

14. Brooks RA, Sank VJ, Di Chiro G, Friauf WS, Leighton SB. Design of a high resolution positron emission tomograph: the Neuro-PET. *J Comput Assist Tomogr* 1980;4:5–13.

15. Brooks RA. Alternative formula for glucose utilization using labeled deoxyglucose. *J Nucl Med* 1982;23:538–9.

16. Damasio H, Damasio AR. *Lesion analysis in neuropsychology.* New York: Oxford University Press, 1989.

17. Clark C, Carson R, Kessler R, et al. Alternative statistical models for the examination of clinical positron emission tomography/fluorodeoxyglucose data. *J Cereb Blood Flow Metab* 1985; 5:142–50.

18. Metter EJ, Riege WH, Kameyama M, Kuhl DE, Phelps ME. Cerebral metabolic relationships for selected brain regions in Alzheimer's, Huntington's, and Parkinson's disease. *J Cereb Blood Flow Metab* 1984;500–6.

19. Winer BT. *Statistical principles in experimental design,* 2nd ed. New York: McGraw Hill, 1971.

20. Fisher RA. On the mathematical foundations of theoretical statistics. *Philos Trans R Soc Lond [A]* 1922;222:309–68.

21. Baxter LR, Phelps ME, Mazziotta JC, Guze BH, Schwartz JM, Selin CE. Local cerebral glucose metabolic rates in obsessive compulsive disorder: a comparison with rates in unipolar depression and normal controls. *Arch Gen Psychiatry* 1987; 44:211–8.

22. Nordahl TE, Benkelfat C, Semple WE, Gross M, King AC, Cohen RM. Cerebral glucose metabolic rates in obsessive compulsive disorder. *Neuropsychopharmacology* 1989;2:23–8.

23. Zametkin AJ, Nordahl TE, Gross M, et al. Cerebral glucose metabolism in adults with hyperactivity of childhood onset. *N Engl J Med* 1990; 323:1361–6.

24. Goldberg G. Supplementary motor area structure and function: review and hypotheses. *Behav Brain Sci* 1985;8:567–616.

25. Sanides F. Representation in the cerebral cortex and its areal lamination patterns. In: Bourne GH, ed. *The structure and function of nervous tissue,* vol 5. New York: Academic Press, 1972.

26. Fuster JM. *The prefrontal cortex,* 2nd ed. New York: Raven Press, 1989.

27. Iverson SD, Mishkin M. Perseverative interference in monkeys following selective lesions of the interior prefrontal convexity. *Exp Brain Res* 1970; 11:376–86.

28. Passingham RE. Visual discrimination learning after selective prefrontal ablations in monkeys (*Macaca mulatta*). *Neuropsychologia* 1972; 10:27–39.

29. Blumer D, Benson DF. Personality changes with frontal and temporal lobe lesions. In: Benson DF, Blumer D, eds. *Psychiatric aspects of neurological disease.* New York: Grune & Stratton, 1975; 151–70.

30. Luria AR. *Higher cortical functions in man.* London: Tavistock, 1966.

31. Rylander G. *Personality changes after operations on the frontal lobes.* London: Oxford University Press, 1939.

32. Witter MP, Groenewegen FH, Lopes Da Silva FH, Lohman AHM. Functional organization of the extrinsic and intrinsic circuitry of the parahippocampal region. *Prog Neurobiol* 1989;33:161–253.

33. Mesulam MM, Mufson E. The insula of Reil in monkey and man: cytoarchitectonics, connectivity and function. In: Peters A, Jones EG, eds. *The cerebral cortex,* vol 4: *Association and auditory cortices.* 1985;179–226.

34. Alexander GE, DeLong MR, Strick PL. Parallel organization of functionally segrated circuits linking basal ganglia and cortex. *Annu Rev Neurosci* 1986;9:357–81.

35. Johnson TN, Rosvold HE, Mishkin M. Projections from behaviorally defined sectors of the prefrontal cortex to the basal ganglia, septum, and dienchephalon of the monkey. *Exp Neurol* 1968; 21:20–34.

36. Chevalier G, Deniau JM. Disinhibition as a basic process in the expression of striatal functions. *Trends Neurosci* 1985;13:277–80.

37. DeLong MR. Cortico-basal ganglia loops. In: Massion J, Paillard J, Schultz W, Weisendanger M, eds. *Neural coding of motor performance. Exp Brain Res Suppl 7.* Berlin: Springer-Verlag, 1983.

38. Rolls ET, Williams GV. Sensory and movement-related neuronal activity in different regions of the striatum of the primate. In: Schneider JS, Lidsky TI, eds. *Sensory considerations for basal ganglia function.* New York: Haber, 1987.

39. Yang CR, Mogenson GJ. Excitatory responses of neurons of nucleus accumbens to hippocampal stimulation and the attenuation of the excitatory responses by the mesolimbic dopaminergic system. *Brain Res* 1984;324:69–84.

40. Heimer L, Wilson R. The subcortical projections of the allocortex: similarities in the neural associa-

tions of the hippocampus, the pririform cortex, and the neocortex. In: Santini M, ed. *Golgi Centennial Symposium.* New York: Raven Press, 1975; 177–93.

41. Haber SN, Groenewegen HJ, Grove EA, Nauta WJH. Efferent connections of the ventral pal-

lidum: evidence of a dual striato-pallidofungal pathway. *J Comp Neurol* 1985;235:322–35.

42. Haber SN, Lynd EL, Mitchell SJ. A comparison between dorsolateral and ventromedial striatal pathways through the monkey basal galglia. *Soc Neurosci Abstr* 1990;16:954.

Advances in Neurology, Vol. 58, edited
by T. N. Chase, A. J. Friedhoff, and
D. J. Cohen. Raven Press, Ltd.,
New York © 1992.

27

PET Studies on the Integrity of the Pre and Postsynaptic Dopaminergic System in Tourette Syndrome

*†David J. Brooks, *†N. Turjanski, *†G. V. Sawle, *E. D. Playford,
and †A. J. Lees

*MRC Cyclotron Unit, Hammersmith Hospital, London, W12 OHS, England
†Institute of Neurology, Queen Square, London, England

Positron emission tomography (PET) provides a noninvasive means of determining the functional integrity of the dopaminergic system in humans. Striatal and cortical dopamine storage capacity, and the density of presynaptic dopamine reuptake and postsynaptic dopamine D-1 and D-2 receptors can be examined. Regional cerebral levels of monoamine oxidase B can also be measured. Table 1 details some of the PET tracers in use for this purpose.

Tourette syndrome (TS) is currently believed to be inherited in an autosomal dominant pattern, chronic tic disease and obsessive–compulsive disorder (OCD) being alternative manifestations of the same genetic diathesis (1). Recombinant DNA technology has to date failed to identify a genetic marker for the disease (2). It has been hypothesized that tic disease may result from supersensitivity of striatal dopamine receptors. This suggestion is largely based on circumstantial evidence such as (a) the beneficial effects of dopamine receptor blocking agents in TS (1) and their ability to cause tardive tic disease (3), (b) reduced levels of the dopamine metabolite homovanillic acid (HVA) in the cerebrospinal fluid of TS patients (4,5), and (c) the aggravation of tics

by amphetamine-like agents (6,7). Currently there is no pathological evidence to support an underlying abnormality of the dopaminergic system in TS, and indeed selective loss of striatal dynorphine projections has been reported in this condition (8). Having said that, tics can be a feature of both Huntington's disease and neurocanthocytosis, which are both associated with profound loss of striatal dopamine D-2 receptors (9).

The locomotor effects of dopamine are primarily transmitted through striatal D-2 sites. The purpose of this study was to examine striatal dopamine storage capacity and D-2 receptor integrity with the PET tracers ^{18}F-dopa and ^{11}C-raclopride in TS and OCD patients. In this way it was hoped to provide additional information on the role of the dopaminergic system in TS.

Three neuroleptic-naive patients fulfilling the *Diagnostic and Statistical Manual*, 3rd ed, revised (DSM-III-R) criteria for TS were selected for ^{18}F-dopa PET. A further three drug-naive TS patients had ^{11}C-raclopride PET. TS patient details are shown in Table 2. TS ^{18}F-dopa and ^{11}C-raclopride findings were compared with those obtained for 30 and 8 normal controls, respectively. Six neuroleptic-naive patients with obsessional

TABLE 1. *PET tracers of the dopaminergic system*

Function	Tracer
Presynaptic	
Dopamine storage	^{18}F-6-fluorodopa
	^{18}F-fluorometatyrosine
Reuptake sites	^{11}C-nomifensine
Postsynaptic	
Dopamine D-1 sites	^{11}C-SCH 23390
	^{11}C-SCH 39166
Dopamine D-2/D-3	^{11}C-raclopride
	^{11}C-methylspiperone
	^{18}F-fluorospiperone
	^{18}F-fluoroethylspiperone
	^{76}Br-bromospiperone
	^{76}Br-bromolisuride

slowness and a compulsive disorder but no tic disease also had ^{18}F-dopa PET. The OCD patient age range was 20–56 years, and clinical disease duration 4–25 years, respectively. Three OCD patients were taking tricyclic antidepressants at the time of PET.

SCANNING DETAILS

PET scans were performed on a CTI 931/08/12 tomograph (CTI, Knoxville, TN) giving 15 simultaneous planes with an axial full-width-half-maximum resolution of 7 mm, and an in-plane resolution of 8.5 × 8.5 mm (10). Correction for tissue attenuation of 511-keV γ-radiation was measured with an external ^{68}Ge ring source. During the hour preceding ^{18}F-dopa scanning, subjects were given a 150-mg oral dose of carbidopa, a peripheral dopa decarboxylase blocker. All subjects were fasted for 12 hours before PET.

^{18}F-dopa

3–5 mCi (mean specific activity 8 mBq/μmol) in 10 ml of N saline were infused intravenously over 2 minutes. Scanning began at the start of tracer infusion with serial 1-minute, increasing to 5-minute, time frames over 90 minutes providing a total of 25 time frames.

^{11}C-raclopride

In 5 ml of N saline, 5–8 mCi was infused intravenously over 2 minutes. Scanning began at the start of tracer infusion with serial 30-second, increasing to 5-minute, time frames over 60 minutes providing a total of 21 time frames.

DATA ANALYSIS

Region of interest (ROI) analysis was performed on SUN 3/60 workstations using image analysis software (ANALYZE 3.0, BRU, Mayo Foundation). In all subjects the positions of striatal, frontal, occipital, and cerebellar structures were defined by summing time frames to create an integrated image representing activity collected 30–90 minutes after ^{18}F-dopa, or over the 60 minutes following ^{11}C-raclopride administra-

TABLE 2. *Untreated Tourette patient details*

Patient	Sex	Age (years)	Duration (years)	Family history	Tics Motor	Tics Vocal	OCD[a]
F-dopa							
1	M	26	21	?Grandfather	+	+	+
2	M	46	41	Paternal	+	+	+
3	M	24	17	−	+	+	+
Raclopride							
1	M	46	36	−	+	+	+
2	M	18	8	−	+	+	−
3	M	37	21	Mother	+	+	−

[a] OCD, obsessive–compulsive disorder.

tion. Although all TS patients exhibited tics during PET, neither the integrated images of striatal ^{18}F nor ^{11}C activity showed evidence of significant degradation due to movement artifact.

ROIs were placed by inspection in a standard template arrangement: one circular region 8.2 mm in diameter was placed over the head of the caudate and three contiguous circular regions 8.2 mm in diameter were lined along the axis of the putamen for each hemisphere in both normal subjects and patients (11,12). One circular region 16.4 mm in diameter was placed over mesial frontal cortex, and one circular region 32.8 mm was placed over the occipital and cerebellar lobes of each hemisphere. This array of ROIs was defined on the integrated images of ^{18}F and ^{11}C activity of the two optimum contiguous 7-mm axial planes for each cerebral structure with reference to the stereotactic atlas of Talairach and Tournoux (13), and then superimposed on individual time frames. Averaged values for each structure (caudate, putamen, occiput, cerebellum) over two planes were then calculated from the individual hemispheric ROI data.

Following decay correction, regional time–activity curves were plotted for [18]F-

dopa and ^{11}C-raclopride. Specific striatal ^{18}F-dopa uptake was determined using a modified multiple time graphical analysis (MTGA) approach with an occipital nonspecific tissue input function for TS patients and a metabolite-corrected plasma input function for OC studies (11,12). This MTGA approach linearizes striatal ^{18}F uptake curves over 30–90 minutes of real time, and the gradients of the plots obtained using this approach can be regarded as composite influx constants (K_i), which reflect the rate of striatal uptake and decarboxylation of ^{18}F-dopa to form ^{18}F-dopamine, and the subsequent breakdown and release of ^{18}F-dopamine as its metabolites dopac and HVA.

Striatal and cerebellar ^{11}C-raclopride uptake were fitted to a two-compartment model providing total and nonspecific striatal volumes of distribution of tracer binding, respectively (14,15). The striatal RAC binding potential (B_{max}/K_d) was calculated from these volumes of distribution.

FINDINGS

Figure 1 shows individual striatal ^{18}F-dopa influx constants (occipital input func-

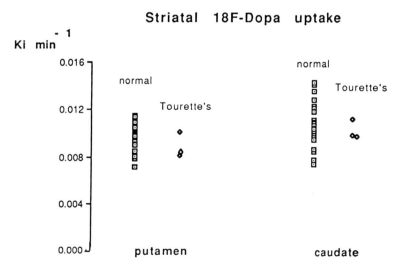

FIG. 1. A scatter diagram showing individual striatal ^{18}F-dopa influx constants (occipital input function) for 30 controls and 3 untreated TS patients.

TABLE 3. *Mean regional striatal ^{18}F-dopa uptake (K_i min^1, mean ± SD)*

	OCD[a] (n = 5)	Control (n = 6)
Left caudate	.0164 ± .0026	.0163 ± .0027
Right caudate	.0159 ± .0037	.0159 ± .0033
Left putamen	.0174 ± .0039	.0152 ± .0025
Right putamen	.0165 ± .0049	.0153 ± .0030
Medial frontal	.0034 ± .0011	.0029 ± .0011

[a] OCD, obsessive–compulsive disorder.

tion) for controls and three neuroleptic-naive TS patients. It can be seen that the three drug-naive patients had striatal ^{18}F-dopa K_i values within the normal range. In Table 3 the mean striatal and frontal ^{18}F-dopa influx constants (plasma input function) of the six neuroleptic-naive OC patients are detailed. It can be seen that these were also normal.

Figure 2 shows individual striatal ^{11}C-raclopride binding potentials for three neuroleptic-naive TS patients. These all fell within the normal range.

We found normal striatal ^{18}F-dopa influx constants for our three TS and six OC neuroleptic-naive patients. ^{18}F-dopa K_i values are determined by a number of composite processes including transport of ^{18}F-dopa

into the striatum, its rate of decarboxylation and storage as fluorodopamine, and the subsequent release of the metabolites ^{18}F-dopac and ^{18}F-HVA. In normal subjects little ^{18}F-dopac or ^{18}F-HVA is formed over the 90 minutes of scanning, and so striatal ^{18}F-dopa uptake primarily reflects the rate of dopa decarboxylation (16). Untreated TS and OCD patients would therefore appear to have normal rates of dopa uptake and decarboxylation. Striatal ^{18}F-dopa uptake is not influenced by tyrosine hydroxylase activity, the enzyme that catalyzes endogenous dopa production from tyrosine. While our findings are suggestive of normal handling of dopa in untreated TS, they do not rule out a defect in endogenous dopa formation from tyrosine. Such impaired endogenous dopa production could also explain the low cerebrospinal fluid (CSF) HVA levels reported by Singer et al. (4) in TS.

We found striatal ^{11}C-raclopride binding potential to be normal in three untreated TS patients, suggesting normal numbers of D-2 sites were present. ^{11}C-raclopride uptake can theoretically be blocked by high levels of endogenous dopamine release (17). If TS patients were releasing micromolar rather than nanomolar dopamine concentrations

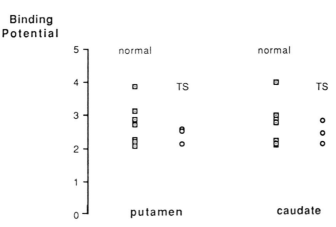

FIG. 2. A scatter diagram showing individual striatal ^{11}C-raclopride binding potentials (B_{max}/K_d) for eight normal controls and three neuroleptic-naive TS patients.

into the synaptic cleft, striatal ^{11}C-raclopride binding could underestimate total D-2 site binding potential. This, however, is unlikely to be the case, as untreated TS patients have been shown to have low, rather than raised, HVA levels in their CSF, suggesting they have a low basal dopamine turnover (4). It is likely, therefore, that striatal D-2 site density is normal in TS. D-2 receptors can adopt high- and low-affinity agonist conformations (18), both of which bind raclopride equally effectively. As a consequence, while the total number of striatal D-2 sites is probably normal in untreated TS, we cannot rule out the presence of abnormal numbers of D-2 sites in either a high or low agonist-affinity conformation. An increased population of high agonist-affinity sites could conceivably lead to involuntary movements.

In summary, we have found normal integrity of striatal dopa metabolism and D-2 site density in untreated TS. To date the only pathological abnormality reported in TS is selective fallout of striatal dynorphine projections (8). Such neurons would be predicted to be D-1 rather than D-2 receptor bearing (19). It will be of interest to see whether future PET studies on TS patients using D-1 antagonists such as ^{11}C-SCH 23390 or ^{11}C-SCH 39166 are able to show a selective loss of striatal D-1 sites.

REFERENCES

1. Kurlan R. Tourette's syndrome: current concepts. *Neurology* 1989;39:1625–30.
2. Kurlan R, Pauls DL, Kidd KK. Linkage analysis approach to hereditary movement disorders. *Int J Neurogenet* 1989;35:161–71.
3. Klawans HL, Falk DK, Nausieda PA, Weiner WJ. Gilles de la Tourette's syndrome after long term chlorpromazine therapy. *Neurology* 1978; 28:1064–8.
4. Singer HS, Butler IJ, Tune LE, Seifert WE, Coyle JT. Dopaminergic dysfunction in Tourette syndrome. *Ann Neurol* 1982;12:361–6.
5. Cohen DJ, Shaywitz BA, Young JG, et al. Central biogenic amine metabolism in children with the syndrome of chronic multiple tics of Gille de la Tourette: norepinephrine, serotonin, and dopamine. *J Am Acad Child Psychiatry* 1979; 18:320–41.
6. Golden GS. Gille de la Tourette's syndrome following methylphenidate administration. *Dev Med Child Neurol* 1974;16:76–8.
7. Meyerhoff JL, Snyder SH. Catecholamine in Gille de la Tourette's disease: a clinical study with amphetamine isomers. *Adv Neurol* 1973;1:123–34.
8. Haber SN, Kowell NW, Vonsattel JP, Bird ED, Richardson EP. Gille de la Tourette's syndrome: a postmortem neuropathological and histochemical study. *J Neurol Sci* 1986;75:225–41.
9. Brooks DJ, Ibanez V, Playford ED, et al. Pre- and post-synaptic striatal dopaminergic function in neuroacanthocytosis: a PET study. *Ann Neurol* 1991;30:166–71.
10. Spinks TJ, Jones T, Gilardi MC, Heather JD. Physical performance of the latest generation of commercial positron scanners. *IEEE Trans Neurol Sci* 1988;35:721–5.
11. Brooks DJ, Ibanez V, Sawle GV, et al. Differing patterns of striatal ^{18}F-dopa uptake in Parkinson's disease, multiple system atrophy, and progressive supranuclear palsy. *Ann Neurol* 1990;28:547–55.
12. Sawle GV, Colebatch JG, Shah A, Brooks DJ, Marsden CD, Frackowiak RSJ. Striatal function in normal aging: implications for Parkinson's disease. *Ann Neurol* 1990;28:799–804.
13. Talairach J, Tournoux P. *Co-planar stereotaxic atlas of the human brain.* Stuttgart: Thieme, 1988.
14. Salmon EP, Brooks DJ, Leenders KL, et al. A two-compartment description and kinetic procedure for measuring regional cerebral ^{11}C]nomifensine uptake using positron emission tomography. *J Cereb Blood Flow Metab* 1990;10:307–16.
15. Farde L, Hall H, Ehrin E, Sedvall G. Quantitative analysis of dopamine-D_2 receptor binding in the living brain by positron emission tomography. *Science* 1986;231:258–61.
16. Firnau G, Sood S, Chirakal R, Nahmias C, Garnett ES. Cerebral metabolism of 6-(^{18}F)fluoro-L-3,4-dihydroxyphenylalanine in the primate. *J Neurochem* 1987;48:1077–82.
17. Seeman P, Guan HC, Niznik HB. Endogenous dopamine lowers the dopamine D_2 receptor density as measured by [^{3}H]raclopride: implications for positron emission tomography of the human brain. *Synapse* 1989;3:96–7.
18. Guttman M, Seeman P. Dopamine D_2 receptor density in parkinsonian brain is constant for duration of disease, age, and duration of L-dopa therapy. *Adv Neurol* 1986;45:51–7.
19. Smith AD, Bolam JP. The neural network of the basal ganglia as revealed by the study of synaptic connections of identified neurones. *TINS* 1990; 13:259–65.

Advances in Neurology, Vol. 58, edited
by T. N. Chase, A. J. Friedhoff, and
D. J. Cohen. Raven Press, Ltd.,
New York © 1992.

28

Positron Emission Tomography Evaluation of Dopamine D-2 Receptors in Adults with Tourette Syndrome

Harvey S. Singer, Dean F. Wong, Janice E. Brown, Jason Brandt,
Laura Krafft, Elias Shaya, Robert F. Dannals, and
Henry N. Wagner, Jr.

*Departments of Neurology, Pediatrics, Nuclear Medicine, and Psychiatry, The
Johns Hopkins University School of Medicine, Baltimore, Maryland 21205*

Clinical pharmacotherapeutic experience and studies of neurotransmitter metabolites have led to speculations that Tourette syndrome (TS) is associated with an imbalance of neurotransmitter systems (1,2). However, the availability of postmortem material for confirmatory neurochemical investigations has been extremely limited (3). Even in those autopsied cases in which neurochemical abnormalities have been noted, it is difficult to determine conclusively whether the observed changes are related to TS itself, to aging, to the use of medications, or to the presence of a systemic disorder.

The development of positron emission tomography (PET) has added a new dimension to the measurement of biochemical, physiological, and hemodynamic processes in humans. Specifically, regional neuropharmacological PET studies have provided an essential link for relating biochemistry within the human brain to measurements of behavior. In this preliminary report, we describe initial results obtained by PET with use of a spiperone derivative, 3-N-[^{11}C]methylspiperone (^{11}C-NMSP), to quantify dopamine receptors in the brains of adults with TS. We also review the potential uses of PET in the assessment of additional markers for dopamine, as well as for other neurotransmitter systems.

POSITRON EMISSION TOMOGRAPHY

One of the distinguishing features of a PET scan is that penetrating radiation originates from within the subject rather than from outside sources. For example, computerized tomography (CT) constructs an image by rotating a source of x-ray completely around the subject and using a detector on the opposite side to record variations in the absorption of radiation after it has passed through intervening tissues. In contrast, imaging with PET relates to the unique physical properties of positron decay. In this technique, a chemical compound with the desired biologic activity is labelled with a radioactive isotope that decays by emitting positrons. Positrons are positively charged electrons that are emitted from unstable nuclei as they decay. The positron emitted from an unstable nucleus travels at most a few millimeters before combining with an electron. When a positron combines with an electron they annihilate each other, i.e., the masses of the electron and positron are converted to electromagnetic radiation and produce a pair of high-energy protons. These two photons are emitted approximately 180° apart, permitting the use of detectors that record the simultaneous arrival of photons on opposite sides of the head. The quality of information obtained by this technique is enhanced by a collimator design that minimizes the acceptance of scattered radiation. Data from multiple sets of detectors are collected over a period of time and through multiple angles around the brain. A computer mathematically processes the spatial distribution of radioactivity and constructs a two-dimensional map of tissue radioactivity concentrations in the appropriate brain section.

The synthesis of ^{11}C-NMSP is a complex task. It involves N-alkylation of spiperone by [^{11}C]methyl iodide, the latter having been produced from ^{11}CO$_2$, which had in turn been made by an in-hospital cyclotron (model RNP-16, Scanditronix Cyclotron, Sweden) (4). Carbon-11 is a positron-emitting isotope with a physical half-life of 20 minutes. Before injection, the product is purified and the specific activity determined by use of a reverse-phase liquid chromatography column. Prior in vivo and in vitro studies have shown that most of the accumulated ^{11}C-NMSP in basal ganglia binds to postsynaptic dopamine receptors, whereas the majority of accumulated ^{11}C-NMSP in cerebral cortex reflects binding to postsynaptic serotonin (S-2) receptors (5).

Quantification of D-2 dopamine receptors in brain is based on a four-compartment model consisting of ligand free in plasma, ligand free in brain, nonspecifically bound ligand, and ligand specifically bound to receptors. After injection of ^{11}C-NMSP, the amount of radioactivity in the striatum is followed over a 90-minute period. Simultaneously, a time–activity curve of the ^{11}C-NMSP concentration in plasma is obtained from a peripheral vessel. The four-compartment model yields a rate constant of binding to the D-2 dopamine receptor, k_3. This rate constant is estimated twice, before and after a blocking dose of haloperidol given 4 hours prior to a second scan. Hence, k_3 is calculated under two conditions; first with receptors unblocked, and then with receptors partially blocked by haloperidol (6–8). D-2 receptor density (B_{max}) is derived from the two k_3 values and the plasma haloperidol concentration. The calculation assumes that the blood–brain partition coefficient and dissociation rate of haloperidol are known in patients and normals.

DOPAMINE RECEPTOR HYPERSENSITIVITY HYPOTHESIS

The dopamine receptor hypersensitivity hypothesis proposes that TS is due to supersensitivity (increased number or increased infinity) of postsynaptic dopamine receptors. Evidence for this postulate is provided by reports of lowered baseline and turnover levels of homovanillic acid (HVA), a major metabolite of brain dopamine (9–10); clinical improvement associated with restoration of cerebrospinal fluid (CSF) HVA levels into the normal range (11); prolonged elevation of CSF HVA levels by haloperidol, which blocks dopamine receptors (11); clinical response of TS patients to low doses of haloperidol (30); and the appearance of a Tourette-like syndrome after withdrawal of chronically used neuroleptic medication in non-TS patients (12,13).

PRESENT STUDY DESIGN

In PET, an increased number of dopamine receptors or an enhancement of receptor affinity would be reflected by increased

[11]C-NMSP binding. In an initial study, based on a simplified mathematical model and a single PET scan, no significant differences were found between adults with TS and controls (14). Nevertheless, advances in PET technology, improved mathematical modeling techniques, and compelling evidence for an abnormality in dopamine receptors, prompted us to repeat the study of ^{11}C-NMSP binding in 19 adults with TS. The specific aims of this study were twofold: to compare striatal D-2 receptor density in TS and healthy controls, and to correlate D-2 dopamine receptor binding with tic severity and other neuropsychological functions.

The study was limited to patients with TS over the age of 18 years. The mean age of the 19 patients, diagnosed by criteria established by Shapiro (15), was 36.2 years, with a range of 19 to 52 years. There were 15 males and 4 females, all with typical age of onset. Family history was positive for TS in 15 of 19, and for obsessive–compulsive disorder (OCD) in 5 of 19. Eleven patients were drug-naive; four had received prior treatment with dopamine receptor antagonists, either haloperidol or thioridazine. The duration of treatment with neuroleptics ranged from 1 week to 10 years, although all patients had been drug-free for at least 6 months prior to the PET scan. (Three patients had not received neuroleptics for at least 3 years prior to this study.) The Frankel Scale for OCD was abnormal (score of greater than 70) in seven subjects. The severity of tics was ranked at the time of PET scan by using both the Johns Hopkins Motor and Vocal Tic Scale (16) and the Shapiro Tourette Syndrome Severity Scale (17). Based on these two scales, seven subjects were rated as mild, five mild to moderate, two moderate, and five moderate to severe.

A battery of neuropsychological tests was administered within a 4-week period prior to scanning (Table 1). Some of these tasks were chosen to assess behaviors associated with frontal and striatal brain function and to identify cognitive deficits previously associated with OCD or TS, that is, impair-

TABLE 1. *Neuropsychological test battery for Tourette syndrome study*

Grooved Pegboard Test (motor speed and dexterity)
  Dominant hand
  Nondominant hand

Symbol Digit Modalities Test (rapid coding)
  Written
  Oral

Wechsler Adult Intelligence Scale—Revised (general verbal and visuoconstructive skill; allows estimation of full-scale IQ)
  Vocabulary subtest
  Block design subtest

Weschler Memory Scale-Revised (comprehensive memory battery)
  Verbal Memory Index
  Visual Memory Index
  General Memory Index
  Attention/Concentration Index
  Delayed Recall Index

Controlled Oral Word Association Test (verbal fluency and productivity)

Design Fluency Test (nonverbal fluency and productivity)

Stylus Maze Test (planning and skill learning)

Standardized Road-Map Test of Directional Sense (personal spatial orientation and route-finding)

Trail Making Test (visual scanning, sequencing, set maintenance)

Wisconsin Card Sorting Test (nonverbal concept formation and problem-solving)

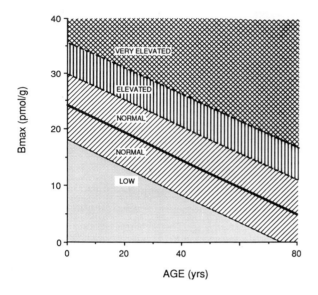

FIG. 1. Diagram illustrating the classification of TS subjects into different categories based upon B_{max} determinations in normals.

ments in visuomotor and visuoconstructional skills, concreteness and mental inflexibility, and difficulties with switching mental sets.

For our PET studies, intravenous injections of 20 μCi of [^{11}C]NMSP (specific activity approximately 2,000 Ci/mmol) were administered while the patient lay supine with eyes closed and head in the PET scanner. Serial PET scans were then obtained over 90 minutes. B_{max} categorization was based upon its relationship to the 95th percent confidence intervals for a B_{max} versus age regression line in normal subjects ranging in age from 18 to 80 years. Since values for D-2 dopamine receptors decline with age (5,18,19), it is necessary to regress the B_{max} values versus age. Subjects within the 95th percent confidence limit who were near or below the lower confidence limit were classified "normal" or "low," respectively. Those at or slightly above the 95th percent confidence limit were considered "elevated" and those clearly above were classified as "very elevated" (Fig. 1).

FINDINGS

Based on the classification of B_{max} values described above, two subjects showed low values, nine normal, two elevated, and six very elevated values. We then determined whether any of the demographic characteristics correlated with B_{max} levels (Table 2). Patients with normal B_{max} levels (n = 9) did not differ significantly from those having very elevated scores (n = 6), in age of the patients, their mean age of onset, family history, tic severity, presence of OCD, or prior neuroleptic exposure. Among the 11 patients completing formal neuropsychological testing, no significant correlations were noted between test scores and B_{max} categories. Although the numbers are small, there was a trend suggesting that the number of perseverative errors on the Wisconsin Card Scoring Test increased in subjects with elevated ^{11}C-NMSP B_{max} determinations. The relationship between severity of symptom and cognitive performance was examined in the 11 patients who underwent neuropsychological testing. Severity of motor tics on the Hopkins Scale significantly correlated with the Block Design subtest of the Wechsler Adult Intelligence Scale-Revised (r = +0.71, p < 0.01), while phonic tics correlated with the Visual Memory Index of the Wechsler Memory Scale-Revised (r = +0.79, p < 0.01). Somewhat paradoxically, more severe tics were associated with better

TABLE 2. *Comparison of B_{max} with other variables[a]*

Characteristic	Groups identified from B_{max} values (Fig. 1)			
	Low	Normal	Elevated	Very elevated
No. of patients	2	9	2	6
Mean age (range)	34.5 yrs (31,38)	35.1 yrs (19–46)	43.5 yrs (42,45)	38 yrs (24–52)
Mean age of onset (range)	6 yrs (5–12)	9.3 yrs (6–14)	8.5 yrs (7–10)	8.2 yrs (6–10)
Family history				
TS Positive	2	7	2	4
OC Positive	0	1	2	2
Tic severity				
Mild	1	4	1	3
Mild–moderate	1	2	0	1
Moderate	0	2	0	0
Moderate–severe	0	1	1	2
OCD	1	3	1	2
Prior neuroleptic treatment	0	2	1	1

[a] OC(D), obsessive–compulsive (disorder); TS, Tourette syndrome.

cognitive performance. Given the small sample, however, this may be the result of sampling artifact. There were no significant correlations between psychological testing and severity of obsessive–compulsive symptoms or overall severity of TS.

CONCLUDING COMMENTS

PET scanning provides a valuable opportunity to compare pathophysiological information with clinical manifestations of TS. The results of our imaging studies of dopamine D-2 receptors in the striatum of adults with TS did not demonstrate a distinct abnormality compared with age-matched normal subjects. Although several patients did have elevated levels of receptor binding, it is unclear whether these individuals represent a distinct subcategory of TS patients. We attempted to determine whether any clinical features were specific for this group by using available demographic information, but found no specific characteristics. Our data, which show no overall significant differences in D-2 receptors, are consistent with preliminary reports of D-2 receptor binding performed on postmortem membranes from the caudate and putamen (20). Hence, the hypothesis that an alteration of

dopamine receptors is the fundamental pathophysiological abnormality in TS does not appear to be supported by available PET or postmortem data.

Abnormalities in many other neurotransmitter systems have been proposed to account for the manifestations in TS, including the serotonergic, noradrenergic, cholinergic, GABAergic, and opioid systems (1,2). In addition, other defects in the dopamine system have been identified, including an increase in dopamine uptake receptor binding (20). Use of newly available radioactive tracers and PET technology permits assessment of many of these hypotheses in patients with TS. For example, it is possible to study presynaptic components of the dopaminergic system. Labeled fluorodopa, a fluorinated derivative of L-dopa similar to its precursor, is taken up into presynaptic terminals, undergoes decarboxylation, and accumulates in vesicles (21). Since accumulation of the tracer has been correlated with presynaptic terminals, labeled fluorodopa has been used to assess neuronal integrity in Parkinson's disease and toxicity after MPTP treatment (22–25). Dopamine reuptake sites, imaged with ^{11}C-nomifensine, were reduced in the striatum of patients with Parkinson's disease (23).

More recently, direct measurement of the presynaptic dopamine transporter site has been carried out by use of the ligands ^{11}C-cocaine (26) and ^{18}F-GBR (27), and a new compound that allows even a higher signal to noise ratio, ^{11}C-WIN 35,428 (28). Further examination of the dopamine transporter is important for the clarification of the role of dopamine hypotheses in both TS (1) and cocaine reinforcement (29).

PET neuropharmacological methods are also available to evaluate other receptors in humans. Currently there are ligands for the study of serotonin, muscarinic cholinergic, opiate, and benzodiazepine binding sites. In addition, new receptor ligands with improved kinetic properties continue to be developed and should be available in the near future. The ability of PET to correlate with in vitro measurements in disease states provides investigators with a valuable alternative to the use of postmortem tissues.

REFERENCES

1. Singer HS, Walkup JT. Tourette syndrome and other tic disorders: diagnosis, pathophysiology, and treatment. *Medicine* 1991;70:15–32.
2. Leckman JF, Riddle MA, Cohen DJ. Pathobiology of Tourette's syndrome. In: Cohen DJ, Bruun RD, Leckman JF, eds. *Tourette's syndrome and tic disorders*. New York: John Wiley & Sons, 1988; 103–16.
3. Richardson EP. Neuropathological studies of Tourette syndrome. In: Friedhoff AJ, Chase TN, eds. *Gilles de la Tourette syndrome*. New York: Raven Press, 1982;83–7.
4. Dannals RF, Ravert HT, Wilson AL, Wagner HN Jr. An improved synthesis of (3-N-[11C]methyl)-spiperone. *Int J Appl Radiat Isot* 1986;37:433.
5. Wong DF, Wagner HN Jr, Dannals RF, et al. Effects of age on dopamine and serotonin receptors measured by positron tomography in the living human brain. *Science* 1984;226:1393–6.
6. Wong DF, Gjedde A, Wagner HN Jr. Quantification of neuroreceptors in the living human brain. Part I. Association rate of irreversibly bound ligands. *J Cereb Blood Flow Metab* 1986;6:137–46.
7. Wong DF, Gjedde A, Wagner HN Jr, et al. Quantification of neuroreceptors in living human brain. Part II. Inhibition studies of receptor density and affinity. *J Cereb Blood Flow Metab* 1986;6:147–53.
8. Wong DF, Wagner HN Jr, Tune LE, et al. Positron emission tomography reveals elevated D_2 dopamine receptors in drug naive schizophrenics. *Science* 1986;234:1558–63.
9. Cohen DJ, Shaywitz BA, Caparulo BK, Young JG, Bowers MB Jr. Chronic multiple tics of Gilles de la Tourette's disease: CSF acid monoamine metabolites after probenecid administration. *Arch Gen Psychiatry* 1978;35:245–50.
10. Butler IJ, Koslow SH, Seifert WE, Caprioli RM, Singer HS. Biogenic amine metabolism in Tourette syndrome. *Ann Neurol* 1979;6:37–9.
11. Singer HS, Butler IJ, Tune LE, Seifert WE, Coyle JT. Dopaminergic dysfunction in Tourette syndrome. *Ann Neurol* 1982;12:361–6.
12. Klawans HL, Falk DK, Nausieda PA, Weiner WJ. Gilles de la Tourette syndrome after long-term chlorpromazine therapy. *Neurology* 1978; 28:1064–6.
13. Singer WD. Transient Gilles de la Tourette syndrome after chronic neuroleptic withdrawal. *Dev Med Child Neurol* 1981;23:518–21.
14. Singer HS, Wong DF, Tiemeyer M, Whitehouse P, Wagner HN. Pathophysiology of Tourette syndrome: a PET and postmortem analysis. *Ann Neurol* 1984;18:416(abst).
15. Shapiro AK, Shapiro ES, Young JG, Feinberg TE. *Gilles de la Tourette Syndrome*, 2nd ed. New York: Raven Press, 1988.
16. Walkup JT, Rosenberg LA, Brown J, Singer HS. The validity of instruments measuring tic severity in Tourette syndrome. *J Am Acad Child Adolesc Psychiatry* 1992;30.
17. Shapiro AK, Shapiro E. Controlled study of pimozide vs placebo in Tourette's syndrome. *J Am Acad Child Psychiatry* 1984;23:161–73.
18. Wong DF, Brousselle E, Villemagne V, et al. D2 dopamine receptor density measured in human brain *in vivo* by positron emission tomography: age and sex differences. In: *Central determinants of age-related declines in motor function. Ann NY Acad Sci* 1988;203–14.
19. Wong DF, Young LT, Pearlson GD, et al. D2 dopamine receptor densities measured by PET are elevated in several neuropsychiatric disorders. *J Nucl Med* 1989;30:731.
20. Singer HS, Hahn I-H, Moran TH. Abnormal dopamine uptake sites in postmortem striatum from patients with Tourette syndrome. *Ann Neurol* 1991; 30:558–62.
21. Garnett RS, Firnau G, Nahmias C. Dopamine visualized in the basal ganglia of living man. *Nature* 1983;305:137–8.
22. Guttman M, Stoessl J, Peppard RF, et al. Correlation between clinical findings and 6-(^{18}F) fluoro-dopa PETs in Parkinson's disease. *Neurology* 1987;37(suppl 1):329.
23. Leenders KL, Aquilonius SM, Bergstrom K, et al. Unilateral MPTP lesion in a rhesus monkey: effects on the striatal dopaminergic system measured *in vivo* with PET using various novel tracers. *Brain Res* 1988;445:61–7.
24. Gjedde A, Reith J, Dyve S, et al. Dopa decarboxylase activity of the living human brain. *Proc Natl Acad Sci* 1991;88:2721–5.
25. Calne DB, Langston JW, Martin WRW, et al. Positron emission tomography after MPTP: observations relating to the cause of Parkinson's disease. *Nature* 1985;317:246–8.

26. Fowler JS, Volkow ND, Wolf AP, et al. Mapping cocaine binding sites in human and baboon *in vivo*. *Synapse* 1989;4:371–7.

27. Kilbourn MR, Carey JE, Koeppe RA, et al. Biodistribution, dosimetry, metabolism and monkey PET studies of [^{18}F]GBR 13119. Imaging the dopamine uptake system *in vivo*. *Int J Rad Appl Instrum* [B] 1989;16:569–76.

28. Scheffel U, Boja JW, Kuhar MJ. Cocaine receptors: *in vivo* labeling with 3H−(−) cocaine, 3H-WIN 35,065-2, and 3H-WIN 35,428. *Synapse* 1989; 4:390–2.

29. Kuhar MJ, Ritz MC, Boja JW. The dopamine hypothesis of the reinforcing properties of cocaine. *Trends Neurosci* 1991;14:299–302.

30. Singer HS, Rabins P, Tune LE, Coyle JT. Serum haloperidol levels in Gilles de la Tourette syndrome. *Biol Psychiatry* 1981;16:79–84.

Advances in Neurology, Vol. 58, edited
by T. N. Chase, A. J. Friedhoff, and
D. J. Cohen. Raven Press, Ltd.,
New York © 1992.

29

Treatment of Tourette Syndrome with Neuroleptic Drugs

Gerald Erenberg

Cleveland Clinic Foundation, Cleveland, Ohio 44195

The modern era of medication treatment of Tourette syndrome (TS) began in 1961 with the first reports of effective treatment of single patients through the use of haloperidol (1,2). Uncontrolled studies through the years have consistently reported that neuroleptic drugs, especially haloperidol, are generally helpful in the treatment of tics. All studies of TS treatment, however, have been hampered by the natural variability of the disorder even in untreated patients. As reported by Shapiro and Shapiro (3), "in evaluating drugs for tic disorders, however, it is important to remember that about 30% of patients improve, 30% remain unchanged, and 30% are worse when treated with placebos; that severity of symptoms spontaneously varies in 97%, type and location of symptoms change in 96%, and 27% report spontaneous remissions lasting one month to more than seven years."

Neuroleptic drugs are generally viewed as the most consistently helpful treatment in the suppression of tics. The neuroleptic agents are presumed to suppress tics because of their dopamine-blocking ability, and haloperidol is felt to be more effective than the phenothiazines because of its ability to bind specifically to D-2 receptors. Haloperidol was approved by the Food and Drug Administration for the treatment of adult patients with Tourette syndrome in 1969. It was approved for treatment of children in 1978. Other neuroleptic agents have been proposed as being capable of providing equal or superior tic-suppressing effects while having fewer side effects (4,5). Major considerations have revolved around the use of pimozide and fluphenazine. Pimozide has specifically been suggested as being a superior neuroleptic agent, but a controlled study of haloperidol, pimozide, and placebo in the treatment of TS did not verify this clinical impression (6). According to this study by Shapiro et al. (6), both haloperidol and pimozide were more effective than placebo, but haloperidol was slightly more effective. There were no statistically significant differences in the adverse affects noted in the 6-week trials of haloperidol or pimozide.

All neuroleptic drugs are used clinically in the same manner. The goal is to find the lowest dosage that will lead to approximately 70% improvement in tics while minimizing side effects. To do so, medication is begun at very low dosage and titrated upward in a slow manner. Haloperidol is typically begun at a low dose, and increased slowly on a weekly basis until major improvements are noticed or there are problems with intolerable side effects. The effect of any given change in dosage is generally noticed within 4 days, but weekly adjustments are usually made for convenience sake. Haloperidol is a long-acting agent, and the dosage can either be given entirely at bedtime or divided into a twice a day schedule. There is no evidence that the concomitant usage of anticholinergic medications is of any value in minimizing side effects when given on a routine basis.

Unfortunately, the incidence of side effects is quite high. Frequent side effects include sedation, dysphoria, weight gain, and movement abnormalities (7). Acute dystonic reactions may occur if dosages are started or increased too rapidly, and there may also be parkinsonian side effects in the form of bradykinesia and akathisia. Other subtle side effects can include depression, poor school performance, and school phobias. Side effects can occur with even low drug dosages in individual patients. The continued use, or even the discontinuation, of these medications can lead to tardive dyskinesia, tardive dystonia, and the withdrawal emergent syndrome (8,9). The risk of these tardive or withdrawal dyskinesias is less in younger patients, but they have been reported at all ages. With rare exceptions, however, these dyskinesias have disappeared in younger patients several months after the medication was discontinued (10). Pimozide has also been found to produce prolongation of the QTc on electrocardiograms (11). Although this did not lead to clinical symptoms, the manufacturer has recommended that periodic electrocardiograms be performed.

There is no doubt that haloperidol and other neuroleptic drugs remain the first agents generally used in the treatment of patients with TS. The 1987 survey of 763 TS patients in Ohio responding to a questionnaire indicated that the majority of patients had been treated with haloperidol at one time or another, and haloperidol was the medication first prescribed in 69% (12). Most reviews on TS have reported that 70–80% of patients treated with haloperidol improve. The report of Shapiro and Shapiro (3) is typical and indicates that 25% of treated patients have at least a 70% reduction of symptoms without significant adverse effects, 50% are significantly improved although with side effects, and 25% are treatment failures because of adverse side effects. Others, however, including our own group, have reported less optimistic results (13,14). In a survey done of our patients who had reached adult age, it was reported that 91% had been treated at one time or another with haloperidol (14). Eighty-four percent reported major side effects, and only 45% felt that the treatment had led to a major improvement in their symptoms.

In our clinical experience, more of our patients are handicapped by the associated behavioral and learning problems of TS rather than the tic aspect of this disorder (14,15). While this is undoubtedly due to ascertainment bias, the reality of clinical practice is such that only a minority of patients have tics of severity so significant that medication to suppress tics is warranted. Since the neuroleptics have no major impact on the behavioral difficulties, and since there is an extremely high incidence of major side effects, there has been an increasing trend in our institution to avoid the use of neuroleptic drugs. While neuroleptic agents can be the sole drug used in patients whose only difficulties are in the area of tics, the majority of our patients requiring treatment will receive behavioral agents alone or in combination with a neuroleptic agent.

The discovery that neuroleptic drugs can help decrease the symptoms of TS represented a major advance in our understanding of this disorder. With the passage of time, however, the usefulness of these medications has diminished somewhat because of side effects and treatment failures. Although there will be continued use of these agents for tic suppression until better chemotherapeutic modalities are discovered, there should be great caution in their use. Diagnosis of TS does not automatically indicate that treatment is necessary. The use of neuroleptics should be limited to use in those whose tics have led to significant physical or emotional stress.

REFERENCES

1. Seignot MJN. Un cas de maladie des tics de Gilles de la Tourette gueri par le R-1625. *Ann Med Psychol* 1961;119:578–9.
2. Caprini G, Melotti V. Un grave sindrome ticcosa guarita con haloperidol. *Riv Sper Freniat* 1961; 85:191–6.
3. Shapiro AK, Shapiro E. Treatment of tic disorders with haloperidol. In: Cohen DJ, Bruun RD, Leckman JF, eds. *Tourette's syndrome and tic disorders*. New York: John Wiley & Sons, 1988;268–80.
4. Singer HS, Gammon K, Quaskey S. Haloperidol, fluphenazine and clonidine in Tourette syndrome: controversies in treatment. *Pediatr Neurosci* 1985-86;12:71–4.
5. Shapiro AK, Shapiro E, Fulop G. Pimozide treatment of tic and Tourette disorder. *Pediatrics* 1987; 79:1032–9.
6. Shapiro E, Shapiro AK, Fulop G, Hubbard M, et al. Controlled study of haloperidol, pimozide and placebo for the treatment of Gilles de la Tourette's syndrome. *Arch Gen Psychiatry* 1989;46:722–30.
7. Bruun RD. Subtle and underrecognized side effects of neuroleptic treatment in children with Tourette's disorder. *Am J Psychiatry* 1988; 145:621–4.
8. Singer HS. Tardive dyskinesia: a concern for the pediatrician. *Pediatrics* 1986;77:553–6.
9. Silverstein FS, Johnston MV: Risks of neuroleptic drugs in children. *Child Neurol* 1987;2:41–3.
10. Golden GS. Tardive dyskinesia in Tourette syndrome. *Pediatr Neurol* 1985;1:192–4.
11. Fulop G, Philips RA, Shapiro AK, Gomes JA, Shapiro E, Nordlie JW. ECG changes during haloperidol and pimozide treatment of Tourette's disorder. *Am J Psychiatry* 1987;144:673–5.
12. Bornstein RA, Stefl ME, Hammond L. A survey of Tourette syndrome patients and their families: the 1987 Ohio Tourette survey. *J Neuropsychiatry* 1990;2:275–81.
13. Cohen DJ, Detlor J, Young JG, Shaywitz BA: Clonidine ameliorates Gilles de la Tourette syndrome. *Arch Gen Psychiatry* 1980;37:1350–7.
14. Erenberg G, Cruse RP, Rothner AD. The natural history of Tourette syndrome: a follow-up study. *Ann Neurol* 1987;22:383–5.
15. Erenberg G, Cruse RP, Rothner AD. Tourette syndrome: an analysis of 200 pediatric and adolescent cases. *Cleve Clin Q* 1986;53:127–31.

Advances in Neurology, Vol. 58, edited by T. N. Chase, A. J. Friedhoff, and D. J. Cohen. Raven Press, Ltd., New York © 1992.

30

Clonidine and Clonazepam in Tourette Syndrome

Christopher G. Goetz

Department of Neurological Sciences, Rush University, Rush-Presbyterian-St. Luke's Medical Center, Chicago, Illinois 60612

Clonidine is a drug that was primarily developed to treat hypertension but has been additionally studied in Tourette syndrome (TS). Clonazepam, a benzodiazepine derivative, has been used in treating other movement disorders like myoclonus and dystonia, but has also been examined in limited studies of TS. Whereas the basic pharmacology of TS is felt to relate to dopaminergic mechanisms, these two drugs appear to act primarily on alternate neurotransmitters. Clonidine is an imidazoline derivative and acts primarily as an agonist at presynaptic α_2-noradrenergic receptors (1,2). Indirect activation of serotonergic and dopaminergic systems has been hypothesized (3–5). Clonazepam acts on γ-aminobutyric acid function and possibly serotonin (6,7).

CLONIDINE

In spite of numerous clinical trials with clonidine, confirmed efficacy has not yet been established. As indicated in Table 1, of 13 open label trials involving more than one subject, 8 have found improvement for 50% or more of enrolled subjects. In the four blinded studies, involving more than one subject, only one trial showed improvement in at least 50% of the group or a statistically significant improvement for the entire group in at least half of assessed variables. Although Leckman et al. (8) concluded that their double-blind placebo-controlled study indicated that clonidine was more effective than placebo, both treatment groups improved significantly compared with baseline function, and the clonidine group improved significantly greater than the placebo group in only 26% of the assessed measures. Numerous single case reports have indicated the same pattern of inconsistent response, with some positive and some negative (9–14). The duration of improvement, if seen, has been inconsistent across trials, with some studies suggesting that positive effects are short-lived (15), and others claiming that benefit only develops gradually (11).

The design and measurement tools used in these studies have varied widely, and efficacy has been based on global impressions, rating scales that combine subjectively and objectively derived data and pure objective measurement. Some series have studied clonidine as monotherapy and others have included patients on neuroleptic medications or clonazepam. Children and adults have been studied, and trials have ranged from weeks to months in duration.

Since no specific pattern of efficacy has emerged, investigators have attempted to identify clonidine-responsive subgroups from the larger series of tiqueurs. Although

TABLE 1. *Clinical trials of clonidine in Tourette syndrome: single case reports not included*

Author (ref. no.)	No. of patients	Monotherapy (M) or with other drugs (W)	Method of assessment[a]	Dose	% of sample improved
Open label					
Cohen et al., 1979	8	M	Neuro. exam & interview	2–3 mg/kg/d	100
Cohen et al., 1980	25	M	TS symptom checklist	0.05–6 mg/d	70
Dorsey, 1980 (23)	12	M	Global assessment	0.3–0.6 mg/d	75
Brunn	20	M,W	Global	0.1–0.4 mg/d	70
Jankovic and Rohaidy, 1987 (17)	27	Not stated	Global	Not stated	66
Leckman	6	M	TSGS	2–3 mg/kg/d	100
Leckman	12	M	TSGS	0.125–0.3 mg/d	83
Marsel-Mershun and Petersen, 1987 (15)	25	M,W	Global	0.1–0.6 mg/d	44% (short-lived)
Shapiro et al., 1983 (18)	68	M	Global	Max = 0.6 mg/d	26
Singer et al., 1985–86 (25)	30	Not stated	Global	0.1–0.8 mg/d	47
Abuzzahab	10	M	Global	0.1–0.6 mg/d	20
Comings et al., 1990 (24)	210	210	Global	¼–2 patch/wk	62
Truong et al., 1988 (27)	16	M,W	Global	0.32 mg/d, mean	38
Controlled					
Double-blind					
Borison et al., 1982 (22)	12	M	15-pt. scale	0.25–0.9 mg/d	58
Goetz et al., 1987 (20)	30	M,W	Objective ratings: motor, vocal tics, psychomotor tests	0.0075–0.015 mg/kg/d	No significant improvements over placebo
Leckman	23	M	TSGS tic counts	Mean, 4.4 + 0.7 mg/kg/d	26% of assessed variables significantly improved over placebo
Single-blind					
Leckman	13	M	TSGS	0.125–3 mg/d	46% improved

[a] TSGS, Tourette syndrome global scale.

numerous observations have been made, investigators have not agreed on accurate predictive features for clonidine response. In a small series, Young et al. (16) reported that although plasma-free 3-methoxy-4-hydroxy-phenyl glycol (MHPG) levels are not consistently low in TS patients receiving clonidine, a low baseline level suggested a positive clinical response. Severity of tics is not discriminative, since Jankovic and Rohaidy (17) found that mild patients responded best to clonidine, Shapiro et al. (18) reported only a minimal clinical effect in mildly affected patients, and Leckman et al.

(8) reported excellent response in moderately and severely affected tiqueurs. In comparing age groups, Leckman's (8,19) series of improved patients were children, Shapiro et al.'s (18) group of not improved patients were adults, but Goetz et al. (20) also found no improvement in either children or adults. Leckman (19,21) followed other biological markers of acute response to single-dose clonidine, measuring MHPG, homovanillic acid (HVA), and human growth hormone but did not find that these indices were useful in predicting clinical efficacy. Borison et al. (22) suggested that a

good response to haloperidol predicted a positive response to clonidine, but Goetz et al. (20) added clonidine to neuroleptics in some patients and used it as monotherapy in others without finding benefit for either subgroup. Whereas some investigators suggested that clonidine ameliorates behavioral aberrations more than motor or vocal tics, others have found all features of the disorder improved (8). Finally, Dorsey (23) reported TS in association with other diagnoses like schizophrenia or histrionic personality respond less well to clonidine than neuroleptics.

Clonidine has also been used in a transdermal patch formulation, designed to administer up to 0.3 mg/day/week. In one study, 8% of patients used ¼ patch, 50% used ½ patch, 30% used 1 patch, and the rest used 2 patches as their weekly dose (24). Comings et al. (24) concluded that improved patient compliance, cost, and lack of interference with school routines made this formulation a highly practical solution to tic management in children. Of 210 TS subjects, they found that 62% showed some improvement in global function, with 40% experiencing improvement of at least 50% of the assessed symptoms. Tics improved as well as behavioral alterations including attentional difficulties, irritability, depression, phobias, and panic disorders. In a comment, the investigators reported patients who experienced rapid deterioration within 30 minutes after the clonidine patch fell off inadvertently. This observation is not easily explained by the half-life of the drug and suggests that at least a partial placebo effect occurred in this population.

One of the guiding stimuli to the studies of clonidine in TS has been the desire to find a medication without the short- and long-term side effects of the neuroleptic medications. Comparative studies between neuroleptics and clonidine have confirmed that clonidine has generally fewer and milder side effects (22,25). Among the common effects, approximate prevalences were drowsiness in 20–90%, insomnia in 10–25%, dry

mouth in 20–60%, and headaches in 20–30%. In a study specifically examining blood pressure changes after acute administration of clonidine, all patients developed postural hypotension (Table 2). Since clonidine is not a neuroleptic dopamine receptor blocker, it has not been associated with tardive dyskinesia.

Of more concern, acute withdrawal effects have been described in some patients who abruptly stop clonidine. Agitation and even manic behaviors have been reported (26); increased agitation (27) and an overshoot sympathetic nervous system crisis with hypertension, tachycardia, and profuse sweating similar to episodes seen with pheochromocytomas have been of serious medical consequence (28). Withdrawal of clonidine is safest when the daily dose is slowly decreased.

In patients receiving clonidine by cutaneous patch, skin rash in the area of the patch has developed in 30% of subjects, and was severe enough to cause cessation of the treatment in 16% (24). This effect has severely limited wider application of this formulation.

Since investigators agree that clonidine is not associated with the threat of tardive dyskinesia, many treating clinicians and investigators are willing to try this medication on mild TS patients prior to suggesting neuroleptic drugs and may add them to neuroleptic-treated patients who need more tic control and cannot take more neuroleptics. In facing such a patient, the author explains the data, and if the patient wishes to take clonidine, the beginning dose is 0.05 mg/day with gradual increases to a usual maintenance dose of 0.3–0.6 mg/day. If the medication is to be stopped, a slow tapering over 2 weeks is preferred.

CLONAZEPAM

Clonazepam, a benzodiazepine derivative, has been examined in very limited settings and has never been studied in a large double-blind trial. Gonce and Barbeau (29)

TABLE 2. *Adverse experiences in clinical trials of clonidine in Tourette syndrome: single case reports not included*[a]

Author (ref. no.)	Sleepiness	Insomnia	Depression, irritability, aggressive behavior, labile affect	Dry mouth	Impotency	Headache, dizziness	Hypotension	Increased saliva	Comment
Cohen et al., 1979	(−)	NM	NM	NM	NM	NM	+	NM	
Cohen et al., 1980	Several	NM	NM	Several	4%	4%	NM	+ Several	
Dorsey, 1980 (23)	NM	NM	NM	NM	NM	NM	NM	NM	58% improved side effect profile compared with haloperidol
Bruun	20%	15%	15%	5%	NM	+	No assessment	NM	
Jankovic and Rohaidy, 1987 (17)	NM	NM	NM	NM	NM	NM	NM	NM	
Leckman	NM	NM	NM	NM	NM	NM	100%	NM	Abdominal pain, nose bleed, glucose intolerance (1 each)
Leckman	24%	24%	NM	NM	NM	24%	8%	NM	
Marsel-Mesulam and Petersen, 1987 (15)	+	NM	NM	NM	NM	NM	+	NM	
Shapiro et al., 1983 (18)	18%	3%	4%	NM	NM	9%	9%	NM	
Singer et al., 1985–86 (25)	+ Frequent	NM	NM	NM	NM	NM	NM	NM	
Abuzzahab	+	NM	NM	NM	NM	+	(−)	NM	
Comings et al., 1990 (24)	NM	NM	+	NM	NM	+	NM	NM	
Truong et al., 1988 (27)	+ Common	+ Common	+ Common	NM	NM	NM	NM	NM	
Borison et al., 1982 (22)	16%	8%	NM	32%	NM	8%	0	NM	
Goetz et al., 1987 (20)	57%	0	27%	37%	0	0	0	0	
Leckman	NM	90%	NM	33%	57%	NM	43%	NM	

[a] NM, not mentioned; +, mentioned, no specific numbers; (−), mentioned as not present.

TABLE 3. *Clinical trials of clonazepam in Tourette syndrome: single case reports not included*

Author (ref. no.)	No. of patients	Monotherapy (M) or with other drugs (W)	Method of assessment	Dose (mg/d)	% of sample improved
Gonce and Barbeau, 1977 (20)	7	M,W	Global	4–6	71
Merikangus, et al., 1985 (30)	19	M	Global	1–6	68
Truong et al., 1988 (27)	28	Not stated	Global	Mean, 4.8	53

reported on seven patients who received clonazepam; five showed improvement, although one had both clonazepam and a neuroleptic drug started simultaneously. They did not give details on other patients in their practice who had received clonazepam without benefit. Truong and colleagues (27) reviewed their open-label experience with 28 TS patients who received trials of clonazepam and had adequate follow-up for evaluation of efficacy and toxicity: 21% had moderate and 32% had marked global improvement (total 53% positive result). In patients benefitting from clonazepam, the mean dose was 4.8 mg/day. Sleepiness, concentrational difficulties, personality change, and weight loss were side effects. Sleepiness and weight loss necessitated cessation of medication in some patients. A small single-blind crossover study compared haloperidol with clonazepam in 12 TS patients and found that clonazepam (dose range, 1–6 mg/day) was superior to neuroleptic treatment in 17%, and equivalent to neuroleptic in 33%. The remaining 50% of

the sample was better controlled on haloperidol (30). Seven additional patients started the trial on clonazepam, but because of good effects, they declined crossover to neuroleptic (Tables 3 and 4).

The usual recommended dose of clonazepam is 0.5 mg/day with gradual increases to a maintenance dose of 2–6 mg/day. This increase may require 3–6 months in order to avoid sedation. If the patient is concurrently receiving a neuroleptic medication when sedation develops, a decrease in the latter drug may improve the side effect and permit the patient to continue on clonazepam. If clonazepam is to be stopped, slow tapering is recommended to avoid withdrawal discomfort and agitation.

CONCLUSIONS AND PRACTICAL APPLICATIONS

The final role of clonidine and clonazepam in the management of TS is unresolved. The data gathered on clonidine so

TABLE 4. *Side effects of clonazepam: single cases not included[a]*

Author (ref. no.)	Sedation	Weight loss	Aggressiveness or personality changes	Forgetfulness	Ataxia
Gonce and Barbeau, 1977 (20)	30%	NM	30%	15%	43%
Merikangus et al., 1985 (30)	NM	NM	NM	NM	NM
Truong et al., 1988 (27)	+	7%	+	+	NM

[a] NM, not mentioned.

far suggest that a positive effect may exist in some patients, but the number of patients improved and the magnitude of that improvement is inconsistent among investigators. Double-blind studies have not uniformally established efficacy, and the marked clinical effect seen even with placebo in one double-blind study casts doubt on much of the open-label work so far accrued (31). For clonazepam, the results remain sketchy; larger and better controlled studies will be essential if efficacy is to be further tested. The sedative effects of clonazepam make a fully blinded study difficult to effect, although a large-scale comparison between a neuroleptic and clonazepam would be feasible to blind. Before further studies on clinical efficacy are designed and executed, however, a reasonable first step would be a careful definition of the patients to be studied, the tools to be used, and a suitable power analysis to determine the number of subjects needed to test for an anticipated mild clinical effect. An implicit problem with any drug trial in TS is the natural waxing and waning nature of the underlying condition. Although multicenter trials have been discussed among investigators, such an effort has not been mounted to date. The newly established Tourette Study Group may contribute in this effort toward collaborative research.

REFERENCES

1. Cedarbaum JM, Aghajanian GK. Catecholamine receptors on locus coeruleus neurons: pharmacological characterization. *Eur J Pharmacol* 1977; 44:375–85.
2. Svensson TH, Bunney BS, Aghajanian GK. Inhibition of both noradrenergic and serotonergic neurons in brain by alpha-adrenergic agonist clonidine. *Brain Res* 1975;92:291–306.
3. Geyer MA, Lee EHY. Effects of clonidine, piperoxane and locus coeruleus lesion on the serotonergic and dopaminergic systems in raphe and caudate nucleus. *Biomed Pharmacol* 1984; 33:3399–404.
4. Maj J, Baran L, Grabowska M, Sowinska H. Effect of clonidine on the 5-hydroxytryptamine and 5-hydroxyindoleacetic acid brain levels. *Biochem Pharmacol* 1973;22:2679–83.
5. Bunney BS, DeRiemer S. Effect of clonidine on dopaminergic neuron activity in the substantia nigra: possible indirect mediation by noradrenergic regulation of the serotonergic raphe system. *Adv Neurol* 1982;35:99–104.
6. Browne R. Clonazepam. *N Engl J Med* 1978; 299:812–6.
7. Fennessy MR, Lee JR. The effect of benzodiazepines on brain amines of the mouse. *Arch Intern Pharmacodyn Ther* 1972;197:37–42.
8. Leckman JF, Detlor J, Harcherik DF, Ort S, Shaywitz BA, Cohen DJ. Short- and long-term treatment of Tourette's syndrome with clonidine: a clinical perspective. *Neurology* 1985;35:343–51.
9. Zarkowska E, Crawley B, Locke AJ. A behavioral intervention for Gilles de la Tourette syndrome in a severely mentally handicapped girl. *J Ment Defic Res* 1989;33:245–53.
10. Dysken MW, Berecz JM, Samarza A, Davis JM. Clonidine in Tourette syndrome. *Lancet* 1980; 2:926–7.
11. McKeith IG, Williams A, Nicol AR. Clonidine in Tourette syndrome. *Lancet* 1981;1:270–1.
12. Lechin F, van der Dijs B, Gomez F, et al. On the use of clonidine and thioproperazine in a woman with Gilles de la Tourette's disease. *Biol Psychiatry* 1982;17:103–8.
13. Max JE, Rasmussen SA. Clonidine in the treatment of Tourette's syndrome exacerbation due to haloperidol withdrawal. *J Nerv Ment Dis* 1986; 174:243–6.
14. Ferre RC. Case report: Tourette's disorder and the use of clonidine. *J Am Acad Child Psychiatry* 1982; 21:294–7.
15. Marsel-Mesulam M, Petersen RC. Treatment of Gilles de la Tourette's syndrome: eight-year, practice-based experience in a predominantly adult population. *Neurology* 1987;37:1828–33.
16. Young JG, Cohen DJ, Hattox SE, et al. Plasma free MHPG and neuroendocrine responses to challenge doses of clonidine in Tourette's syndrome: preliminary report. *Life Sci* 1981;29:1467–75.
17. Jankovic J, Rohaidy H. Motor behavioral and pharmacologic findings in Tourette's syndrome. *J Can Sci Neurol* 1987;14(Suppl 3):541–6.
18. Shapiro AK, Shapiro E, Eisenkraft GJ. Treatment of Gilles de la Tourette's syndrome with clonidine and neuroleptics. *Arch Gen Psychiatry* 1983; 40:1235–40.
19. Leckman JF, Detlor J, Harcherik DF, et al. Acute and chronic clonidine treatment in Tourette's syndrome: a preliminary report on clinical response and effect on plasma and urinary catecholamine metabolites, growth hormone, and blood pressure. *J Am Acad Child Psychiatry* 1983;22 5:433–40.
20. Goetz CG, Tanner CM, Wilson RS, Carroll VS, Garron PG, Shannon KM. Clonidine and Gilles de la Tourette's syndrome: double-blind study using objective rating methods. *Ann Neurol* 1987; 21:307–10.
21. Leckman JF, Cohen DJ, Gertner JM, Ort S, Harcherik DF. Growth hormone response to clonidine in children ages 4–17: Tourette's syndrome vs. children with short stature. *J Am Acad Child Psychiatry* 1984;23,2:174–81.

22. Borison RL, Ang L, Chang S, Dysken M, Comaty JE, Davis JM. New pharmacological approaches in the treatment of Tourette syndrome. *Adv Neurol* 1982;35:377–82.

23. Dorsey R. Clonidine and Gilles de la Tourette syndrome. *Arch Gen Psychiatry* 1980;37:1350–7.

24. Comings DE, Comings BG, Tacket T, Li, S. The clonidine patch and behavior problems. *J Am Acad Child Adolesc Psychiatry* 1990;29:4 667–8.

25. Singer HS, Gammon K, Quaskey S. Haloperidol, fluphenazine and clonidine in Tourette syndrome: controversies in treatment. *Pediatr Neurosci* 1985–86;12:71–4.

26. Tollefson GD. Hyperadrenergic hypomania consequent to the abrupt cessation of clonidine. *J Clin Psychopharmacol* 1981;1:L93–5.

27. Truong DD, Bressman S, Shale H, Fahn S. Clonazepam, haloperidol, and clonidine in tic disorders. *South Med J* 1988;81:1103–4.

28. Hansson L. Blood pressure crisis following withdrawal of clonidine with special reference to arterial and urinary catecholamine levels, and suggestions for acute management. *Am Heart J* 1973; 85:605–10.

29. Gonce M, Barbeau A. Seven cases of Gilles de la Tourette's syndrome: partial relief with clonazepam: a pilot study. *Can J Neurol Sci* 1977; 4:279–83.

30. Merikangas JR, Merikangas KR, Koop U, Hanin I. Blood choline and response to clonazepam and haloperidol in Tourette's syndrome. *Acta Psychiatr Scand* 1985;72:395–9.

31. Leckman JF, Hardin MT, Riddle MA, et al. Clonidine treatment of Tourette's syndrome. *Arch Gen Psychiatry* (in press).

Advances in Neurology, Vol 58, edited
by T. N. Chase, A. J. Friedhoff, and
D. J. Cohen. Raven Press, Ltd.,
New York © 1992.

31

Neuroendocrine and Behavioral Effects of Naloxone in Tourette Syndrome

*Phillip B. Chappell, *James F. Leckman, *Mark A. Riddle,
*George M. Anderson, †S. J. Listwack, *S. I. Ort, *M. T. Hardin,
*L. D. Scahill, and *Donald J. Cohen

*Child Study Center, Clinical Research Centers, and the Departments of
Psychiatry and Pediatrics, Yale University School of Medicine, New Haven,
Connecticut 06515 and †Clinical Neuroendocrinology Branch, National Institute of
Mental Health, Bethesda, Maryland 20892*

Tourette syndrome (TS) is an inherited neuropsychiatric disorder of childhood onset that is characterized by multiform motor and phonic tics and a spectrum of behavioral problems, including obsessive–compulsive disorder (OCD). Variability of severity over time is a hallmark of the disorder, and tics are often exacerbated by stress and fatigue (1–3). Neuropharmacological data have implicated dopaminergic, serotonergic, and noradrenergic systems as playing a significant role in the pathophysiology of TS and related disorders (1,4–11). A substantial body of data (reviewed in ref. 11) derived from neuroanatomical, neuroimaging, and neurochemical studies has singled out the basal ganglia and related cortical and thalamic structures as the most likely site of the underlying lesion. Moreover, recent pathophysiological hypotheses have suggested that disinhibition of cortico-striato-thalamo-cortical "minicircuits," which subserve a wide range of motor, sensorimotor, cognitive, and limbic processes, may underlie the protean symptomatology of TS and related forms of OCD (12).

Long associated with a variety of abnormal movement disorders, the basal ganglia contain high concentrations of endogenous opioid peptides (EOP) such as dynorphin and met-enkephalin (13). Opioid peptides are known to interact with dopaminergic (14–16), serotonergic (17,18), noradrenergic (19,20), and γ-aminobutyric acid (GABA)ergic neurons (21), and have been implicated in a wide range of biological processes, including the gating of sensorimotor functions (15,21) and the modulation of neuroendocrine responses (22). In human brain significant levels of opiate receptor binding have been detected in such regions as the amygdala, hypothalamus, thalamus, neostriatum, and substantia nigra (23).

Opioid peptides have been directly implicated in the pathophysiology of Parkinson's disease (24), Huntington's disease (25), schizophrenia (26), and (recently) TS (27). In a postmortem immunohistochemical study of a single TS brain, Haber et al. (27) demonstrated a marked attenuation of dynorphin A(1-17)-like immunoreactivity in striatal fibers projecting to the globus pallidus. This observation, taken with the neuroanatomic distribution of dynorphin, its motor and behavioral effects, and its modulatory interactions with dopaminergic neurons, suggested that dynorphin might be involved in the pathoetiology of TS.

In a preliminary study of a small group of TS patients, many of whom had prominent OC symptoms, we found that cerebrospinal fluid (CSF) levels of dynorphin A(1-8) were increased in comparison with controls and were significantly correlated with severity of OCD symptoms (10). This finding, taken with the neuropathological report of Haber et al. (27), suggested that regional alterations in processing of the prohormone might underlie some aspects of the pathophysiology of TS, such as the mechanisms involved in the obsessive–compulsive features of the syndrome.

Anecdotal evidence for a role of opioids in TS has been provided by clinical descriptions of the unmasking or exacerbation of TS symptoms after sudden withdrawal of chronic opiate therapy (28–30) and by uncontrolled reports of dramatic, though inconsistent, effects of the opiate antagonists naloxone and naltrexone on both tics and obsessive–compulsive symptoms (31,32). Moreover, in a recent controlled trial of propoxyphene and naltrexone in ten medicated adult TS subjects, Kurlan et al. (33) found that naltrexone produced a statistically significant but mild improvement in tic severity and attentional ability.

In addition, recent uncontrolled observations of abnormal growth hormone, cortisol, and luteinizing hormone (LH) responses to naloxone in some TS patients have prompted speculation that opioid modulation of endocrine function may be dysregulated in TS and that the hypothalamus may be involved in TS-related pathology (34–36).

To evaluate the role of opioid peptides in TS and to test the specific hypothesis that there may exist a defect in opioid modulation of endocrine function in TS, we performed a dose–response study of the neuroendocrine and behavioral effects of naloxone in TS subjects and normal controls. The rationale for the study was based on the fact that different opioid mechanisms, with different sensitivities to naloxone, are involved in modulation of the release of adrenocorticotropic hormone (ACTH) and gonadotropins from the anterior pituitary. While low doses of naloxone significantly increase resting levels of LH (by blocking sensitive μ receptors), 10- to 20-fold higher doses are required to elevate plasma levels of ACTH and cortisol significantly (by blocking resistant κ and δ receptors) (37–39). Hence the demonstration of a significant shift in the LH, ACTH, or cortisol dose response in TS subjects in comparison with controls would be consistent with a change in sensitivity of opioid receptors and would be suggestive of a functional alteration in activity of hypothalamic opioid circuits.

STUDY DESIGN

Five adult male TS patients and five adult male normal controls participated in this study. Four of the TS subjects had been medication free for periods ranging from 1 month to many years. The remaining patient was receiving atenolol, a peripherally active β-blocker, for borderline hypertension at the time of the study. There were no significant differences in age, height, and weight between the two groups.

All subjects were in good health and received physical and neurological examinations and laboratory studies to rule out the presence of any medical disorder. Urine drug screens were also performed. Both patients and controls received a rigorous psychiatric evaluation to establish the appropriate *Diagnostic and Statistical Manual*, 3rd ed, revised (DSM-III-R) lifetime diagnosis or, in the case of the controls, to rule out the presence or history of any psychiatric disorder, including substance abuse. All patients met DSM-III-R criteria for TS, and in addition three met criteria for obsessive–compulsive personality. The TS patients were all moderately to severely affected as determined by baseline clinician

TABLE 1. *Clinical characteristics of five TS patients given naloxone[a]*

	Mean	± SD	Range
Age (years)	29.4	6.9	23–40
Height (cm)	174.9	5.0	173–183
Weight (kg)	80.0	20.2	70.4–118.6
Baseline YGTSS tic ratings			
Total tic score	21.7	5.9	14.5–29.0
Motor tic score	13.8	0.9	11.0–14.5
Phonic tic score	10.0	5.9	0–18.0
Baseline YGTSS impairment rating	27.0	7.5	20–40

[a] TS, Tourette syndrome; YGTSS, Yale Global Tic Severity Scale.

ratings using the Yale Global Tic Severity Scale (YGTSS) (40). All subjects gave informed consent. Clinical characteristics are given in Table 1.

All naloxone infusions were performed at 1800 hours in a randomized, double-blind fashion at intervals of not less than 3 days. On each test day subjects fasted (except for water ad libitum) for at least 6 hours prior to and during the infusion. Subjects were not permitted to sleep. Blood pressure and pulse were monitored at baseline and at regular postdrug intervals. The doses of naloxone were 10, 30, 100, and 300 µg/kg, and a single saline placebo infusion was also given. Blood samples were obtained at 15-minute intervals for 1 hour before and 1 hour after each infusion for measurement of LH, ACTH, and cortisol.

Concurrent self-ratings, clinician ratings, and videotape records were obtained at baseline (−30 to 0) and over two postdrug intervals (+30 to +60 and +90 to +120). Immediately before and at 60 and 120 minutes after the dose, TS subjects completed visual analog scales designed to evaluate their ability to suppress tics, the intensity of their urge to have tics, and the amount of time spent performing tics over the previous 30-minute period. Motor and phonic tics were rated separately. During the same half-hour intervals, bedside clinician ratings of motor and phonic tics were performed using the YGTSS (40). In addition, concurrent 15-minute videotape recordings of patients were also obtained (i.e., at −15 to 0, +45 to +60, and +90 to +105) from which

counts of total motor and phonic tics were made in a blinded fashion.

Blood samples were collected through a stopcock in the IV and immediately placed on ice. Plasma for ACTH and cortisol and serum for LH were separated in a refrigerated centrifuge and frozen at −70°C until analyzed.

Plasma ACTH concentrations were determined by a previously described (41) specific radioimmunoassay using a commercially available antiserum (anti-ACTH-1 from IgG Corporation, Nashville, TN). For this study four separate assays were done. The typical detection limit was 4.0 pg/ml. The intra- and interassay coefficients of variation (CV) for three ACTH dose levels (spanning the standard curve) were 13.6% and 16.0% at 12.6 pg/ml, 5.3% and 4.7% at 30.3 pg/ml, and 1.4% and 5.4% at 85.0 pg/ml, respectively.

Plasma cortisol was measured with the GammaCoat [^{125}I] Cortisol RIA kit from Baxter Travenol Diagnostics, Inc. (Cambridge, MA). Five assays were performed. The sensitivity of the assay was 1.4 ng/ml. The interassay CV was 9.1%, while the intraassay variability ranged from 4.0% to 1.0%.

Serum LH concentrations were determined using the LH Double Antibody [^{125}I] RIA kit from Diagnostic Products Corporation (Los Angeles, CA). The detection limit of this assay is approximately 2 mIU/ml. The intraassay CV ranged from 7.0% to 2.2%, and the interassay CV from 7.9% to

6.2%. Three assays were performed for this study.

Hormone measurements and clinical ratings were analyzed using standard repeated measures analysis of variance (ANOVA) (42). Both parametric and nonparametric tests were utilized. Post hoc testing was performed with Duncan's multiple range test or paired t tests as appropriate (at $\alpha = 0.05$). Standard Pearson's correlation coefficients were computed for the self-ratings, clinician ratings, and videotape tic counts.

Preinfusion mean serum LH levels were calculated from the five basal samples, and preinfusion mean plasma ACTH and cortisol levels from the -15 and 0 timepoint samples. For each dose, the difference between the mean hormone concentration before and after naloxone was calculated (i.e., mean change), as well as the difference between the preinfusion mean and the postinfusion maximum (i.e., maximum or peak change). The results were analyzed for main effects of diagnosis and dose.

Subject's clinical ratings and vital signs were subjected to repeated measures ANOVA to assess main effects of dose and time.

NEUROENDOCRINE RESPONSES

In contrast to previous reports (34–36), there were no significant between-group differences in the neuroendocrine responses of the TS patients and the normal controls. In addition, there were no significant between- or within-group differences in mean baseline levels of ACTH, cortisol, or LH.

As shown in Fig. 1C, the LH dose–response curves of the TS patients and the controls were quite similar despite an elevated placebo response by the TS subjects. There was a significant effect of dose on both the change in mean serum LH levels [$F(4,32) = 5.53$, $p < 0.002$] and the maximum rise [$F(4,32) = 3.06$, $p < 0.03$]. However, no significant effects of diagnosis or of the interaction of diagnosis and dose were de-

tected. In the combined group of subjects, individual dose comparisons showed that every dose from 10 to 300 μg/kg caused a significant and similar increase in serum LH in comparison with the placebo infusion. Our observation that the lowest dose of naloxone (10 μg/kg) significantly elevated serum LH is concordant with previous work implicating naloxone-sensitive μ receptors in the regulation of gonadotropin secretion (37–39).

In contrast to a previous uncontrolled report in which TS subjects were found to have an abnormal cortisol response to low-dose naloxone (35), in the present study the cortisol dose–response curves of the TS patients and the normal controls were essentially identical (Fig. 1B). Not surprisingly, the ANOVA revealed a highly significant dose effect for both the change in mean cortisol levels [$F(4,32) = 21.3$, $p < 0.0001$] and the maximum rise [$F(4,32) = 21.8$, $p < 0.0001$]. In the combined group of subjects, individual dose comparisons indicated that the 30, 100, and 300 μg/kg doses significantly elevated the plasma cortisol in comparison with the control infusion. In addition, the effect of the 300 μg/kg dose was significantly more robust than the 30 and 100 μg/kg doses, an observation consistent with previous reports that have implicated naloxone-resistant κ and δ receptors in the modulation of ACTH and cortisol secretion (37–39).

A highly significant effect of dose also was shown for the change in mean plasma ACTH [$F(4,32) = 21.7$, $p < 0.0001$] and the maximum rise [$F(4,32) = 13.6$, $p < 0.0001$]. Interestingly, there emerged a significant diagnosis-by-dose interaction for the maximum rise in plasma ACTH [$F(4,32) = 2.52$, $p < 0.05$]. However, the analysis of the mean change in plasma ACTH failed to reveal any significant effect of diagnosis or diagnosis-by-dose interaction. Moreover, while inspection of the dose–response curves of the two groups (Fig. 1A) shows that the TS subjects had a smaller response on average to the highest naloxone dose,

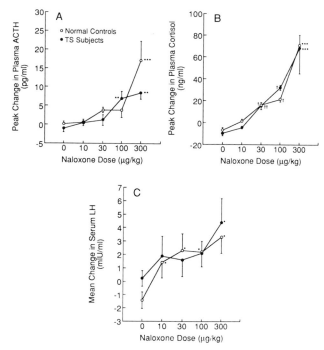

FIG. 1. Hormonal responses to naloxone of TS subjects (n = 5) and normal controls (n = 5). Each point represents the mean ± SEM. Individual dose comparisons were made with the Duncan multiple range test at α = 0.05. *, significantly different from placebo but not one another. **, significantly different from 0, 10, and 30 μg/kg but not one another. ***, significantly different from 0, 10, 30, and 100 μg/kg. +, significantly different from 0, 10, and 300 μg/kg but not one another. + +, significantly different from 0 and 300 μg/kg.

neither the difference in peak rise nor in mean change between the two groups at the 300 μg/kg dose was significant by post hoc testing. Individual dose comparisons in the combined group of subjects indicated that the 30, 100, and 300 μg/kg dose significantly elevated the plasma ACTH in comparison with the control infusion.

EFFECTS OF NALOXONE ON BEHAVIOR

The most provocative clinical findings from this study were provided by the videotape tic counts. In contrast to previous reports, naloxone was not associated with any dramatic effects on tic symptoms. However, analysis of the videotape tic counts suggested a tendency for motor tics to increase in response to low doses (i.e., 10 and 30 μg/kg) of naloxone.

In the overall analysis of the tic count data, there emerged only trends for an effect of time [$F(2,8) = 4.25$, $p < 0.06$] on phonic tics and an effect of dose on motor tics [$F(4,16) = 2.47$, $p < 0.09$]. However, inspection of the data revealed that there appeared to be a dose-related increase in motor tics (Fig. 2) over the first postdrug interval in response to the two low doses of naloxone. By contrast, phonic tics showed a clear tendency to increase over both postdrug intervals regardless of the dose (with a 114% average increase from baseline). When an analysis was performed of this subset of the data (i.e., doses = 0, 10, and 30 μg/kg), a significant effect of dose [$F(4,8) = 6.05$, $p < 0.02$] on motor tics was detected. Post hoc testing confirmed that the

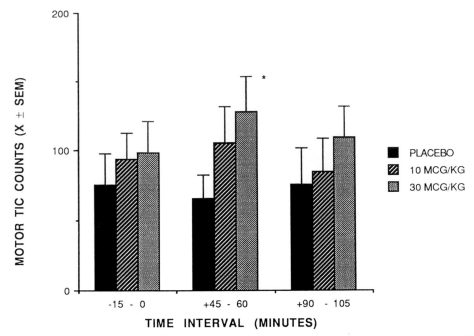

FIG. 2. Average (± SEM) motor tic counts following placebo and low-dose naloxone. ANOVA revealed a significant dose effect ($F(2,8) = 6.05$, $p < 0.02$), and post hoc pairwise tests showed that the 30 μg/kg dose was significantly different from placebo in the first postdrug interval ($p < 0.05$).

30 μg/kg dose of naloxone produced a significant ($p < 0.05$) increase in motor tics (26% on average) in comparison with placebo.

In terms of the individual responses, two subjects (nos. 101 and 102) showed no appreciable change in tic frequencies following the 30 μg/kg dose of naloxone. The remaining three subjects showed increases in motor tics ranging from 27% to 140% of baseline and in phonic tics ranging from 137% to 488% of baseline. All five subjects had more (from 9% to 348%) frequent motor tics during the first postdrug interval following 30 μg/kg of naloxone than following placebo.

By contrast, the analyses of the patients' self-ratings and the clinician ratings were generally unremarkable. Consistent with these results, the videotape motor tic counts were found to correlate poorly with the self- and clinician ratings of motor symptoms. No clinically significant side effects occurred in any subject at any dose.

POSSIBLE ROLE OF ENDOGENOUS OPIOIDS

In view of the small number of subjects studied, these results must be regarded as preliminary and interpreted with caution. It is apparent, however, that our findings contrast with previous reports of abnormal neuroendocrine responses to naloxone in some TS patients and of dramatic effects of naloxone both to increase and decrease TS symptoms. The absence of any between-group differences in the hormonal responses of the TS patients and the controls suggests that hypothalamic opioid circuits that modulate endocrine responses are probably unaffected in TS. On the other hand, the observation that low-dose naloxone was associated with a significant, though modest and transitory, increase in motor tic symptoms does appear to provide some additional support for a role for opioids in the pathobiology of TS.

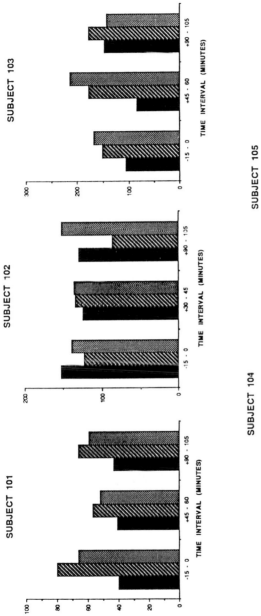
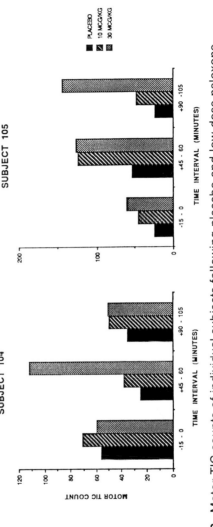

FIG. 3. Motor TIC counts of individual subjects following placebo and low-dose naloxone.

It also is likely that the effect of low-dose naloxone to increase motor tics is mediated primarily by naloxone-sensitive μ receptors rather than by κ or δ receptors, which are relatively resistant to blockade by naloxone (37–39). Additional evidence for involvement of μ receptors is provided by our neuroendocrine results, since the doses of naloxone that produced significant increases in motor tics were also quite effective in elevating LH (which is modulated by μ receptors), but not ACTH or cortisol (which are modulated by κ and δ receptors).

If substantiated in future studies, it would appear that an inhibitory opioid input mediated by μ receptors may be important for the suppression of motor tics in some TS patients. Alternatively, these results could be interpreted as providing evidence for overactivity of endogenous opioids in TS, with low doses of naloxone inducing a transitory withdrawal state through antagonism of μ receptors that contributes to exacerbation of tics. This hypothesis would be consistent with recent case reports of exacerbations of TS symptoms by withdrawal of chronic opiate therapy (28–30) and also is supported by animal studies showing that opiate withdrawal produces increased synthesis and turnover of dopamine in nigrostriatal pathways (43).

Involvement of μ receptors in TS is not inconsistent with previous findings that have implicated dynorphin in this disorder. The smaller forms of dynorphin, such as dynorphin A(1–8), have been shown to have appreciable affinity at both μ and κ receptors (44,45). Moreover, both pharmacological and behavioral studies have shown that chronic stimulation or blockade of one opioid receptor subtype can lead to up- or downregulation of other subtypes (46,47). For example, chronic administration of morphine, a μ agonist, has been shown to result in upregulation of striatal κ opioid receptors without affecting μ or δ receptors (48). Thus it is possible that functional alterations of both μ and κ receptors may be involved in some aspect of the pathophysiology of TS.

Along with κ and δ receptors, μ receptors are highly concentrated in the basal ganglia (13,49) and are among the earliest prenatal neurochemical markers to appear in the dorsal striatum, where they develop in register with striatal dopamine systems (49). Moreover, μ receptors are known to be localized on both dopaminergic and noradrenergic nerve terminals and cell bodies and to mediate opiate effects on catecholaminergic neurotransmission (19,49,50). In addition, prenatal stress, which is associated with severity of TS symptoms (51), in animal studies has been shown to cause a long-term decrease in striatal μ opiate receptors (52).

Future studies should be directed at replicating this preliminary finding in a larger sample size. Additional challenge strategies also should be developed utilizing specific opiate agonists and antagonists, as they become clinically available. If further evidence for involvement of μ receptors in TS accumulates, a neurochemical assessment of β-endorphin, which is known to have effects on μ receptors (53), and in vivo quantification of μ receptors with positron emission tomography should be undertaken (54).

REFERENCES

1. Leckman JF, Walkup JT, Riddle MA, Towbin KE, Cohen JD. Tic disorders. In: Meltzer HY, Coyle JT, Kopin IJ, et al., eds. *Psychopharmacology: the third generation of progress*. New York: Raven Press, 1987;1239–46.
2. Jagger RL, Prusoff BA, Cohen DJ, Kidd KK, Carbonari CM, John K. The epidemiology of Tourette syndrome: a pilot study. *Schizophr Bull* 1982; 8:267–8.
3. Surwillo WW, Shafti M, Barrett CL. Gilles de la Tourette: a 20-month study of the effects of stressful life events and haloperidol on symptom frequency. *J Nerv Ment Dis* 1978;166:812–6.
4. Shapiro AK, Shapiro ES, Young JG, Feinberg TE. *Gilles de la Tourette syndrome*. New York: Raven Press, 1988.
5. Ross MS, Moldofsky H. A comparison of pimozide and haloperidol in the treatment of Gilles de la Tourette syndrome. *Am J Psychiatry* 1978; 135:585–7.
6. Klawans HL, Falk DK, Nausieda PA, Weiner WJ. Gilles de la Tourette syndrome after long-term chlorpromazine therapy. *Neurology* 1978; 28:1064–6.

7. Golden GS. Gilles de la Tourette syndrome following methylphenidate administration. *Dev Med Child Neurol* 1974;16:76–8.

8. Cohen DJ, Shaywitz BA, Caparulo BK, Young JG, Bowers MB. Chronic, multiple tics of Gilles de la Tourette's disease: CSF acid monoamine metabolites after probenecid administration. *Arch Gen Psychiatry* 1978;35:245–50.

9. Cohen DJ, Shaywitz BA, Young JG, et al. Central biogenic amine metabolism in children with the syndrome of chronic multiple tics of Gilles de la Tourette syndrome: norepinephrine, serotonin, and dopamine. *J Am Acad Child Psychiatry* 1979; 18:320–41.

10. Leckman JF, Riddle MA, Berrettini WH, et al. Elevated CSF dynorphin A[1-8] in Tourette's syndrome. *Life Sci* 1988;43:2015–23.

11. Chappell PB, Leckman JF, Pauls D, Cohen DJ. Biochemical and genetic studies of Tourette's syndrome. In: Deutsch SI, Weizman A, Weizman R, eds. *Application of basic neuroscience to child psychiatry.* New York: Plenum, 1990;241–55.

12. Leckman JF, Knorr AM, Rasmussen AM, Cohen DJ. Basal ganglia research and Tourette's syndrome [Letter]. *TINS* 1991;14:94.

13. Nieuwenhuys R. *Chemoarchitecture of the brain.* New York: Springer-Verlag, 1985.

14. Quirion R, Gaudrea P, Martel JC, St. Pierre S, Zamir N. Possible interactions between dynorphin and dopaminergic systems in rat basal ganglia and substantia nigra. *Brain Res* 1985;331:358–62.

15. Herrera-Marschitz M, Christensson-Nylander I, Staines W, et al. Striato-nigral dynorphin and substance P pathways in the rat. *Exp Brain Res* 1986; 64:193–207.

16. Li S, Sivam SP, Hong JS. Regulation of the concentration of dynorphin A1-8 in the striatonigral pathway by the dopaminergic system. *Brain Res* 1986;398:390–2.

17. Kiefel JM, Paul D, Bodner RJ. Reduction in opioid and non-opioid forms of swim analgesia by 5-HT2 receptor antagonists. *Brain Res* 1989;500:231–40.

18. Gurtu S. Mu receptor-serotonin link in opioid induced hyperactivity in mice. *Life Sci* 1990; 46:1539–44.

19. Mulder AH, Hogenboom F, Wardeh G, Schoffelmeer ANM. Morphine and enkephalins potently inhibit [³H]noradrenaline release from rat brain cortex synaptosomes: further evidence for a presynaptic localization of mu-opioid receptors. *J Neurochem* 1987;48:1043–7.

20. Werling LL, Brown SR, Cox BM. Opioid receptor regulation of the release of norepinephrine in brain. *Neuropharmacology* 1987;26:987–96.

21. Matsumoto RR, Lohof AM, Patrick RL, Walker JM. Dopamine-independent motor behavior following microinjection of rimorphin in the substantia nigra. *Brain Res* 1988;444:67–74.

22. Delitala G, Motta M, Serio M, eds. *Opioid modulation of endocrine function.* New York: Raven Press, 1984.

23. Kuhar MJ, Pert CB, Snyder SH. Regional distribution of opiate receptor binding in monkey and human brain. *Nature* 1973;245:447–50.

24. Taquet H, Javoy-Agid F, Giraud P, Legrand JC, Agid Y, Cesselin F. Dynorphin levels in parkinsonian patients: Leu-enkephalin production from either proenkephalin A or prodynorphin in human brain. *Brain Res* 1985;341:390–2.

25. Seizinger BR, Liebisch DC, Kish SJ, Arendt RM, Hornykiewicz O, Herz A. Opioid peptides in Huntington's disease: alterations in prodynorphin and proenkephalin systems. *Brain Res* 1986; 378:405–8.

26. Iadarola MJ, Ofri D, Kleinman JE. Enkephalin, dynorphin, and substance P in postmortem substantia nigra from normals and schizophrenic patients. *Life Sci* 1991;48:1919–30.

27. Haber SN, Kowall NW, Vonsattel JP, et al. Gilles de la Tourette's syndrome: a postmortem neuropathological and immunohistochemical study. *J Neurol Sci* 1986;75:225–41.

28. Lichter D, Majumdar L, Kurlan R. Opiate withdrawal unmasks Tourette's syndrome. *Clin Neuropharmacol* 1988;11:559–64.

29. Bruun R, Kurlan R. Opiate therapy and self-harming behavior in Tourette's syndrome [Letter]. *Mov Disord* 1991;6:184.

30. Walters AS, Hening W, Chokroverty S. Opioid therapy in the management disorders. *Mov Dis* 1990;5:89–90.

31. Gillman MA, Sandyk R. Tourette syndrome and the opioid system [Letter]. *Psychiatry Res* 1985; 15:161–2.

32. Sandyk R. Naloxone abolishes obsessive compulsive behavior in Tourette's syndrome. *Intern J Neuroscience* 1987;35:93–4.

33. Kurlan R, Majumdar L, Deeley C, Mudholkar GS, Plumb S, Como PG. A controlled trial of propoxyphene and naltrexone in patients with Tourette's syndrome. *Ann Neurol* 1991;30;19–23.

34. Sandyk R, Bamford CR, Iacono RP, Crinnian CT. Abnormal growth hormone response to naloxone challenge in Tourette's syndrome. *Int J Neurosc* 1987;37:191–2.

35. Sandyk R, Bamford CR. Opioid modulation of gonadrotropin release in Tourette's syndrome. *Int J Neurosci* 1988;39:233–4.

36. Sandyk R, Bamford CR. Heightened cortisol response to administration of naloxone in Tourette's syndrome. *Int J Neurosci* 1988;39:225–7.

37. Grossman A, Moult PJA, Cunnah D, Besser M. Different opioid mechanisms are involved in the modulation of ACTH and gonadotrophin release in man. *Neuroendocrinology* 1986;42:357–60.

38. Spiler IJ, Molitch ME. Lack of modulation of pituitary hormone stress response by neural pathways involving opiate receptors. *J Clin Endocrinol Metab* 1980;50:516–20.

39. Grossman A, Besser GM. Opiates control ACTH through a noradrenergic mechanism. *Clin Endocrinol* 1982;17:287–90.

40. Leckman JF, Riddle MA, Hardin MT, et al. The Yale Global Tic Severity Scale: initial testing of a clinician-rated scale of tic severity. *J Am Acad Child Adolesc Psychiatry* 1989;28:566–73.

41. Chrousos GP, Shulte HM, Oldfield EH, Gold PW, Cutler GB, Loriaux DL. The corticotropin releasing factor stimulation test: an aid in the evaluation

of patients with Cushing's syndrome. *N Engl J Med* 1984;310:622–6.

42. Weisberg S. *Applied linear regression analysis.* New York: John Wiley & Sons, 1985.

43. Lee JM, Fields JZ, Ritzmann RF. Cyclo(Leu-Gly) attenuates the striatal dopaminergic supersensitivity induced by chronic morphine: agonist binding to D_2 dopamine receptors correlates with stereotype behavior. *Life Sci* 1983;33:405–8.

44. James IF, Fischli W, Goldstein A. Opioid receptor selectivity of dynorphin gene products. *J Pharmacol Exp Ther* 1984;228:88–93.

45. Mulder AH, Wardeh G, Hogenbloom F, Frankhuyzen AL. Selectivity of various opioid peptides towards delta-, kappa-, and mu-opioid receptors mediating presynaptic inhibition of neurotransmitter release in the brain. *Neuropeptides* 1989; 14:99–104.

46. Walker MJK, Le AD, Poulos CX, Cappell H. Chronic selective blockade of mu opioid receptors produces analgesia and augmentation of the effects of a kappa agonist. *Brain Res* 1991;538:181–6.

47. Bhargava HN, Gulati A, Ramarao P. Effect of chronic administration of U-50, 488H on tolerance to its pharmacological actions and on multiple opioid receptors in rat brain regions and spinal cord. *J Pharmacol Exp Ther* 1989;251:21–6.

48. Gulati A, Bhargava HN. Up-regulation of brain and spinal cord kappa opioid receptors in morphine tolerant-dependent mice. *Fed Am Soc Exp Biol* 1988;2:A368.

49. Edley SM, Herkenham M. Comparative development of striatal opiate receptors and dopamine revealed by autoradiography and histofluorescence. *Brain Res* 1984;305:27–42.

50. Schwartz JC. Opiate receptors on catecholaminergic neurones in brain. *TINS* 1979;2:137–9.

51. Leckman JF, Dolnansky ES, Hardin MT, et al. Perinatal factors in the expression of Tourette's syndrome: an exploratory study. *J Am Acad Child Adolesc Psychiatry* 1990;29:220–6.

52. Insel TR, Kinsley CG, Mann PE, Bridges RS. Prenatal stress has long-term effects on brain opiate receptors. *Brain Res* 1990:93–7.

53. Spanagel R, Herz A, Shippenberg TS. Identification of the opioid receptor types mediating beta-endorphin-induced alterations in dopamine release in the nucleus accumbens. *Eur J Pharmacol* 1990; 190:177–84.

54. Mayberg HS, Sadzor B, Meltzer CC, et al. Quantification of mu and non-mu opiate receptors in temporal lobe epilepsy using positron emission tomography. *Ann Neurol* 1991;30:3–11.

Advances in Neurology, Vol. 58, edited by T. N. Chase, A. J. Friedhoff, and D. J. Cohen. Raven Press, Ltd., New York © 1992.

32

Therapeutics of Tourette Syndrome New Medication Approaches

Peter A. LeWitt

The Clinical Neuroscience Program, Sinai Hospital, and The Department of Neurology, Wayne State University School of Medicine, Detroit, Michigan 48235

Some of the strongest insights into the biological basis of Tourette Syndrome (TS) have come from the dramatic improvements that several classes of medications can produce. This responsiveness, in turn, has focused attention on those neurochemical systems known to mediate movement and behaviors pertinent to the phenomenology of TS (1,2). The most influential experiences in this still unfolding chapter of therapeutics have been the improvements occurring from drug interventions lessening dopaminergic neurotransmission. Regardless of how tics manifest, they can be greatly diminished in both severity and frequency through the use of haloperidol and similar drugs blocking dopamine receptors. Neuroscientists pondering the mysteries of TS have looked to hyperactivity in dopamine pathways as prime candidates for explaining virtually all aspects of motor and behavioral control (3).

There are several reasons, however, why such an assumption may fail to explain the full range of TS symptomatology, just as disturbance of dopaminergic neurotransmission has been inadequate to explain the pathophysiology of schizophrenia and Parkinson disease. With TS, not all patients benefit from the use of neuroleptics, and they sometimes achieve symptomatic control from drugs (such as clonidine and clona-zepam) that act upon other neurochemical systems. The variety of medications capable of suppressing the tics and other features of TS would suggest that more than a single neurochemical mechanism is linked to this disorder's pathophysiology. Furthermore, pharmacological studies have shown that augmented dopaminergic neurotransmission does not always enhance TS features. Other clues for the neurochemical origins of TS may emerge from further study of the TS brain. An example of this is a regional decrease in dynorphin receptors (4), a finding that awaits pharmacological investigation with appropriate ligands to learn if this abnormality is related to modulation of tics or other TS features. Taken together, the few clues we have regarding the neurochemical pathology of TS emphasize both the lack of a coherent picture for the disorder as well as the important role that pharmacological investigation has played and will continue to offer for future progress.

Following the initial report of haloperidol ameliorating tics (5), a search for additional therapies has continued through the ensuing three decades. Studies of alternatives to haloperidol and other neuroleptics have dealt with most classes of centrally acting medications [even including drugs with an illicit status, such as LSD (6) and marijuana (7)]. Several reviews have reported on the range of medications that have undergone various sorts of testing (8–11). In a few instances, controlled clinical trials have been conducted that have documented their results using rating scales or other objective means. In other instances, appraisals of drug effect have been by clinical impressions without the benefit of placebo control. Many observations reported in the literature are at best limited case experiences, inconclusive for establishing the pharmacological questions they set out to answer. Factors that have made TS extremely difficult to study include the heterogeneity of its features and the marked variability that can occur from day to day in its expression. Even efforts at controlled clinical trials often have been thwarted by inadequate periods of observation, nonvalidated rating methods, or drugs whose actions include sedation or otherwise preclude "blinding" for purposes of study. A systematic evaluation directed at many classes of medications known to modulate important systems of the central nervous system (CNS) is lacking. While at first glance it would seem that virtually all of the available psychotropic medications have been used on some occasion to treat TS patients, it appears from the scanty literature on TS therapeutics that many commonly used neuropharmacological agents (for example, buspirone, clorazepate, or reserpine) have not undergone assessment.

There is a continuing need for alternative treatment options for TS. Many patients fail to respond to any of the drugs known to be effective against TS, such as haloperidol, pimozide, other neuroleptics, clonazepam, and clonidine. Even when effective against tics, these drugs have limited actions against the broader range of problems TS can present. Drugs are needed that lack sedating or tranquilizing effects, or the propensities of neuroleptics for producing tardive movement disorders. Unfortunately, research into novel therapeutic interventions has not had many targets to choose from. Several trials have been linked to a

rationale based on known pathophysiology in TS, such as alteration in dopaminergic (12) or opiate (13) systems. Other hypotheses have explored neuropharmacological systems known to have an activating role in cortical operations, such as the noradrenergic system (14). Based on this reasoning, clonidine came into clinical trials (15) and has become one of the most widely used alternatives to neuroleptic medication for TS. While its utility against tics has been called into question by a placebo-controlled clinical trial (16), clonidine continues to be widely used for lessening tics and behaviors associated with TS. Its pharmacology is reviewed elsewhere in this book, as are the actions of clonazepam (see Goetz, *this volume*).

The sections below review a number of pharmacological studies into therapeutics of tics in TS. In some instances, the drugs tested have served as probes of discrete neurochemical systems. Anecdotal experience abounds in the reports of treatments of TS, much of it inadequate for the purposes of answering important pharmacological issues. Hence, many of the comments published as brief letters or single experiences in patient care cannot stand as definitive statements on the benefits or inefficacy of the drugs reported upon.

LITHIUM

Lithium's pharmacological actions are diverse, among them alteration of dopamine receptor sensitivity and other effects on the monoamine neurotransmitter systems (17). While the drug has not been subjected to a controlled clinical trial in TS, several studies have been published regarding the results of prolonged periods of treatment. In one case report, a patient with multiple tics achieved resolution of this problem by use of lithium carbonate, 500 mg/day (18). Another study found that five of ten patients with TS and bipolar symptomatology showed various types of improvement with lithium treatment, especially with respect to behavior (19). These authors concluded that lithium improved those TS patients with features of grandiosity or bipolar symptomatology. Other reports have concluded that lithium can either improve or exacerbate TS symptomatology, or have no effect at all (20–23).

CARBAMAZEPINE

In addition to its anticonvulsant properties, carbamazepine has been useful for treating manic and impulsivity problems (24). Apart from accounts that six patients experienced an amelioration of tics from carbamazepine (25,26), there have been no controlled studies to indicate that this drug is useful for TS. In fact, three reports have indicated that carbamazepine can induce or exacerbate tics in addition to producing other movement disorders such as dystonia, orofacial dyskinesias, myoclonus, and asterixis (27–29).

NICOTINE AND CANNABINOIDS

Both nicotine and cannabinoids, plant alkaloids with a long history of use in humans for their psychotropic properties, possess complex neuropharmacological effects. A few studies have assessed their effects upon TS. One report claimed amelioration of tics from regular use of marijuana (6). Among their many CNS actions, cannabinoids exert effects on the nonpyramidal motor system via a cholinergic (nicotinic) mechanism (30). There have been other claims that nicotine might be of benefit for TS (31). Evidence has been presented that nicotine potentiates the effects of haloperidol in alleviating symptomatology of TS (32). In this trial, a significant decrease of tic severity and improvement in attention span occurred for eight of ten TS subjects who made regular use of Nicorette chewing gum (which contains 2 mg nicotine/piece). An earlier account by these investigators (33)

reported details of two TS boys treated with Nicorette. One, aged 6, achieved only a slight improvement of behavior and tics with use of up to 1.5 mg/day of haloperidol, which caused drowsiness. Adjunctive use of the nicotine chewing gum led to improvements lasting throughout the duration of gum effect, including fewer disruptive behaviors. The second boy gained only transient effects from haloperidol, 0.75 mg/day, against TS features. Addition to this regimen of Nicorette twice daily markedly enhanced the effect, with more calmness and fewer tics lasting for about 1 hour after chewing. It may be that gum chewing alone has some effectiveness in suppressing tics (34), as has also been suggested from experience in managing other types of oral-facial involuntary movement disorders.

Studies of nicotine's pharmacological actions in rats provides some clues as to its actions: given alone, it produced no change of motility, though the same dose potentiated hypokinesia induced by haloperidol treatment (30). This effect appears to have been mediated via a nicotinic cholinergic mechanism, since the neuroleptic-potentiating effect can be blocked by administering the nicotinic antagonist mecamylamine. Other actions of nicotine include dopaminergic properties that may link to its addictive properties (35).

CALCIUM CHANNEL BLOCKERS

Drugs that inhibit the entry of calcium ions through voltage-sensitive channels of cell membranes have had a number of medical applications. Calcium-mediated mechanisms in the CNS are found among several classes of neuronal systems (36), including those medicating motor activities. Myoclonic–dystonic movements have been reported with use of both verapamil (37) and nifedipine (38). Other adverse effects such as parkinsonism have been described from use of several of these compounds, presumably on the basis of their ability to block dopamine D-2 receptors. Neuroleptic drugs like haloperidol possess properties of calcium channel inhibition, although their mode of action against tics is likely to be primarily on the basis of their D-2 receptor dopaminergic blockade.

As this class of drugs became available, several trials have been carried out with calcium channel blockers to assess possible benefits against tics. With the use of nifedipine, 25 mg/day, one patient (39) experienced fewer involuntary vocalizations and internal urges for tics, as well as a reduction in other motor tics. Another case report mentioned that 10 mg of nifedipine three times daily led to improvements in tics and other behavioral indices of TS (40). Two additional patients with tics were reported to have sustained improvements with the use of calcium channel blockers (41). In one, a boy with TS, verapamil 20 mg three times daily gave continuing control of motor and vocal tics, along with improvements in irritability and compulsive features. A woman with a tic disorder responsive to haloperidol also showed improvements with nifedipine (10 mg three times daily) but because of flushing and persistent tachycardia, she switched to another calcium channel blocker, diltiazem (180 mg/day). Diltiazem was ineffective, and so the previous dose of nifedipine was resumed with the same symptom control as before.

Additional reports have dealt with the results of calcium channel blockers in TS (42). In one study, the calcium channel blocker flunarizine was administered to seven TS subjects. In this open-label placebo-controlled trial, the sustained use of flunarizine was associated with improvements in tics for six of the seven subjects, who experienced little in the way of side effects (43). Previously testing with a single 10-mg test dose of nifedipine for three of the subjects had shown no effect. Another clinical trial raised the possibility of a synergism between calcium channel inhibition and neuroleptic therapy. In a 9-year-old boy with TS, the trial use of nifedipine appeared to augment the effects of haloperidol in reducing tics and features of hyperactivity associated with attention deficit disorder (44,45).

In summary, calcium channel blocking compounds (especially nifedipine) may offer the potential for relief of TS features. Whether these drugs share a mechanism in common with neuroleptic drugs deserves further attention. Sedation or other nonspecific effects do not seem to be the basis for the claimed benefits, but, as is the case for any medications not yet subjected to controlled studies, further clinical investigations are warranted.

CHOLINERGIC STRATEGIES

The physiological antagonism of striatal dopaminergic neurotransmission by acetylcholine has prompted trials to increase its effect pharmacologically. One strategy to increase striatal CNS synthesis of acetylcholine has been administration of precursors such as lecithin, choline chloride, or deanol. With these, improvements have been claimed in some (46–48) but not all (8,49,50) reports. Such studies may have included selected patients, such as those not previously responding to neuroleptics (50). Another way to increase acetylcholine, with physostigmine by the intravenous route, has prominent effects of short duration. Nonetheless, several studies have been carried out to assess qualitative and quantitative effects on tics. Two studies of physostigmine injections in TS found two of five (8) and six of six (46) subjects manifesting improvements in tics for up to several hours. Another investigation found that scopolamine acutely produced a decrease of motor tics for ten TS subjects, whose benefits reversed (sometimes dramatically) with physostigmine injections (51). Among those subjects with prominent vocal tics, different patterns of response were found, such as worsening with scopolamine, which was reversed by physostigmine. In the only other investigation of physostigmine challenges, two of five subjects so treated in an open trial showed mild improvement, while the others showed no change (52).

A placebo-controlled double-blind crossover study was conducted in five TS subjects using a direct-acting muscarinic compound, 2-ethyl-8-methyl-2, 8-diazospiro-[4.5]-decane-1,3-dione hydrobromide (also known as RS-86) (53). The drug was administered for 4 weeks, and, after crossover, results were compared with an equivalent period of placebo treatment (54). Three of five patients were improved in motor tic counts and severity ratings, and three subjects also improved in regard to vocal tics (an additional subject worsened in vocal tics). This small-scale study suggests some promise for muscarinic compounds in treatment of TS. Though RS-86 was cancelled from further development, other cholinergic-enhancing compounds are under development for the symptomatic treatment of primary progressive dementia, and may come to be available for TS research.

GABAergic STRATEGIES

Clonazepam can be highly effective against tics (55–58) (see Goetz, *this volume*) for reasons that may be related to its γ-aminobutyric acid (GABA) receptor-stimulating properties. GABA has widespread actions on CNS neurotransmission, among them inhibitory effects on cholinergic, dopaminergic, and serotonergic neurotransmission (59,60). There have been a few trials with other drugs stimulating GABA receptors in attempts to learn if agonism might result in inhibition of tics. In one trial, a synthetic precursor to GABA, progabide, was administered to 17 patients with hyperkinetic movement disorders, among them 4 subjects with TS (61). Two were claimed to benefit more than 25% in tic control, with few or no side effects. Another investigation used an analog of GABA, γ-vinyl-GABA, which was not effective for TS (62).

MISCELLANEOUS TREATMENTS

As mentioned earlier, various ways of modulating the dopaminergic system can be effective in lessening tics. Treatments that decrease dopaminergic neurotransmission such as reserpine, tetrabenazine, and alpha-methyl-para-tyrosine have been shown to be clinically useful (52,63). Neuroleptic drugs that block striatal D-2 receptors can be expected to block tics (64). The only exception has been the "atypical" neuroleptic clozapine, whose action may be mediated through other classes of dopamine receptors (65). In a trial of clozapine treatment for seven TS patients (six of whom previously responded to haloperidol), control of tics seemed to occur for only one of them (65). Other studies with medications acting on the dopaminergic system include a trial with amantadine (66) and the selective D-1 dopamine receptor agonist SK&F 38393 (67), neither of which showed efficacy.

A recent report suggests that inosine might offer control of tics (68). This purine compound, which may act indirectly to lessen dopaminergic neurotransmission, was administered in daily oral doses of 50–90 mg/kg. Of 36 subjects (11 of them participating in a double-blind placebo-controlled crossover trial), 27 achieved good tic control lasting for months afterwards.

Other pharmacological effects on monoaminergic neurotransmission have been studied. The β-adrenergic blocker propranolol, tested for effects against tics, showed no effects (69,70). However, one case report deals with an instance of neuroleptic-induced akathisia in a TS patient that was controlled convincingly by addition of propranolol treatment (71). Another report describes the use of the serotonin precursor 5-hydroxytryptophan, 1,600 mg/day with carbidopa (72). A case of TS showed marked improvement of both tics and self-injurious behavior.

A few reports have made claims of effects from hormonal interventions, such as corticosteroids (73,74), estrogen (75), and clomiphene (76). Efforts to modulate tics from the use of the opiate antagonist naloxone, though claimed by anecdotal reports, have not been substantiated by careful trials (77,78). However, a TS patient's self-injurious behavior was reported to decrease under the influence of the orally active opiate antagonist naltrexone (79). Another trial found self-reporting of tics to decrease in ten adults treated with naltrexone, though clinical ratings of tic frequency did not change (13).

CONCLUSIONS

Most reports of TS therapeutics range from single case observations to rather limited clinical trials. Even reports documenting lone instances of unequivocal improvements [for example, a case in which marked improvement of tics occurred during lorazepam withdrawal (80)], can be difficult to interpret as to their pharmacological basis. Methodologies for evaluating TS have been extremely problematic in the absence of a consensus as to what constitutes representative and objective methods for rating the disorder. Fortunately, efforts to create a Unified Tourette Syndrome Rating Scale have resulted in rating instruments now under development for use in therapeutics research (81).

Even with the issues of definitions and adequate period of observation resolved, many problems face small-scale drug studies. There is sufficient heterogeneity in the features and disabilities of TS that patient groups of adequate size are necessary in studies designed to detect clinical utility from a new treatment. The design of studies investigating new therapies can benefit from review of methods and results that have been used in the few controlled clinical trials investigating drugs for TS (e.g., refs. 16,82)].

While most of the studies reviewed above have negative results or were limited in scope, several point to new therapeutic strategies that might be tried for TS. In particular, calcium channel blockers (including others than those cited in the reports above) merit further study. Other classes of drugs also show promise. Findings of decreased dynorphin receptors in globus pallidus in the TS brain (4) would make studies of compounds acting upon the dynorphin receptor of particular interest. Other candidates for investigation in the therapeutics of TS are drugs acting upon NMDA receptors, since glutaminergic pathways have profound effects on motor control. In neonatal rats, the NMDA antagonist MK-801 suppressed adventitious movements that normally occur during development (83). Although these paroxysmal muscle jerks have been tentatively classified as a developmental myoclonus, they might share more than a superficial similarity to tic disorders, and so the role for NMDA antagonists remains intriguing. The effectiveness of certain antidepressant drugs in moderating features of obsessive–compulsive disorder (see Leonard, *this volume*), a problem often associated with TS, indicates that strategies for managing the full spectrum of TS may need to incorporate several classes of medication into optimal therapy.

REFERENCES

1. Devinsky O. Neuroanatomy of Gilles de la Tourette syndrome: possible midbrain involvement. *Arch Neurol* 1983;40:508–13.
2. Caine ED. Gilles de la Tourette syndrome. A review of clinical and research studies and consideration of future directions for investigation. *Arch Neurol* 1985;42:393–7.
3. Snyder SH, Taylor KH, Coyle JT, et al. The role for brain dopamine in behavioral regulation and the actions of psychotropic drugs. *Am J Psychiatry* 1970;127:199–207.
4. Haber SN, Kowall NW, Vonsattel JP, Bird ED, Richardson EP. Gilles de la Tourette's syndrome. A post mortem neuropathological and immunological study. *J Neurol Sci* 1986;75:225–41.
5. Seignot MJN. Un cas de maladie des tics de Gilles de la Tourette gueri par le R1625. *Annu Med Psychol* 1961;119:578–9.
6. Smith CG. Gilles de la Tourette syndrome treated with LSD. *Irish J Med Sci* 1969;2:269–71.
7. Sandyk R, Awerbuch G. Marijuana and Tourette's syndrome. *J Clin Psychopharmacol* 1988;8:444–5.
8. Shapiro AK, Shapiro E, Sweet RD. Treatment of

tics and Tourette syndrome. In: Barbeau A, ed. *Disorders of movement*. Philadelphia: J.B. Lippincott, 1981;105–32.

9. Shapiro AK, Shapiro E, Young JG, Feinberg TE. *Gilles de la Tourette Syndrome*. New York: Raven Press, 1988.

10. Cohen DJ, Bruun RD, Leckman JF. *Tourette's syndrome and tic disorders: clinical understanding and treatment*. New York: John Wiley & Sons, 1988.

11. Messiha FS. Biochemical pharmacology of Gilles de la Tourette's syndrome. *Neurosci Biobehav Rev* 1988;12:295–305.

12. Singer HS, Tune LE, Butler IJ, Zaczek R, Coyle JT. Clinical symptomatology, CSF neurotransmitter metabolites, and serum haloperidol levels in Tourette syndrome. *Adv Neurol* 1982;35:177–83.

13. Kurlan R, Majumdar L, Deeley C, Mudholkar GS, Plumb S, Como PG. A controlled trial of propoxyphene and naltrexone in patients with Tourette's syndrome. *Ann Neurol* 1991;30:19–23.

14. Cohen DJ, Shaywitz BA, Young JG, et al. Central biogenic amine metabolism in children with the syndrome of chronic multiple tics of Gilles de la Tourette: norepinephrine, serotonin, and dopamine. *J Am Acad Child Psychiatry* 1979; 18:320–41.

15. Leckman JF, Walkup JT, Cohen DJ. Clonidine treatment of Tourette's syndrome. In: Cohen DJ, Bruun RD, Leckman JF, eds. *Tourette's syndrome and tic disorders: clinical understanding and treatment*. New York: John Wiley & Sons, 1988; 292–301.

16. Goetz CG, Tanner CM, Wilson RS, Carroll VS, Como PG, Shannon KM. Clonidine and Gilles de la Tourette syndrome: double-blind study using objective rating methods. *Ann Neurol* 1987; 21:307–10.

17. Bunney WE, Garland-Bunney BL. Mechanisms of action of lithium in affective illness: basic and clinical implications. In: Meltzer HY, ed. *Psychopharmacology: the third generation of progress*. New York: Raven Press, 1987;553–65.

18. Hamra BJ, Dunner FH, Larson C. Remission of tics with lithium therapy: case report. *J Clin Psychiatry* 1983;44:73–4.

19. Kerbeshian J, Burd L. A clinical pharmacological approach to treating Tourette syndrome in children and adolescents. *Neurosci Biobehav Rev* 1988;12:241–5.

20. Messiha FS, Erickson HM Jr, Goggin JE. Lithium carbonate in Gilles de la Tourette's disease. *Res Commun Chem Pathol Pharmacol* 1976; 15:609–12.

21. Erickson HM Jr, Goggin JE, Messiha FS. Comparison of lithium and haloperidol therapy in Gilles de la Tourette syndrome. *Adv Exp Med Biol* 1977; 90:197–205.

22. Borison RL, Ang L, Chang S, Dysken M, Comaty JE, Davis JM. New pharmacological approaches in the treatment of Tourette syndrome. *Adv Neurol* 1982;35:377–82.

23. Yassa R, Ananth J. Lithium carbonate in the treatment of movement disorders. A critical review. *Int Pharmacopsychiatry* 1980;15:301–18.

24. Evans RW, Gualtieri CT. Carbamazepine: a neuropsychological and psychiatric profile. *Clin Neuropharmacol* 1985;8:221–41.

25. Zawadzki A. Treatment of maladie des tics with carbamazepine. *Pediatr Pathol* 1972;47:1105–10.

26. Lutz EG. Alternative drug treatment in Gilles de la Tourette syndrome. *Am J Psychiatr* 1977; 134:99–100.

27. Gualtieri CT, Evans RW. Carbamazepine-induced tics. *Dev Med Child Neurol* 1984;26:546–8.

28. Neglia JP, Glaze DG, Zion TE. Tics and vocalizations in children treated with carbamazepine. *Pediatrics* 1984;73:841–4.

29. Kurlan R, Kersun J, Behr J, et al. Carbamazepine-induced tics. *Clin Neuropharmacol* 1989; 12:298–302.

30. Moss DE, Manderscheid PZ, Montgomery SP, Norman AB, Sanberg PR. Nicotine and cannabinoids as adjuncts to neuroleptics in the treatment of Tourette syndrome and other motor disorders. *Life Sci* 1989;44:1521–5.

31. Devor EJ, Isenberg KE. Nicotine and Tourette's syndrome. *Lancet* 1989;2:1046.

32. Sanberg PR, McConville BJ, Fogelson HM, et al. Nicotine potentiates the effects of haloperidol in animals and in patients with Tourette syndrome. *Biomed Pharmacother* 1989;43:19–23.

33. Sanberg PR, Fogelson HM, Manderscheid PZ, Parker KW, Norman AB, McConville BJ. Nicotine gum and haloperidol in Tourette's syndrome. *Lancet* 1988;1:592.

34. Brill CB. Gum chewing as therapy for Tourette syndrome. *Pediatr Neurol* 1988;4:128.

35. Lapin EP, Maker HS, Sershen H, Hurd Y, Lajtha A. Dopamine like action of nicotine: lack of tolerance and reverse tolerance. *Brain Res* 1987; 407:351–6.

36. Snyder SH, Reynolds IJ. Calcium antagonist drugs. *N Engl J Med* 1985;313:995–1002.

37. Hicks CB, Abraham K. Verapamil and myoclonic dystonia. *Ann Intern Med* 1985;103:154.

38. De Medina A, Biasini O, Rivera A, Sampera A. Nifedipine and myoclonic dystonia. *Ann Intern Med* 1986;104:125.

39. Berg R. A case of Tourette syndrome treated with nifedipine. *Acta Psychiatr Scand* 1985;72:400–1.

40. Goldstein JA. Nifedipine treatment of Tourette's syndrome. *J Clin Psychiatry* 1984;45:360.

41. Walsh TL, Lavenstein B, Licamele WL, Bronheim S, O'Leary J. Calcium antagonists in the treatment of Tourette's disorder. *Am J Psychiatry* 1986;143:1467–8.

42. Bhatia MS, Balkrishna, Singhal PK, Kaur N. Tourette syndrome treated with nifedipine. *Indian J Pediatr* 1989;56:300–1.

43. Micheli F, Gatto M, Lekhuniec E, et al. Treatment of Tourette's syndrome with calcium antagonists. *Clin Neuropharmacol* 1990;13:77–83.

43. Alessi NE, Walden ME, Hsieh PS. Nifedipine augments haloperidol in the treatment of Tourette syndrome. *Pediatr Neurol* 1988;4:191.

44. Alessi NE, Walden M, Hsieh PS. Nifedipine-haloperidol combination in the treatment of Gilles de

la Tourette's syndrome: a case study. *J Clin Psychiatry* 1989;50:103–4.

45. Barbeau A. Cholinergic treatment in the Tourette syndrome. *N Engl J Med* 1980;302:1310–1.

46. Stahl SM, Berger PA. Physostigmine in Tourette syndrome: evidence for cholinergic underactivity. *Am J Psychiatry* 1981;138:240–2.

47. Finney JW, Christophersen ER, Ziegler DK. Deanol and Tourette syndrome. *Lancet* 1981;2:989.

48. Pinta ER. Deanol in Gilles de la Tourette syndrome: a preliminary investigation. *Dis Nerv Syst* 1977;38:214–5.

49. Polinsky RJ, Ebert MH, Caine ED, Ludlow C, Bassich CJ. Cholinergic treatment in the Tourette syndrome. *N Engl J Med* 1980;302:1310.

50. Moldowsky H, Sandor P. Lecithin in the treatment of Gilles de la Tourette syndrome. *Am J Psychiatry* 1983;140:1627–9.

51. Tanner CM, Goetz CG, Klawans HL. Cholinergic mechanisms in Tourette syndrome. *Neurology* 1982;32:1315–7.

52. Sweet RD, Bruun R, Shapiro E, Shapiro AK. Presynaptic catecholamine antagonists as treatment for Tourette syndrome. Effects of alpha methyl para tyrosine and tetrabenazine. *Arch Gen Psychiatry* 1974;31:857–61.

53. Spiegel R. Effects of RS-86, an orally active cholinergic agonist, on sleep in man. *Psychiatry Res* 1984;11:1–13.

54. LeWitt PA, Kesaree N, Berchou RC, Kareti D, Schlick P. Treatment of Tourette syndrome with the muscarinic agonist RS-86. *Neurology* 1988; 38(suppl 1):361.

55. Gonce M, Barbeau A. Seven cases of Gilles de la Tourette's syndrome: partial relief with clonazepam: a pilot study. *Can J Neurol Sci* 1977; 4:279–83.

56. Merikangas JR, Merikangas KR, Kopp U, Hanin I. Blood choline and response to clonazepam and haloperidol in Tourette's syndrome. *Acta Psychiatr Scand* 1985;72:395–9.

57. Erenberg G. Pharmacologic therapy of tics in childhood. *Pediatr Ann* 1988;17:395–404.

58. Golden GS. Tourette syndrome: recent advances. *Neurol Clin* 1990;8:705–14.

59. Scatton B, Zivkovic B, Dedek J, et al. Gamma-aminobutyric acid (GABA) receptor stimulation (III). Effect of progabide (SL 76002) on norepinephrine, dopamine, and 5-hydroxytryptamine. *J Pharmacol Exp Ther* 1982;220:678–88.

60. Scatton B, Bartholini G. Gamma-aminobutyric acid (GABA) receptor stimulation (IV). Effect of progabide (SL 76002) and other GABAergic agents on acetylcholine turnover in rat brain areas. *J Pharmacol Exp Ther* 1982;220:689–95.

61. Mondrup K, Dupont E, Braendgaard H. Progabide in the treatment of hyperkinetic extrapyramidal movement disorders. *Acta Neurol Scand* 1985; 72:341–3.

62. Stahl SM, Thornton JE, Simpson ML, Berger PA, Napoliello MJ. Gamma-vinyl-GABA treatment of tardive dyskinesia and other movement disorders. *Biol Psychiatry* 1985;20:888–93.

63. Jankovic J, Glaze DG, Frost JD. Effect of tetra-

benazine on tics and sleep of Gilles de la Tourette's syndrome. *Neurology* 1984;34:688–92.

64. Uhr SB, Pruitt B, Berger PA, Stahl SM. Improvement of symptoms in Tourette syndrome by piquindone, a novel dopamine-2 receptor antagonist. *Int Clin Psychopharmacol* 1986;1:216–20.

65. Caine ED, Polinsky RJ, Kartzinel R, Ebert MH. The trial use of clozapine for abnormal involuntary movement disorders. *Am J Psychiatry* 1979; 136:317–20.

66. Borison RL, Davis JM. Amantadine in Tourette syndrome. *Curr Psychiatr Ther* 1983;22:127–30.

67. Braun A, Mouradian MM, Mohr E, Fabbrini G, Chase TN. Selective D-1 dopamine receptor agonist effects in hyperkinetic extrapyramidal disorders. *J Neurol Neurosurg Psychiatry* 1989; 52:631–5.

68. Cheng Y, Jiang DH. Therapeutic effect of inosine in Tourette syndrome and its possible mechanism of action. *Chung-Hua Ching Ching Shen Ko Tsa Chih* 1990;23:90–3.

69. Sverd J, Kupietz S. Effects of high dose propranolol in Tourette syndrome. *J Clin Psychopharmacol* 1984;4:359–61.

70. Sverd J, Cohen S, Camp JA: Brief report: effects of propranolol in Tourette syndrome. *J Autism Dev Disord* 1983;13:207–13.

71. Chandler JD: Propranolol treatment of akathisia in Tourette's syndrome. *J Am Acad Child Adolesc Psychiatry* 1990;29:475–7.

72. Van Woert MH, Yip LC, Balis ME. Purine phosphoribosyltransferase in Gilles de la Tourette syndrome. *N Engl J Med* 1977;296:210–2.

73. Kondo K, Kabasawa T. Improvement in Gilles de la Tourette syndrome after corticosteroid therapy. *Ann Neurol* 1978;4:387.

74. Geschwind N, Kondo K. Corticosteroid therapy and Tourette syndrome. *Ann Neurol* 1979;5:495.

75. Sandyk R, Bamford CR. Estrogen as adjuvant treatment of Tourette syndrome. *Pediatr Neurol* 1987;3:122.

76. Sandyk R, Bamford CR, Laguna J. Clomiphene citrate in Tourette's syndrome. *Postgrad Med J* 1987;63:510–1.

77. Berecz JM, Dysken MW, Davis JM. Naloxone effect in Tourette syndrome. *Neurology* 1979; 29:1316–7.

78. Gadoth N, Gordon CR, Streifler J. Naloxone in Gilles de la Tourette's syndrome. *Ann Neurol* 1987;21:415.

79. Herman BH, Hammock MK, Arthur-Smith A, et al. Naltrexone decreases self-injurious behavior. *Ann Neurol* 1987;22:550–2.

80. Wright S, Peet M. Gilles de la Tourette's syndrome. Amelioration following acute akinesia during lorazepam withdrawal. *Br J Psychiatry* 1989; 154:257–9.

81. Kurlan R. Tourette's syndrome: current concepts. *Neurology* 1989;39:1625–30.

82. Shapiro AK, Shapiro E. Controlled study of pimozide vs. placebo in Tourette's syndrome. *J Am Acad Child Psychiatry* 1984;23:161–73.

83. Pranzatelli MR. Antimyoclonic effect of MK-801: a possible role for NMDA receptors in developmental myoclonus of the neonatal rat. *Clin Neuropharmacol* 1990;13:329–38.

Advances in Neurology, Vol. 58, edited by T. N. Chase, A. J. Friedhoff, and D. J. Cohen. Raven Press, Ltd., New York © 1992.

33

Methylphenidate in Hyperactive Boys with Comorbid Tic Disorder

I. Clinic Evaluations

Jeffrey Sverd, Kenneth D. Gadow, Edith E. Nolan, Joyce Sprafkin, and Stacy N. Ezor

Department of Psychiatry and Behavioral Science, State University of New York at Stony Brook, Stony Brook, New York 11794

Attention deficit hyperactivity disorder (ADHD) is frequently present in children with Tourette syndrome (TS) (1–9). Prevalence rates of ADHD in samples of TS patients vary from 35% to 80% and higher (1–9). ADHD symptoms often predate the onset or recognition of tics by an average of 2.5 years (1–9). In one study, 48% of TS patients received a diagnosis of ADHD before a diagnosis of TS (4).

In addition to the high rate of ADHD in children with TS, tics and TS are frequently present in children referred for evaluation of ADHD. For example, Comings and Comings (4) observed that in the children they evaluated for ADHD, one-half either had tics or a family history of tics or TS, and Sverd and colleagues (8) reported that 9 of 82 (11%) boys referred for evaluation of behavioral disturbance actually had undiagnosed TS. This figure did not include those boys without tics in whom a family history of tics or TS, might have been present. Similarly, other investigators reported the presence of tics in 30% to 35% of the ADHD children that they evaluated (10–12).

Because chronic motor tic disorder and TS are genetically related and some cases of transient tic disorder may be a result of

familial TS (1,2), a significant portion of children with ADHD may actually be expressing symptoms of a genetic diathesis for TS. This consideration, combined with the report that the carrier frequency of the TS gene may be as high as 18% (14) and that a high rate of family members of TS patients have ADHD, suggests that ADHD is a variant expression of the TS gene and that TS constitutes a major etiologic subgroup of ADHD (1,13–16).

Psychostimulants are the drugs of choice for the treatment of children with ADHD, have been prescribed to millions of school-aged children in the United States (17), and are considered to be among the safest psychoactive agents in current use in child psychiatry. Although clinical reports indicate that they ameliorate ADHD symptoms in TS patients (1–4,6,9,15,18,19), their use has been associated with the onset or exacerbation of tics (1–4,6,9,18–21), leading some clinicians to discourage their use in TS patients or in hyperactive children with family histories of tics or TS (10,20,21). The proscription against stimulant use in TS patients is a result of the theory that hyperdopaminergic dysfunction in the central nervous system underlies the TS disorder

and that administration of dopamine agonists would result in symptom exacerbation
(1,2,19).

Other evidence suggests, however, that
stimulant drugs do not cause TS and that
their effects on tic symptoms are not always negative. For example, some patients
appear to experience tic amelioration
(1–4,6,9,18,19,22,23). Comings and Comings suggested that stimulant treatment
might delay the onset of tics (3), and Price
et al. (22) and Waserman et al. (23) suggested that stimulants might reduce the
long-term severity of TS symptoms by de-
sensitizing catecholamine receptor sites
(24). Although surveys of medication histories show that 13% to 33% of TS patients
are reported to have experienced stimulant-
associated tic exacerbation (1,2,6,22), Shapiro et al. (2) argued that the worsening of
tics in such patients may be a result of the
natural waxing phase of the TS disorder and
that ascertainment bias in surveys may account for the increased percentage of patients thought to have experienced stimu-
lant-induced tics. Bias in reporting cases of
stimulant-associated tic exacerbation or
onset might also contribute to the belief that
stimulants cause or exacerbate tics (1). Furthermore, the positive association between
severity of tic disorder and severity of
behavior disorder in some instances
(1,4,8,19,25,26), combined with the observation that behavior disorder often predates
the emergence of tics (1–9), suggests that
tic onset or exacerbation associated with
stimulant use may be coincidental in a significant portion of cases (1–4,8,9,15,19).

In spite of the aforementioned evidence
and considerations to the contrary, it is generally accepted that stimulants are contra-
indicated for child patients with TS
(1,2,6–10,15,19,22,23). Interestingly, there
are few cases in which there is unequivocal
evidence to support this belief and little experimental research that addresses this
issue.

Establishing the efficacy and safety of
methylphenidate in the treatment of TS chil-

dren is of importance for the following reasons: (a) a significant number of TS children
may not require neuroleptic treatment of
their tics but may require pharmacologic
treatment of their associated behavioral and
attentional problems (1,3,4,6,18,19); (b)
some children treated with neuroleptics
may require the addition of stimulants to alleviate neuroleptic side effects and ameliorate symptoms of ADHD (1,2,19); and (c)
TS patients treated with neuroleptics primarily for the control of learning and behavior problems may be at risk for tardive and
withdrawal dyskinesia.

Given the controversy surrounding the
use of stimulant medication for the treatment of ADHD in children with tic disorders, the authors conducted a single-blind
placebo-controlled investigation of the effects of methylphenidate on tic status and
behavioral disturbance in four boys diagnosed as having TS and ADHD (19). Clinical ratings and playroom observations
showed amelioration of ADHD symptoms
with methylphenidate and no untoward effects on tic status. In all four boys, the highest dose resulted in improved classroom ratings of tics compared with initial placebo
treatment. In three children, mild tic exacerbation was reported for a lower dose. The
findings suggested that tic response was independent of clinical doses of methylphenidate but were also consistent with the theory that methylphenidate might affect tic
status by altering dopamine receptor sensitivity. The authors concluded that methylphenidate alone might prove to be a safe
and effective treatment for many ADHD-
TS patients. Other investigators who have
conducted controlled studies have reached
similar conclusions (27,28).

To further evaluate the safety and efficacy of methylphenidate for the treatment
of ADHD children with comorbid tic disorder, a double-blind placebo-controlled
study was undertaken. This study was divided into two distinct components: (a) clinic-based evaluations that involved direct
observations of child behavior in a simu-

lated classroom setting and physician and parent ratings of symptom severity, and (b) school-based evaluations that involved direct observations of child behavior in the classroom, lunchroom, and playground and teacher ratings of symptom severity. This report pertains to the clinic evaluations. A companion article by Gadow et al. (29) describes the findings from the school evaluation.

STUDY DESIGN

The subjects were 11 boys between the ages of 6.1 and 11.9 years old (mean, 8.3 years; SD, 1.96), who were referred for evaluation by a clinician who specialized in the treatment of patients with tic disorders (J.Sv.) or to a child psychiatry outpatient service. All subjects met *Diagnostic and Statistical Manual*, 3rd ed., revised (DSM-III-R) diagnostic criteria for ADHD and either chronic motor tic disorder or Tourette disorder (established on the basis of a clinical interview with the parent) and were above cutoff on two out of three parent- and teacher-completed hyperactivity/ADHD behavior rating scales. The ADHD measures were the Abbreviated Teacher Rating Scale (ATRS) (30), the IOWA Conners Teacher's Rating Scale (31), the Conners (48-item) Parent Rating Scale (32), the Primary Secondary Symptom Checklist (PSSC) (33) completed by the mother, and the parent and teacher versions of the Stony Brook Child Psychiatric Checklist-3R (34).

Each child met research diagnostic criteria (Tourette Syndrome Association) for Tourette syndrome, definite (n = 7) or by history (n = 3), or chronic multiple motor or phonic tic disorder, definite (n = 1). The terms "definite" and "by history" are defined as follows: Definite means that "motor and/or phonic tics must be witnessed by a reliable examiner directly at some point in the illness or be recorded by videotape or cinematography." The term "by history" is used when the tics have not

been witnessed by a reliable examiner but were witnessed by reliable family member or close friend and "the description of tics as demonstrated are accepted by reliable examiner." Our application of these criteria was more rigorous in that we required that *both* motor and vocal tics had to be witnessed by *two* or more reliable examiners, each on the basis of behavior exhibited in a different setting to be considered definite. (At least one reliable examiner witnessed motor and vocal tics in all of our subjects.) The extent to which their tics interfered with normal daily living is best characterized by their Overall Impairment Rating scores from the Yale Global Tic Severity Scale (35): none (n = 2), minimal (n = 4), mild (n = 4), and severe (n = 1). Their Global Severity Scores from the same instrument ranged from 16 to 79 (mean, 40.6; SD, 16.6).

Children who exhibited one or more of the following were excluded from consideration for the study: children who were believed to be too severely ill (dangerous to self or others; tics were the major clinical management concern), psychotic, or mentally retarded (IQ < 75), or who had a seizure disorder, major organic brain dysfunction, major medical illness, medical or other contraindication to medication (other than tics), or pervasive developmental disorder. However, children were not excluded from participation in the study if they had prior experience with stimulant drug therapy or if such therapy had purportedly exacerbated their tics. Six of the boys had a prior history of drug therapy for either TS (n = 2), hyperactivity (n = 3), or both disorders (n = 1). Five of these boys were receiving medication at time of referral. In the case of stimulants (n = 4), the minimum washout period was 1 week. The washout period for the one boy who was receiving a neuroleptic (pimozide) was 3 weeks.

A family history of tics and psychiatric disturbance was ascertained via clinical interview with the mother of the proband. One boy was adopted, and there was no information on his biological relatives. In 80%

of the cases, the proband had a first-degree relative who also had a tic disorder. Almost all of the families had a history of psychiatric disturbance, which included obsessive–compulsive behaviors, ADHD, drug and alcohol abuse, antisocial behaviors, bad temper, physical abusiveness, hypersexual behavior, gambling, chronic psychosis, psychotic depression, depression, suicide, and eating disorders.

Planning the most appropriate design for a methylphenidate study with TS patients is complicated by (a) the possible adverse reaction on TS symptoms, (b) the ground-breaking nature of group studies in this area, and (c) the unknown risks of premature exposure to higher therapeutic doses. On the one hand, there is much to recommend a fixed-dose increment design with pre- and postplacebo periods, given (a) the potential risk of tic exacerbation, which has been reported to be dose-related in some patients; (b) that the dependent measures are not sensitive to order effects; and (c) that this procedure closely simulates clinical practice. On the other hand, randomized dosage schedules, which control for order effects, are the norm in methylphenidate studies of ADHD children. Our response to this dilemma was to employ randomly assigned, counterbalanced dosage schedules, which permitted 3–5-day build-up periods for 10-, 15-, and 20-mg doses. The actual doses employed were 0.1, 0.3, and 0.5 mg/kg and placebo. For any given 0.1 mg/kg dose, the minimum was 2.5 mg. The maximal individual dose for any child was 20 mg. Medication was administered morning and noon, 7 days a week. School-day doses were given approximately 3.5 hours apart. Clinician, parent, child, teacher, observers, and laboratory aides were blind to the identity of the specific treatment conditions. Placebo and all drug conditions were identical in appearance, and each dose was placed in a dated envelope. Parents and school nurses were asked to return unused medication envelopes to assess compliance.

Prior to enrollment in the study, parents were repeatedly warned of the possible risk of transient and irreversible tic exacerbation as a result of stimulant treatment and were required to sign a written statement consenting to their participation. Once enrolled in the study, each child was monitored very closely. Parents had telephone access to clinicians (home and office) day and night for the duration of the drug evaluation, and the school was alerted to the possibility of tic exacerbation and the importance of immediate notification of changes in clinical status.

Once the medication evaluation began, the ADHD boys and their mothers were required to come to the clinic at 2-week intervals for clinical evaluation and to receive the next 2-week allotment of medication. During the clinical evaluation the mother was interviewed by the clinician (J.Sv.), and the child's clinical status was determined. The mother was asked to complete separate rating scales for her son's ADHD and tic symptoms. The clinician also briefly interviewed the child and observed him for tics.

The child was required to complete work activities in a simulated classroom during which time he was video recorded for 15 minutes through a one-way window. Clinic observations were conducted 1.25 hours after drug ingestion.

In addition to the rating scales that the parent completed as part of the clinic interview, parents were also asked to provide behavioral, side effect, and tic ratings for each weekend. Parents completed one set of ratings for their son's behavior during the morning and early afternoon on Saturday and Sunday.

Various measures were used to assess the impact of treatment.

Physician Evaluations

The tic measures (completed by J.Sv.) included the Yale Global Tic Severity Scale (YGTSS) (35) and, at the request of the Tourette Syndrome Association, the Tourette Syndrome Unified Rating Scale (36). The YGTSS generates 20 scale scores, several of which are recommended for clinical use. In this study we used the Total Motor Tic Score, Total Phonic Tic Score, Overall Impairment Rating, and the Global Severity Score. We used six scale scores from the TS Unified Rating Scale: the Shapiro Symptom Checklist (total number of tics), Examiner's Ratings of Motor and Phonic Tic Severity Rating (motor and phonic tics are rated separately), Tic Count (number of tics observed in 2 minutes during quiet conversation), Shapiro Interference Index (a three-point scale assessing the degree to which tics interfere with daily functioning), and the LeWitt Disability Scale. The latter is a global symptom severity-interference scale that assesses tics and Tourette-related features (compulsive actions, obsessive thoughts, ritualistic behaviors, anxiety spells, etc.). We interpreted this to include, with regard to children, disruptive behavior disorders and attention deficits.

Clinic Observations

The playroom procedure developed by Routh and Schroeder (37) and modified by Roberts and Loney and their colleagues (38,39) was used to assess drug effects. In this study, we used only the 15-minute restricted academic period. In the restricted academic setting the child is instructed to complete worksheets and not to play with toys on an adjacent table. Worksheet items are similar to those on the coding subtest of the WISC-R. Clinic sessions are video recorded to facilitate ease of scoring. The behaviors coded by observers during these periods are those traditionally associated with ADHD and include activity level and attention to task. Observer-coded playroom data have been found to be highly reliable and to discriminate between ADHD children and nonreferred children (38) and to differentiate subgroups of hyperactive children (40). Hyperactivity scores from the playroom have been demonstrated to correlate significantly with ratings of hyperactivity obtained from clinical charts, to be independent of measures of aggression, and to display significant stability over a 2-year period. The tapes were coded by a trained observer who had acquired literally hundreds of hours of experience using the observation code on a regular basis over a 7-year period.

Parent Rating Scales

The Abbreviated Parent Rating Scale (APRS) (30), is one of the most widely used drug evaluation instruments in studies of ADHD. The APRS contains ten items, rated on a four-point scale (not at all = 0; very much = 3), which are summed to generate a total score.

The Primary Secondary Symptom Checklist (PSSC) contains 32 hyperactivity/ADHD symptoms arranged in a checklist format. The mother simply checks whether or not each item characterizes her child (checked = 1; unchecked = 0). PSSC generates a hyperactivity scale score and an aggression scale score, which correlate significantly with chart ratings of hyperactivity and aggression, respectively (convergent validity), but do not correlate significantly with chart ratings of aggression and hyperactivity, respectively (divergent validity).

The occurrence of TS symptoms was rated on the Global Tic Rating Scale (GTRS) (41). The GTRS contains five items on the frequency of motor tics of the head (e.g., eye blinking, head jerking), neck, shoulder, and torso (e.g., shoulder shrugs), and arms, hands, legs, and feet (e.g., arm thrusting, clapping, touching objects or other people), nonverbal sound tics (e.g., coughing, grunting), and verbal tics (e.g., repetitive phrases). Four additional items pertain to the severity of tics (i.e., noticeable to others, embarrassing for the child, interfere with school/home functioning, lead to social rejection). All items are rated on a four-point scale (0 = not at all; 3 = very much).

The scores for the three motor tic items and the two vocal tic items are summed to form a Motor Tic Index and a Vocal Tic Index, respectively. The four tic severity items are summed to form a Tic Severity Index. Our own experience with the GTRS suggests that it is sensitive to drug effects, easily completed by care providers, and of potentially significant value in everyday clinical management.

Side effects were systematically monitored using the Stimulant Side Effects Checklist (SSEC) (42). The SSEC contains 13 side effect items rated on a four-point scale (0 = not at all; 3 = very much). Individual items are grouped to form three indices of drug effects: Mood Index, Attention-Arousal Index, and Somatic Complaints Index. One item pertains to unusual motor movements. We have employed the SSEC in several drug studies and have found it to be a useful device for obtaining side effects information.

FINDINGS

Each group of dependent measures was first analyzed using a two-way (behavior by dose) repeated measures ANOVA. Both behavior (the type of behavior assessed by each instrument) and dose (placebo, 0.1 mg/kg, 0.3 mg/kg, 0.5 mg/kg) were within-subjects factors. Because a significant main effect of behavior simply indicates that the rate of occurrence/score for specific behaviors differed from one another, we report here only the main effect of dose. Follow-up repeated measures ANOVAs were performed for each behavior category when

there was a main effect of dose. To localize additionally the source of statistically significant dose effects, post hoc Newman-Keuls tests were performed to assess differences between doses on dependent measures.

Clinic Observations of Behavior

Observations of child behavior in the structured academic setting were first analyzed using a 3 × 4 (behavior by dose) repeated measures ANOVA. These analyses revealed a significant main effect of dose, $F(3,30) = 4.76$, $p < 0.01$. Follow-up ANOVAs indicated dose effects for the amount of time spent attending to task and the number of worksheet items completed (Table 1). Post hoc analyses indicated statistically significant differences between placebo and all three doses of methylphenidate on both measures (Table 2). Inspection of the group means (Table 1) shows that the biggest degree of behavioral improvement occurred on the 0.1 mg/kg dose, but the 0.3 mg/kg dose also resulted in additional gains in attending to task and work output.

Physician Evaluations

A 10 × 4 (behavior by dose) repeated measures ANOVA conducted on the tic scale scores did not reveal a main effect of dose. However, given the modest sample size and the number of different tic scales, we were concerned about making a type II error (i.e., erroneously concluding that methylphenidate did not have an adverse effect on tics). Therefore, we conducted fol-

TABLE 1. *Means (standard deviations) and analyses of variance for direct observations by dose of methylphenidate*

| Category | Placebo | Methylphenidate (mg/kg) | | | F ratio | p |
		0.1	0.3	0.5		
On task (%)	56.5 (31.4)	76.5 (25.3)	85.4 (11.2)	88.0 (13.0)	8.02	0.0005
Fidgeting (%)	45.3 (18.4)	31.2 (23.3)	29.5 (17.9)	30.1 (30.1)	2.03	0.1313
Worksheets (no.)	152.3 (110.0)	204.3 (97.6)	223.4 (112.1)	230.4 (131.9)	4.75	0.0079

TABLE 2. *Mean group differences between treatment conditions for direct observations and behavioral rating scales*[a]

Measure	Placebo vs. (mg/kg)		
	0.1	0.3	0.5
Observations (SOAPS)			
On task	19.9**	28.8**	31.4**
Worksheets	52.0*	71.1*	78.1**
Parent ratings			
APRS	9.1**	3.67	8.12*
Peer conflict scale	3.41*	2.98*	4.35*
Mood index (SSEC)	2.29*	0.74	1.96

[a] SOAPS, Systematic Observation of Academic and Play Settings; APRS, Abbreviated Parent Rating Scale; SSEC, Stimulant Side Effects Checklist.
* *p* < 0.05.
** *p* < 0.01.

low-up ANOVAs on each measure. The results of these analyses and the means and standard deviations for each tic scale are presented in Table 3. With the exception of the LeWitt Disability Scale, increasing mean values indicate a worsening in tic status. On the YGTSS, there was no evidence

that methylphenidate exacerbated tics. In fact, the most favorable ratings were reported for the 0.1 mg/kg drug condition. Further, the mean scale score for the 0.5 mg/kg dose was at or below placebo levels. The strongest indication of improvement in tic status was for one of the YGTSS subscales not included in our primary analyses, the Number of Phonic Tics exhibited during the previous week, $F(3,30)$ = 2.92, p = 0.05. The mean score for the placebo and dose conditions were as follows: placebo (2.00), 0.1 mg/kg (1.27), 0.3 mg/kg (1.55), and 0.5 mg/kg (1.91).

The findings for the TS Unified RS scores are fairly consistent with the YGTSS with two notable exceptions. There was a tendency (p = 0.10) for the boys to exhibit more tics during a 2-minute interaction with the physician (Tic Count) on medication compared with placebo. Elevated Tic Count scores for the 0.3 and 0.5 mg/kg doses were evident in eight children. For four boys, the Tic Count on the 0.5 mg/kg dose was more

TABLE 3. *Means (standard deviations) for physician ratings of tics by dose of methylphenidate*[a]

Scale	Placebo	Methylphenidate (mg/kg)			F ratio	p
		0.1	0.3	0.5		
YGTSS						
Total motor tics	13.1 (4.72)	13.1 (4.74)	13.4 (5.2)	12.9 (4.48)	0.07	0.9757
Total phonic tics	10.6 (4.30)	7.8 (7.26)	8.6 (2.9)	9.9 (4.61)	1.35	0.2779
Overall impairment rating	13.6 (11.20)	12.7 (7.86)	16.4 (11.2)	12.7 (11.04)	0.58	0.6310
Global severity score	37.4 (18.12)	33.0 (16.82)	38.4 (15.9)	35.5 (16.80)	0.50	0.6830
TS Unified RS						
Shapiro Symptom Checklist	14.1 (11.12)	13.2 (10.11)	12.4 (7.57)	14.6 (10.02)	0.40	0.7557
Examiners' rating						
Motor tic severity	12.9 (5.05)	11.1 (3.86)	12.0 (3.87)	13.4 (7.41)	0.75	0.5312
Phonic tic severity	3.9 (4.41)	3.2 (4.71)	4.4 (3.83)	3.6 (2.81)	0.36	0.7824
Tic count	5.1 (3.24)	6.6 (7.09)	12.4 (16.50)	14.2 (16.16)	2.27	0.1007
Shapiro Interference Index	0.6 (0.50)	0.7 (0.47)	0.9 (0.54)	0.7 (0.47)	1.13	0.3523
LeWitt Disability Scale	61.8 (12.50)	66.4 (11.20)	69.1 (11.36)	70.0 (8.94)	2.61	0.0695

[a] YGTSS, Yale Global Tic Severity Scale; TS Unified RS, Tourette Syndrome Unified Rating Scale.

TABLE 4. *Means (standard deviations) and analyses of variance for parent-completed rating scales by dose of methylphenidate[a]*

Scale	Placebo	Methylphenidate (mg/kg)			F ratio	p
		0.1	0.3	0.5		
Behavior						
APRS	13.5 (8.64)	5.7 (2.72)	11.5 (7.74)	7.9 (7.18)	3.61	0.0244
Peer Conflict Scale	6.7 (3.62)	3.3 (4.92)	3.7 (4.20)	2.3 (3.75)	5.83	0.0046
Hyperactivity (PSSC)	2.6 (1.64)	2.4 (1.65)	2.6 (1.57)	2.3 (1.64)	0.23	0.8761
Aggression (PSSC)	2.9 (2.33)	2.0 (1.98)	2.6 (1.86)	1.4 (1.78)	1.67	0.1976
Tics (GTRS)						
Motor tic index	2.6 (2.09)	1.8 (1.42)	2.6 (2.96)	2.7 (2.71)	0.61	0.6162
Vocal tic index	1.3 (0.79)	1.1 (0.64)	1.1 (0.86)	1.1 (1.17)	0.13	0.9385
Tic severity index	2.0 (1.84)	1.5 (1.28)	2.6 (2.96)	2.7 (2.71)	0.33	0.8013
Side effects (SSEC)						
Mood index	3.4 (2.09)	1.1 (0.70)	2.7 (1.83)	1.4 (1.24)	4.89	0.0086
Attention-arousal index	0.6 (0.10)	0.5 (0.55)	0.4 (0.51)	0.4 (0.53)	0.08	0.9681
Somatic complaints index	1.4 (1.48)	0.9 (0.66)	1.2 (1.34)	1.4 (1.18)	0.66	0.5819
Unusual motor movements	1.1 (0.74)	0.6 (0.66)	0.9 (0.88)	0.9 (1.00)	1.26	0.3094

[a] APRS, Abbreviated Parent Rating Scale; PSSC, Primary Secondary Symptom Checklist; GTRS, Global Tic Rating Scale; SSEC, Stimulant Side Effects Checklist.

than twice the score for the placebo condition. The second exception to the general pattern of tic findings was the LeWitt Disability Scale, which showed a dose-related improvement in overall tic status, Tourette-related features, and disruptive behaviors as a function of increasing dose of methylphenidate.

Parent Ratings

The subject sample for the APRS and Peer Conflict Scale was 11 and 8, respectively. Analyses of these data revealed a significant main effect of dose, $F(3,18) = 4.55$, $p < 0.05$. Follow-up repeated measures ANOVAs were performed on each of the parent rating scale scores (Table 4). Dose effects were significant for the APRS and the Peer Conflict Scale (which were based on behavior exhibited on the weekend during peak hours of drug efficacy) but not for the PSSC. The latter was completed by the parent during their biweekly clinic visit and was based on behavior exhibited during the previous week (primarily evenings). Although post hoc analyses revealed significant differences between placebo and medication (see Table 2), the dose–response profile was unusual and unexpected. The ratings showed dramatic improvement on the 0.1 and the 0.5 mg/kg dose, with only modest improvement on the 0.3 mg/kg dose. Further, this pattern of drug response was fairly characteristic of the majority of the boys.

Analyses of parent ratings of tic frequency and severity as measured on the GTRS did not reveal a main effect of dose (see Table 4). Mean ratings for the 0.1 and 0.3 mg/kg doses were generally lower than for placebo.

The analysis of the main effect of dose for the SSEC ratings was significant, $F(3,24) = 3.41$, $p < 0.05$. Follow-up repeated measures ANOVAs indicated significant dose effects for only the Mood Index, $F(3,24) = 4.89$, $p < 0.01$. The mean rating for the 0.1 mg/kg dose was significantly lower than placebo. In other words, parents perceived methylphenidate treatment to result in an improvement in mood. Similar to the APRS and Peer Conflict Scale ratings, improvement on the 0.3 mg/kg dose (compared with placebo) was less than the other two doses. For the remaining three side effect indices, the mean ratings were more favorable for methylphenidate conditions than for placebo.

EFFICACY OF METHYLPHENIDATE

The findings from this clinic-based investigation provide fairly compelling evidence that methylphenidate is an effective treatment for ADHD in children with tic disorder. Observations of child behavior in a simulated academic setting revealed dramatic changes in child behavior as a function of drug dose. For example, the overall rate of on task behavior increased 56% on the 0.5 mg/kg dose of methylphenidate compared with placebo. Even more gratifying was the finding of comparable improvement in work output. Although improvements in behavior increased in linear fashion with increasing dose of methylphenidate, treatment with the 0.5 mg/kg dose produced only trivial gains over the 0.3 mg/kg dose. These improvements in clinical status pursuant to methylphenidate treatment were associated with similar changes in school behavior (29).

A truly unexpected finding was the sensitivity of parent ratings to treatment effects. Prior research, including our own (43), indicates that parent rating scales such as the ones used in this study, are not particularly sensitive to treatment effects. We believe that one likely explanation for the dose effects evidenced in this study is the relatively higher level of emotional lability in our sample of ADHD boys with tic disorder (as indicated by the higher SSEC Mood Index rating on placebo) compared with other samples of hyperactive boys (43). This observation that methylphenidate treatment improved mood in ADHD boys with tic disorder was first reported by us in our initial study (19). Many others, of course, have reported that stimulants elevate mood in ADHD children (10,44–46). Children with tic disorders who are referred for psychiat-

ric evaluation appear to be at greater risk for mood and anxiety disorders (1,26) and our findings suggest that methylphenidate's salutary effects may extend beyond the suppression of ADHD symptoms. These findings suggest further study of methylphenidate and mood disturbance in children with ADHD and tics. The unusual finding that parent ratings of symptom severity were more favorable for the 0.1 and 0.5 mg/kg dose compared with the 0.3 mg/kg dose is odd, and is not consistent with teacher ratings or direct observations of school behavior of these same children (29) or the findings from other studies (43). For these reasons, we are refraining from speculating on the significance of these findings until more children have been evaluated.

In general, the findings from this investigation do not support the claim that treatment with methylphenidate results in an exacerbation of tics, although individual children may experience a worsening of tics at certain doses. The tic rating scales used in this study were in uniform agreement (group data) that methylphenidate treatment did not produce a deterioration in tic symptoms. The only divergence from this general pattern were actual counts of tics conducted by the examiner. The Number of Phonic Tics score (rating scale format) from the YGTSS indicated a decrease in tic frequency for methylphenidate compared with placebo, a finding that is consistent with our direct observation study (29). Conversely, the 2-minute Tic Count score from TS Unified RS indicated an increased frequency of tics particularly in four boys (two of whom had prior neuroleptic treatment for tic disorder) while receiving methylphenidate compared with placebo. Because the Tic Count scores are based on 8 minutes of observation of each child across the four treatment conditions, we question their reliability. For example, our direct observation data from the public schools, which are based on more than 20 hours of observation of each child, indicate that the frequency of motor tics actually decreased when the child was receiving medication compared with placebo. Further, in one boy whose Tic Count score was three times higher on the 0.5 mg/kg dose (compared with placebo), tics were less frequently observed on this dose during school observations compared with the placebo condition. This observation suggests that a natural fluctuation in the tic disorder might account for the increased number of tics observed during the tic count period. Another possible explanation is that some patients receiving higher doses of methylphenidate may be vulnerable to transient tic exacerbation during periods of stress. Nevertheless, scores on the LeWitt Disability scale and on the YGTSS Overall Impairment Rating indicate that transient tic exacerbations are relatively nonsignificant clinically.

With the exception of one child who exhibited extreme oppositional/defiant behavior, we were able to identify a dose of medication that produced clinically significant behavioral improvement without causing worsening in motor or vocal tics (29). In fact, the majority of our sample experienced somewhat lower rates of tic occurrence on methylphenidate compared with placebo. Why this should be is not clear at the present time. It is important to emphasize that most of our subjects met the diagnostic criteria for Tourette syndrome, the expression of tics was substantiated by multiple observers and under controlled conditions, and in 80% of the cases, at least one first-degree relative also had a tic disorder. Further, with the exception of only one family, there was evidence of psychiatric disturbance. Indeed, the spectrum of psychiatric disorders and tics on both sides of the patients' families was remarkably similar to those reported for other samples of TS patients (1,16). Based upon these findings, we do not believe that our sample of ADHD-tic disorder children was atypical with regard to familial risk factors.

REFERENCES

1. Comings DE. *Tourette syndrome and human behavior.* Duarte, CA: Hope Press, 1990.

2. Shapiro AK, Shapiro ES, Young JG, Feinberg TE. *Gilles de la Tourette syndrome.* New York: Raven Press, 1988.

3. Comings DE, Comings BG. Tourette's syndrome and attention deficit disorder with hyperactivity: are they genetically related? *J Am Acad Child Psychiatry* 1984;23:138–46.

4. Comings DE, Comings BG. A controlled study of Tourette syndrome. I. Attention deficit disorder, learning disorders, and school problems. *Am J Hum Genet* 1987;41:701–41.

5. Cohen DJ, Detlor J, Young JG, Shaywitz BA. Clonidine ameliorates Gilles de la Tourette syndrome. *Arch Gen Psychiatry* 1980;37:1350–7.

6. Erenberg G, Cruse RP, Rothner AD. Gilles de la Tourette's syndrome: effects of stimulant drugs. *Neurology* 1985;35:1346–8.

7. Erenberg G, Cruse RP, Rothner AD. Tourette syndrome: analysis of 200 pediatric and adolescent cases. *Cleve Clin Q* 1986;53:127–31.

8. Sverd J, Curley AD, Jandorf L, Volkersz L. Behavior disorder and attention deficits in boys with Tourette syndrome. *J Am Acad Child Adolesc Psychiatry* 1988;27:413–7.

9. Singer HS, Wallkup JT. Tourette syndrome and other tic disorders: diagnosis, pathophysiology, and treatment. *Medicine* 1991;70:15–32.

10. Barkley RA, McMurray MB, Edelbrock CS, Robbins K. Side effects of methylphenidate in children with attention deficit hyperactivity disorder: a systematic, placebo-controlled evaluation. *Pediatrics* 1990;86:198–2.

11. Munir K, Biederman J, Knere D. Psychiatric comorbidity in patients with attention deficit disorder: a controlled study. *J Am Acad Child Adolesc Psychiatry* 1987;26:844–8.

12. Conners CK. Symptom patterns in hyperkinetic, neurotic, and normal children. *Child Dev* 1970; 41:667–82.

13. Comings DE, Hines JA, Comings BG. An epidemiologic study of Tourette's syndrome in a single school district. *J Clin Psychiatry* 1990;51:563–9.

14. Comings DE, Comings BG. A controlled family history study of Tourette's syndrome. I: Attention-deficit hyperactivity disorder and learning disorders. *J Clin Psychiatry* 1990;51:275–80.

15. Gadow KD, Sverd J. Stimulants for ADHD in child patients with Tourette's syndrome: the issue of relative risk. *J Dev Behav Pediatr* 1990;11:269–71.

16. Sverd J. Clinical presentations of the Tourette syndrome diathesis. *J Multihandicapped Person* 1989; 2:311–26.

17. Gadow KD. *Children on medication*, vol. 1: *Hyperactivity, learning disabilities, and mental retardation.* Austin, TX: PRO-ED, 1986.

18. Rapoport JL, Nee L, Mitchell S, Polinsky MR, Ebert M. Hyperkinetic syndrome and Tourette syndrome. In: Friedhoff AJ, Chase TN, eds. *Gilles de la Tourette syndrome.* New York: Raven Press, 1982;423–6.

19. Sverd J, Gadow KD, Paolicelli LM. Methylphenidate treatment of attention-deficit hyperactivity disorder in boys with Tourette syndrome. *J Am Acad Child Adolesc Psychiatry* 1989;28:574–9.

20. Golden GS. Letter to the editor. *JAMA* 1982; 248:1063.
21. Lowe TL, Cohen DJ, Detlor J, Kremenitzer MW, Shaywitz BA. Stimulant medications precipitate Tourette's syndrome. *JAMA* 1982;247:1729–31.
22. Price RA, Leckman JF, Pauls DL, Cohen DJ, Kidd KK. Gilles de la Tourette's syndrome: tics and central nervous system stimulants in twins and nontwins. *Neurology* 1986;36:232–7.
23. Waserman J, Lal S, Gauthier S. Gilles de la Tourette's syndrome in monozygotic twins. *J Neurol Neurosurg Psychiatry* 1983;46:75–7.
24. Friedhoff AJ. Receptor maturation in pathogenesis and treatment of Tourette syndrome. In: Friedhoff JA, Chase TN, eds. *Gilles de la Tourette syndrome.* New York: Raven Press, 1982;133–40.
25. Singer HS, Rosenberg LA. Development of behavioral and emotional problems in Tourette syndrome. *Pediatr Neurol* 1989;5:41–4.
26. Sverd J, Gadow KD, Nolan E. Psychiatric symptoms and Tourette syndrome: a study of their relationship. Presented at the annual meeting of the American Academy of Child and Adolescent Psychiatry, San Francisco, 1991.
27. Borcherding BG, Keysor CS, Rapoport JL, Elia J, Amass J. Motor/vocal tics and compulsive behaviors on stimulant drugs: is there a common vulnerability? *Psychiatry Res* 1990;33:83–94.
28. Konkol RJ, Fischer M, Newby RF. Double-blind placebo-controlled stimulant trial in children with Tourette's syndrome and attention-deficit hyperactivity disorder. *Ann Neurol* 1990;28:424(abst).
29. Gadow KD, Nolan EE, Sverd J. Methylphenidate in hyperactive boys with comorbid tic disorder: II. Short-term behavioral effects in school settings. J Am Acad Child Adolesc Psychiatry 1992; 31:462–71.
30. Conners CK. Rating scales for use in drug studies with children. *Psychopharmacol Bull* 1973;24–84.
31. Loney J, Milich R. Hyperactivity, inattention, and aggression in clinical practice. In: Wolraich M, Routh DK, eds. *Advances in developmental and behavioral pediatrics*, vol. 3. Greenwich, CT: JAI Press, 1982;113–47.
32. Conners CK. The Conners Rating Scales: instruments for the assessment of childhood psychotherapy. Unpublished manuscript, Children's Hospital National Medical Center, Washington, DC, 1985.
33. Loney J. A short parent scale for subgrouping childhood hyperactivity and aggression. Presented at the annual meeting of the American Psychological Association, Toronto, 1984.
34. Gadow KD, Sprafkin J. *Stony Brook Child Psychiatric Checklist-3R.* Department of Psychiatry, State University of New York, Stony Brook, 1987.
35. Leckman JF, Riddle MA, Hardin MT, et al. The Yale Global Tic Severity Scale: initial testing of a clinic-rated scale of tic severity. *J Am Acad Child Adolesc Psychiatry* 1989;28:566–73.
36. Kurlan R, Riddle M, Como P. Tourette Syndrome Unified Rating Scale. Bayside, NY: Tourette Syndrome Association, Inc, 1988.
37. Routh DK, Schroeder CS. Standardized playroom measures as indices of hyperactivity. *J Abnorm Child Psychol* 1976;4:199–207.
38. Roberts MA, Ray RS, Roberts RJ. A playroom observational procedure for assessing hyperactive boys. *J Pediatr Psychol* 1984;9:177–91.
39. Milich R, Loney J, Landau S. Independent dimensions of hyperactivity and aggression: a validation with playroom observational data. *J Abnorm Psychol* 1982;91:183–98.
40. Roberts MA. A behavioral observation method for differentiating hyperactive and aggressive boys. *J Abnorm Child Psychol* 1990;18:131–42.
41. Gadow KD, Paolicelli L. *Global Tic Rating Scale.* Department of Psychiatry, State University of New York, Stony Brook, 1986.
42. Gadow KD. *Stimulant Side Effects Checklist.* Department of Psychiatry, State University of New York, Stony Brook, 1986.
43. Gadow KD, Nolan EE, Sverd J, Sprafkin J, Paolicelli L. Methylphenidate in aggressive-hyperactive boys: I. Effects on peer aggression in public school settings. *J Am Acad Child Adolesc Psychiatry* 1990;29:710–8.
44. Klorman R, Brumaghim JT, Fitzpatrick PA, Borgstedt AD. Clinical effects of a controlled trial of methylphenidate on adolescents with attention deficit disorder. *J Am Acad Child Adolesc Psychiatry* 1990;29:702–9.
45. Nolan EE. The effects of methylphenidate on aggression in ADD boys. Unpublished doctoral dissertation, Department of Psychology, State University of New York, Stony Brook, 1988.
46. Walker MK, Sprague RL, Sleator EK, Ullmann RK. Effects of methylphenidate hydrochloride on the subjective reporting of mood in children with attention deficit disorder. *Issues Mental Health Nursing* 1988;9:373–85.

Advances in Neurology, Vol. 58, edited by T. N. Chase, A. J. Friedhoff, and D. J. Cohen. Raven Press, Ltd., New York © 1992.

34

Psychopharmacology of Obsessive–Compulsive Disorder in Tourette Syndrome

*Robert A. King, *Mark A. Riddle, and †Wayne K. Goodman

*Yale Child Study Center, Yale University School of Medicine, New Haven, Connecticut 06510 and †Department of Psychiatry, Yale University School of Medicine, New Haven, Connecticut 06510

In the decade since the first International Tourette Syndrome Scientific Symposium, the pharmacotherapy of obsessive–compulsive disorder (OCD) has been revolutionized by the development and clinical availability of potent serotonin reuptake inhibitors, which, alone or in combination with other drugs, have provided dramatic relief for a large proportion of children and adults with OCD. These practical advances reflect equally dramatic advances in the neurobiology of OCD. Despite these impressive developments, however, many practical and theoretical questions remain unanswered about the treatment of the obsessive–compulsive features of Tourette syndrome (TS).

Very little of the burgeoning OCD literature specifically addresses patients with TS; indeed, the presence of TS is an exclusion criterion for many studies. Although evidence suggests that OCD may be a heterogeneous disorder, much work is needed to define: (a) to what extent TS-related OCD has distinctive clinical and neurobiological features, and (b) whether it differs from other forms of OCD in its pattern of response to various psychopharmacologic agents. In addition, there is a relative pau-city of studies of antiobsessional drugs in childhood and adolescence, the age groups that comprise the bulk of TS patients seeking clinical attention. This lack is especially serious, as developmental factors may affect both the therapeutic efficacy and toxicity of these agents (1).

SEROTONIN REUPTAKE INHIBITORS

On the basis of open and double-blind studies, several serotonin reuptake inhibitors appear effective in relieving the symptoms of a substantial proportion of patients with OCD and have proved superior to placebo and/or other tricyclic antidepressants that lack these agents' specific serotonergic effects. Currently, only clomipramine (Anafranil) and fluoxetine (Prozac) are available for general clinical use in the United States; however, clinical trials of fluvoxamine, paroxetine, and sertraline (Zoloft) are now planned or under way.

Clomipramine

Clomipramine, the most extensively studied antiobsessional drug, is a tricyclic antidepressant (TCA) structurally similar to imipramine. While sharing properties of the other TCAs, clomipramine and its principal active metabolite, desmethylclomipramine (DMCMI), differ from other tricyclics in potently inhibiting serotonin reuptake. In double-blind, controlled studies in both children and adults, clomipramine has been shown to produce marked improvement or even complete suppression of OCD symptoms in as many as 50% of subjects (3). The role serotonin plays in clomipramine's antiobsessional efficacy is underlined by crossover studies demonstrating that clomipramine is superior in its antiobsessional effects to other tricyclics such as desipramine, which are not potent inhibitors of serotonin reuptake (3,4). Indeed, when crossed over to desipramine, most clomipramine responders relapse within a few weeks (3).

The clinical and biological predictors of clomipramine response have not been well defined. A positive antiobsessional response to clomipramine appears to be correlated with higher baseline cerebrospinal fluid (CSF) levels of 5-hydroxyindoleacetic acid (5-HIAA) (5), higher baseline platelet serotonin (5-HT) (6), and greater clomipramine-induced decrements in these measures. The significance of blood levels of clomipramine and its principal metabolites (such as desmethylclomipramine) in different age groups is unclear. Mavissakalian et al. (2,7) found that adult responders had significantly higher plasma clomipramine levels and a trend toward lower desmethylclomipramine/clomipramine ratios. In children and adolescents with primary OCD, however, Leonard et al. (3) found plasma clomipramine levels did not predict clinical response. Attempts to find other predictors of response have also produced conflicting findings. Thus, Hollander et al. (8) found that old age, male sex, severity of depression or obsessions, high number of neurological soft signs, and a distinctive pattern of response to various neurobiologic probes predicted a poor antiobsessional response to clomipramine or fluoxetine. In a

small double-blind study of adolescents with OCD, clomipramine was ineffective in two patients with learning disability, low-normal IQ, and (in one case) chronic tics (9). In other studies, however, neither gender, age of onset, duration or severity of illness, symptom type, or presence or absence of depression appeared to be reliable predictors of response to clomipramine (3,10). Although, as with the other serotonin reuptake inhibitors, a significant therapeutic response may be seen within 2 weeks of beginning clomipramine, antiobsessional effects may take as long as 10 weeks to develop fully (11).

Many of the side effects of clomipramine resemble the predominantly anticholinergic side effects of other tricyclics—dry mouth, constipation, sweating, somnolence, electrocardiographic (EKG) changes, and orthostatic hypotension; other frequent common side effects of clomipramine—nausea, tremor, and anorgasmia—are shared in common with the other serotonin reuptake inhibitors. These difficulties lead to discontinuation of treatment in up to 20% of adult patients, and perhaps a larger proportion of children. Seizures appear to be dose- and duration related, with a cumulative incidence at 1 year of 1.45% in patients exposed to doses of up to 300 mg/day (12).

The tricyclic antidepressants have a range of cardiovascular effects, including prolongation of PR and QT interval (13). Furthermore, children may be at greater risk for these cardiotoxic effects than adults (14). These potentially cardiotoxic effects of the tricyclic antidepressants are particularly worrisome in light of the recent report of three cases of sudden death in children receiving desipramine (1,13,15–17). Baseline and periodic EKGs are necessary especially during the initial titration of clomipramine dosage.

Because of concerns over cardiotoxicity and seizures, the usual current limit for clomipramine is usually 250 mg/day for adults or 3 mg/kg/day for children (18). Once an optimal therapeutic response has been obtained, however, it is often possible to reduce the dose substantially without increasing symptoms (19).

Clomipramine has not been studied systematically in patients with TS-related OCD. Clinical experience and scattered case reports suggest that clomipramine may be useful for the OCD symptoms of TS patients. For example, Ratzoni et al. (20) described a 16-year-old boy with late-onset TS and OCD whose dramatic response to clomipramine included remission of both his tic and OCD symptoms. Although the TCA's initial propensity to increase noradrenergic activity might be theoretically expected to increase tic activity in TS patients early in the course of treatment, the actual effects of clomipramine (and other TCAs) on tics have not been well studied. A few patients have been reported to experience exacerbation of tics on clomipramine, imipramine, or desipramine (21,22). The majority of patients with TS, however, appear to tolerate the tricyclic antidepressants well without increased tics (21,23), and a few subjects even respond with an improvement in their tic symptoms (20,24,25).

Fluoxetine, fluvoxamine, paroxetine, and sertraline are among the newer generation of serotonin reuptake blockers with more selective effects on serotonin than CMI.

Fluoxetine

Fluoxetine (Prozac) is a highly selective blocker of serotonin reuptake, with little affinity for dopaminergic, noradrenergic, histaminergic, muscarinic cholinergic, or other receptor sites (26). Several, but not all, open trials have found fluoxetine effective and relatively well tolerated in adults, adolescents, and children with OCD (27–31). The manufacturer's large double-blind, placebo-controlled study in adults is still unpublished but reportedly confirms fluoxetine's antiobsessional efficacy.

Ongoing studies at the Yale Child Study Center are examining the use of fluoxetine in children, adolescents, and adults with OCD, both in the presence and absence of TS (27,31,32). In an open trial of fluoxetine, 10–40 mg/day, in ten children and adolescents, half of the subjects showed substantial improvement in OCD symptoms, with comparable response rates among subjects who had primary OCD and those who had both OCD and TS (27). Subsequent clinical experience and data from a double-blind, placebo-controlled study now being analyzed confirm the usefulness of fluoxetine for the OCD features of TS, but suggest that fluoxetine has little effect, positive or negative, on the tic symptoms per se (Riddle et al., unpublished data, 1991). Even in the absence of any objective change in tic severity, however, several patients felt better because of improvement in these comorbid depressive and OCD features.

The commonest behavioral side effects of fluoxetine—nervousness, anxiety, insomnia, or restlessness—are estimated to occur in 10–25% of adults (33). Among 24 children aged 8 to 16 years who received fluoxetine 20–40 mg/day, half of the subjects showed motor restlessness, sleep disturbance, social disinhibition, or subjective sensations of excitation; such activation symptoms occurred in three of the nine children with TS in the sample (31). Reduction or discontinuation of fluoxetine led to the disappearance of these symptoms. In order to avoid or minimize these side effects, many clinicians now begin children on much smaller initial doses of fluoxetine, perhaps as little as 2.5 mg/day, a procedure facilitated by the recent introduction of a liquid formulation of Prozac. The activating effects of fluoxetine may be disorganizing for some vulnerable individuals. Although sporadic accounts of suicidality occurring in conjunction with fluoxetine continue to appear, the causal role of fluoxetine remains unclear (32). In a series of six such cases among children and adolescents receiving fluoxetine for OCD, we described one 17-year-old nondepressed boy with TS and OCD who acutely developed intense, de novo, ego-dystonic suicidal ideation after his fluoxetine was briefly increased to 60 mg/day; these symptoms remitted following discontinuation of the medication (32).

Fluvoxamine

Fluvoxamine (marketed in Canada under the name of Luvox) is currently available in the United States only on an investigational basis. Multicenter, double-blind, placebo-controlled clinical trials in support of the manufacturer's New Drug Application to the Food and Drug Administration (FDA) have been completed in adults with reportedly promising results, and studies in children are now beginning. Unfortunately, TS will be one of the exclusion criteria for children eligible to receive fluvoxamine in this multisite study. In double-blind studies in adult OCD patients, fluvoxamine has proved effective in reducing OCD symptoms in as many as half of subjects and is superior to placebo (34,35) and desipramine (36).

Fluvoxamine is generally very well tolerated and lacks the anticholinergic-like side effects of clomipramine; the commonest reported side effects of fluvoxamine—sedation, nausea, anorexia, tremulousness, and sexual dysfunction—resemble those of fluoxetine with the exception that sedation appears more common than insomnia (34,37).

The antiobsessional effects of other serotonin reuptake inhibitors have been less extensively studied than those of clomipramine, fluoxetine, and fluvoxamine, but show some evidence of promise. In double-blind, placebo-controlled studies, sertraline has proved to be more effective than placebo; in a multisite, parallel study, sertraline produced "much" or "very much" improvement in 25% of 43 adult OCD patients receiving up to 200 mg/day (38). Another smaller double-blind study, however, failed to find sertraline effective (39). If sertraline, a more specific inhibitor of serotonin reuptake than clomipramine, fluoxetine, and flu-

voxamine, is indeed a less effective antiobsessional agent than these drugs, the observation raises important questions about whether it is serotonergic activity alone that is required to relieve OCD symptoms (39). Sertraline's most frequent side effects were nausea, dyspepsia, and ejaculatory failure; stimulant-like adverse effects such as nervousness, agitation, or anxiety were reportedly rare. Application to market sertraline for depression is pending, and controlled studies of the use of the drug in children and adolescence for OCD are about to start.

OTHER ANTIOBSESSIONAL AGENTS

In addition to the specific serotonin reuptake inhibitors, several other agents that influence serotonin transmission have been tried in the treatment of OCD.

Buspirone

Buspirone (Buspar) is a relatively short-acting partial agonist at the 5-HT la receptor site. Used extensively for the treatment of generalized anxiety disorder, buspirone enhances serotonin transmission (39) while blocking dopaminergic transmission. Used alone as a treatment for OCD, buspirone has produced conflicting results, with Pato et al. (40) finding it as effective as clomipramine, while Jenike and Baer (41) judged it ineffective.

Clonazepam

Clonazepam (Klonopin) is a novel high-potency benzodiazepine, which, in addition to its affinity for the γ-aminobutyric acid (GABA) receptor, appears to increase synaptic serotonin (42). In the small number of cases of OCD in which it has been used in open trials, clonazepam appears to be effective in reducing OCD symptoms (43,44). The drug's principal side effects are sedation, ataxia, appetite changes, slurred speech, diarrhea, habituation, and dependence. Clonazepam is of particular interest for patients with TS-related OCD because a small number of open trials suggest that, in addition to its anticonvulsant, anxiolytic, and apparent antiobsessional effects, clonazepam has potentially beneficial effects on tic symptoms per se (45–48).

AUGMENTATION TECHNIQUES

As many as half of OCD patients do not respond adequately to trials of individual serotonin reuptake inhibitors. One approach to such nonresponders has been to try to enhance these patients' response to serotonergic agents by means of adding adjunctive agents such as buspirone (49,50), lithium (51), tryptophan, or fenfluramine.

Although, when used alone, buspirone's antiobsessional effects are equivocal, buspirone has proved useful in augmenting the antiobsessional effects of fluoxetine. In 50–81% of adult OCD patients initially treated with fluoxetine alone, addition of buspirone 10 mg tid produced a better therapeutic response than had been achieved on fluoxetine alone (49,50). In addition, in open trials with patients with fluoxetine-resistant OCD, addition of buspirone appears to be effective and well tolerated (McDougle et al., unpublished data). In contrast, however, a small uncontrolled study found buspirone augmentation of fluoxetine or clomipramine ineffective (52).

Despite a plausible theoretical rationale, promising anecdotal accounts, and lithium's proven effectiveness in augmenting antidepressant effects in otherwise treatment refractory patients, recent double-blind, placebo-controlled studies of lithium augmentation of fluvoxamine show no clinically significant improvement in the OCD symptoms of patients unresponsive to fluvoxamine or clomipramine alone (51,53).

When used alone, neuroleptics have generally not proved particularly useful in unse-lected groups of OCD patients (54). However, a small number of studies suggest that these agents may have a useful adjunctive role in TS-related OCD. In a single-case, double-blind, sequential discontinuation study, Delgado and colleagues (55) described a 25-year-old man with both TS and OCD, whose OCD responded to the combined use of pimozide and fluvoxamine. Neither drug alone was satisfactory; pimozide alone decreased the subject's tics but did not affect his OCD, while fluvoxamine alone had no effect on his OCD and exacerbated his tics. McDougle and colleagues (56) recently reported that in 55% of OCD patients, addition of a neuroleptic (i.e., pimozide, thioridazine, or thiothixene) enhanced their antiobsessional response to fluvoxamine (with or without lithium). The presence of a tic disorder or schizotypal personality was associated with a positive response to neuroleptic augmentation.

The underlying mechanism of neuroleptic augmentation remains unclear. Although serotonergic activity appears to be essential for antiobsessional efficacy, it is plausible that both the pathophysiology of OCD and the action of antiobsessional agents may involve an interaction between the serotonergic and dopaminergic systems (51).

IMPLICATIONS FOR THE TREATMENT OF TS-RELATED OCD

Marked interindividual differences in OCD patients are apparent in the failure of half of OCD patients to respond favorably to any given antiobsessional agent and the diversity of individuals' patterns of preferential response to different agents. It is unclear to what extent these divergent treatment responses reflect a deeper underlying biological diversity to OCD based on heterogeneous forms of dysregulation of serotonin and other neurotransmitter systems.

TS-related OCD provides a model of an identifiable OCD subtype that might serve as a natural starting point for assessing the possible biological diversity of OCD (and its relationship to treatment response). For example, one strategy might be to dichotomize OCD patients into two groups: OCD patients with chronic tics (or a family history of chronic tics) (OCD/T) and those without tics or family history of tics (OCD/NT). The two groups might then be studied with respect to distinctive phenomenology, imaging findings, and neurobiological factors, including the response to antiobsessional agents and pharmacologic probes.

Surprisingly few such comparative data are available. Indeed, there are not even reliable estimates of what proportion of OCD cases appear to be genetically related to TS. In terms of clinical phenomenology, several studies suggest that, compared with age- and gender-matched OCD patients without tics, OCD patients with a lifetime history of chronic tic disorder have more touching, repeating, tapping, staring, blinking, and rubbing compulsions, as well as more obsessions with symmetry and fewer obsessions with contamination (57,58). Leonard (59) found that on follow-up, a large proportion of patients with childhood-onset OCD subsequently met the criteria for a chronic tic disorder; however, the pattern of initial OCD symptomatology (including type of obsession or compulsion) did not differentiate those who subsequently developed a tic disorder (59).

Whether TS-related OCD is associated with a distinctive profile of response to various antiobsessional agents is an unanswered question with important theoretical and practical implications and deserves systematic study. For example, it remains to be determined whether TS-related OCD shows the same pattern and degree of response to the various serotonin reuptake inhibitors. McDougle and colleagues (56) found that the presence of a tic disorder in OCD patients was associated with a positive antiobsessional response to neuroleptic augmentation of fluvoxamine. This same research group at Yale is now embarked on a systematic double-blind randomized study to determine whether TS-spectrum and non-TS-spectrum OCD patients who are refractory to fluvoxamine alone differ in their response to buspirone or neuroleptic augmentation (McDougle, personal communication).

A PRACTICAL APPROACH TO CHOICE OF MEDICATION FOR TS-SPECTRUM OCD

Pending rigorous comparative studies, how can the clinician best approach the choice of antiobsessional medication for TS-related OCD? The physician must balance several considerations, including (a) comparative efficacy studies, (b) profile of side effects (including age-specific properties), and (c) impact on tics and comorbid conditions (such as attention deficit disorder).

Although there are few systematic studies of response selectivity, clinicians often observe that individuals refractory to one antiobsessional medication may respond well to a trial of a different antiobsessional agent. In a randomized crossover comparison of clomipramine (up to 250 mg/day) versus fluoxetine (up to 80 mg/day) in 11 adult OCD patients, 5 patients responded preferentially to clomipramine, 2 responded preferentially to fluoxetine, and 4 responded similarly to both drugs (60). Predictors of preferential response have not yet been identified.

Direct studies of the comparative efficacy of the various antiobsessional agents are difficult. Because of power considerations, unattainably large sample sizes are needed to demonstrate significant differences between active agents (61). Meta-analyses by Jenike et al. (35,62) compared the effect size of clomipramine, fluoxetine, fluvoxamine, and sertraline and concluded that clomipramine seemed to produce a greater therapeutic effect. The implications of these studies, however, are not clear in light of the relatively small magnitude of differences and the numerous methodological difficulties with which such meta-analytic studies are fraught (37).

Distinctive patterns of side effects provide another basis for choice of agent. Compared to clomipramine, with its mixture of anticholinergic and serotonergic effects, fluvoxamine and fluoxetine appear to have fewer troublesome side effects and appear to be less dangerous in case of overdose (60,62,63).

Compared with adults, children may have distinctive vulnerabilities and patterns of side effects that influence drug choice. For example, the tricyclic antidepressants' idiosyncratic pharmacokinetics and potential cardiotoxicity in children make divided doses and careful monitoring of EKG and blood levels advisable, at least during the initial titration of the drug (1,16). In the course of clinical trials of new drugs for approval by the FDA, more systematic studies in children are necessary. Unfortunately, once a drug has been approved by the FDA as safe and effective in adults, it often becomes widely used in children without any mandatory or systematic study of its therapeutic or adverse effects.

The pharmacological treatment of children and adults with TS-related OCD often poses an especially difficult clinical challenge. In addition to treating these patients' obsessive–compulsive symptoms, the clinician must be concerned with ameliorating (or at least not exacerbating) comorbid tics, attentional difficulties, depression, emotional lability, or developmental immaturities (such as enuresis). These considerations may strongly influence the choice of antiobsessional medication. For example, the presence of a comorbid attention deficit hyperactivity disorder (ADHD) may suggest the use of clomipramine which, like the other tricyclics (23), appears to be useful for ADHD (64) and lacks the activating effects of fluoxetine. Whether clomipramine is more likely than other serotonin reuptake inhibitors to exacerbate tics in some TS patients remains to be clarified. Given their apparent usefulness in suppressing tics, clo-

nazepam (65) or neuroleptic augmentation (55,56) may be useful in TS patients with both OCD and poorly controlled tics.

IMPLICATIONS FOR THE FUTURE

The increasing availability of receptor subtype-specific serotonergic agents promises to increase our understanding of the pathophysiology of OCD while broadening our therapeutic armamentarium. At the same time, our growing insight into the complex interaction between the serotonin system and other neurotransmitter systems may provide a more refined approach to the development of various augmentation techniques.

Finally, future antiobsessional drug studies need to examine the therapeutic response of patient with TS-related OCD. Subtyping of OCD patients by tic history is important in order to improve the treatment of patients with TS and to explicate the biological diversity of OCD. In this way, rather than remaining the neglected stepchild of antiobsessional pharmacotherapy research, the study of TS-related OCD can play an important role in advancing our understanding and clinical mastery of two puzzling and disabling disorders.

REFERENCES

1. Riddle MA, Nelson JC, Kleinman CS, et al. Sudden death in children receiving Norpramin: a review of three reported cases and commentary. *J Am Acad Child Adolesc Psychiatry* 1991;30:104–8.
2. Mavissakalian MR, Jones B, Olson S, Perel JM. Clomipramine in obsessive–compulsive disorder: clinical response and plasma levels. *J Clin Psychopharmacol* 1990;10:261–8.
3. Leonard HL, Swedo SE, Rapoport JL, et al. Treatment of obsessive–compulsive disorder with clomipramine and desipramine in children and adolescents: a double-blind crossover comparison. *Arch Gen Psychiatry* 1989;46:1088–92.
4. Zohar J, Insel TR. Obsessive–compulsive disorder: psychobiological approaches to diagnosis, treatment, and pathophysiology. *Biol Psychiatry* 1987;22:667–87.
5. Thoren P, Asberg M, Cronholm B, Jorenstedt L, Traskman L. Clomipramine treatment of obses-

sive–compulsive disorder: I. A controlled clinical trial. *Arch Gen Psychiatry* 1980;37:1281–5.

6. Flament M, Rapoport J, Murphy D, Berg CJ, Lake R. Biochemical changes during clomipramine treatment of childhood obsessive–compulsive disorder. *Arch Gen Psychiatry* 1987;44:219–5.

7. Mavissakalian M, Jones B, Olson S, Perel JM. The relationship of plasma clomipramine and N-desmethylclomipramine response in obsessive–compulsive disorder. *Psychopharmacol Bull* 1990; 26:119–22.

8. Hollander E, DeCaria CM, Saoud JB, Liebowitz MR. Predictors of treatment outcome in OCD. *Poster Presented at American College of Neuropsychopharmacology, Annual Meeting*, 1990;194 of Abstracts.

9. March JS, Johnston H, Jefferson JW, Kobak KA, Greist JH. Do subtle neurological impairments predict treatment resistance to clomipramine in children and adolescents with obsessive–compulsive disorder? *J Child Adolesc Psychopharmacol* 1990;1:133–40.

10. DeVeaugh-Geiss J, Katz R, Landau P, Goodman W, Rasmussen S. Clinical predictors of treatment response in obsessive–compulsive disorder: exploratory analyses from multicenter trials of clomipramine. *Psychopharmacol Bull* 1990;26:45–9.

11. DeVeaugh-Geiss J. Pharmacologic treatment of obsessive–compulsive disorder. In: J Zohar, T Insel, S Rasmussen, eds. *The psychobiology of obsessive compulsive disorder*. New York: Springer, 1991;187–207.

12. Anafranil (clomipramine HCR) package insert.

13. Elliott GR, Popper CW. Editorial: tricyclic antidepressants: the QT interval and other cardiovascular parameters. *J Child Adolesc Psychopharmacol* 1991;1:187–91.

14. Ryan ND. Heterocyclic antidepressants in children and adolescents. *J Child Adolesc Psychopharmacol* 1990;1:21–31.

15. The Medical Letter: sudden death in children treated with a tricyclic antidepressant. *Med Lett Drug Ther* 1990;32:53.

16. Popper CW, Elliott GR. Sudden death and tricyclic antidepressants: clinical considerations for children. *J Child Adolesc Psychopharmacol* 1990; 1:125–32.

17. Biederman J. Sudden death in children treated with a tricyclic antidepressant: a commentary. *Biol Ther Psychiatry Newslett* 1991;14:1–4.

18. Leonard HL, Rapoport JL. Pharmacotherapy of childhood obsessive–compulsive disorder. *Psychiatr Clin North Am* 1989;12:963–70.

19. Pato MT, Hill JL, Murphy DL. A clomipramine dosage reduction study in the course of long-term treatment of obsessive–compulsive disorder patients. *Psychopharmacol Bull* 1990;26:211–4.

20. Ratzoni G, Hermesh H, Brandt N, Lauffer M, Munitz H. Clomipramine efficacy for tics, obsessions, and compulsions in Tourette's syndrome and obsessive–compulsive disorder: a case study. *Biol Psychiatry* 1990;27:95–8.

21. Caine ED, Polinsky RJ, Ebert MH, Rapoport HL, Mikkelsen EJ. Trial of chlorimpramine and desipramine for Gilles de la Tourette syndrome. *Ann Neurol* 1979;6:305–6.

22. Fras I, Karlavage J. The use of methylphenidate and imipramine in Gilles de la Tourette's disease in children. *Am J Psychiatry* 1977;134:195–7.

23. Riddle MA, Hardin MT, Cho SC, Woolston JL, Leckman JF. Desipramine treatment of boys with attention-deficit hyperactivity disorder and tics: preliminary clinical experience. *J Am Acad Child Adolesc Psychiatry*, 1988;27:811–4.

24. Yaryura-Tobias JA. Clomipramine in Gilles de la Tourette disease. *Am J Psychiatry* 1975;132:1221.

25. Hoge SK, Biederman J. A case of Tourette's syndrome with symptoms of attention deficit disorder treated with desipramine. *J Clin Psychiatry* 1986; 47:478–9.

26. Fuller RW, Wong DT. Serotonin reuptake blockers in vitro and in vivo. *J Clin Psychopharmacology* 1987;7:36S–43S.

27. Riddle MA, Hardin MT, King RA, Scahill L, Woolston JL. Fluoxetine treatment of children and adolescents with Tourette's and obsessive–compulsive disorders: preliminary clinical experience. *J Am Acad Child Adolesc Psychiatry*, 1990; 29:45–8.

28. Liebowitz MR, Hollander E, Schneier F, et al. Fluoxetine treatment of obsessive–compulsive disorder: an open clinical trial. *J Clin Psychopharmacol* 1989;9:423–7.

29. Jenike MA, Buttolph L, Baer L, Ricciardi J, Holland A. Open trial of fluoxetine in obsessive–compulsive disorder. *Am J Psychiatry* 1989; 146:909–11.

30. Levine R, Hoffman JS, Knepple ED, Kenin M. Long-term fluoxetine treatment of a large number of obsessive–compulsive patients. *J Clin Psychopharmacol* 1989;9:281–3.

31. Riddle MA, King RA, Hardin MT, et al. Behavioral side effects of fluoxetine in children and adolescents. *J Child Adolesc Psychopharmacol* 1991; 1:193–8.

32. King RA, Riddle MA, Chappell PB, et al. Emergence of self-destructive phenomena in children and adolescents during fluoxetine treatment. *J Am Acad Child Adolesc Psychiatry* 1991;30:179–86.

33. Lipinski JF, Mallya G, Zimmerman P, Pope HG. Fluoxetine-induced akathisia: clinical and theoretical implications. *J Clin Psychiatry* 1989; 50:339–42.

34. Goodman WK, Price LH, Rasmussen SA, Delgado PL, Heninger GR, Charney DS. Efficacy of fluvoxamine in obsessive–compulsive disorder: a double-blind comparison with placebo. *Arch Gen Psychiatry* 1989;46:36–44.

35. Jenike MA, Hyman S, Baer L, et al. A controlled trial of fluvoxamine in obsessive–compulsive disorder: implications for a serotonergic theory. *Am J Psychiatry* 1990;147:1209–15.

36. Goodman WK, Price LH, Delgado PL, et al. Specificity of serotonin reuptake inhibitors in the treatment of obsessive–compulsive disorder: comparison of fluvoxamine and desipramine. *Arch Gen Psychiatry* 1990;47:577–85.

37. Goodman WK, McDougle CJ, Price LH. Choice of serotonin reuptake inhibitors for obses-

sive–compulsive disorder: comparative efficacy and tolerability. Unpublished manuscript, 1990.

38. Chouinard G, Goodman WK, Greist J, et al. Results of a double-blind placebo controlled trial of a new serotonin uptake inhibitor, sertraline, in the treatment of obsessive–compulsive disorder. *Psychopharmacol Bull* 1990;26:279–84.

39. Jenike MA, Baer, Summergrad P, Minichiello WE, Holland A, Seymour R. Sertraline in obsessive–compulsive disorder: a double-blind comparison with placebo. *Am J Psychiatry* 1990; 147:923–8.

40. Pato MT, Pigott TA, Hill JL, Grover GN, Bernstein S, Murphy SL. Controlled comparison of buspirone and clomipramine in obsessive–compulsive disorder. *Am J Psychiatry* 1991;148:127–9.

41. Jenike MA, Baer L. An open trial of buspirone in obsessive–compulsive disorder. *Am J Psychiatry* 1988;145:1285–6.

42. Pratt J, Jenner P, Reynolds EH, Marsden CD. Clonazepam induces decreased serotoninergic activity in the mouse brain. *Neuropharmacology* 1979; 18:791–9.

43. Hewlett WA, Vinogradov S, Agras WS. Clonazepam treatment of obsessions and compulsions. *J Clin Psychiatry* 1990;51:158–61.

44. Bodkin JA, White K. Clonazepam in the treatment of obsessive–compulsive disorder associated with panic disorder in one patient. *J Clin Psychiatry* 1989;50:265–6.

45. Truong DD, Bressman S, Shale H, Fahn S. Clonazepam, haloperidol, and clonidine in tic disorders. *South Med J* 1988;81:1103–5.

46. Merikangas JR, Merikangas KR, Kopp U, Hanin I. Blood choline and response to clonazepam and haloperidol in Tourette's syndrome. *Acta Psychiatr Scand* 1985;72.395–9.

47. Gonce M, Barbeau A. Seven cases of Gilles de la Tourette syndrome: partial relief with clonazepam: a pilot study. *Can J Neurol Sci* 1977;4:279–83.

48. Kaim B. A case of Gilles de la Tourette's syndrome treated with clonazepam. *Brain Res Bull* 1983;11:213–4.

49. Jenike MA, Baer L, Buttolph L. Buspirone augmentation of fluoxetine in patients with obsessive–compulsive disorder. *J Clin Psychiatry* 1991; 52:13–4.

50. Markovitz PJ, Stagno SJ, Calabrese JR. Buspirone augmentation of fluoxetine in obsessive–compulsive disorder. *Am J Psychiatry* 1990;147:798–800.

51. McDougle CJ, Price LH, Goodman WK, Charney DS, Heninger GR. A controlled trial of lithium augmentation in fluvoxamine-refractory obsessive–compulsive disorder: lack of efficacy. *J Clin Psychopharmacol* 1991;11:175–84.

52. L'Heureux, Pigott TA, Yoney TH, et al. New Research Abstract #93, American Psychiatric Association 143rd Annual Meeting, New York, 1990; 81.

53. Pigott TA, Pato MT, Grover GN, et al. New Research Abstract #94. American Psychiatric Association Annual Meeting, New York, May, 1990.

54. Towbin et al., 1987.

55. Delgado PL, Goodman WK, Price LH, Heninger GR, Charney DS. Fluvoxamine/pimozide treatment of concurrent Tourette's and obsessive–compulsive disorder. *Br J Psychiatry* 1990; 157:762–5.

56. McDougle CJ, Goodman WK, Price LH, et al. Neuroleptic addition in fluvoxamine-refractory obsessive–compulsive disorder. *Am J Psychiatry* 1990;147:652–4.

57. Holzer JC, Boyarsky BK, McDouble CJ, Lee N, Price LH, Goodman WK. Differential symptoms in OCD with and without a tic disorder. Poster Presented at American College of Neuropsychopharmacology, 29th Annual Meeting, Puerto Rico, 1990;195 of Abstracts.

58. Pittman RK, Green RC, Jenike MA, Mesulam MM. Clinical comparison of Tourette's disorder and obsessive–compulsive disorder. *Am J Psychiatry* 1987;144:1166–71.

59. Leonard HL. Overlap of OCD and TS: childhood primary OCD. Presented at Second International Scientific Symposium on Tourette Syndrome, Boston, June, 1991.

60. Pigott TA, Pato MT, Bernstein SE, et al. Controlled comparisons of clomipramine and fluoxetine in the treatment of obsessive–compulsive disorder: behavioral and biological results. *Arch Gen Psychiatry* 1990;47:926–32.

61. Montgomery SA, Fineberg N, Montgomery DB. The efficacy of serotonergic drugs in OCD: power calculations compared with placebo. In: MA Montgomery, WK Goodman, N Goeting, eds. *Current approaches: obsessive–compulsive disorder.* 1990;54–63.

62. Jenike MA, Baer L, Greist JH. Clomipramine versus fluoxetine in obsessive–compulsive disorder: a retrospective comparison of side effects and efficacy. *J Clin Psychopharmacol* 1990;10:122–4.

63. Riddle MA, Brown N, Dzubinski D, Jetmalani AJ, Law Y, Woolston JL. Fluoxetine overdose in an adolescent. *J Am Acad Child Adolesc Psychiatry* 1989;25:587–8.

64. Garfinkle BD, Wender PH, Sloman L, O'Neill. Tricyclic antidepressant and methylphenidate treatment of attention deficit disorder in children. *J Am Acad Child Psychiatry* 1983;22:343–8.

65. Hewlett WA, Vinogradov S, Agras S. Lack of efficacy of clonidine in the treatment of obsessive–compulsive disorder with and without vocal/motor tics. Research Poster Presented at Second International Scientific Symposium on Tourette Syndrome, Boston, June, 1991.

Advances in Neurology, Vol. 58, edited
by T. N. Chase, A. J. Friedhoff, and
D. J. Cohen. Raven Press, Ltd.,
New York © 1992.

35

Effects of Foods on the Brain

Possible Implications for Understanding and Treating Tourette Syndrome

Richard J. Wurtman

*Department of Brain and Cognitive Sciences and Clinical Research Center,
Massachusetts Institute of Technology, Cambridge, Massachusetts 02139*

Anecdotes abound concerning ways that food intake might affect or be affected by Tourette Syndrome (TS). Some caregivers and patients are certain that the neurological or behavioral abnormalities associated with the disease are exacerbated whenever particular foods are consumed; others are just as convinced that the disease causes unusual patterns of food intake, like cravings for chocolates or other sweets, or for carbohydrates in general.

Should these anecdotes be taken seriously, and if so, do they help us to understand and even treat the disease? Should certain foods be avoided, or does the tendency of the patient to choose these foods provide clues as to possible deficiencies (or excesses) in the brain neurotransmitters they affect? Unfortunately, there is at present no scientific basis for answering these questions, because there have never been adequate epidemiologic or experimental studies on TS patients to provide the necessary data base.

However both types of effects certainly

are *possible*. Certain foods very definitely *can* enhance the production of particular brain neurotransmitters (1), and thereby, at least theoretically, modify behaviors that are mediated in part by those transmitters (2). Moreover, other disease states—for example, carbohydrate-craving obesity (3), seasonal affective disorder (4), the premenstrual syndrome (5), and the nicotine-withdrawal syndrome (6)—clearly *are* associated with aberrant patterns of eating, in which the subject apparently chooses to eat certain foods, at certain times, precisely because those foods, by affecting neurotransmitter synthesis, make him feel better.

This article, modified from one published earlier in *NIPS* (7), summarizes available information on the effects of nutrients on brain neurotransmitters. It includes no data on TS because, as lamented above, such data are unavailable. It is published in the hope that it may encourage physicians who care for TS patients to conduct scientific studies on *what* the patients eat, and on *whether* eating certain foods causes characteristic neurological or behavioral responses.

That there can be wide variations in the amounts of acetylcholine, serotonin, and

---

Portions of this manuscript have been adapted from Wurtman, R.J. Presynaptic control of release of amine neurotransmitters by precursor levels. *NIPS* (Am. Physiol. Soc.) 3:158–63, 1988 (Ref. 7)

the catecholamines that neurons release, spontaneously or by firing, is now well established. One process that causes such variations involves receptors on the neurons' own presynaptic terminals. When activated by neurotransmitter molecules that the neuron has released into a synapse, by concurrently released neuromodulators (like adenosine), or by transmitters (like the enkephalins) secreted by different neurons at axoaxonal synapses, these receptors initiate intracellular events that diminish subsequent transmitter release.

An additional type of process can modulate the release of amine neurotransmitters: changes in their rates of synthesis, caused by variations in the availability of the precursor substances whose concentrations control these rates. The precursors themselves are nutrients, and their concentrations in blood and neural tissue can be raised or lowered physiologically (by eating certain "real" foods) or experimentally (by administering the pure nutrients). Such variations in precursor levels may uniformly affect the outputs of all of the neurons that release a particular aminergic transmitter (like serotonin) or, in the case of dopamine and norepinephrine, only those particular neurons that happen at the time to be undergoing prolonged periods of physiological activity.

Unlike the receptor-mediated modulations of transmitter release, this type of modulation depends primarily on metabolic events that occur *outside* the brain and that are influenced by a particular type of behavior, i.e., *eating*. Indeed, the primary physiological role of this dependency may be sensory, i.e., to provide the omnivore's brain with information about what has been eaten, so that the animal can then decide what and when to eat next. However, because precursor-dependent neurotransmitters are involved in a wide variety of normal (and pathological) brain mechanisms besides those controlling the intake and utilization of nutrients, this relationship may have broad physiological and medical implications.

FOOD CONSUMPTION, TRYPTOPHAN AVAILABILITY, AND BRAIN SEROTONIN SYNTHESIS

The initial observation that physiological changes in precursor availability (i.e., after food consumption) could affect neurotransmitter synthesis was made in studies on rats performed in 1971 (8). Animals were allowed to eat a test diet that contained carbohydrates and fat but lacked protein. Soon after the start of the meal, brain levels of the essential (and scarce) amino acid tryptophan were found to have risen, thus increasing the substrate saturation of the enzyme tryptophan hydroxylase, which controls serotonin synthesis. The resulting increase in brain serotonin levels was associated with an increase in brain levels of serotonin's metabolite 5-hydroxyindoleacetic acid (5-HIAA), suggesting that serotonin release had also been enhanced. [Direct evidence that physiological variations in brain tryptophan concentrations affect serotonin release was not obtained, however, until 1987 (9).]

The rise in brain tryptophan levels after consumption of this test diet was accompanied by a small increase (rats) or no change (humans) in plasma tryptophan levels. Both of these changes had been unanticipated, since the insulin secretion elicited by dietary carbohydrates was known to lower plasma levels of most of the other amino acids. However, the unusual response of plasma tryptophan to insulin was soon recognized as resulting from the amino acid's unusual propensity to bind loosely to circulating albumin. Insulin causes nonesterified fatty acid (NEFA) molecules to dissociate from albumin and to enter adipocytes. This dissociation increases the protein's capacity to bind circulating tryptophan; hence whatever reduction insulin causes in "free" plasma tryptophan levels is compensated for by a rise in the tryptophan bound to albumin, yielding, in humans, no net change in total plasma tryptophan levels (10). Because this binding is of low affinity, the albumin-bound tryptophan is almost as able as free tryptophan to be taken up into the brain.

Considerably more difficult to explain were the data obtained subsequently on what happened to brain tryptophan and serotonin levels after rats consumed a meal rich in protein. Although plasma tryptophan levels rose, reflecting the contribution of some of the tryptophan molecules in the protein, brain tryptophan and serotonin levels either failed to rise or, if the meal contained sufficient protein, actually fell (11). The explanation for this paradox was found to lie in the transport systems that carry tryptophan across the blood–brain barrier (12) and into neurons. The endothelial cells that line central nervous system capillaries contain various macromolecules that shuttle specific nutrients or their metabolites between the blood and the brain's extracellular space. One such macromolecule mediates the transcapillary flux (by facilitated diffusion) of tryptophan and other large neutral amino acids (LNAA); others move choline, basic or acidic amino acids, hexoses, monocarboxylic acids, adenosine, adenine, and various vitamins. The amount of any LNAA transported by the macromolecule depends on its ability to compete with the other circulating LNAA for binding sites. Thus the ability of circulating tryptophan molecules to enter the brain is increased when plasma levels of the other LNAA fall (as occurs after insulin is secreted) and is diminished when the other LNAA rise, even if plasma tryptophan levels remain unchanged. Since all dietary proteins are considerably richer in the other LNAA than in tryptophan (only 1.0–1.5% of most proteins), consumption of a protein-rich meal decreases the plasma tryptophan ratio (the ratio of the plasma tryptophan concentration to the summed concentrations of its major circulating competitors for brain uptake: tyrosine; phenylalanine; the branched-chain amino acids leucine, isoleucine, and valine; and methionine). This, in turn, decreases tryptophan's transport into

the brain and slows its conversion to serotonin. (Similar plasma ratios predict brain levels of each of the other LNAA, including drugs like L-dopa, after meals or other treatments that modify plasma amino acid patterns.)

The fact that giving pure tryptophan could increase brain serotonin synthesis and could thereby affect various serotonin-dependent brain functions (e.g., sleepiness, mood) had been known at least since 1968. What was novel and perhaps surprising about the above findings was their demonstration that brain tryptophan levels, and serotonin synthesis, normally undergo important variations in response, for example, to the decision to eat a carbohydrate-rich versus a protein-rich breakfast. It remained possible, however, that mechanisms might exist external to the serotonin-releasing neuron that kept such food-induced increases in serotonin's synthesis from causing parallel changes in the amounts released into the synapses. Indeed, it was known that if rats were given very large doses of tryptophan, sufficient to raise brain tryptophan levels well beyond their normal range, the firing frequencies of their serotonin-releasing raphe neurons decreased markedly; this was interpreted as reflecting the operation of a feedback system designed to keep serotonin release within a physiological range. [Similar decreases in raphe firing had also been observed in animals given drugs, like monoamine oxidase (MAO) inhibitors or serotonin-reuptake blockers, that cause persistent increases in intrasynaptic serotonin levels.] However, if rats were given small doses of tryptophan, sufficient to raise brain tryptophan levels but not beyond their normal peaks, or if they consumed a carbohydrate-rich meal, which raised brain tryptophan levels physiologically, no decreases in raphe firing occurred. Hence food-induced changes in serotonin synthesis *are* able to affect the amounts of serotonin released per firing without slowing the neuron's firing frequencies, and thus *are* "allowed" to modulate the net output of information from serotoninergic neurons.

BRAIN SEROTONIN, NUTRIENT CHOICE, AND CARBOHYDRATE CRAVING

If rats are allowed to pick from foods in two pans, presented concurrently, which contain differing proportions of protein and carbohydrate, they choose among the two so as to obtain fairly constant (for each animal) amounts of these macronutrients. However, if before "dinner" they receive either a carbohydrate-based snack or a drug that facilitates serotoninergic neurotransmission, they quickly modify their food choice, selectively diminishing their intake of carbohydrates. These observations support the hypothesis that the responses of serotoninergic neurons to food-induced changes in the relative concentrations of plasma amino acids allow these neurons to serve a special function as sensors in the brain's mechanisms governing nutrient choice (3). Perhaps they participate in a feedback loop through which the composition of breakfast (that is, its proportions of protein and carbohydrate) can, by increasing or decreasing brain serotonin levels, influence the choice of lunch.

A similar mechanism may operate in humans. Subjects housed in a research hospital were allowed to choose from six different isocaloric foods (containing varying proportions of protein and carbohydrate but constant amounts of fat) at each meal, taking as many small portions as they liked; they also had continuous access to a computer-driven vending machine, stocked with mixed carbohydrate-rich and protein-rich isocaloric snacks. It was observed (e.g., ref. 4) that the basic parameters of each person's food intake (total number of calories, grams of carbohydrate and protein, number and composition of snacks) tended to vary only within a narrow range, day to day, and to be unaffected by placebo administration.

To assay the involvement of brain serotonin in maintaining this constancy of nutrient intake, pharmacological studies were undertaken in individuals in whom the feed-

back mechanism might be impaired. These were obese people who claimed to suffer from carbohydrate craving, manifested as their tendency to consume large quantities of carbohydrate-rich snacks, usually at a characteristic time of day or evening (4). (Too few protein-rich snacks were consumed by the subjects to allow assessment of drug effects on this source of calories.) Other drugs also thought to enhance serotonin-mediated neurotransmission selectively (for example, the antidepressants zymelidine, fluvoxamine, and fluoxetine) also have been found to cause weight loss; this contrasts with the weight gain (and carbohydrate craving) often associated with less chemically specific antidepressants, such as amitriptyline. It has not yet been determined whether these drugs also selectively suppress carbohydrate intake in humans.

Severe carbohydrate craving is also characteristic of patients suffering from seasonal affective disorder syndrome (SADS), a variant of bipolar clinical depression associated with a fall onset, a higher frequency in populations living far from the equator, and concurrent hypersomnia and weight gain. A reciprocal tendency of many obese people to suffer from affective disorders (usually depression) has also been noted. Since serotoninergic neurons apparently are involved in the actions of both appetite-reducing and antidepressant drugs, they might constitute the link between a patient's appetitive and affective symptoms. Some patients with disturbed serotoninergic neurotransmission might present to their physicians because of a problem with obesity, reflecting their overuse of dietary carbohydrates to treat their dysphoria. (The carbohydrates, by increasing intrasynaptic serotonin, would mimic the neurochemical actions of bona fide antidepressant drugs, like the MAO inhibitors and tricyclic compounds.) Other patients might complain of depression, and their carbohydrate craving and weight gain would be perceived as secondary problems. Another group might include women with the premenstrual syndrome, who have late luteal phase mood disturbances, weight gain, carbohydrate craving (6), and sometimes fluid retention. Yet another includes people attempting to withdraw from nicotine—a "drug" that releases nicotine. The participation of serotoninergic neurons in a large number of brain functions besides nutrient choice regulation might have the effect of making such functions hostages to eating (seen in the sleepiness that can, for example, follow carbohydrate intake) just as it could cause mood-disturbed individuals to consume large amounts of carbohydrates for reasons related neither to the nutritional value nor taste of these foods. In support of this view, we have recently found that the serotoninergic drug d-fenfluramine can be an effective treatment for both the affective and the appetitive symptoms of SADS (5), PMS (6), and smoking withdrawal (7).

UNDER WHAT CIRCUMSTANCES WILL NUTRIENT INTAKE AFFECT NEUROTRANSMISSION?

On the basis of the tryptophan–serotonin relationship, one can formulate a sequence of biochemical processes that would have to occur in order for any nutrient precursor to affect the synthesis and release of its neurotransmitter product.

1. Plasma levels of the precursor (and of other circulating compounds, such as the LNAA that affect tryptophan's availability to the brain) must be allowed to increase after its administration (or after its consumption as a constituent of foods), that is, plasma levels of tryptophan or the other LNAA or of choline cannot be under tight homeostatic control comparable to, for example, plasma calcium or osmolarity. In actuality, plasma levels of tryptophan, tyrosine, and choline do vary several fold after the consumption of normal foods, and those of the branched-chain

amino acids may vary by as much as five- or sixfold.

2. The brain level of the precursor must be dependent on its plasma level, i.e., there must not be an absolute blood–brain barrier for circulating tryptophan, tyrosine, or choline. In fact, such absolute barriers do not exist; rather, facilitated diffusion mechanisms operate that allow these compounds to enter the brain at rates that depend on the plasma levels of these ligands.

3. The rate-limiting enzyme within presynaptic nerve terminals that initiates the conversion of the precursor to its neurotransmitter product must, similarly, be unsaturated with this substrate so that when presented with more tryptophan, tyrosine, or choline it can accelerate synthesis of the neurotransmitter. [Tryptophan hydroxylase and choline acetyltransferase (CAT) do indeed have very poor affinities for their substrates tryptophan and choline. As discussed below, tyrosine hydroxylase activity becomes tyrosine-limited when neurons containing the enzyme have been activated and the enzyme has been phosphorylated.]

4. The activity of this enzyme cannot be subject to local end-product inhibition, i.e., the products of tryptophan's hydroxylation, 5-hydroxytryptophan and serotonin itself, may not appreciably suppress tryptophan hydroxylase activity nor may acetylcholine levels within cholinergic nerve terminals affect CAT activity. Tyrosine hydroxylase activity probably is subject to some end-product inhibition when the enzyme protein is in its nonphosphorylated state; however, once the enzyme is phosphorylated, when the nerve cells containing it become active, it apparently is freed from this constraint.

Available evidence suggests that only some of the neurotransmitters present in the human brain are subject to such precursor control, principally the monoamines mentioned above (serotonin; the catecholamines dopamine, norepinephrine, and epinephrine; acetylcholine) and, possibly, histidine and glycine. Pharmacological doses of the amino acid histidine do elevate histamine levels within nerve terminals, and the administration of threonine, a substrate for the enzyme that normally forms glycine from serine, can elevate glycine levels within spinal cord neurons. One large family of neurotransmitters, the peptides, almost certainly is *not* subject to precursor control. Brain levels of these compounds have never been shown to change with variations in brain amino acid levels; moreover, there are sound theoretical reasons why it is unlikely that brain peptide synthesis would respond. The immediate precursor for a brain protein or peptide is not an amino acid per se, as is the case for some of the monoamine neurotransmitters, but the amino acid molecule attached to its particular species of tRNA. In brain tissue, the known enzymes that catalyze the coupling of an amino acid to its tRNA have very high affinities for their amino acid substrates, such that their ability to operate at full capacity in vivo is probably unaffected by amino acid levels (except possibly in pathological states, such as phenylketonuria, which are associated with major disruptions in brain amino patterns).

Little information is available concerning the possible precursor control of the nonessential amino acids, such as glutamate, aspartate, and γ-aminobutyric acid (GABA), even though these are probably the most abundant neurotransmitters in the brain, for the reason that it is very difficult to do experiments on these relationships. Even though glutamate and aspartate can be formed at various organs in the body via many different biochemical pathways, the precise pathways that synthesize these compounds within the terminals of neurons are not well established. In the case of GABA, although its precursor glutamate is well established, brain levels of that amino acid apparently cannot be raised experimentally without sorely disrupting normal brain functions. The macromolecule that transports acidic amino acids like glutamate and aspartate across the blood–brain barrier is unidirectional and secretes these compounds by an active-transport mechanism from the brain into the blood (12). Hence administration of even an enormous dose of monosodium glutamate will not affect brain glutamate levels unless it elevates plasma osmolarity to the point of disrupting the blood–brain barrier.

TYROSINE EFFECT ON DOPAMINE AND NOREPINEPHRINE SYNTHESIS

Because tyrosine administration had not been shown to increase brain dopamine or norepinephrine levels in otherwise untreated animals, it was assumed until fairly recently that the catecholamine neurotransmitters were not under precursor control, in spite of the fact that plasma tyrosine levels do increase several fold after protein intake or tyrosine administration; that the LNAA transport system does ferry tyrosine, like tryptophan, across the blood–brain barrier; and that tyrosine hydroxylase, which catalyzes the rate-limiting step in catecholamine synthesis, is unsaturated in vivo (2). It seemed possible that a pool of neuronal dopamine or norepinephrine might exist whose synthesis did depend on tyrosine levels, but that was of too small a size, in relation to total catecholamine levels, to be detected.

Hence studies were performed to determine whether catecholamine synthesis or release could be affected by changes in brain tyrosine concentrations. Catecholamine synthesis was estimated by following the rate at which dopa, the product of tyrosine's hydroxylation, accumulated in brains of rats treated acutely with a drug that blocks the next enzyme in catecholamine formation (aromatic L-amino acid decarboxylase); tyrosine administration increased dopa accumulation, whereas other LNAAs decreased both dopa accumulation and brain tyrosine levels (2). Catecholamine release was then estimated by measuring brain levels of metabolites of dopamine [homovanillic acid (HVA); dihydroxyphenylacetic acid (DOPAC)] or norepinephrine [methoxyhydroxyphenylglycol sulfate (MHPH-SO$_4$)]. Administration of even large doses of tyrosine had no consistent effect on these metabolites. However, if the experimental animals were also given an additional treatment designed to accelerate the firing of dopaminergic or noradrenergic tracts (e.g., dopamine receptor blockers; cold exposure; partial lesions of dopaminergic tracts; reserpine), the supplemental tyrosine now caused a marked augmentation of catecholamine release (2). These initial observations formed the basis for the hypothesis that catecholaminergic neurons become tyrosine-sensitive when they are physiologically active and lose this capacity when they are quiescent.

The biochemical mechanism that couples a neuron's firing frequency to its ability to respond to supplemental tyrosine involves phosphorylation of the tyrosine hydroxylase enzyme protein, a process that occurs when the neurons fire. This phosphorylation, which is short-lived, enhances the enzyme's affinity for its cofactor (tetrahydrobiopterin) and makes the enzyme insensitive to end-product inhibition catechols; these changes allow its net activity to depend on the extent to which it is saturated with tyrosine. An additional mechanism underlying this coupling may be an actual depletion of tyrosine within nerve terminals, as a consequence of its accelerated conversion to catecholamines. If slices of rat caudate nucleus are superfused with a standard Krebs' Ringer's solution (which lacks amino acids) and are depolarized repeatedly, they are unable to sustain their release of dopamine; concurrently, their contents of tyrosine but not of other LNAA, decline markedly. The addition of tyrosine to the superfusion solution enables the tissue to continue releasing dopamine at initial rates,

and also protects it against depletion of its tyrosine. The concentrations of tyrosine needed for these effects are proportional to the number of times the neurons are depolarized. (Of course, the intact brain is continuously perfused with tyrosine-containing blood, making it highly unlikely that tyrosine levels fall to a similar extent, even in continuously active brain neurons. However, they might decline somewhat, since tyrosine is poorly soluble in aqueous media, and diffuses relatively slowly.)

More recently, in vivo dialysis techniques have been used to assess tyrosine's effects on dopamine release from the rat's corpus striatum. When otherwise untreated animals receive the amino acid systematically, there is, after 20–40 minutes, a substantial increase in dopamine output, unaccompanied by detectable increases in dopamine's metabolites DOPAC or HVA. However, this effect is short-lived, and dopamine release returns to basal levels after 20–30 minutes. This latter response probably reflects receptor-mediated decreases in the firing frequencies of the striatal neurons (to compensate for the increase in dopamine release that occurs per firing) or perhaps local presynaptic inhibition. If animals are given haloperidol, a dopamine-receptor blocking agent, before or along with the tyrosine, the supplemental tyrosine continues to amplify dopamine output for prolonged periods (13).

Tyrosine has now been shown to enhance the production and release of dopamine or norepinephrine in a variety of circumstances, and this amino acid may ultimately have considerable utility in treating catecholamine-related diseases or conditions. However it is important to remember that, when it (or any other amino acid) is given by itself—and not in the form of dietary protein, where it is accompanied by all of the other 21 amino acids—its fate in the body is entirely different. The use of tyrosine (or any other amino acid) to promote a physiological or behavioral process must be considered as a *drug*; as such it must be supported by the same quality of safety,

efficacy, and purity data as would be required for any other drug.

EFFECTS OF CHOLINE ON SYNTHESIS
OF ACETYLCHOLINE AND
PHOSPHATIDYLCHOLINE

The amounts of acetylcholine released by
physiologically active cholinergic neurons
depend on the concentrations of choline
available. In the absence of supplemental
free choline, the neurons will continue to
release constant quantities of the transmitter, especially when stimulated (14). However, when choline *is* available (in concentrations bracketing the physiological range),
a clear dose relationship is observed between its concentration and acetylcholine
release (14,15). When no free choline is
available, the source of the choline used for
acetylcholine synthesis is the cells' own
membranes (14,16). Membranes are very
rich in endogenous phosphatidylcholine
(PC), and this phospholipid serves as a res-
ervoir of free choline, much as bone and
albumin serve as reservoirs for calcium and
essential amino acids. It has been suggested
that a prolonged imbalance between the
amounts of free choline that are available to
a cholinergic neuron and the amounts
needed for acetylcholine synthesis might
alter the dynamics of membrane phospholipids to the point of interfering with normal
neuronal functioning ["autocannibalism"
(15,17)]. In that event, providing the brain
with supplemental choline would serve two
purposes: it would enhance acetylcholine
release from physiologically active neurons,
and it would replenish the choline-contain-
ing phospholipids in their membranes.

Neurons can draw on three sources of
free choline for acetylcholine synthesis:
that stored as PC in their own membranes;
that formed intrasynaptically from the hy-
drolysis of acetylcholine (and taken back up
into the presynaptic terminal by a high-af-
finity process estimated to be 30–50% efficient in the brain); and that present in the

blood stream (and taken into the brain by a
specific blood–brain barrier transport system). PC in foods (e.g., liver, eggs) is rapidly hydrolyzed to free choline in the intestinal mucosa (or broken down more slowly
after passage into the lymphatic circula-
tion). Consumption of adequate quantities
of PC can lead to several fold elevations in
plasma choline levels, thereby increasing
brain choline levels and the substrate saturation of CAT.

The PC molecules consumed in the diet,
as well as those formed endogenously in
neuronal membranes, are very heterogeneous with respect to their fatty acid composi-
tions. Some PCs (e.g., those in soy beans
and nerve terminals) are relatively rich in
polyunsaturated fatty acids; others (e.g., in
eggs) are highly saturated. PCs are also heterogeneous with reference to their mode of
synthesis. Brain neurons produce PC by
three distinct biochemical pathways: the sequential methylation of phosphatidylethanolamine (PE), the incorporation of preexisting free choline via the CDP–choline
cycle, or the incorporation of free choline
via the base-exchange pathway [in which a
choline molecule substitutes for the etha-
nolamine in the PE or the serine in phosphatidylserine (PS)]. Quite possibly, the different varieties of PC may survive distinct
functions; for example, one type of PC, distinguished by its fatty acid composition or
its mode of synthesis, could be preferentially utilized to provide a choline source for
acetylcholine synthesis, or could be formed
preferentially during the processes of cell
division or synaptic remodeling, or it might
be involved in the pathogenesis of particular
degenerative diseases afflicting cholinergic
neurons (e.g., Alzheimer's disease).

Supplemental choline or PC has been
used with some success in the treatment of
tardive dyskinesia. A summary of related
publications (18) concluded that choline and
the cholinesterase-inhibitor physostigmine
were about equally efficacious and that choline was less toxic. Most patients exhibited
some improvement in the frequency of ab-

normal movements, but in only a few was there complete cessation of the movements. Choline sources have also been tried in the treatment of Alzheimer's disease. Most well-controlled studies have treated subjects for relatively short intervals (6–8 weeks) and have focused on younger subjects, with little or no success. A single double-blind study administered the PC for 6 months (19). Improvement was noted in about one-third of the subjects; the average age of the responders was 83 and that of nonresponders 73, a relationship thought to be compatible with evidence that Alzheimer's disease may be more restricted to cholinergic neurons in subjects who become symptomatic at a later age. Occasional reports have also described useful effects of choline or PC in treating mania, ataxis, myasthenic syndromes, and TS. Very recently it has been observed (20) that brains of people dying of Alzheimer's disease (but not Down's syndrome) contain reduced levels of PC and of free choline, but major increases in those of the PC metabolites glycerophosphocholine (GPC). These changes were not restricted to regions containing plaques, tangles, or amyloid.

REFERENCES

1. Wurtman RJ, Hefti F, Melamed E. Precursor control of neurotransmitter synthesis. *Pharmacol Rev* 1980;32:315.
2. Wurtman RJ. Behavioural effects of nutrients. *Lancet* 1983;1:145–7.
3. Wurtman JJ, Wurtman RJ, Mark S, Tsay R, Gilbert W, Growdon J. D-fenfluramine selectively suppresses carbohydrate snacking by obese subjects. *Int J Eating Disord* 1985;4:89–99.
4. O'Rourke D, Wurtman J, Wurtman R, Chebli R, Gleason R. Treatment of seasonal depression with d-fenfluramine. *J Clin Psychiatry* 1989;50:343–7.
5. Brzezinski AA, Wurtman JJ, Wurtman RJ, Gleason R, Nader T, Laferrere B. D-fenfluramine sup-

presses the increased calorie and carbohydrate intakes and improves the mood of women with premenstrual syndrome. *Obstet Gynecol* 1990; 76:296–301.
6. Spring B, Wurtman J, Gleason, Kessler R, Wurtman RJ. Weight gain and withdrawal symptoms after smoking cessation: a preventive intervention using d-fenfluramine. *Health Psychol* 1991; 10:216–23.
7. Wurtman RJ. Presynaptic control of release of amine neurotransmitters by precursor levels. *NIPS (Am Physiol Soc)* 1988;3:158–63.
8. Fernstrom JD, Wurtman RJ. Brain serotonin content: physiological dependence on plasma tryptophan levels. *Science* 1971;173:149–52.
9. Schaechter J, Wurtman RJ. Tryptophan availability modulates serotonin release from rat hypothalamic slices. *J Neurochem* 1989;53:1925–33.
10. Madras BK, Cohen EL, Messing R, Munro HN, Wurtman RJ. Relevance of serum-free tryptophan to tissue tryptophan concentrations. *Metabolism* 1974;23:1107–16.
11. Fernstrom JD, Wurtman RJ. Brain serotonin content: physiological regulation by plasma neutral amino acids. *Science* 1972;178:414–6.
12. Pardridge WM. Regulation of amino acid availability to the brain. In: Wurtman RJ, Wurtman JJ, eds. *Nutrition and the brain*, vol 7. New York: Raven Press, 1977;141–204.
13. During MJ, Acworth IN, Wurtman RJ. Dopamine release in rat striatum: physiological coupling to tyrosine supply. *J Neurochem* 1989;52:1449–54.
14. Maire J-C, Wurtman RJ. Effects of electrical stimulation and choline availability on release and contents of acetylcholine and choline in superfused slices from rat striatum. *J Physiol (Paris)* 1985; 80:189–95.
15. Blusztajn JK, Wurtman RJ. Choline and cholinergic neurons. *Science* 1983;221:614–20.
16. Blusztajn JK, Liscovitch M, Richardson UI. Synthesis of acetylcholine from choline derived from phosphatidylcholine in a human neuronal cell line. *Proc Natl Acad Sci USA* 1987;84:5474–8.
17. Wurtman RJ. Alzheimer's disease. *Sci Am* 1985; 252:62–75.
18. Nasrallah HA, Dunner FL, Smith RE, McCalley-Whitters M, Sherman AD. Variable clinical response to choline in tardive dyskinesia. *Psychol Med* 1984;14:697–700.
19. Little A, Levy R, Chaqui-Kidd P, Hand D. A double-blind placebo controlled trial of high-dose lecithin in Alzheimer's disease. *J Neurol Neurosurg Psychiatry* 1985;48:736–42.
20. Nitsch R, Pittas A, Blusztajn JK, Slack BE, Growdon JH, Wurtman RJ. Evidence for a membrane defect in Alzhemier's disease. *Proc Nat Acad Sci USA* 1992;89:1671–5.

Advances in Neurology, Vol. 58, edited
by T. N. Chase, A. J. Friedhoff, and
D. J. Cohen. Raven Press, Ltd.,
New York © 1992.

36

Is There a Role for Megavitamin Therapy in the Treatment of Attention Deficit Hyperactivity Disorder?

Robert H. A. Haslam

*Departments of Pediatrics and Medicine (Neurology), University
of Toronto and Department of Pediatrics, Hospital for Sick Children, Toronto,
Ontario M5G 1X8, Canada*

The routine use of vitamins in the pediatric population appears to be increasing (1). A common belief holds that if a little vitamin is good, more may be better. In a recent study of Canadian children, as many as 70% received regular vitamin supplementation. Only 10% of this group had not been given vitamin polypharmacy at some time (2). During the past decade, with the increased emphasis on holistic medicine and a growing reluctance to accept traditional and scientifically proven methods of medical care, there has been a movement to unorthodox methods of treatment. Megavitamin therapy is no exception!

Megavitamin therapy may be defined as treatment with quantities of one or more vitamins in amounts ten or more times the recommended dietary allowance (3). A number of diseases warrant large doses of vitamins based upon abnormalities of enzyme activity or receptor responsiveness (e.g., vitamin D-resistant rickets and pyridoxine-dependency seizures). These conditions have been thoroughly investigated, and there is ample evidence to support the use of large doses of specific vitamins to overcome the basic physiological or biochemical abnormalities in these diseases. In contrast, there

is an increasing group of conditions that are treated by some physicians with megavitamin therapy in which scientific efficacy for their use is totally lacking. These include mental retardation, especially Down syndrome (4), autism (5), learning disorders, schizophrenia, epilepsy, colds (6), cancer (7), wound healing, poor sexual performance, premenstrual discomfort, the process of aging, and arthritis. When these therapies are subjected to rigorous scientific scrutiny, the lack of positive effect from megavitamin therapy becomes readily apparent (8–11). Furthermore, serious side effects resulting from megavitamin treatment have been identified. There have been no reports in peer-reviewed journals of the use of megavitamin therapy in children or adults with Tourette syndrome (TS).

Several studies have reported the efficacy of megavitamins for the management of attention deficit hyperactivity disorder (ADHD) (5,12,13). Unfortunately, in each case, the study was poorly designed and lacked appropriate controls and the conclusions were based on faulty data. This study was designed to determine whether megavitamin therapy has a positive effect on children with ADHD by monitoring physical, behavioral, and biochemical parameters (14).

STUDY DESIGN

Forty-one children (35 boys and 6 girls) with ADHD as defined in the *Diagnostic and Statistical Manual*, 3rd ed (DSM III) (15) were accepted into the clinical trial. The diagnostic criteria included developmentally inappropriate inattention, impulsivity, and hyperactivity with an onset before 7 years and a duration of greater than 6 months. Additional inclusion factors consisted of average intelligence, absence of primary affective disorders, and a baseline rating of 15 or greater on the Hyperactivity Index of the Conner's Parent or Teacher Questionnaire (16). Seventy-five children (36 boys and 39 girls) served as controls for normative serum ascorbic acid and pyridoxine values. Informed consent was obtained from parents, and assent from the subjects

when appropriate, prior to the enrollment of children into the study.

The clinical study was designed in two stages. Stage 1 consisted of an open clinical period in which each subject was treated with megavitamin therapy for 3 months. Stage 2, a double-blind crossover trial, was reserved for those subjects who were positive responders to megavitamin therapy during stage 1. Stage 2 was initiated following a 6-week washout period and consisted of four trial periods, each 6 weeks in duration. Drug (vitamin V) or placebo (P) was assigned randomly during the 24-week study period of stage 2 as DPDP or PDPD (Fig. 1). Parents, teachers, investigators, and the children were blinded to the treatment order. It was determined that a sample size of seven children during stage 2 would be sufficient to detect a mean difference equal to 1 SD of the parameter under consideration with $\alpha = 0.10$ and $\beta = 0.15$.

Each subject underwent psychological testing during the baseline period including

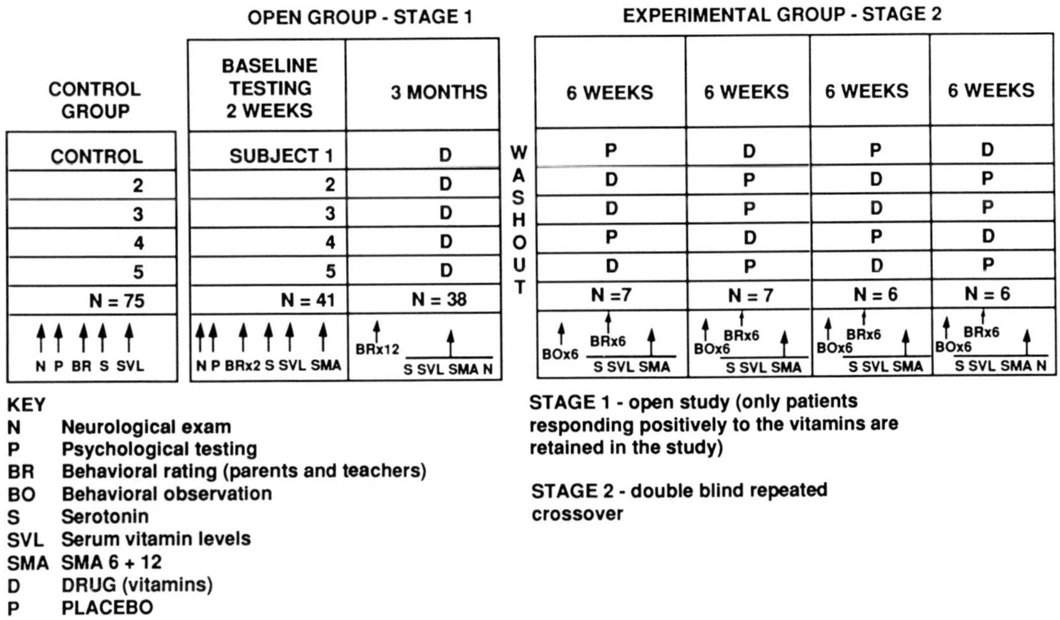

KEY
N   Neurological exam
P   Psychological testing
BR Behavioral rating (parents and teachers)
BO Behavioral observation
S   Serotonin
SVL Serum vitamin levels
SMA SMA 6 + 12
D   DRUG (vitamins)
P   PLACEBO

STAGE 1 - open study (only patients responding positively to the vitamins are retained in the study)

STAGE 2 - double blind repeated crossover

FIG. 1. The megavitamin protocol consisted of a control group (n = 75) and subjects (n = 41). Following baseline testing, 38 subjects were enrolled in the open clinical trial. Following a 6-week washout period, seven positive responders entered the double-blind repeated crossover study. From ref. 14 with permission.

the Weschler Intelligence Scale for Children (WISC-R) and the Wide Range Achievement Test (WRAT); the family was administered a test of socioeconomic status (SES) (17). A series of blood tests were obtained throughout the study as shown in Fig. 1. Serum was obtained for pyridoxine and ascorbic acid levels during baseline testing and at the completion of stages 1 and 2. All medications, including stimulants, had been discontinued at least 1 week prior to entry into the study.

Behavioral changes of the subjects were monitored throughout the study. Parent and teacher ratings were recorded weekly in both stages 1 and 2. During stage 2 a highly skilled and well-trained behavioral observer visited each subject's classroom for a 30-minute period at the same time each week with the cooperation of the child's teacher. The Stony-Brook Observational Code, which measures nine disruptive classroom behaviors, was used by the behavioral observer for each subject (18). During stage 1, each subject was assigned a behavioral response while taking vitamins. A positive response was defined as a decrease for 2 consecutive weeks in the mean Conner's hyperactivity ratings by 20% compared with baseline; a nonresponse occurred when the mean behavior ratings did not increase or decrease by at least 20% from the baseline, and a negative response was defined by an increase in behavior ratings by at least 20% for 2 consecutive weeks with no positive response at any point during the trial (Fig. 2).

The megavitamin regimen utilized during the study was selected because of its widespread use and reported efficacy (13). A combination of water-soluble vitamins including niacinamide 250 mg, ascorbic acid 250 mg, pyridoxine 50 mg, and calcium pantothenate 100 mg were packaged in each capsule. The vitamin and placebo capsules were indistinguishable by taste and color. At the onset of stage 1, the subject received 4 capsules each day divided evenly between morning and evening. During the 3-month period, the dosage was gradually increased

to a maximum of 12 capsules daily. If side effects developed, the vitamin dosage was decreased to the last dose tolerated by the subject. The vitamin dosage prescribed during stage 2 was equivalent to the least dosage that provided the greatest observed benefit during stage 1. The drug schedule initiated at the onset of stage 2 was maintained throughout the remainder of the study. Parents were instructed to follow a schedule of drug treatment that was outlined on a weekly calendar and to return the vitamin bottles on a regular basis. The study coordinator was always available to respond to parent concerns and to check vitamin dose changes and count capsules on return of the empty vitamin containers.

OBSERVATIONS

The clinically relevant data comparing subjects and control children is presented in Table 1. The most significant differences included intelligence testing, the performance, reading, spelling, and arithmetic percentiles, and hyperactivity rating by mother and teacher. There was no difference in serum pyridoxine and ascorbic acid levels between the two groups. Three subjects could not complete stage 1 and were withdrawn from the study because of excessive vomiting, abdominal pain, or inability to swallow the capsule. A comparison of laboratory data during baseline testing and at the completion of stage 1 is shown in Table 2. The most significant abnormality was an elevation in serum transaminase levels, all of which returned to baseline values within 4–6 weeks. Forty-two percent of the subjects exceeded the upper limits of transaminase levels, with values reaching 171 μm/L. There was also a significant increase in serum bilirubin levels, but none exceeded the upper range of normal. Although some patients complained of nausea and vomiting, no subject developed jaundice or hepatomegaly. There were no significant changes in serum transaminase or bilirubin

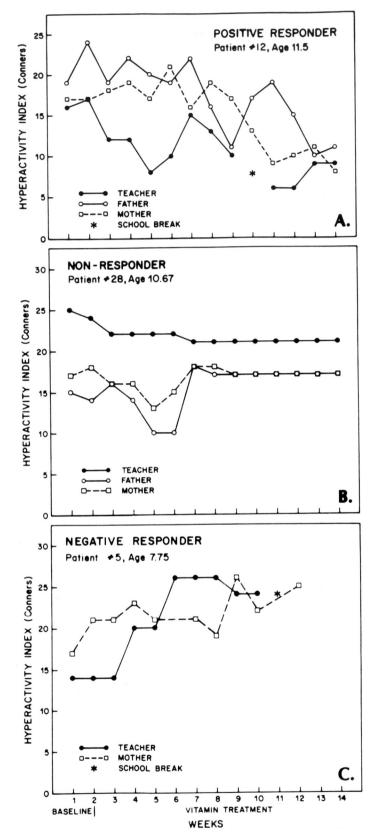

FIG. 2. Behavioral responses to megavitamin therapy during stage 1. **A:** Positive response. **B:** Nonresponse. **C:** Negative response. From ref. 14 with permission.

TABLE 1. Clinical data and vitamin levels, controls and subjects (mean ± SD)

	Control children (n = 75)	Subjects (n = 41)
Age (yr)	9.94 ± 1.87	9.31 ± 1.99
Height (cm)	140.47 ± 12.44	134.08 ± 13.82
Weight (kg)	33.58 ± 8.96	30.78 ± 11.02
Head circumference (cm)	53.50 ± 1.55	52.26 ± 1.90**
Verbal IQ	**114.49 ± 11.56**	**101.33 ± 12.85***
Performance IQ	**114.80 ± 11.84**	**101.26 ± 11.44***
Full-scale IQ	**116.07 ± 11.70**	**101.33 ± 11.38***
Reading percentile	**83.19 ± 17.47**	**47.81 ± 31.36***
Spelling percentile	**75.53 ± 21.78**	**40.09 ± 29.19***
Arithmetic percentile	**52.72 ± 21.98**	**35.51 ± 23.85***
Present grade level	4.59 ± 1.94	3.41 ± 1.96**
Abnormal pregnancy or delivery (by history)	20%	39%*
Soft neurologic signs (≥1)	12%	34%**
Socioeconomic status (SES) rating	**60.56 ± 13.71**	**50.26 ± 14.19***
Hyperactivity rating (by mother)	**4.81 ± 3.99**	**20.02 ± 4.34***
Hyperactivity rating (by teacher)	**3.99 ± 4.17**	**14.85 ± 6.68***
Serum pyridoxine (ng/mL)	9.58 ± 5.33	11.60 ± 6.01
Serum ascorbic acid (µmmol/L)	61.11 ± 16.79	67.50 ± 19.72

* $p < 0.05$.
** $p < 0.01$.
*** $p < 0.001$.

levels while the children were taking placebo. As expected, a significant elevation of serum ascorbic acid and pyridoxine was documented at the termination of stage 1.

Twelve children (29%) had a positive behavioral response during stage 1. There was no difference in baseline pyridoxine and ascorbic acid levels in positive responders as compared with nonresponders or negative responders. Five of the positive responders declined to participate in stage 2, primarily due to undesirable side effects during the open clinical period. Seven subjects, all boys with a mean age of 8.9 years, entered stage 2. Four of these positive responders had the most beneficial behavioral response taking 8 capsules daily, one on 10 capsules, and two on the maximum of 12 capsules per day.

During the crossover phase, four subjects

TABLE 2. Laboratory data for study subjects (maximum n = 38)

	Pre-stage 1	Post-stage 1
Creatinine (µmol/L)	58.12 ± 9.51	61.38 ± 9.31
Total protein (g/L)	67.57 ± 3.86	68.37 ± 4.22
Albumin (g/L)	44.63 ± 2.29	45.06 ± 2.89
Calcium (mmol/L)	2.51 ± 0.09	2.44 ± 0.11**
Inorganic phosphate (mmol/L)	1.49 ± 0.16	1.47 ± 0.24
Total bilirubin (µmol/L)	**5.67 ± 2.55**	**8.01 ± 3.23***
Alkaline phosphatase (U/L)	280.46 ± 84.96	289.40 ± 99.22
Creatine kinase (U/L)	122.29 ± 74.52	173.15 ± 161.26*
Lactate dehydrogenase (U/L)	251.29 ± 31.25	258.00 ± 46.98
Aspartate transaminase (U/L)	**27.14 ± 7.71**	**48.81 ± 29.08***
Serum pyridoxine (ng/mL)	11.60 ± 5.35	60.47 ± 53.35***
Serum ascorbic acid (µmol/L)	67.50 ± 19.59	85.48 ± 33.70*

* $p < 0.05$.
** $p < 0.01$.
*** $p < 0.001$.

TABLE 3. F *statistics for comparison of drug and placebo in stage 2 of study for seven subjects*

Scale	F statistic	p value (2-tailed test)	Coefficient (SE)
Teacher (df = 1 and 89)			
Overall	0.35	NS*	2.64 (4.46)
Conduct problem	**6.10**	**0.01 < p < 0.025**	**4.04 (1.63)**
Hyperactivity	2.48	NS	3.20 (2.04)
Inattentive/passive	**15.9**	**p < 0.001**	**−4.60 (1.15)**
Mother (df = 1 and 125)			
Overall	2.66	NS	5.25 (3.22)
Conduct problem	0.73	NS	1.14 (1.33)
Learning problem	**18.64**	**p < 0.001**	**2.60 (0.60)**
Psychosomatic complaints	**14.85**	**p < 0.001**	**−2.55 (0.66)**
Hyperactivity	**7.79**	**0.005 < p < 0.01**	**3.78 (1.35)**
Anxiety	1.64	NS	0.28 (0.22)
Father (df = 1 and 68)			
Overall	3.22	NS	8.91 (4.96)
Conduct problem	0.63	NS	1.61 (2.02)
Learning problem	**10.23**	**0.001 < p < 0.005**	**2.93 (0.92)**
Psychosomatic complaints	1.69	NS	−1.28 (0.98)
Hyperactivity	**5.44**	**0.01 < p < 0.025**	**5.19 (2.23)**
Anxiety	1.18	NS	0.49 (0.41)
Behavioral observation	7.30	0.005 < p < 0.01	24.91 (9.22)

* NS, $p > 0.05$.

were assigned to the PDPD order and three to DPDP, as shown in Fig. 1. One subject was withdrawn midway through stage 2 because of unacceptable behavior. On breaking the code, that child was found to have been assigned drug (D) followed by placebo (P). The parents were certain that placebo had been prescribed from the onset. Analysis of the parent, teacher, and behavioral observer scores for this child showed no difference between drug and placebo.

Table 3 highlights the statistical comparison of drug and placebo during stage 2 of the study. The overall score is the sum of subscales calculated separately for teacher, mother, and father. Subscales (e.g., conduct problem, hyperactivity) were derived from the extended Conner's questionnaire. The hyperactivity subscale of the questionnaire most closely correlates with the definition of ADHD. The *F* statistic is a test of differences between drug and placebo, adjusted for carryover effects of the drug. Also shown is the partial regression coefficient for drug effect. A positive coefficient indicates a better response for placebo, whereas

a negative coefficient is a positive response for vitamin. The differences between drug and placebo as recorded by the behavioral observer were also analyzed.

Inspection of Table 3 shows there were no significant differences in overall scales for teacher, mother, and father comparing drug and placebo. Certain components of the overall scale did show significant differences. For example, conduct problems documented by the teacher and learning problems and hyperactivity noted by the mother and father showed significant improvement while on placebo. Inattentive and passive behavior recorded by the teacher and psychosomatic complaints observed by the mother responded more favorably to vitamin. The data indicate that the behavioral observer documented significant worsening of behavior and classroom performance while on vitamins.

GENERAL COMMENTS

Data from this study do not support the suggestion that children with ADHD have pyridoxine or ascorbic acid vitamin deficiency. There was no significant difference in baseline serum pyridoxine and ascorbic acid levels in the subjects compared with controls. Furthermore, there was no difference between the vitamin levels in positive responders during stage 1, as compared with nonresponders and negative responders.

Megavitamin therapy produced an elevation of serum transaminase levels in 42% (17/41) of the children during the open clinical trial. In some cases, the transaminase levels did not return to normal for 4–6 weeks following the removal of the drug. There was also a significant rise in the serum bilirubin levels, but in no case did the value exceed the upper limits of normal. Clinical signs of liver injury including jaundice and hepatomegaly were not observed. Niacinamide was likely responsible for the elevation of the liver enzymes in the present study. Animals fed diets with high concentrations of nicotinic acid may develop fatty livers (19). Several reports in humans have implicated prolonged use of nicotinic acid as a cause of liver failure (20,21). Of equal concern is the potential toxicity following high doses of pyridoxine. A toxic neuropathy may develop following long-term ingestion of 200 mg pyridoxine/day. These patients develop an unsteady gait, have abnormalities of touch and pain perception with impaired coordination, and complain of numbness in the hands and feet. It may take months for the symptoms to regress once the vitamin has been discontinued (22). Excessive vitamin C may also produce harmful side effects in humans. Doses of 1–1.5 g may cause diarrhea and kidney stones of the oxalate type. The proponents of megavitamin therapy commonly prescribe drug doses exceeding those reported in the literature to cause severe side effects.

The most critical finding of the study is related to the comparison of drug and placebo effects in the seven subjects during the crossover phase. There were no significant differences in behavior between drug and placebo when overall scores of the teacher, mother, and father scales were compared. The majority of the differences observed in the individual component scores noted by the parent and teacher raters involved improved behavior while on placebo. The hyperactivity scale, which most closely resembles the principal diagnostic component of ADHD, was found to favor the placebo-treated group significantly as rated independently by the mother, father, and teacher. It is of particular note that the ratings by the independent behavior observer documented a negative effect of vitamin therapy as compared with placebo on nine specific disruptive classroom behaviors.

It is highly unlikely that megavitamin therapy would prove beneficial in Tourette syndrome, unless a specific vitamin deficiency or vitamin-dependent enzyme system is proved to be the cause. Megavitamins have no beneficial effect for children with ADHD and should not be used because of their ineffectiveness and potential serious side effects.

In summary, this study was designed to determine the effectiveness of megavitamin therapy in children with ADHD. Forty-one ADHD children were enrolled in a two-stage drug trial. Stage 1 consisted of a 3-month clinical trial of vitamins (niacinamide, ascorbic acid, pyridoxine, and calcium pantothenate). Twenty-nine percent of the 41 subjects had a positive behavioral response to the vitamin regimen. Seven of the 12 positive responders entered stage 2, which consisted of four 6-week, double-blind repeated crossover periods.

There was no statistical difference in the serum ascorbic acid and pyridoxine levels comparing subjects and 75 controls. Furthermore, there was no difference in the vitamin levels between positive responders, nonresponders, and negative responders during stage 1. Using analysis of variance methods for crossover studies, there was no significant difference (p > 0.05) in most behavior scores comparing vitamin and placebo during stage 2 of the trial. In general, positive behavioral responses, particularly those associated with ADHD, were more apparent during placebo as compared with vitamin therapy. A behavioral observer documented 25% more disruptive classroom behavior during vitamin therapy as compared with placebo ($p < 0.01$).

Forty-two percent of the subjects had a significant elevation of serum transaminase levels during stage 1. There was also a significant increase in serum bilirubin levels compared with baseline values, but none exceeded the upper limits of normal. It is concluded that megavitamins are ineffective in the management of ADHD and should not be utilized because of their potential hepatotoxicity.

REFERENCES

1. Staton JL. Vitamin usage: rampant or reasonable? *Vitam Issues Series*. Nutley NJ: Hoffman-La-Roche, 1983;3:1–3.
2. Issenman RM, Slack R, MacDonald L, Taylor W. Children's multiple vitamins: overuse leads to overdose. *Can Med Assoc J* 1985;132:781–4.
3. Committee on Dietary Allowances, Food and Nutrition Board, National Research Council. *Recommended dietary allowances*, 8th ed. Washington DC: National Academy of Sciences, 1974.
4. Harrell RF, Capp RH, Davis DR, Peerless J, Ravitz LR. Can nutritional supplements help mentally retarded children? An exploratory study. *Proc Natl Acad Sci USA* 1981;78:574–8.
5. Rimland B, Callaway E, Dreyfus P. The effect of high doses of vitamin B_6 in autistic children: a double-blind crossover study. *Am J Psychiatry* 1978;135:472–5.
6. Pauling L. *Vitamin C and the common cold*. San Francisco: Freeman 1976.
7. Cameron E, Pauling L. Supplemental ascorbate in the supportive treatment of cancer: prolongation of survival times in terminal human cancer. *Proc Natl Acad Sci USA* 1976;73:3685–9.
8. Smith GF, Spiker D, Peterson CP, Cicchetti D, Justine P. Use of megadoses of vitamins with minerals in Down's syndrome. *J Pediatr* 1984;105:228–34.
9. Shaywitz B, Siegel NJ, Pearson HA. Megavitamins for minimal brain dysfunction. A potentially dangerous therapy. *JAMA* 1977;238:1749–55.
10. Chalmers TC. Effects of ascorbic acid on the common cold. An evaluation of the evidence. *Am J Med*. 1975;58:532–6.
11. Moertel CG, Fleming TR, Creagan ET. High dose vitamin C versus placebo in the treatment of patients with advanced cancer who have had no prior chemotherapy: a randomized double-blind comparison. *N Engl J Med* 1985;312:137–41.
12. Cott A. Megavitamins: the orthomolecular approach to behavioral disorders and learning disabilities. *Acad Ther* 1972;7:245.
13. Cott A. *The orthomolecular approach to learning disabilities*. San Rafael, CA: Academic Therapy Publications, 1977;26–9.
14. Haslam RHA, Dalby JT, Rademaker AW. Effects of megavitamin therapy on children with attention deficit disorders. *Pediatrics* 1984;74:103–11.
15. *Diagnostic and statistical manual of mental disorders*, 3rd ed. Washington, DC: American Psychiatric Association, 1980.
16. Goyette CH, Conners CK, Ulrich RF. Normative data on revised Conners Parent and Teacher Rating Scales. *J Abnorm Child Psychol* 1978;6:221–36.
17. Blishen BR. A socioeconomic index for occupation in Canada. *Can Rev Social Anthropol* 1967;4:41.
18. O'Leary KD, Becker WC, Evans MB, et al. A token reinforcement program in the public school: a replication and systematic analysis. *J Appl Behav Ann* 1969;2:3.
19. Rikans LL, Arata D, Cederquist D. Fatty livers produced in albino rats by excess niacin in high fat diets. *J Nutr* 1965;85:107–12.
20. Mosher LR. Nicotinic acid side effects and toxicity: a review. *Am J Psychiatry* 1970;126:124–30.
21. Winter SL, Boyer JL. Hepatic toxicity from large doses of vitamin B_3 (nicotinamide) *N Engl J Med* 1973;289:1180–2.
22. Schaumberg H, Kaplan J, Windebank N, et al. Sensory neuropathy from pyridoxine abuse. *N Engl J Med*. 1983;309:445–8.

Advances in Neurology, Vol. 58, edited
by T. N. Chase, A. J. Friedhoff, and
D. J. Cohen. Raven Press, Ltd.,
New York © 1992.

37

Educational Management of Children with Tourette Syndrome

*Larry Burd and †Jacob Kerbeshian

*Child Evaluation and Treatment Program, Medical Center Rehabilitation Hospital
and Clinics, Departments of Neuroscience and Pediatrics, and the Center for
Teaching and Learning, University of North Dakota, Grand Forks, North Dakota
58202 †Department of Neuroscience, University of North Dakota,
Grand Forks, North Dakota 58202*

In the past decade major strides have been made in the conceptualization of developmental disorders. In 1982 Cohen et al. (1) set the stage for this change in thinking with a framework to encourage inquiry into the interaction of genetic, behavioral, and environmental factors in the emergence and expression of these disorders, e.g., the recent findings suggesting that the putative gene for Tourette syndrome (TS) can be expressed either as chronic multiple tics, TS or as obsessive–compulsive disorder (2,3). While the syndromal defining boundaries of TS are as yet unknown, what is clear is that TS is a highly complex disorder that at a minimum is associated at a high frequency with conditions such as obsessive–compulsive disorder and attention deficit-hyperactivity disorder (2,3). Earlier research has suggested that approximately 50% of children with TS also have a learning disability (4–7). A review of the literature produces limited data about this relationship, and very few case reports describe the results of interventions in schools. Yet children with TS who also have academic, social, or behavioral difficulties comprise fully two-thirds of children referred to the authors TS program (5,8–21).

In this chapter we will present strategies for the management of children with TS and learning disabilities and then suggest further research for children with the more severe developmental disabilities and TS.

In a recent study of children with TS with IQs above 70, in North Dakota, we found that 51% met criteria for a 1.5 standard deviation IQ/specific academic skill discrepancy in one subject area, 21% met criteria in two or more areas, and 11% in three or more areas (22). Using a 2.0 standard deviation discrepancy, 21% met criteria for a learning disability in one area, 9.5% in two areas, and 2.4% in all three areas.

In our experience less than 25% of children with TS and a learning disability are diagnosed in their school setting. This is consistent with the work of Shaywitz and Shaywitz (23) in a population of school aged children with learning disabilities and suggests that many children with TS may require evaluations in centers outside of the school setting (5,24,25).

We have noted elsewhere that in some children with TS the onset of learning problems coincides with the onset of their tics (5,25). These children were doing well in school and with the onset of tics also had the onset of significant learning problems. Interestingly, in some cases, this included letter and number reversals that had not been present previously (3,5,25). We have observed that this specific finding occurs as late as the end of the third grade.

EDUCATION OF CHILDREN WITH TS AND LEARNING DISABILITIES

The single most important element of a successful educational program is accommodation to meet the child's individual needs (25). These efforts are primarily focused on the development of effective compensation skills for the child, responsive intervention by the teacher, and acceptance by the child's peers.

We recommend management strategies in school that emphasize the use of long-term, positive reinforcement behavior management programs targeting individual behaviors we wish to see increase in frequency. Surprisingly, this is not a routine component in many individual education plans (IEPs) for children with TS. In our interventions, positive reinforcement is a mainstay of the IEP since a small, but significant, number of children react to cost response or punishment-dependent behavioral programs with an exacerbation of tics and related behavior problems (26).

Social skill deficiencies are common in children with TS and are often overlooked as a focus of intervention programs in schools for children with TS and accompanying learning and behavioral disturbances. Our goal is to identify skills in which the children are lacking and then teach those skills first, as we have found that many of the negative behaviors seen in TS result from a lack of an alternative positive social repertoire.

Children with TS are frequent victims of teasing in school and in other social settings. Teasing can become a chronic problem that may limit children's opportunities for social acceptance and interaction. We believe that teasing by peers should not be tolerated and must be dealt with by adults in positions of authority. Children must have a safe and ac-cepting environment in which to learn and develop socially. It is important for adults to consider empathically how teasing affects children. Imagine if teachers were publically taunted at work or while shopping. Homework assignments are a source of conflict for children both at home and at school. Problems with homework assignments are frequently managed by loss of privileges, physical punishment, or restriction of social activities. These actions do not improve the child's academic skills or improve motivation, both of which are essential to complete homework assignments successfully.

We have utilized a standard homework plan that begins by baselining the average amount of homework the child can do successfully, followed by gradually increasing the amount. For example, rather than have the child work at 20 math problems and complete only 2, with the focus of attention being on the 18 that are not done, we begin with 2 math problems and develop a work environment so that they may be completed. Then we work to complete three problems, then four, and so on.

Significant handwriting problems are a frequent complaint of teachers who have children with TS in their classrooms. We recommend typing and after the 4th grade a word-processing program, preferably one with a Spell-Check capability.

For children with math difficulties, a calculator can be a very effective aid. It provides nearly immediate success, is economical, and eliminates the need for the child having to work outside the classroom.

Having the child sit close to the door so that as necessary he or she may get up and walk down the hall to get a drink or to go into the bathroom to discharge accumulated tics seems helpful for many.

Children with TS usually require multidisciplinary management since their educational and treatment needs are frequently complex. More than two-thirds of our patients required intervention from outside the school setting. As in other developmental disorders, children with TS will benefit from the availability of a full range of

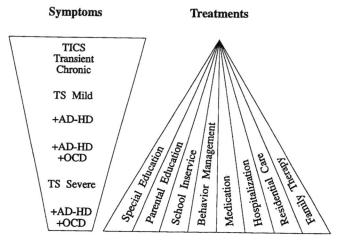

FIG. 1. The milder the symptoms, the fewer treatments are necessary. As symptoms become more severe, the number of people requiring treatment, as well as the number of treatment options required increase.

both diagnostic and therapeutic interventions.

Further research and practitioner training need to focus on learning disorders, which may be the most frequent element of comorbidity in children with TS. This work should parallel the efforts to understand and manage the co-occurrence of TS and attention deficit hyperactivity disorder (ADHD) when several treatment options are available.

MANAGEMENT SUGGESTIONS FOR CHILDREN WITH TS AND OTHER HANDICAPS

There is a population of multiply handicapped children with TS who in comparison with children with TS and learning disabilities are largely unrecorded in the medical, developmental, or educational literature. In our study of learning disabilities we reviewed the records of all children with TS

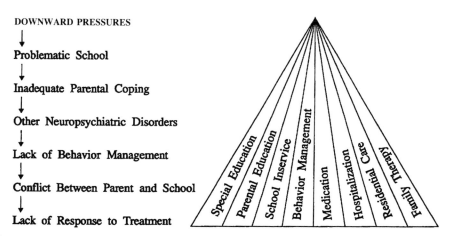

FIG. 2. Factors that increase the severity of symptomatology in subjects with Tourette syndrome and the increase in interventions required to provide successful intervention.

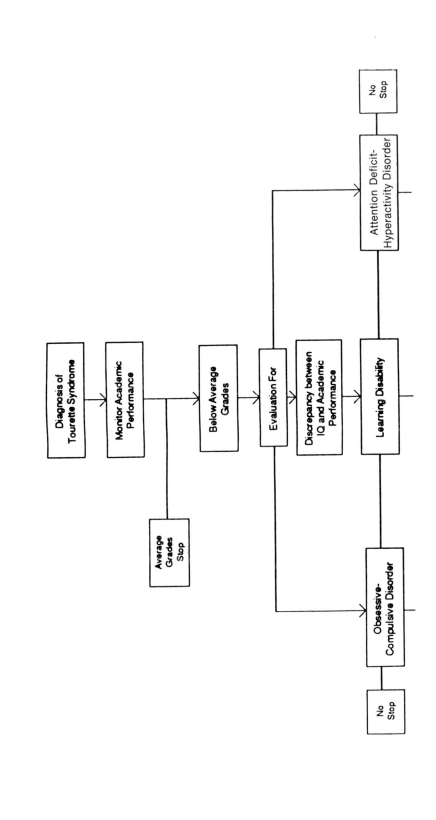

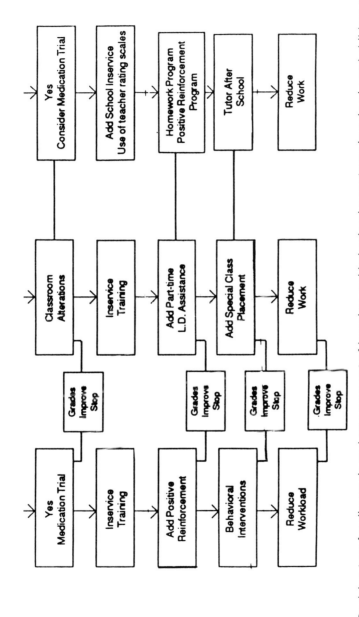

FIG. 3. Decision tree for diagnosis and management of learning and behavioral symptoms in school-aged children with Tourette syndrome. From ref. 25 with permission.

whom we had seen. We excluded children who had IQs below 70 (26 children) and children with severe sensory impairment, i.e., blindness (9), or deafness (3). Children who were nonverbal were also excluded (10). Children with such severe school phobias that their opportunities for traditional academic instruction had been severely limited were excluded (8). Children with an additional diagnosis of bipolar disorder (2) or schizophrenia (3) were also excluded from this study. Several children met more than one of these exclusionary criteria. Since we care for most children from North Dakota with severe TS or children with TS and other developmental disorders, the patients who were excluded from the learning disabilities studies may have had more severe developmental disorders than would typically be found in a general population of children with TS. If we include other disorders commonly associated with TS including ADHD and obsessive–compulsive disorder (OCD), comorbidity among multiply handicapped children with TS is substantial. Is this population of children with TS atypical? In North Dakota these are the children that parents, schools, and physicians struggle to manage (5,16,18,25). These children have long-term problems that require the most specialized care. As a component of our ongoing epidemiologic surveillance of neuropsychiatric disorders, we have described the prevalence rates and the natural history of TS occurring with schizophrenia and bipolar disorder (8–21). The long-term follow-up of this population has been the major impetus for our increased concern for the children who have TS and associated conditions.

IMPLICATIONS

When we completed our early prevalence studies of TS we were quite surprised at the frequency of comorbid conditions in our population (8–21). As we followed these patients and expanded our studies to adults, we also found high rates of comorbidities in adults with TS. In the absence of a cure and given the limitations of pharmacologic interventions, we must expand our research into the appropriate management of these most vulnerable persons with TS.

Figure 1 gives a comparison of children with TS and a range of associated disorders. While the numbers of these children compared with the mildly affected TS child are small in our state, they consume a large portion of the dollars expended on children with TS in our state.

The demands for services for this population of children with multiple disorders are extensive and are presented in Fig. 2 (8–21,24,25). The need for such a wide range of services rapidly excludes local public schools as the sole service provides for these children. This has led to residential placement for many of these children, rather than less restrictive and less expensive community care and education.

The literature available to develop educational management programs for these children is quite limited. Children with TS and multiple developmental disorders are seen as atypical, yet in our work, many children with TS who present for care have other developmental disorders (8–21,24,25).

The capability to diagnose, treat, and manage TS in children must encompass all TS children. In order to accomplish this goal we need to expand the scope of research in this population (27). In addition, research is needed to improve diagnostic, treatment, and management paradigms to care for children with TS and ADHD, TS and OCD, and learning disability, and for children with other combinations of developmental disorders. An example is presented in Fig. 3 (25).

The research goal is to evaluate critically the safety, efficacy, and durability of these interventions before they are applied to populations of children with TS.

REFERENCES

1. Cohen DJ, Detlor J, Shaywitz BA, Leckman JF. Interaction of biological and psychological factors

in the natural history of Tourette syndrome: a paradigm for childhood neuropsychiatric disorders. In: Friedhoff AJ, Chase TN, eds. *Gilles de la Tourette syndrome*, New York: Raven Press, 1982;31–40.

2. Pauls DL, Leckman JF. The inheritance of Gilles de la Tourette syndrome and associated behaviors: evidence for autosomal dominant transmission. *N Engl J Med* 1986;315:993–7.

3. Comings DE. *Tourette syndrome and human behavior*. Duarte, CA: Hope Press, 1990.

4. Golden GA. Psychologic and neuropsychologic aspects of Tourette's syndrome. *Neurol Clin* 1984; 2:91–102.

5. Burd L, Kerbeshian J, Cook J, Bornhoeft DM, Fisher W. Tourette disorder in North Dakota. *Neurosci Biobehav Rev* 1988;12:223–8.

6. Hagin RA, Beecher R, Pagano G, Kreeger H. Effects of Tourette syndrome on learning. In: Friedhoff AJ, Chase TN, eds. *Gilles de la Tourette syndrome*, New York: Raven Press, 1982;323–33.

7. Hagin RA, Kugler J. School problems associated with Tourette's syndrome. In: Cohen DJ, Brunn RD, Leckman JF, eds. *Tourette's syndrome and tic disorders: clinical understanding and treatment*, New York: John Wiley & Sons, 1988; 223–36.

8. Kerbeshian J, Burd L. Familial pervasive development disorder, Tourette disorder and hyperlexia. *Neurosci Biobehav Rev* 1988;12:233–4.

9. Kerbeshian J, Burd L. Tourette disorder and schizophrenia in children. *Neurosci Biobehav Rev* 1988;12:267–270.

10. Kerbeshian J, Burd L. Tourette disorder and mutational falsetto. *Neurosci Biobehav Rev* 1988; 12:271–4.

11. Fisher W, Burd L, Kerbeshian J. Comparisons of DSM-III defined pervasive developmental disorders in North Dakota children. *J Am Acad Child Adolesc Psychiatry* 1987;26:704–10.

12. Kerbeshian J, Burd L. Are schizophreniform symptoms present in attenuated form in children with Tourette disorder and other developmental disorders? *Can J Psychiatry* 1987;32:123–35.

13. Burd L, Kerbeshian J, Fisher W, Barcome D. Pseudohemiparesis and Tourette syndrome. *J Child Neurol* 1986;1:369–71.

14. Kerbeshian J, Burd L. Asperger's syndrome and Tourette syndrome. *Br J Psychiatry* 1986; 148:781–6.

15. Kerbeshian J, Burd L. A second case of Tourette syndrome, atypical pervasive developmental disorder and Ganser syndrome: diagnostic classification and treatment. *Int J Psychiatry Med* 1986; 16:67–75.

16. Kerbeshian J, Burd L, Fisher W, Martsolf J, Wilkenheiser M. Gilles de la Tourette disorder in multiply disabled children. *Rehab Lit* 1985;46:255–8.

17. Kerbeshian J, Burd L. Auditory hallucinosis and atypical tic disorder. *J Clin Psychiatry* 1985; 46:398–9.

18. Burd L, Kerbeshian J. Tourette syndrome, atypical pervasive developmental disorder, and Ganser syndrome in a 15-year-old, visually impaired, mentally retarded boy. *Can J Psychiat* 1985;30:74–6.

19. Kerbeshian J, Burd L, Martsolf J. Fragile X syndrome associated with Tourette symptomatology in male with moderate mental retardation and autism. *J Dev Behav Pediatr* 1984;5:201–3.

21. Burd L, Kerbeshian J. Tourette syndrome and bipolar disorder. *Arch Neurol* 1984;41:1236.

23. Shaywitz SE, Shaywitz BA, Fletcher JM, Escobar MD. Prevalence of reading disability in boys and girls. *JAMA* 1990;264:998–1002.

24. Burd L, Kerbeshian J. Tourette syndrome and learning disabilities. (*submitted.*)

25. Burd L, Hearle T, eds. Educational needs of children with Tourette syndrome: In: Children with Tourette syndrome. *A parents guide*. Rockville, Maryland: Woodbine House, 1992:169–205.

26. Burd L, Kerbeshian J. Treatment generated side effects from the use of behavior modification in Tourette syndrome. *Dev Med Child Neurol* 1987; 29:831–2.

27. Leckman JF. *Research on children and adolescents with mental, behavioral and developmental disorders*. Washington, DC: Institute of Medicine National Academy Press, 1989.

Advances in Neurology, Vol. 58, edited
by T. N. Chase, A. J. Friedhoff, and
D. J. Cohen. Raven Press, Ltd.,
New York © 1992.

38

The Family in Tourette Syndrome

Gordon Harper

*Departments of Psychiatry and Medicine, Children's Hospital, Boston, and the
Judge Baker Children's Center, Boston, Massachusetts, 02115*

The decade of the 1980s was, as the decade
of the 1990s promises to be, a period of dramatic increase in our knowledge of Tourette
Syndrome (TS) from the genetic, physiological, and pharmacological points of view (1).
In such periods, along with the biology of
the disorder, there is a need to study the
experience of the individual with TS (2) and
the experience of the *family* whose child has
TS. The familiar role of the family in the
upbringing of the child takes on particular
meanings when a child has a neuropsychiatric disorder like TS.

It is in the family that children with TS,
like all children, first learn about themselves
and the world. It is the family that gives children their first meanings—including the
meaning of the illness and symptoms. It
is in the family that children develop those
aspects of the self most affected by
Tourette's—the self's boundaries, efficacy, impulse control, confidence, and
responsibility, as well as self-esteem. In the
family children will be held, or not, when
they are hurt; will see how others manage
impulses, including impulses that aren't
manageable; and will acquire the most abid-
ing sense of who they are and what they are
worth.

This paper reviews the experience of the
family with a TS child and the ways that the
clinician can support the family.

In addition to the well-known variability
in the expression and course of TS (1), there
is equally great variability in the family and
social environment in which the child grows
up. Historically, children with tics and odd
behavior have been more likely to encounter stigma and punishment than understanding, a fate most often unrecorded, but occasionally described in the lives of famous
individuals, like the Roman Emperor Claudius, whose handicap, including multiple
tics, might well have resulted in death in
childhood had he not been a son of the impe-
rial household. Even as a prince, he grew
up amid scorn and verbal abuse (3).

The persistence of such conditions in
modern times is illustrated by reports like
one a few years ago from Saudi Arabia, of
a girl with motor and verbal tics, including
coprolalia, from a family described as very
religious (4). Physically abused by older
brothers at home, she was teased at school,
called "lizard," and made to stand before
the class for her coprolalic tics, even when,
terrified, she wet herself; eventually she
was excluded from school and confined at
home.

Nowadays there are children whose families recognize they have a medically treatable disorder and whose physicians prescribe
medication, but whose families remain unaware of the children's associated behavior
and learning problems and the high toll
taken in self-esteem and social adjustment
(5). In a recent report from Halifax, school
children ranked their peers' social standing;

of the children with Tourette's, 35% were ranked the least popular in their classes—a rank not predicted by the severity of their tics (6).

At the most fortunate end of the continuum, obviously, are those families able to provide, with their physicians and other treaters, comprehensive services including assessments, special services, and pharmacology, who can advocate for their children, and who understand the need to balance the needs of the child with TS with the needs of others in the family.

Such responses are influenced both by the level of scientific understanding and clinical practice available in a community and by processes within the family, processes that can be described on the family level, just as the child's development of a stable, cohesive, effective, and loved self can be described in the individual.

THE TASKS OF THE FAMILY

The family of the child with TS faces a series of tasks, occurring in a certain sequence but with a good deal of overlap.

The first phase is prediagnosis, when tics begin and are noticed or not noticed, or when the children's greater difficulty in managing themselves (problems with impulsivity and affect regulation) makes them stand out from peers.

Diagnosis, the next stage, constitutes an injury, or the confirmation of an injury. With the wound fresh, parents may seek repeated consultations in visits to centers far and wide, so-called doctor-shopping or second-opinion shopping in pursuit of what has been lost, the "way we thought things would be."

The next stage is that of wound healing. This can only start when the doctor-shopping stops, since healing requires that the broken part be still, that the parents feel psychologically "held" by one clinician—usually a physician—and a family can't be held while on the move seeking new

opinions. Clinicians provide more than a diagnosis and information. Equally important, they sit with and receive the parents' hurt, their grief, their anger (including the necessary reproaches against physicians), and their guilt. With the children, clinicians listen and then speak in a voice that is knowledgable about the disorder and its treatment; at the same time they size up the child's overall development and model for the parents an attitude that considers the child, though a patient, still a child, and a growing child at that.

In the phase of adaptation, families of children with "dys-volitional" disorders—that is, disorders that make them do things they don't "want" to do—face a special task, a variant on the need of every family to help a child learn to take responsibility. The family of the child with TS has to help the child live with ambiguities of volition and with problems in impulse control and emotional regulation quite unexpected by both child and parent (7). Learning and attention problems, and difficulties in becoming organized—the kind of difficulties that lie behind the peer problems reported from Halifax—can cause child and parents more trouble than the tics themselves.

HOW TO UNDERSTAND THE FAMILY

What *language* to choose for clinical inquiry and discourse? Despite the wish to reduce what is mysterious and hard to control to one-factor models, clinicians are well advised to steer clear of reductionistic phrases like, "It's this," or "It's that," and to speak rather of *all* the factors that contribute to a problem. In contrast to the one-factor psychological models that prevailed for many years, contemporary knowledge describes TS as a neuropsychiatric disorder, genetically determined but variable in expression, with a course varying both spontaneously and in response to stress (1). This model can inform clinicians' language. Children who are trying to make something of themselves, to preserve self-esteem and a sense of efficacy while experiencing tics, and the families that are trying to support the children, are well served by language that is both circumspect and inclusive.

To understand the experience of the family, clinicians can draw on several models. The model of *stress* considers the burdens of TS like the burdens of other chronic illnesses. The model of *grieving* identifies for the family and child, as with any handicap, a necessary task of mourning—acknowledging, bearing, and sharing the pain. Mourning begins with diagnosis and recurs as the growing child encounters life's milestones—school entry, puberty, graduation, home leaving.

The model of *emotional adaptation* considers the vicissitudes of the emotions aroused by the phenomena of TS—impulse disinhibition, poorly differentiated excitement, and scatology—phenomena that have profound meaning to everyone. This model also addresses the feelings inevitable in a severe, chronic disorder with a genetic basis, including guilt, the blow to parental self-esteem, and the loss of faith that the child can manage as expected. Some parents have particular vulnerabilities; they have low self-esteem, or are unusually anxious about their progeny, or are diffusely anxious about dangers emanating from a world where things "just happen."

The model of *family functioning* examines the effects of the illness on the family's accustomed ways of loving and working, the so-called family system. The illness affects the couple's working together and activates buried rancor and wishes for what might have been. Today's models of genetic inheritance can induce guilt and stimulate blame-casting just like the psychogenic models of yesteryear.

The *functional* model examines the part within the family that the child's symptoms come to play, as well as the child's use of the parents, and of the silently acquired understanding of where he/she stands between them, in order to foster growing up.

An *adaptive* model examines the built-in need of child and parent to cope, to manage, to get on with growing and with life, and the irrepressible tendency of all human beings to make meaning out of events, and to master fate by assimilating events into existing meanings while sometimes taking in information to make new meanings.

When a child is caught in the middle, and says, "Look, Ma, Dad is frustrating me. If I start to feel tense, I'll have a tic," the clinician can approach the child and parent with one eye on the child's ambivalence about taking responsibility, as well as the excitement that can be felt in the oedipal triangle, and the other eye on the marital schism, and the ambivalence about control, in which the excitement grows.

And then, what can the clinician do?

WHAT THE CLINICIAN DOES

No conditions require clinicians to carry out a broader range of professional activities than does TS. These functions, most often provided by physicians, will often be met as well by psychiatric nurses, social workers, psychologists, or special educators.

1. Clinicians diagnose the disorder, provide information, and help parents begin to live with this change in their lives.
2. They absorb parents' anger, hear their guilt.
3. They help parents break the doctor-shopping habit, to get some relief from the cycle of increasing disappointment–anger–guilt that goes along with the habit, with no relief while it continues.
4. They help parents to assess their learning needs, and give them information as requested and as indicated.
5. They coordinate the variety of evaluations needed by the child—special education, psychological, reading.
6. After the evaluations, clinicians help

parents make sense of the findings and decide what to do with the recommendations.

7. They help parents in decisions about pharmacotherapy. When parents are active in the Tourette Syndrome Association, and otherwise keep up to date on scientific progress, clinicians help them sort out the latest developments and bear the painful waiting until the next drug, the "really good one," is available for their child.

8. They help parents struggle with the ambiguities of personal responsibility, when the child protests "it just happened" or "I couldn't stop it, it's a tic", and to develop criteria that work for them and for the child, to find a way both to acknowledge that something is "out of control" and to help the child grow in responsibility.

9. They help parents identify and find words to express, or other ways to manage, the tensions that arise.

10. They provide, or arrange with colleagues to provide, a range of psychosocial therapies: family support, family or couples or individual therapy for specific problems, tension management, and other behavioral interventions.

11. They help parents advocate for the child and for themselves—with other clinicians, and with schools, camps, and insurance carriers.

12. They respond to crises: with listening, with special appointments, with psychological intervention, with medication, or with hospitalization, as needed.

13. They help parents keep an eye on the child's overall growth, including self-esteem, self-confidence, and ability to feel safe, to be active, and to make friends away from home.

14. They help parents strike a balance between the needs of the affected child and the needs of the rest of the family—including their needs as a couple.

15. Throughout, they support a positive view of child and parents—they are interested in the family's strengths, the things they like about themselves, their accomplishments and foibles—as a necessary counterpoint to all of their experiences with TS.

These are some of the factors that form the tapestry of life with TS, and some of the ways that clinicians help families recognize the patterns and help to weave them into a fabric supportive of their child and the others in the family.

REFERENCES

1. Cohen DJ, Leckman JF, Riddle M. Tourette's syndrome and tic disorders. In: Noshpitz J, et al, eds. *Basic handbook of child psychiatry*. New York: Basic Books, 1992.
2. Cohen DJ. Finding meaning in one's self and others: clinical studies of children with autism and Tourette's syndrome. In: Kessel F, Bornstein M, Sameroff A, eds. *Contemporary constructions of the child: essays in honor of William Kessen*. Hillsdale, NJ: Lawrence Erlbaum Associates, 1991.
3. Graves R. *I, Claudius*. New York: Random House, 1932.
4. El-Assra A. A case of Gilles de la Tourette Syndrome in Saudi Arabia. *Br J Psychiatry* 1987; 51:397–8.
5. Silver AA. Intrapsychic processes and adjustment in Tourette's syndrome. In: Cohen DJ, Bruun RD, Leckman JF, eds. *Tourette's syndrome and tic disorders: clinical understanding and treatment*. New York: John Wiley & Sons, 1988;197–206.
6. Stokes A, Bawden HN, Camfield PR, et al. Peer problems in Tourette's disorder. *Pediatrics* 1991; 87:936–42.
7. Bruun RD, Cohen DJ, Leckman JF. *Guide to the diagnosis and treatment of Tourette syndrome*. Bayside, NY: Tourette Syndrome Association, 1990.

Advances in Neurology, Vol. 58, edited by T. N. Chase, A. J. Friedhoff, and D. J. Cohen. Raven Press, Ltd., New York © 1992.

39

Social Adaptation of Tourette Syndrome Families in Japan

Yoshiko Nomura, Michiko Kita, and Masaya Segawa

Segawa Neurological Clinic for Children, Tokyo, 101, Japan

Tourette syndrome (TS) is a neuropsychobehavioral disorder occurring during the process of development that is modified by environmental factors. It is useful to explore features of TS in different sociocultural conditions to examine the role of environmental factors. This approach would not only help to understand aspects of pathophysiology but also may lead to new effective interventions for helping individuals with TS adapt to their disorder.

Ten years ago at the first International Symposium on TS (1), we presented clinical studies on 100 cases of TS in Japan. We noted that the clinical characteristics of TS in Japan are essentially the same as in western countries. The only differences we reported were a greater male predominance and a reduced frequency of coprolalia. Because of the mildness of most of our cases of coprolalia, which may reflect cultural differences in the expression of strong emotions, we suggested that the symptom in Japan might better be referred to as quasicoprolalia.

Over the last decade, we have continued to study the clinical features, social functioning, and adaptation of patients with TS and their families in Japan. Our goals are to clarify the socioenvironmental factors that might influence the clinical features of TS and to use this knowledge to help to improve medical and environmental management.

THE JAPAN TS SURVEY

To evaluate the social status of individuals with TS, a survey by questionnaire was conducted. Seventy-one individuals with TS above age 12 years and 106 family members, mostly parents of TS patients, who consecutively visited our clinic during January 1991–April 1991, were involved in this study. Before the questionnaire was administered, the purpose of the study was explained to the patients and family members. Their willingness to enter the study was confirmed.

The patients were divided into three groups (I–III) by age and clinical status. Group I consisted of 53 patients (46 men and 7 women) attending either middle school or high school. Their ages ranged between 12 and 18 years except for two (aged 23 years) who were attending college. Group II consisted of 15 patients (12 men and 3 women) who were above 18 years of age and were employed either full-time or part-time. Group III was composed of 3 unemployed men; their ages ranged from 24 to 26 years.

The 106 family members consisted of 93 mothers, 12 fathers, and one aunt who is a

TABLE 1. *Questions on individual profile*

1. Do you think your problem is a disease?
   1. Yes
   2. No
2. Do you feel troubled by your tic symptoms?
   1. Yes
   2. No
3. Do other people point at your symptoms (tics)?
   1. Yes
   2. No
4. Do you feel hurt when other people point at your symptoms?
   1. Very much
   2. Slightly
   3. No
5. Do people treat you unfairly?
   1. Yes
   2. No
6. What is the reason for the unfair treatment?
   1. Tics and OCD
   2. Others

guardian of a patient. There were seven pairs of parents. We tried to recruit both patients and their parents to enter the study; in some cases the patient was not able to participate in the study. Also, fathers were generally not available for the study.

The questionnaire consisted of two parts. The first part contained questions about the current social status of the patient, past visits to medical and related professionals, and their diagnosis or impression. We also inquired about the patient's own view of TS,

(e.g., if it is a disease or not, if one is inconvenienced by the symptoms, how others relate to the TS, etc.) (see Table 1). The second part of the survey was modified from Social Adjustment Scale II (2) and consisted of a series of questions about the patient's life style in regard to school or work, relationship with friends and family members, and personal life in the preceding two weeks. The life style questions were multiple choice, graded to 5 (see Table 2). The total number of questions ranged from 30 to 37 depending on the social status of the patient in groups I–III.

SOCIAL AND PERSONAL ADAPTATION

The results of the questionnaire were summarized according to the patient's social status (groups I, II, and III) and family members. Fifty-six % of group I, 85% of group II, 100% of group III, and 78% of family members believed that TS symptoms are a disease. Older patients answered affirmatively more than younger patients. However, there were no differences in the rate of affirmative answers among family members according to age or social status of the patients.

About 60% of groups I and II, and all of

TABLE 2. *Questions on individual life style[a]*

Choose one that is applicable to your life for the past 2 weeks

A. School (work) life[b]

Question (Q)	1. How many days were you absent from school (work)?
Answer (A)	1. None
	2. 1–3 days
	3. About half the time
	4. More than half but attended at least one day
	5. All (2 weeks)
Q	2. Did you do well at school (work)?
A	1. Very well
	2. Fairly well, but there was a small problem
	3. Did not do well about half the time and needed help
	4. Did not do well most of the time
	5. Did not do well all the time
Q	3. Was there any embarrassing thing at school (at work)?
A	1. None
	2. Yes, once or twice
	3. Yes, there was sometimes
	4. Yes, most of the time, felt embarrassed
	5. Yes, all the time

TABLE 2. *Continued.*

A. School (work) life[b] (*Continued*)

Q 4. Did you have trouble with somebody at school (work)?
A 1. None
2. Did fairly well except on a few occasions
3. More than a few times
4. Often
5. Always

Q 5. Was there any worry or problem in class (work)?
A 1. None
2. Once or twice
3. About half the time
4. Most of the time
5. All the time

Q 6. Did you enjoy class (work)?
A 1. Always
2. Most of the time
3. Moderately
4. Did not enjoy most of the time
5. Did not enjoy at all

B. Relationship with friends

Q 7. Have you met or talked with friends in the past 2 weeks?
A 1. More than 9 friends
2. 5–8 friends
3. 2–4 friends
4. 1 friend
5. None

Q 8. Were you able to talk to at least one friend about your feelings or your problems?
A 1. Always
2. Most of the time
3. About half the time
4. On most occasions was not able to speak of one's own feelings
5. Not at all

Q 9. How many times did you go out with friends, for example, visiting them, playing sports, going to restaurants, going to movies with them, or inviting them to your home?
A 1. More than four times
2. Three times
3. Twice
4. Once
5. None

Q 10. Did you have trouble with your friends?
A 1. None
2. Did well most of the time except on a few occasions
3. More than a few occasions
4. Often
5. Always

Q 11. Were you hurt by friends, if so how severely?
A 1. There was no such occasion or if there was, it had no effect on me
2. It took 2 or 3 hours to overcome
3. It took 2 or 3 days to overcome
4. It took 1 week to overcome
5. It may take several months to overcome

C. About oneself

Q 12. How much time did you spend on hobbies, for example, going to the movies, on sports, reading, or club activities?
A 1. Almost every day; most of the free time was spent on hobbies
2. Some days, most of the free time was spent on hobbies
3. Part of the free time was spent on hobbies
4. Did not spend any free time on hobbies or watching TV

(*Continued*)

TABLE 2. *Continued.*

C. About oneself (*Continued*)

Q 13. Did you feel nervous being with people?
A   1. Not at all, and always felt relaxed
    2. Felt nervous sometimes but soon felt relaxed
    3. Felt nervous about half the time
    4. Felt nervous most of the time
    5. Always felt nervous

Q 14. Have you felt lonesome and wished to be with friends?
A   1. Not at all
    2. On a few occasions
    3. Half the time
    4. Most of the time
    5. Always

Q 15. Have you felt bored during your free time?
A   1. Not at all
    2. On a few occasions
    3. Half of the time
    4. Most of the time
    5. Always

D. Relationship with the family

Q 16. Do you think you have discouraged or treated your family unfairly?
A   1. Not at all
    2. On a few occasions
    3. Half the time
    4. Most of the time
    5. Always

Q 17. Do you think you were discouraged or treated unfairly by your family?
A   1. Not at all
    2. On a few occasions
    3. Half the time
    4. Most of the time
    5. Always and felt hurt very much

Q 18. Have you had trouble with your family?
A   1. Not at all, always did well
    2. Did fairly well except for a few small troubles
    3. More than two troubles with at least one member of the family
    4. Very often
    5. Always

Q 19. Were you able to speak of your feelings or problems with at least one member of your family?
A   1. Always
    2. On most occasions
    3. Half the time
    4. Not most of the time
    5. Not at all

Q 20. Did you avoid your family?
A   1. Not at all
    2. Sometimes
    3. Waited for my family to approach me
    4. Avoided them, but they approached me
    5. Did not have any contact with them

Q 21. Did you feel need for help, advice, or moral support from your family?
A   1. Not at all
    2. Not most of the time
    3. Half the time
    4. Most of the time
    5. Always

Q 22. Have you objected to your family strongly, to the point of making them angry?
A   1. Not at all
    2. Once or twice
    3. Half the time
    4. Most of the time
    5. Always

Q 23. Were you worried about your family more than necessary?
A   1. Not at all
    2. Once or twice
    3. Half the time
    4. Most of the time
    5. Always

[a] The same questions were given to the family, asking "if the patient . . ."
[b] This question is not applicable to unemployed patients.

group III, experienced inconveniences because of TS symptoms.

The ratio of affirmative answers to the question if others pointed at their TS symptoms went up from group I (62%) to groups II (80%) and III (100%). About 65% of family members believed that others pointed at the TS patient. An increasing number of patients from groups I (50%), II (67%), and group III (100%) felt hurt when others pointed at the TS symptoms, with 85% of families feeling that such experiences were emotionally upsetting for the patient. Yet only about 6% of the younger group (group I) and 36% of group II felt they were treated unfairly. All of group III felt they were treated unfairly. Twenty-six percent of family members felt the patient was treated unfairly. The patients and family members who answered "yes" to the previous question were asked if the reason for the unfair treatment was due to the TS symptoms, to obsessive–compulsive disorder (OCD), or to other causes. Most felt the treatment was the result of TS and OCD (group I, 50%; II, 86%; and III, 100%). Most of the family members (96%) felt the cause of the unfair treatment was due to the TS and OCD.

LIFE STYLE

Groups I and II were asked about conditions at school and work (see Table 2, Q1 to 6). The results of four questions are presented in Fig. 1: if one was absent from school or work, if one did well at school or at work. Most of the patients attended school or work. The feeling of accomplishment at school or work differed slightly, but overall, patients felt they had done fairly well. Also, the majority of patients did not have major trouble with other people at school or work.

The patients' relationship with friends are summarized in Fig. 2, which plots the following questions, from top to bottom: if one has seen or talked by phone with friends, if one has gone out with friends to enjoy one-

self, and if one felt hurt by friends. The group I patients seemed to have seen or talked with friends more than the other two groups. More than half of both groups I and II went out with friends for enjoyment. Group III patients associated much less with friends. To the question if one was hurt by friends, the majority of groups I and II answered similarly that they were not. In group III, one patient reported not being hurt, one was hurt, and one patient did not answer.

Questions about oneself are summarized in Fig. 3, including, from top to bottom: if one spent time on hobbies, if one felt lonely, and if one felt bored. More patients in group I spent time on hobbies, group III patients did not do so, and group II patients were in between. The feeling of loneliness was most noticeable in group III, less in group II, and least in group I. Groups I and II felt bored in a moderate degree, and group III felt bored most of the time.

Patients' relationships with family members are summarized in Fig. 4, from top to bottom: if one had trouble with the family, if one could depend on the family, and if one was able to speak frankly to the family about feelings. The majority of groups I and II showed similar features, that is, they did fairly well with their families and could depend on them. Group III's answers revealed negative features. The answers to the question if one is able to speak frankly to the family showed that groups I and II responded variously, and group III was mostly unable to speak to the family.

The answers of the family members to these three questions tended to be different from the patients. They felt there were more problems than groups I and II, but not to the extent of group III.

CASE HISTORIES

The following case histories exemplify patients followed at the Segawa Clinic.

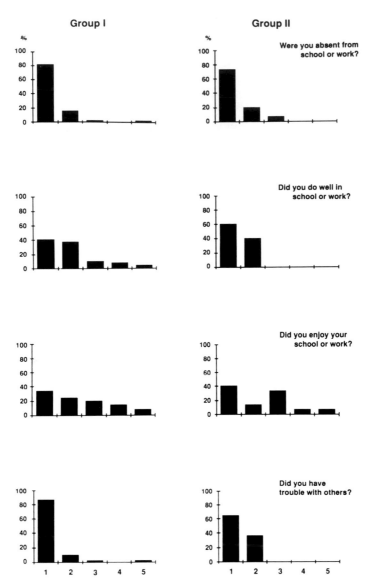

FIG. 1. Status at work or school. *Abscissa:* 1–5 represents the grade of answers in Table 2 part A. *Ordinate:* applicable patients by percentage. *Group I,* school age; *group II:* employed.

Mr. A., 25-Year-Old Man

Family history:
  Father—tics and stuttering
  Sister—school refusal

Past history
  2 y—epilepsy started
  5 y—traffic accident

Present illness:

Infancy—tended to put fingers into mouth and shake body
5 y—stuttering, head nodding
6 y—facial grimacing, blinking, hand shaking, tongue protrusion, spitting, speaking to himself
8 y—jumping while walking, vocal tics, "ah"
9 y—coprolalia
10 y—raising arms and shaking hips

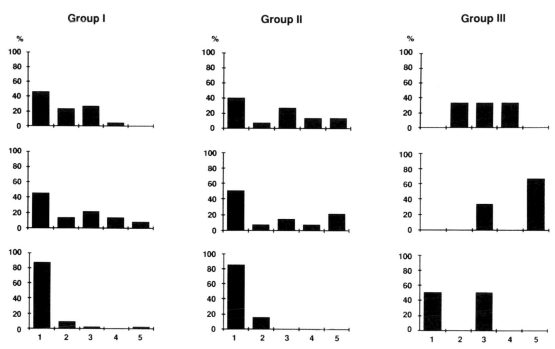

FIG. 2. Relationship with friends. *Abscissa:* 1–5 represents the grade of answers in Table 2 part B. *Ordinate:* applicable patients by percentage. *Group I*, school age; *group II*, employed; *group III*, unemployed.

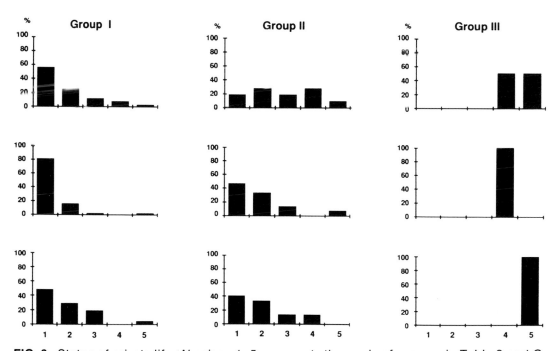

FIG. 3. Status of private life. *Abscissa:* 1–5 represents the grade of answers in Table 2 part C. *Ordinate:* applicable patients by percentage. *Group I*, school age; *group II*, employed; *group III:* unemployed.

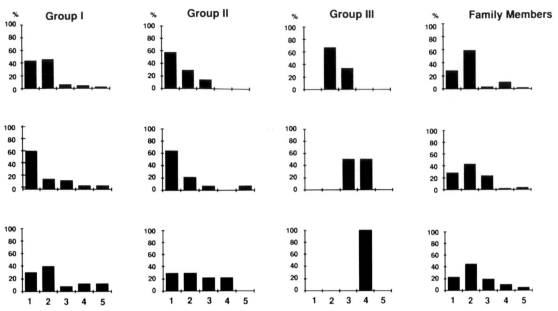

FIG. 4. Relationship with family. *Abscissa:* 1–5 represents the grade of answers in Table 2 part D. *Ordinate:* applicable patients by percentage. *Group I*, school age; *group II*, employed: *group III*, unemployed.

12 y—tongue protrusion

13 y—spitting

14 y—first visit to Segawa Clinic: severe multiple motor tics, vocal tics, coprolalia, restlessness, OCD tics gradually improved by treatment

Social aspects:

14 y—family problems due to the TS symptoms of this patient

15 y—hospitalized for 7 months when mother died, because family could not manage

16 y—high school (night); part-time work during the day

20 y—began working; lives in his own apartment

Mr. Y., 22-Year-Old Man

Family history:

No tics, sister with hypochondria

Neonatal period:

Neonatal jaundice, moderate

Past history:

6–7 y—suffered head trauma twice

Present illness:

6 y—blinking

10 y—shaking neck, jumping, licking lips, multiple tics, vocal tics, tics wax and wane and worsened

21 y—first visit to Segawa Clinic; multiple motor and vocal tics, severe OCD

Social aspects:

18 y—graduated from high school

18 y—preparatory school

19 y—entered college; absence from school for 1 y due to severe tics

20 y—restarted college; lives by himself

Mr. I., 27-Year-Old Man

Family history:

No tics, no OCD

Present illness:

4–5 y—opening and closing legs

6 y—eye blinking, facial grimacing, neck shaking

7 y—tics spread to arms and legs, stuttering

10 y—vocal tics, "ah"

13 y—coprolalia

14 y—put stimulating ointment into eyes, hit eyes

15 y—"traumatic cataracts" operated on, tics wax and wane, hit eyes

19 y—retinal detachment

22 y—throwing objects

23 y—coprolalia, split, tapping legs, hitting ears

24 y—first visit to Segawa Clinic; severe multiple motor tics, vocal tics, coprolalia severe OCD

Social aspects:

Primary school—often refused

Middle school—graduated from the regular class

Unable to enter high school

Stayed at home

Rehabilitation center—attended for a short period, unable to continue

Vocational aid center—attended for a short period, unable to continue

These three patients all suffer from severe symptoms of TS and OCD. Mr. A. has been improving markedly and has adjusted fairly well to work; Mr. Y. goes to college, and Mr. I. is the most seriously affected and has difficulties in all aspects of life.

ADAPTATION TO TS IN JAPAN

The awareness of TS in the Japanese medical and lay society is limited, and mild cases often remain unrecognized. Simple tics are considered mostly as habits or of psychological origin and are not brought to medical attention. Furthermore, when tics are diagnosed, the mother's way of bringing up the child is often blamed, and both the child and mother are sent to a psychologist for counseling. Adequate judgment and management are often lacking. It is rather rare that patients with tics are brought to medical specialists, except some of the most severely affected cases of TS, who are usually under the care of psychiatrists. We have done the first study on social aspects of TS patients in Japan.

The severity of TS symptoms was similar among groups I and II, and was most severe with group III. The ratio of understanding TS as a disease went up with age. Almost two-thirds of TS patients in groups I and II, and all of group III patients experienced inconveniences in daily life because of TS symptoms. With increasing age, patients with TS experienced increased frequency of having their tics pointed out by other people. This increase with age may also reflect the increasing severity of tics with age. Mild tics among younger children are often regarded as part of normal behavior. On the other hand, the symptoms of group III are most severe, and the social status of being unemployed because of severe TS symptoms cause more emotional burden. Older patients felt they were not treated fairly. This may reflect increasing severity of symptoms with age and the increased social visibility with work and advanced schooling.

Many factors other than TS influence the life style of individuals. It would not be possible to judge all the features of social adaptation of TS from our survey alone; however, it seems to give some idea of the daily life style of TS patients in Japan. The majority of patients are able to attend and do well at school or work, but they do not seem to enjoy school or work as much. Some patients had severe symptoms of TS, which hindered attendance at school or work. On the other hand, some patients with the most severe TS are attending school in spite of the symptoms and are trying to cope with their problems.

Relationships with friends seem to be fair for groups I and II, but many TS patients seem unable to make close friendships. There were some patients in group II who did not associate much with friends because of TS symptoms. The social state of being employed and lacking the opportunity of enjoying friendship might be present. Relationships with friends were markedly damaged for group III.

This feeling of being hurt by friends was minimal in all groups. This was an unexpected finding, particularly in group III, whose symptoms of TS were most severe. This finding appears to contradict the fact that the symptoms of TS were pointed out more frequently among severely affected patients. This discordance may reflect a Japanese characteristic: people do not talk about other peoples' physical or mental matters among acquaintances but they may do so among unknown people.

The features of private life also seem to reflect the severity of TS symptoms. Less severe cases or younger patients lead an ordinary life, in contrast to the severe cases, who did not spend time at hobbies and were isolated, feeling lonely and bored.

All groups experienced difficulties with their families. There were some differences between the patient groups and family members in different aspects of the family relationship; family members seemed to have felt more difficulty than the patients themselves. Troubles within families may relate to the feeling of guilt on the part of family members, who erroneously interpret the tics as the result of an aberrant way of raising the child.

In summary, aspects of the life style and social adaptation of TS patients in Japan seem to reflect mostly the severity of the symptoms. Our previous study (1) suggested that the clinical characteristics of TS in Japan were essentially the same as those of western countries. However, comparison of the severity of TS symptoms between the two cultures is still not defined.

One of the characteristics of Japanese society is its homogenous nature, in many aspects including the value of sense in the life style. TS patients as a whole seem to blend into society, but in a rather passive way. Efforts to publicize an understanding of this disorder are still lacking, yet, as was seen in the case histories, even the severest cases can be managed when diagnosed early and approached by a multidisciplinary team at an early stage of the disorder. It is likely that early and adequate intervention can modify not only the development and progression of the disease process but also the behavioral aspects and social interactions of the individual.

REFERENCES

1. Nomura Y, Segawa M. Tourette syndrome in oriental children: clinical and pathophysiological considerations. In: Friedhoff AJ, Chase TN, eds. *Advances in neurology*, vol 35, *Gilles de la Tourette syndrome*. New York: Raven Press, 1982;277–280.
2. Schooler NR, Hogarty GE, Weissman MM. Social Adjustment Scale II (SAS). In: Hargreaves WA, Attkinson CC, Sorensen JE, eds. *Resource materials for community mental health program evaluation*, 2nd ed. Washington, DC: U.S. Department of Health, Education and Welfare; Public Health Service, Alcohol, Drug Abuse and Mental Administration, 1977.

Advances in Neurology, Vol. 58, edited by T. N. Chase, A. J. Friedhoff, and D. J. Cohen. Raven Press, Ltd., New York © 1992.

40

Behavior Therapy for Obsessive–Compulsive Disorder and Trichotillomania

Implications for Tourette Syndrome

Lee Baer

Department of Psychiatry, Harvard Medical School, and Director of Research, OCD Clinic and Research Unit, Massachusetts General Hospital, Boston, Massachusetts 02114

Behavior therapy is a directive form of psychotherapy that uses principles of learning to change specific problem behaviors. In obsessive–compulsive disorder (OCD), its goal is to teach the patient how to alter his or her compulsive rituals directly. The behavior therapy techniques consistently found effective in reducing compulsive behaviors (and related obsessive thoughts) are exposure to the feared situation, and response prevention, in which the patient is then helped to resist the urge to perform a compulsion to reduce discomfort (1).

The procedure of exposure and response prevention is straightforward in the case of a patient with compulsive handwashing and showering related to contamination fears of cancer "germs." In this case exposure consists of gradually bringing the patient into contact with objects believed to be contaminated, such as a magazine or chair in the waiting area of an outpatient cancer clinic. The OCD patient is then encouraged to remain in contact with the "contaminated" object for as long as possible (Exposure), and next to refrain from handwashing or showering for a period of time afterward (Response Prevention).

The procedures of exposure and response prevention are implicitly based on the learning process of habituation, or extinction, of an emotional response; that is, if a person is actively prevented from engaging in escape behaviors from a feared situation, then the aversive emotion reaction will habituate, or extinguish, on its own (1).

Although less obvious, the same principles of exposure and response prevention apply to patients with other kinds of compulsive rituals. For example, a patient who retraces his path while driving to ensure that he has not struck a pedestrian is accompanied for a ride by the therapist or family member; while driving, the patient is encouraged to engage in the feared behaviors, such as driving on a bumpy road, or passing

---

Parts of this chapter have been adapted from: Jenike MA, Baer L. Obsessive–compulsive disorder: Treatment with behavior therapy. *Psychiatric Times*, August, 1988, and from Baer L, Osgood-Hynes D, Minichiello WE. Trichotillomania, in Ammerman RT, Last CG, Hersen M, eds. *Handbook of Prescriptive Treatments for Children and Adolescents*. Needham Heights, MA: Allyn & Bacon. (In press)

pedestrians in the road (Exposure), while resisting the urge to turn the car around to check that no one has been injured (Response Prevention).

Behavior therapy produces its largest changes in behavioral rituals, such as compulsive cleaning or checking as described above, whereas changes in obsessive thoughts are less predictable. This is in contrast to traditional psychotherapy, in which any changes are mainly in obsessional thoughts, with little effect seen in rituals (2). This difference reflects the specific effects of behavioral treatment, in which behaviors themselves are the targets of treatment. Consequently behavior therapy is now regarded as the treatment of choice when behavioral rituals predominate. For patients in whom obsessive thoughts predominate (i.e., no or few rituals) pharmacotherapy is the therapy of choice. In many cases a combination of behavioral and drug treatments is most efficient (3).

HISTORY OF BEHAVIORAL TREATMENTS FOR OCD

A century ago Janet (4) gave a remarkably accurate description of what is now termed exposure therapy, including the name itself:

> The guide, the therapist, will specify to the patient the action as precisely as possible. He will analyse it into its elements if it should be necessary to give the patient's mind an immediate and proximate aim. By continually repeating the order to perform the action, that is, exposure, he will help the patient greatly by words of encouragement at every sign of success, however insignificant, for encouragement will make the patient realize these little successes and will stimulate him with the hopes aroused by glimpses of greater successes in the future. Other patients need strictures and even threats and one patient told 'Unless I am continually being forced to do things that need a great deal of effort I shall never get better. You must keep a strict hand over me.'

This outline of the behavioral treatment of OCD remains accurate today, and expo-

sure therapy as described by Janet remains the major behavioral treatment of OCD almost a century later. Yet, despite the fact that behavioral techniques were successfully employed a century or more ago, it was not until the late 1960s that these techniques were widely and effectively employed in the treatment of this disorder. The reason lies with the impact of the new psychoanalytic theory at the turn of this century; soon after Janet described exposure therapy, Freud published his analysis of the patient known as the Rat Man, and interest turned toward the meaning of obsessions and compulsions, and away from considering the compulsive behaviors as treatment targets in and of themselves.

Although the presentation of many OCD patients appears to coincide with psychodynamic themes, and psychodynamic formulations have descriptive value, they have not yielded reliable techniques for modifying obsessions and compulsions (2).

COMMON MISCONCEPTIONS ABOUT BEHAVIOR THERAPY FOR OCD

We have found that some patients with OCD are not given behavior therapy because of long-standing misconceptions about this form of treatment. Corrections of the most common misconceptions [1] follow: (a) behavior therapy does not lead to the formation of substitute symptoms, (b) interrupting compulsive rituals is not in any way dangerous to the patient, (c) the patient's thoughts and feelings are not ignored in behavior therapy, (d) behavior therapy no longer assumes that all maladaptive behavior is learned through simple conditioning processes, (e) the use of medication is not incompatible with behavior therapy, and (f) behavior therapists recognize that their methods are not equally effective for all patients.

OUTCOME STUDIES IN OCD

Controlled outcome studies of exposure and response prevention for OCD over the past 15 years, involving more than 200 patients in various countries, have found that 60–70% of patients with ritualistic behaviors were much improved after behavioral treatment (3,4). Approximately 20–30% of the patients were resistant to the treatment, and the dropout rate averaged 20%. Treatment was carried out over a relatively short period averaging 3–7 weeks, with a ten-session treatment program most common. At follow-up of 2 years or more, improvements in rituals were maintained in most patients. The majority of patients included in these studies have been adults, and had mainly cleaning and checking rituals; patients with only obsessive thoughts, without ritualistic activity, have been studied separately, with less predictable results (3).

There have as yet been no controlled studies of behavior therapy specifically for other types of OCD rituals and obsessions, such as hoarding, slowness, counting, repeating, superstitions, symmetry or ordering; anecdotal experience indicates that behavior therapy is also helpful in these disorders. There are no controlled trials of behavior therapy for OCD in children or adolescents, although case reports (see ref. 1 for review) indicate that if the family is involved, the outcome can be equal to that with adult patients.

The use of the following cognitive techniques in the treatment of obsessions and compulsions is less predictable than the treatments of exposure plus response prevention: Although the technique of thought-stopping is widely used to treat obsessive thoughts, clear empirical support for its usefulness remains lacking. Because OCD patients engage in obvious cognitive errors in inference and assessing the probability of danger, the application of cognitive therapy techniques to change these cognitive processes directly would seem to be useful. However, the only controlled study in this area found that cognitive therapy did not add significantly to the therapeutic effects of exposure in vivo (3).

In summary, although obsessive and compulsive symptoms are usually greatly reduced with behavioral treatment, and interference with occupational and social functioning is reduced, ritualistic behavior is rarely totally eliminated. Marks (4) has observed:

> Although most patients who are cooperative (and those are the great majority) improve with exposure in vivo, few of them are totally cured. Patients are generally told that they need to acquire a coping set to deal with tendencies to ritualize that might recur after discharge. Occasionally brief booster treatment is needed, but this is minimal apart from explicit advice about regular homework, which may be needed for many months after discharge.

PREDICTORS OF TREATMENT FAILURE IN OCD

Despite these advances, certain patients still do not respond to treatment. Predictors of failure in behavior therapy are noncompliance with treatment, concomitant severe depression, absence of rituals, fixed beliefs in rituals, presence of concomitant personality disorder, and type of compulsive ritual (3,5). Patients with schizotypal and possibly other severe personality disorders [axis II in *Diagnostic and Statistical Manual*, 3rd ed, revised (DSM-III-R)] may also do poorly with pharmacotherapy. These poor predictors are considered below.

Poor Compliance

Outcome studies indicate that poor compliance with a behavioral treatment program is the most common reason for treatment failure (4). Behavior therapy is more demanding of patients than many other forms of psychotherapy, and the patient must comply with behavioral instructions, both during treatment sessions and also during "homework" assignments. If the patient is inconsistent in doing this, treatment is unlikely to be successful. The aid of a family member or friend in carrying out homework assignments is often critical to ensure compliance. In addition, the concomitant use of antidepressant medication often increases patients' compliance with exposure treatments. We are currently investigating new methods of improving compliance with behavioral treatment, including use of a portable computer, which assists the patient in carrying out homework assignments.

Severe Depression

Severe depression has also been found in most studies to be a negative predictor for improvement with behavior therapy of OCD. In patients with severe depression (e.g., neurovegetative signs), the behavioral processes of physiological habituation to the feared stimuli do not occur, regardless of the length of exposure. Patients with severe depression often respond well to behavior therapy procedures after depression is controlled with medication.

No Rituals

If a patient has only obsessive thoughts without rituals, behavior therapy is less likely to succeed. For example, some patients experience disturbing intrusive sexual or aggressive thoughts that prevent normal social functioning, but they do not engage in behavioral rituals. In these cases pharmacotherapy is the treatment of first choice.

Overvalued Ideas

Patients who strongly hold the belief that their compulsive rituals are necessary to forestall future catastrophes [i.e., "overvalued ideas" (6)] have been found to have a poorer outcome with behavioral treatments. For example, a patient who truly believes that a family member will die if he does not wash his entire house every day is unlikely to give up the rituals with behavior therapy

alone. In some cases we have found treatment with antidepressant medication produces changes in a patient's fixed beliefs, and behavior therapy may then be successful in eliminating rituals.

Schizotypal Personality and OCD

As noted above, our preliminary data indicates that patients meeting DSM-III-R criteria for both OCD and schizotypal personality disorder do not respond well to either behavior therapy or pharmacotherapy. The idea of concomitant schizotypal personality disorder as a poor prognostic indicator in OCD appears valid in light of the other literature on treatment failure, since this personality disorder encompasses several of the poor predictive factors reviewed above. Most noticeably, these patients have strongly held beliefs that their rituals are necessary to prevent some terrible event. Also, these patients have a difficult time complying with treatment and assigned record-keeping. Rachman and Hodgson (7) have similarly found that the presence of an "abnormal personality" is a negative predictor of outcome in behavior therapy for OCD. More recently, Solyom et al. (8) have reported on a subcategory of patients with "obsessional psychosis" similar to our schizotypal subgroup, who also respond poorly to both behavior therapy and pharmacotherapy.

Checking Rituals

Patients with contamination fears and cleaning rituals appear to respond best to behavioral treatment, while patients with checking rituals and primary obsessional slowness do not respond as rapidly or completely. Several characteristics of patients with checking rituals may explain this difference: (a) they may check hundreds of times per day, (b) they frequently check only in their home when alone, making exposure and response prevention difficult, and (b) they are typically afraid of catastrophic events that will never occur, such as a death or disaster to which they cannot be exposed in real life. As a result Foa et al. (9) found that treatment of checking rituals may require a combination of exposure to feared events in imagination, plus response prevention.

BEHAVIOR THERAPY FOR TRICHOTILLOMANIA

Trichotillomania is a disorder of chronic hairpulling that predominantly affects females, usually beginning in the teenage years, resulting in alopecia (10). The major clinical features of trichotillomania include pulling of hair from the scalp, eyebrows, and eyelashes (which may be totally or partially lost), usually symmetrically, and occasionally pulling of pubic hair and other bodily hair (11). It is common for the self-inflicted nature of the hair loss to be denied, with the rate as high as 84% in one sample of 19 patients (12).

Trichotillomania is categorized in the DSM-III-R as an impulse control disorder, with the following diagnostic criteria:

1. Recurrent failure to resist impulses to pull out one's own hair, resulting in noticeable hair loss
2. Increasing sense of tension immediately before pulling out the hair
3. Gratification or a sense of relief when pulling out the hair
4. No association with a preexisting inflammation of one's skin, and not a response to a delusion or hallucination

Although there has been increased discussion recently regarding the similarities between trichotillomania and OCD (which is classified as an anxiety disorder in DSM-III-R) in their response to clomipramine (13), trichotillomania is likely to remain as a distinct disorder, remaining classified under impulse control disorders in DSM-IV (MA Jenike, personal communication, 1991).

There are at least two important differences between OCD rituals (which sometimes also involve grooming) and trichotillomania: First, patients with OCD usually can provide a logical explanation of why they are washing excessively, or engaging in excessive grooming rituals (e.g., to prevent contamination, to prevent social ridicule, or to forestall catastrophic events). Patients with trichotillomania, however, rarely justify their hairpulling; it is described solely as a tension-reducing behavior (14).

Second, and more importantly for treatment, as noted above, if patients with OCD are prevented from engaging in their rituals, their urges to perform these rituals gradually decrease, or extinguish. Conversely, patients with trichotillomania often find that their urge to pull their hair often increases if the habit is blocked, as with the use of gloves or a scarf. One of our patients described a feeling of "electricity in her body that kept building up and up," until she discharged it with a bout of hairpulling. In this respect, trichotillomania can be seen as intermediate between an OCD grooming ritual and a complex motor tic (in which an uncomfortable sensation may sometimes precede or provoke tics) (15). Because of this difference between OCD and trichotillomania, standard exposure and response prevention methods have not proved sufficient in eliminating hairpulling (10). As a result, a behavior therapy method developed by Azrin and Nunn (16) for the treatment of complex motor tics, habit reversal, has been applied to trichotillomania, along with a variety of other behavioral techniques.

Our review of the adult literature (10) found six single case reports of successful treatment (e.g., usually complete control of hairpulling) with a variety of behavioral methods: thought-stopping; self-monitoring, including saving the pulled hairs and bringing them to the therapist weekly; increasing awareness of the habit and use of a competing response (e.g., grasping an object or fist-tightening) to the urge; relaxation training and systematic desensitization to the situations that elicit hairpulling; increasing awareness of the habit; and coping self-instructions (reviewed in ref. 10). In addition to these successful adult single case reports, the literature contains three multiple case comparisons of the method of habit reversal for adult hairpullers, with elimination of hairpulling in as little as one treatment session (10).

Although these findings suggest at least the short-term efficacy of behavior therapy for adult hairpullers, what are their implications for the treatment of children and adolescents with trichotillomania? Among the group studied by Rosenbaum and Allyon (17) was a 10-year-old girl, who, like the adults, responded rapidly to the habit reversal method, and maintained complete control of the habit at 12-month follow-up. Similarly, among Azrin et al.'s (18) group were a 14-year-old adolescent boy and two 14- and one 17-year-old adolescent girls; like the adults in this report, all four adolescents showed complete control of their hairpulling after habit control training, and maintained these gains at 4-week follow-up. Although these authors report that 67% of subjects followed at 22 months maintained no hairpulling, no details are provided about the ages of these patients.

Adding to the evidence for the efficacy of behavior therapy (especially habit reversal) for child and adolescent trichotillomania are a number of successful single case reports that have recently appeared in the literature. These reports have used a variety of behavioral methods (10).

Habit reversal has been the most studied effective behavior therapy method for trichotillomania, and its multimodal approach encompasses most of the effective behavioral interventions for hairpulling. The 13 major components of habit reversal, as specified by Azrin et al. (18), are: (a) competing response training—the subject learns the competing and preferably inconspicuous response of grasping or clenching the hands for 3 minutes whenever hairpulling has occurred or is likely to occur; (b)

awareness training—the subject learns to be aware of the specific movements involved in hairpulling; this is helped by observing herself in a mirror; (c) identifying response precursors—a common response that is a precursor to hairpulling is face touching or hair straightening; (d) identifying habit prone situations—the subject learns to identify which situations lead to hairpulling, such as watching TV, studying, or being alone; (e) relaxation training; (f) prevention training—the subject practices the competing reaction for 3 minutes, grasping or clenching whenever nervousness, a response precursor, or a habit-prone situation exists; (g) habit interruption—the subject practices using the competing grasping or clenching reaction to interrupt the hairpulling immediately; (h) positive attention/overcorrection—the subject practices positive hair care, such as combing or brushing the hair, after each episode of pulling; (i) daily practice of competing reaction—the subject practices the competing response before a mirror at home; (j) self-recording—the subject records each instance of hairpulling and each compulsion to hairpulling to provide greater awareness and give feedback for progress in hairpulling; (k) display of improvement—the subject seeks out those situations previously avoided; (l) social support—a significant other is taught how to encourage and remind, in a positive manner, the person to stop pulling hair; and (m) annoyance review—the subject lists and discusses the various problems caused by hairpulling, serving to increase motivation for treatment and to identify sources of reinforcement for controlling hairpulling. In our clinical practice, our focus is primarily on elements a and b.

IMPLICATIONS FOR USE OF BEHAVIOR THERAPY IN TOURETTE SYNDROME

Many patients with Tourette syndrome (TS) also have obsessions and compulsions, both adults (19) and children (20). Although there are as yet no controlled trials of exposure and response prevention for these comorbid problems, our anecdotal clinical experience is that patients with TS can reduce their comorbid obsessions and compulsions with behavior therapy. Because there is preliminary evidence that the type of obsessions and compulsions present in combination with tic disorders differs from those in OCD patients without tic disorders (21), the response of these comorbid symptoms to behavior therapy awaits controlled investigation.

In addition, since alternate behavioral techniques such as habit reversal have helped control trichotillomania, an impulse control disorder that shares phenomenological features with complex motor tics [e.g., tension-reducing, semivoluntary, not performed in response to an obsession (10)], there has been much interest in the role of behavioral therapy in the direct treatment of the tics of TS. A variety of behavior therapy techniques have been applied to TS in case study reports: massed negative practice, contingency management, relaxation training habit reversal, and self-monitoring. However, only habit reversal has been shown to be effective in a semicontrolled trial with more than three subjects (22). Azrin and Peterson (22) used a waiting list control group comparison of two groups of five patients with TS and demonstrated a 93% reduction in tic frequency during 8–11 months of treatment (22). These findings with habit reversal have yet to be replicated or applied to larger patient samples. In our clinical experience in the OCD Unit at Massachusetts General Hospital, we have had less success in applying habit reversal to patients with TS, apparently due to poor compliance with practice, which appears to be related to strong urges to tic [described by Bliss (23) as an almost intolerable urge requiring gratification]; although the components of the habit reversal technique reduce this urge sufficiently for some patients to comply with this self-control method, it may

not be sufficient for all. As a result, we are currently investigating the combined effect of habit reversal and clonazepam in the treatment of TS and other chronic motor tics. Our clinical model is OCD, in which the combination of behavior therapy and anticompulsive medications such as clomipramine can enhance outcome in patients with very strong urges to ritualize (1).

In summary, behavior therapy, consisting of exposure to the feared situation (Exposure), and prevention of the ritual (Response Prevention) is highly effective in the treatment of OCD rituals, either used alone, or in combination with anticompulsive medications. In the treatment of trichotillomania, the behavior therapy method of habit reversal has been found effective in controlled clinical trials. Habit reversal includes techniques to decrease actively the tension produced by resisting the hair pulling. Since many patients with TS also have OCD rituals, exposure and response prevention may be effective in providing relief for these comorbid problems; our limited clinical experience suggests this is so. In addition, habit reversal methods, as used in trichotillomania, may provide a method for directly controlling the complex motor and vocal tics of TS, either alone or in combination with medications.

REFERENCES

1. Baer L, Minichiello WE. Behavior therapy for obsessive-compulsive disorder. In: Jenike MA, Baer L, Minichiello WE, eds. *Obsessive-compulsive disorders: theory and management*, 2nd ed. Chicago: Year Book Medical Publishers, 1990;203–32.
2. Jenike MA. Psychotherapy of obsessive-compulsive personality disorder. In: Jenike MA, Baer L, Minichiello WE, eds. *Obsessive-compulsive disorders: theory and management*, 2nd ed. Chicago: Year Book Medical Publishers, 1990;295–305.
3. Baer L, Minichiello WE. Behavioral treatment (BT) for obsessive-compulsive disorder. In: Noyes R, Roth M, Burrows GD, eds. *Handbook of anxiety*, vol 4: *The treatment of anxiety*. Amsterdam: Elsevier Science Publishers, 1990;363–87.
4. Marks IM. Review of behavioral psychotherapy. I: Obsessive-compulsive disorders. *Am J Psychiatry* 1981;138:584–92.
5. Jenike MA. Predictors of treatment failure. In:

Jenike MA, Baer L, Minichiello WE, eds. *Obsessive-compulsive disorders: theory and management*, 2nd ed. Chicago: Year Book Medical Publishers, 1990;306–11.

6. Foa EB. Failure in treating obsessive-compulsives. *Behav Res Ther* 1979;17:169–76.
7. Rachman SJ, Hodgson RJ. *Obsessions and compulsions*. Englewood Cliffs, NJ: Prentice-Hall, 1980.
8. Solyom L, DiNicola VF, Phil M, et al. Is there an obsessive psychosis? Aetiological and prognostic factors of an atypical form of obsessive compulsive neurosis. *Can J Psychiatry* 1985;30:372–80.
9. Foa EB, Steketee G, Milby JB. Differential effects of exposure and response prevention in obsessive compulsive washers. *J Clin Consult Psychol* 1980;48:71–9.
10. Baer L, Osgood-Hynes D, Minichiello WE. Trichotillomania. In Ammerman RT, Last CG, Hersen M, eds. *Handbook of prescriptive treatments for children and adolescents*. Needham Heights, MA: Allyn & Bacon (in press).
11. Muller SA. Trichotillomania. *Dermatol Clin* 1987;5:595–601.
12. Greenberg HR, Sarner CA. Trichotillomania. *Arch Gen Psychiatry* 1965;12:482–9.
13. Swedo SE, Leonard HL, Rapoport JL, Lenane MC, Goldberger EL, Cheslow DL. A double-blind comparison of clomipramine and desipramine in the treatment of trichotillomania (hair-pulling). *N Engl J Med* 1989;321:497–501.
14. Christenson GA, Mackenzie TB, Mitchell JE.

Characteristics of 60 adult chronic hair pullers. *Am J Psychiatry* 1991;148:365–70.
15. Singer HS, Walkup JT. Tourette syndrome and other tic disorders: diagnosis, pathophysiology, and treatment. *Medicine* 1991;70:15–32.
16. Azrin NH, Nunn RG. Habit reversal: a method of eliminating nervous habits and tics. *Behav Res Ther* 1973;11:619–28.
17. Rosenbaum MS, Allyon T. The habit reversal technique in treating trichotillomania. *Behav Ther* 1981;12:473–81.
18. Azrin NH, Nunn RG, Frantz SE. Treatment of hair-pulling (trichotillomania): a comparative study of habit reversal and negative practice training. *J Behav Ther Exp Psychiatry* 1980;11:13–20.
19. Pitman RK, Green RC, Jenike MA, Mesulam MM. Clinical comparison of Tourette's disorder and obsessive-compulsive disorder. *Am J Psychiatry* 1987;144:1166–71.
20. Grad LR, Pelcovitz D, Olson M, Matthews M, Grad GJ. Obsessive-compulsive symptomatology in children with Tourette's syndrome. *J Am Acad Child Adolesc Psychiatry* 1987;26:69–73.
21. Holzer JC, Price L, McDougle CJ, Boyarsky BK, Goodman WK. Symptoms in OCD with and without a tic disorder. Paper presented at American Psychiatric Association Meeting, May, 1991.
22. Azrin NH, Peterson AL. Treatment of Tourette syndrome by habit reversal: a waiting list control group comparison. *Behav Ther* 1990;21:305–18.
23. Bliss J. Sensory experiences of Gilles de la Tourette syndrome. *Arch Gen Psychiatry* 1980;37:1343–7.

Advances in Neurology, Vol. 58, edited
by T. N. Chase, A. J. Friedhoff, and
D. J. Cohen. Raven Press, Ltd.,
New York © 1992.

41

Tourette Syndrome

Extending Basic Research to Clinical Care

Donald J. Cohen, Arnold J. Friedhoff, James F. Leckman, and
Thomas N. Chase

*Child Study Center, Yale University School of Medicine, New Haven,
Connecticut 06510*

From a relatively obscure status three decades ago at the junction between neurology and psychiatry, Tourette syndrome (TS) has emerged as a model neuropsychiatric disorder that is diagnosed throughout the world and is the object of intense scientific investigation. TS is now recognized to be among the more common, childhood onset, genetically transmitted behavioral disorders. In addition, methods and findings from studies of TS are relevant to the understanding of other psychiatric disorders. A major factor in the increasing awareness and study of TS has been the work of the Tourette Syndrome Association (TSA) in educating clinicians, informing the public, advocating, providing research funding, and convening investigators in forums such as (1980 see ref. 1) and 1991 International Scientific Symposiums on TS.

In 1980, there was a paucity of research directly bearing on the biology, genetics, and treatment of TS, but there was marked optimism for the future. At that time, the first population-based genetic studies had only recently appeared; treatment response to haloperidol and studies of cerebrospinal fluid (CSF) metabolites had implicated monoaminergic systems, and there was a good deal of speculation suggesting involvement of basal ganglia and other brain regions in the pathogenesis. In many ways, this optimism was well warranted, as suggested by the reports in this current volume using methods and technologies that had not been utilized one decade ago, e.g., sophisticated genetic analyses, brain imaging techniques, and neurochemical analyses of brain tissue. Along with new data, however, complexities and controversy have appeared. In many areas of TS research, including some that seemed clear a decade ago, we are faced with open questions and conflicting findings indicative of the vitality and the scientific challenges for the field.

PHENOMENOLOGY

The broader recognition of TS and related tic disorders in afflicted individuals and family members has been coupled with a renewed interest in defining both the clinical phenotype and the spectrum of these disorders. Since the first publications by Georges Gilles de la Tourette more than a century ago, there has been broad agreement on characteristic features of TS: multiple, ever-changing, spasmodic, rapid "tic" movements and sounds; distinctive motor and linguistic phenomena (complex movements, echopraxia, echolalia, coprolalia, etc.); and mental or psychological symptoms (obsessions, compulsions, "disinhibition"). Individuals fitting the vivid descriptions provided by Gilles de la Tourette may be seen today, providing testimony to his clinical acumen and to the relative stability and reliable diagnosis of the syndrome across ethnic and national boundaries and over an epoch of major social change. Moreover, Tourette's early suggestion of constitutional and familial contributions has been more than amply documented during the past decade with data supporting a genetically transmitted, neurobiological vulnerability.

Based on accumulated clinical experience, and particularly the pioneering work of Arthur and Elaine Shapiro (2,3), in 1980 the Diagnostic and Statistical Manual of the American Psychiatric Association (DSM-III) provided clinical criteria for TS that continue to guide research and clinical diagnosis. These included an age of onset during childhood and up through late adolescence (age 15); recurrent, rapid, involuntary, purposeless motor movements affecting multiple muscle groups; multiple vocal tics; ability to suppress movements voluntarily for minutes to hours; variations in the intensity of the symptoms over weeks to months (waxing and waning); and a duration of more than 1 year (see Jancovic, *this volume*). The revision of DSM-III (DSM-III-R) in 1987 extended the age of onset to age 21 and reduced the number of vocal tics from "multiple" to "one or more." It thus became "easier" to have TS in 1987 than 1980.

There is an enormous variety among the phenomena that are lumped together as tics: rapid, rhythmic, "involuntary" movements of individual muscles; tensing of muscle groups; paroxysms of movements; meaningless, little sounds; and explosive, meaningful utterances. These differences are conveyed by such distinctions as "simple" versus "complex" tics, but boundaries are blurred, and one video is worth a thousand words. Also, it is sometimes hard to define

the border between tics (especially complex tics, such as hopping, jumping, or orchestrated movements of several body parts) and other compulsive actions (such as hair pulling, mannerisms, nail biting, or the stereotypic actions or self-injuries of patients with pervasive disorders).

The criteria provided in the Diagnostic and Statistical Manuals serve as a useful guide to diagnosis; yet, as with virtually all disorders in DSM-III-R, judgment is needed when applying the criteria in specific cases. Further, the diagnostic criteria are essentially a summary of current clinical consensus or convention. Changes should be anticipated with new knowledge.

Diagnostic Criteria

During the past several years, clinical experience and rigorous research have confirmed and augmented the core features of TS (see ref. 4 and Bruun and Budman, *this volume*). The study of relatives of patients and the diagnosis of TS by more physicians have helped shape the current concept that there is a tremendous range of severity or impairment associated with TS, from inconsequential to debilitating, from harmless "motor habits" to self-mutilating and life-threatening acts. Because of broadened experience we no longer feel that TS is always severe, terribly impairing, or lifelong. However, this raises the question of just how mild the symptoms can be and still deserve the specific diagnosis.

By the strict letter of current criteria, any individual with two motor tics and one vocal tic, over more than 1 year, may be diagnosed as having TS. The least afflicted patients may have only a few tics—"nervous habits"—when they are tired or tense and they may be completely unaware of having any problem. For them, a diagnostic label such as "Tourette syndrome" may overstate their symptoms and burden them unnecessarily with a diagnosis that may arouse worries. Yet, the field remains without agreement about how to define impairment and, indeed, whether substantial impairment should be required for diagnosis. The Tourette Syndrome Association has organized a work group to help clarify research criteria, but clinical diagnostic issues remain in need of further study. Surely, if severity and impairment are not considered in conferring a diagnosis, and only a few tics are required, many times the number of individuals would be diagnosed as having TS than would be considered as *clinical cases* of a tic disorder. In family genetic studies, such individuals are often identified. The provision of a diagnosis to nonimpaired individuals may be useful for certain research purposes but unsuitable in the context of clinical care. On the other side, the most severely afflicted TS patient may have disruptive bouts of 30–100 tics/min and medleys of maddening obsessions and compulsions; he or she may be unable to function in the mainstream of society. For such a patient, the diagnostic label TS may fail to convey the extent of handicap adequately (see Robertson, *this volume*).

Research on Phenomenology

Four areas of phenomenology have been of special interest to clinical researchers.

First, it is now appreciated that many adult patients, and perhaps the majority, experience subtle but distinctive, premonitory tensions or sensations that precede some motor and phonic tics. For these patients, the tic behavior (movement or sound) may feel like a capitulation to an ineradicable urge and symptoms may thus occur in a psychological domain between "volitional" and "involuntary" (see Lang, *this volume* and Leckman et al., *this volume*). The sensory aspects of tics, and attempts at their control, shape the individual's internal experience of the disorder and the sense of disturbed self-regulation (5,6).

The second elaboration of the clinical portrait of TS involves the increased appreciation of obsessional and compulsive symptoms and obsessive–compulsive disorder (OCD) as aspects of TS (see Cath et al. *this volume*, and Leonard et al., *this volume*). Many patients, particularly adults with the disorder, may be more burdened by these or other psychiatric or behavioral difficulties than by the tics as such (see Kerbeshian and Burd, *this volume*). Indeed, in the majority of cases, some of the most troublesome tics wane during adolescence and adulthood, and most patients improve. Yet for those with the most severe difficulties, the non-tic symptoms may be the greatest source of impairment.

The third area of investigation involves the delineation of the close linkages among disorders that are treated as separate categories in the classification system of DSM-III-R and in textbooks (e.g., chronic motor tic versus TS). Associations among these disorders are revealed by the natural history of many patients, e.g., children may first have several episodes of transient tics, over the course of months or years, and then move on to TS. They are also revealed by the finding of genetic continuities, e.g., there is an increased prevalence of chronic motor tics and OCD in families of individuals with TS. There is broad consensus that recurrent episodes of transient tics, chronic motor or vocal tics, persistent motor and vocal tics (TS), and OCD are closely related clinical phenomena. In some families, they seem to reflect separate manifestations of the same underlying genetic vulnerability. In isolated cases, however, we do not yet know when recurrent episodes of transient tics, chronic motor tics, or OCD are associated with or will be followed by full-blown TS.

Fourth, there has been increasing study of the factors that influence the development and social functioning of individuals with TS (7). While there is some degree of correlation between the severity of core tic symptoms and overall clinical impairment, the relation between these domains is not as tight as might be expected. Remarkably, individuals with relatively minor tic symptoms may sometimes have serious social difficulties, while others with more severe symptomatology may be less impaired. The development of individuals with TS appears to be influenced by various factors: the attitudes, behavior, and emotional climate of the family; interactions with peers and teachers; the disruptiveness of tics; other aspects of the TS diathesis (such as dysfunctions involving attention and other neurocognitive processes); and modes of psychological defense and adaptation to the intrusions of tic phenomena into consciousness and behavior.

Comorbidity

Within clinic populations, up to 50% of patients with TS have behavioral difficulties that satisfy the diagnostic criteria for other psychiatric conditions, including attention deficit hyperactivity disorder (ADHD), learning disorders, anxiety disorders, personality disorders, affective disorders, and, as noted above, OCD. There are various pathways that may lead to *comorbidity*—the apparent association between two conditions in the same individual or in a group of patients.

Developmental and Emotional Sequelae

Any chronic, medical illness (such as cystic fibrosis) may make an individual vulnerable to other psychiatric problems (such as depression).

Medical Consequences

One condition may be the result of or a "complication" of another disease, e.g., retinitis and peripheral neuropathy (disorders in their own right) are complications of diabetes.

Sampling or Ascertainment Bias

A patient with more than one disorder (such as a child with a learning disability + severe conduct disorder or an adult with obesity + hypertension) is more likely to come for treatment than an individual with only one condition (such as obesity alone). Similarly, a visible or disruptive problem (such as a severe behavioral difficulty) is likely to bring a patient for treatment; at the time of evaluation, a second, less noticeable problem (such as a mild tic) may be detected that otherwise would have escaped notice. Finally, individuals with the worst overall problems—such as life-threatening asthma—are more likely to come to medical attention than those with milder problems, such as exercise-induced bronchospasm. The sicker individuals are more likely to have other problems, including diagnosable disorders.

Thus, for various reasons, complicated, multi-problem patients are over-represented in clinic samples as compared with community surveys. This type of phenomenon was described by Berkson in 1946 (8) and is often referred to as *ascertainment bias*.

Pleiotropic or Variant Manifestations

Two distinctive conditions may be manifestations of the same pathophysiological process, expressed in different systems or organs. For examples, endocarditis and arthritis are variant manifestations of rheumatic fever; kidney disease and central nervous system (CNS) vasculitis are variants of lupus. In a disorder with variant manifestations, such as AB syndrome, disorder B is not a consequence of A nor simply something that is more likely to bring a patient with A to medical attention; also, a patient with AB syndrome may present with either A or B or with both A + B.

Tic disorders are found to be associated with other conditions (such as OCD or

ADHD) at a far higher rate than chance and there appears to be intrinsic connections between the etiology of TS and these other conditions. Patients can be found with either tics or OCD alone, or with both tics + OCD. It has been argued that tics and OCD can be considered to be variant expressions of the same underlying diathesis.

The relation between tics and ADHD is somewhat less clear. In some respects, the symptoms of ADHD are similar to nonspecific medical symptoms such as "malaise," "lethargy," "fatigue," and "weight loss." Symptoms such as these may bring a child for evaluation and serve as a starting point for a process that may lead to a specific psychiatric diagnosis, such as depression, or a medical diagnosis, such as mononucleosis. At times, though, nothing more specific is found. The symptoms may then be labeled a disorder in their own right, e.g., "chronic fatigue syndrome."

Analogously, the cluster of symptoms found in ADHD—overactivity, inattentiveness—occur with high frequency in normal populations. In community surveys, up to one-third of all mothers will endorse at least some of the symptoms for their sons, e.g., that they are easily distracted. These ADHD symptoms, just like fatigue, may be the starting point of a process leading to a more specific diagnosis, such as mania, schizophrenia, fragile X syndrome, or a neurological disease, or the ADHD symptoms may stand on their own. When these symptoms are found in association with TS, they may be a prodrome or consequence of the underlying TS diathesis or an additional, associated disorder. It is still a matter of scientific study whether or how often ADHD, when found in isolation, may represent a variant manifestation of TS.

Defining the Phenotype

It is intuitively obvious why clinicians may see patients with the most serious tic problems and with more than one domain of difficulty: these individuals are more likely to be impaired, to be noticed, and to be brought or to come for care. To sort out the different types of deeper relations among comorbid conditions, however, is an interesting and important area of clinical and preclinical research.

We are still unsure about the homogeneity of even "classically defined" TS populations. The more that is learned about other medical conditions, the clearer it becomes that (a) different genotypes (underlying processes) may lead to the same phenotype (clinical syndrome) and that (b) a single genotype may have varying phenotypic expressions.

Phenocopies

When a genetic disorder is mimicked by another condition whose clinical expression is identical or similar to it but whose mode of transmission is different, the mimic is called a phenocopy of the disorder of interest. We do not know how many phenocopies there are of TS, nor what proportion of diagnosed TS cases represent phenocopies. If experience with other genetic disorders holds true, it is probable that there is more than one type of TS and at least some phenocopies. For example, tics are quite common among schoolchildren, with up to 8% of all children having tics at some time in their lives. With such a high "base" or "population" rate, it seems likely that there are varied etiologies for tic disorders in addition to TS. Similarly, given the breadth of the diagnostic category, it would not be surprising to find more than one "cause" of TS. Similar conclusions are suggested for OCD, which may be diagnosed in perhaps 3–4% of all adolescents and adults. In general medicine, we rely on laboratory tests to clarify the differential diagnosis of clinically indistinguishable forms of infections, joint diseases, and the like. To date, there is no laboratory test for "authentic" TS, no way to separate the "real disorder" from possible, but not proven, counterfeits.

Range and Severity of Expression

A genetic disorder may be expressed in many organ systems, in different parts of the same organ, or with different severity. Not every patient with muscular dystrophy or Down syndrome, for example, has identical problems, although they may have the same genetic abnormality. Similarly, infectious agents (such as streptococcus) may cause different types of illnesses, from minor skin infections to life-threatening septicemia. Thus, we should anticipate that the underlying vulnerability to TS, even if it is a single gene, may be expressed in a variety of tic and behavioral symptoms.

One hypothesis for the range of symptoms in TS is that the genetic vulnerability—the TS "gene"—is manifested as dysregulation of the parallel cortico-striato-thalamo-cortical circuits, which are involved in sensory, motor, emotive, and cognitive processes and their integration (see ref. 9 and Leckman et al., *this volume*). If the disturbance in regulation involves a fundamental process such as neuromodulation or disinhibition within these circuits, one can envision a quite broad range of functional difficulties—short-circuits, cross-talk, reverberations, static, and echoes—that could lead to the medley and the ever-changing nature of symptoms seen in TS. The range and severity of expression of TS may also be influenced by the age of onset, by other genes that modify the expression of the vulnerability to TS, and by other types of "host factors" that make one individual relatively more susceptible or resistant than another. As we will suggest, the status of the dopaminergic system may be one type of "host factor" that influences the severity of TS.

New strategies of investigation may help define the boundaries of the TS diagnostic category and reveal underlying associations among apparently quite disparate conditions (see Comings and Comings, *this volume*). We may find new ways of subdividing "typical" TS into more biologically or behaviorally discrete conditions, which would help us understand the differences among patients in severity, impairment, natural history, or response to medication. The strategies that may be useful include genetic and twin studies, brain imaging, pharmacological probes, and neuropsychological measures (see Reader and Denckla, *this volume*). Brain-imaging methods are already beginning to focus on regions involved in the parallel brain circuits proposed by Leckman et al. (9) as being possibly involved in TS. The study of unaffected, young offspring and first-degree relatives of TS patients will clarify the developmental and social context for the emergence of tics and associated symptoms during childhood and the progression of symptoms over time, in specific environments. Similarly, the long-term follow-up of patients, on and off of medication, will help define those patients who are at highest risk for continued difficulty and those with more self-limited conditions.

Because of the interaction between severity, types of symptoms, and use of varied treatments, the study of the natural history of TS is complicated and will require large numbers of patients and families. An important issue is the way in which comorbid conditions (ADHD, OCD, learning difficulties, adjustment problems) affect the severity of tic symptoms over time and the ultimate adult outcome. Also, there is a remarkable paucity of hard information on the short- and long-term impact of medication, of behavioral and psychological interventions, and of family functioning and psychosocial supports. Thus, many issues that are critical for making clinical decisions remain in need of study. In this area of work there is a dialectical process between diagnostic concepts and other types of research. Findings from basic research are likely to alter the definition of the phenotype and its core features; in turn, diagnostic clarification will shape other types of research. Also, it is essential to keep in mind the interactions between biological preconditions and vulnerabilities, on the one hand, and environmental influences, on the other. For disorders which have their onset early in development, the ultimate shape of the illness and the functioning of the individual are most likely the result of multiple, interacting processes (10).

GENETICS

Probably the most dramatic advances in understanding TS during the past decade have come from studies of genetic transmission (see Pauls, *this volume*). The familial nature of TS was first observed in 1885 by Gilles de la Tourette himself. However, it was not until the late 1970s that studies demonstrated an increased frequency of a positive family history of tics in the families of TS patients. Subsequent work in the United States and elsewhere has replicated those observations and has shown that the risk to relatives is significantly elevated over what would be expected by chance (see Heutinck et al., *this volume*).

After the first reports in the late 1970s and early 1980s, a number of studies tested specific genetic hypotheses regarding the inheritance of TS and chronic, multiple tic syndromes (CMT). Most studies reported that the pattern of inheritance within families is consistent with a genetic hypothesis postulating the existence of a single gene of major effect that conferred susceptibility to TS and/or CMT. In all but one study, the patterns of transmission are consistent with an autosomal dominant mode of inheritance. One group (see Comings and Comings, *this volume*) has hypothesized that the mode of inheritance for TS is not strictly dominant or recessive and has suggested that the inheritance of TS may best be described as "semi-dominant, semi-recessive." This hypothesis is based on a broader diagnostic convention and the inclusion of a wide range of other behaviors as manifestations of the genetic susceptibility for TS. More work is needed to help clarify the range of phenotypes that constitute the TS spectrum, and rigorous genetic studies will provide very useful information to help with this process.

Since published reports of genetic analyses suggest that TS and associated disorders are inherited as a single gene, genetic linkage studies have been warranted as the next step in clarifying the inheritance of this syndrome (see Devor, *this volume*). Genetic linkage investigations provide a powerful method for confirming the conclusions of segregation analysis, since linkage results can demonstrate the existence of a major locus and help clarify the pattern of inheritance even in the absence of a known association between a biological abnormality and TS. The Tourette Syndrome Association has organized an international collaborative network of researchers involved with the genetics of TS and similar disorders. This network has been pooling information on high-density and other families for linkage studies. Using restriction fragment length polymorphisms (RFLPs), over 80% of the human genome has already been searched for possible linkage with the vulnerability to TS. To date, no linkage has been defined.

Methodological Considerations

If no genetic linkage is discovered after the entire genome has been excluded, it will be necessary to challenge some of the basic assumptions underlying the genetic studies of TS, such as the diagnostic criteria, diagnostic assessment of probands and family members, mode of inheritance, structure of the high-density pedigrees, and statistical models.

Phenotypic Specificity

The success of genetic linkage studies is dependent upon an appropriate understanding of the range of phenotypic expressions of TS. If an individual without TS is diagnosed as having the syndrome (false-positive diagnosis), the statistical analyses involved in linkage studies are likely to lead to a negative conclusion even if there is a linkage. In the absence of laboratory tests, and with a reasonably high population rate for tics and associated problems, there is some likelihood of heterogeneity. If so, ongoing studies may be comprised methologically by individuals with phenocopies of TS being diagnosed as having TS. Thus, it is imperative that work continue that will lead to a better understanding of the spectrum of behaviors constituting the core symptoms of TS.

For the most conservative approach to linkage analysis, it would seem wisest to use strict, narrow diagnostic criteria. The heterogeneity of a sample would be reduced by further diagnostic specificity, such as substantial impairment, onset between 6 and 10 years, a typical progression or natural history, coprolalia, response to medication, etc.

There are trade-offs in the search for diagnostic purity. By increasing the apparent clinical homogeneity through stricter criteria, investigators will almost certainly reduce the number of individuals who can be considered to be "affected," that is, increasing diagnostic specificity comes at the cost of decreasing diagnostic sensitivity. When there are too few affected individuals in a family, linkage studies become more difficult or are precluded.

Also, requiring major disability as a criterion might not serve as a good method for reducing heterogeneity. An individual with tics might be burdened, in addition, by depression, obsessions, and social isolation, and thus have a high degree of "clinical caseness" and require treatment. Yet this individual might not be clearly or specifically affected with TS. Indeed, the higher the degree of comorbidity, the more one might wonder about specificity.

There is no unassailable gold standard for TS. The discovery of a laboratory test would thus add immeasurably to the performance of valid genetic linkage studies.

Prevalence

Another clinical area of relevance to linkage studies is the estimation of the prevalence of the syndrome. Linkage analysis is, essentially, a statistical approach to defining an association between a clinical manifestation (such as a tic syndrome) and a biological marker (such as a specific site on a chromosome). The Lod score is a measure of probability of chance association, similar to the significance level of a correlation. The statistical models for linkage analysis require specification of the frequency of the condition in the general population. Most genetic analyses have estimated that fullblown TS occurs in about 1 in every 1,500 individuals and that the gene occurs in one in every several hundred individuals (see Apter et al., *this volume*). Some investigators have recently suggested a frequency that is magnitudes higher. If the prevalence of the disorder is as high as 1 in every 30 or 40 individuals, as has been suggested, then genetic analyses need to be reevaluated (see Comings and Comings, *this volume*). More rigorous epidemiological studies will help to clarify these issues (see Fallon and Schwab-Stone, *this volume*, and Kurlan, *this volume*).

Family Structure

A third area of relevance to current linkage studies is the nature of the families being studied. These families with "high density" of several generations of tic disorders seem ideally suitable for linkage studies. However, they tend to come from geographically isolated communities. The high density of TS may reflect inbreeding or other factors. If there is transmission of the vulnerability to TS from both parents (bilineality), available methods are not suitable for detecting linkage.

Advances in Genetic Studies

At present, investigators are making use of newly developed techniques for linkage (see Wilkie et al., *this volume*). Over the next few years, methods will be coming on line that will provide more informative markers for linkage and also allow for more rapid screening of the human genome. Concurrently, investigators are reviewing the diagnostic methodologies that have been used in defining cases of TS. The convergence of greater diagnostic rigor and new molecular approaches leads to realistic optimism that the genetic locus for TS will be identified relatively soon. When this is accomplished, methods are already available for cloning the gene and defining the gene product. Usually the steps between localization of the gene and cloning are relatively straightforward, although there have been some disorders in which this has been a challenging and lengthy process.

The localization and availability of a gene or genes responsible for the expression of TS would, of course, be a major step forward in understanding the genetic/biological risk factors important for the expression of TS. The identification of a linked marker will permit the design of much more incisive studies to illuminate the physiological/biochemical etiology of TS by examination of the gene product and its impact on the manifestation of the syndrome. In addition, the identification of the gene(s) would allow the potential identification of nongenetic factors associated with the manifestation or the amelioration of the symptoms of the disorders. By controlling for genetic factors (e.g., by studying siblings with and without the gene) it will be possible to examine gene–environment interactions—the ways in which environmental and nongenetic factors affect the expression of the TS spectrum.

Genetic Counseling

The current status of genetic knowledge about TS already allows for clinical genetic counseling. Based on available knowledge about transmission and recurrence risk, individuals with TS, as well as their parents and siblings, can be given information about the risk of recurrence. Roughly speaking, if the mode of transmission is that of an autosomal dominant trait, one-half of all children born to a parent with TS are likely to inherit the same genetic vulnerability. Current estimates suggest that about 70% of individuals with the inherited vulnerability will have some degree of clinical expression or symptomatology. While the likelihood of transmission and expression is thus reasonably high, families can find some reassurance in two facts: first, there is a broad range of severity (from mild in most cases to severe in perhaps only 10% of affected individuals) and, second, the natural course is generally one of diminishing severity. Thus, even if a child is born with the vulnerability gene, it is far more likely than not that he or she will not have a seriously impairing case of TS. While the estimates are very broad, perhaps only 1 in 10–20 children in a vulnerable family is likely to develop very impairing TS. Another source of optimism is the rapid rate of advancement in knowledge and treatment of TS. The availability of molecular methods for diagnosis will improve the specificity of genetic counseling, but a great deal more will have to be learned about the biological and environmental factors that affect expression and severity.

NEUROCHEMISTRY AND NEUROENDOCRINOLOGY

Much of the neurochemical research on TS has focused on the monoamine neurotransmitters and the endogeneous opioid peptides. Among the monoamines studied are the catecholamines, norepinephrine (NE) and dopamine (DA), and the indoleamine, serotonin or 5-hydroxytryptamine (5-HT). Among the neuropeptides, the dynorphin family of endogenous opioids has received the most attention. Neuroendocrinological research is just beginning and has focused on the effects of sex hormones on brain function.

Monoamines

The catecholamines have been implicated in the pathogenesis of TS since the first reports of the efficacy of haloperidol, a DA-blocking compound, almost three decades ago (2,3). The hypothesis that TS represents a syndrome of dopaminergic oversensitivity with resultant disturbances involving inhibitory processes was the central, biologically heuristic hypothesis at the time of the first TS International Symposium (1). Over the past decade, monoamines have continued to be of great interest to investigators concerned with the pathobiology of TS and associated disorders. Intriguing findings have emerged from various lines of basic and pharmacological research.

As demonstrated by several decades of psychopharmacological research in animals and humans, DA, NE, and 5-HT play many important roles in brain–behavior relations and in the action of drugs that affect behavior. The beneficial effects of DA-blocking agents in the treatment of TS, the elicitation or worsening of tics in some children by stimulant medications, reductions in CSF homovanillic acid, (HVA), the major metabolite of DA in some TS patients, and the physiological role of dopaminergic systems in the basal ganglia and the regulation of movement highlight a pathophysiological role for increased dopaminergic activity in tic syndromes. An alternative proposal for the role of DA is that it is the neurotransmitter mediator of a compensatory system that serves a restitutive function in disturbances in which neuroleptic dopamine D_2 receptor antagonists are therapeutically effective (including TS, schizophrenia, bipolar illness, organic psychoses). Thus, individuals who may be carriers of a gene for TS but who also have a relatively "strong" compensatory system might be free of symptoms, while those with a less effective system would have clinical TS. This could lead to a large number of "false-negative" determinations of carriers of the TS gene (11,12).

Additional hypotheses have been put forth concerning the possibility of alterations in central 5-HT and NE in TS. An involvement for 5-HT has been suggested, theoretically, on the basis of the rich innervation of the basal ganglia by serotonergic fibers, 5-HT's general inhibitory role in DA neurotransmission, and the functioning of serotonin in sensory gating and inhibitory processes (e.g., pain and temperature perception). Most recently, the role of serotonergic mechanisms in TS and associated disorders has become of much greater interest with the demonstration of the therapeutic benefit in the treatment of OCD of medications that reduce serotonin reuptake. Consistent with a role for serotonin in TS has been the observation of reduced CSF 5-hydroxyindoleacetic acid (5-HIAA) the major 5-HT metabolite, in some patients with TS.

NE has been implicated in TS due to its major role in arousal, its modulation of behavioral systems such as the startle reflex, and the beneficial effects in TS (as well as in attentional disorders) of clonidine, a medication that reduces noradrenergic functioning (see below).

In addition to the theoretical considerations and drug-behavior findings, neurochemical research on TS has emphasized monoamines because of their implication in other psychiatric and neurological disorders (e.g., depression, Huntington's disorder, and Parkinson's disease), yet there are methodological difficulties involved in the study of monoamine systems in humans. Among these are the following: the measurement of monoamines, and their precursors and metabolites in peripheral fluids including CSF, can be expected to detect only robust or global changes in neurotransmitter metabolism; medications may lead to long-term alterations; it is difficult to obtain normal control samples, especially for children; and there is lack of clarity about the relations between monoamine metabolites and clinical state or trait. Also, the functional activity of specific neurotransmitter systems may be related as much to dimensions of behavior (such as inhibitory processes) as to a specific diagnostic category.

Although there are limitations to approaching central neurotransmitter functioning through peripheral measures, further study of CSF neurochemicals is clearly warranted. Studies of various compounds in the CSF need to be more carefully designed with respect to issues of diagnosis, comorbidity, and dimensions of behavior. They also need to be expanded to include the measurement of important neuropeptides such as arginine vasopressin, dynorphin, and enkephalin (see below).

Opioids

In recent years a number of approaches have been used to study endogenous opioid peptides in TS and related disorders. Endogeneous opioids such as dynorphin and met-enkephalin are highly concentrated in structures of the basal ganglia, are known to interact with central dopaminergic, serotonergic, and γ-aminobutyric acid (GABAergic neurons), and are likely to be involved in the gating of motor functions (see Lavoie et al., *this volume*). Pilot neuropathological (postmortem) studies (see Haber and Wolfer, *this volume*) found decreased levels of dynorphin A(1–17) immunoreactivity in striatal fibers projecting to the globus pallidus in some patients. In a preliminary study of a small group of TS patients, many of whom had prominent OC symptomatology, CSF levels of dynorphin A(1–8) were increased in comparison with controls and were significantly correlated with severity of OC symptoms (see ref. 13 and Chappell et al., *this volume*). This finding suggested that some aspects of the pathophysiology of TS might be associated with regional alterations in processing of the prodynorphin pro-

hormone. Additional evidence for a role for opioids in TS has been provided by clinical descriptions of the unmasking or exacerbation of TS symptoms after sudden withdrawal of chronic opiate therapy and by uncontrolled reports of dramatic, though inconsistent, effects of the opiate antagonists naloxone and naltrexone on tics and obsessive–compulsive symptoms (see Chappell et al., *this volume*).

A controlled trial of propoxyphene (Darvon) and naltrexone in TS subjects reported that naltrexone was associated with a statistically significant but mild improvement in tic severity and attentional ability, while propoxyphene had no effect (14). Pilot dose–response studies of the behavioral and neuroendocrine effects of both the opiate antagonist naloxone and the selective κ-opioid agonist spiradoline mesylate (U-62,066E, Upjohn Company) have been performed (see Chappell et al., *this volume*). Low doses of naloxone were associated with an increase in motor tics. Taken together, preliminary studies suggest a modulatory role of opioids in the pathobiology of TS.

Future studies are needed to replicate these preliminary findings and explore coordinated, functional alterations in multiple opioid systems. An array of additional challenge strategies should be developed utilizing receptor-selective opiate agonists and antagonists targeted at each subtype of opioid receptor localized to the basal ganglia (i.e., μ, κ, and δ). As further evidence for involvement of endogeneous opioids in TS accumulates, in vivo quantification of opioid receptors with positron emission tomography (PET) may be undertaken.

Neuroendocrinology

Neuroendocrine research may prove to be helpful in better understanding the clinical features and disease mechanisms of TS, as well as in devising novel treatment strategies for the disorder. For instance, the male predominance of TS has long been recognized but has been difficult to reconcile with the autosomal dominant models that are currently favored for its genetic transmission, since that mechanism should equally predispose males and females to the disorder. These sex-specific prevalence differences could derive from numerous potential nongenetic influences on the expression of the putative TS vulnerability gene. Sex-specific hormone differences are known modulators of both gene expression and nerve cell function, and are good candidates for the differential modulation of TS disease expression between the sexes.

Although this hypothesis of hormone-dependent variability in gene expression is attractive, the large number of sex-specific hormones and the complexity of the brain regions and neurochemical systems that are responsive to them make testing and elaboration of the hypothesis difficult. Moreover, structural features laid down in utero may cause the male and female CNS to respond differently to the same steroid hormone. In adult men, for instance, many of the "masculinizing" effects of androgens on behavior often are mediated by their conversion first to estrogens, which then act on brain regions that differ structurally and functionally from corresponding regions in female brains, ultimately causing different behavioral responses to the same class of hormones.

Despite these complexities, some clinical evidence supports the idea that gonadal hormones may influence symptom expression in TS. In particular, androgens appear likely to provoke TS symptoms. Case reports of symptom exacerbation in androgen-abusing athletes anecdotally implicate these agents in modulating disease expression (15). Additional case reports of symptom improvement in two men and a woman following androgen-receptor blockade with flutamide (Eulexin) also support the view that androgens are provocative in TS (16). Antiandrogen therapy has also appeared effective in several cases of OCD (17).

Further study will be required to define better which hormones, if any, are influencing TS symptom severity, and in which patient populations. Safely provoking and blocking the effects of androgens and estrogens in both men and women, and perhaps in boys and girls, will help to determine whether these agents have different effects on CNS functioning and TS symptoms of male and female and pre- and postpubertal individuals. These studies could play an important role in developing safer and more effective treatment modalities as well as in clarifying basic mechanisms of endocrine modification of gene expression.

Postmortem Studies

Neurochemical and anatomical studies of brains that are obtained following the deaths of patients with TS offer great promise for clarifying structural and neurochemical alterations in the pathobiology of TS. Specific, suggestive differences have already been seen in the small number of postmortem neurochemical studies that have been done to date. These preliminary findings (see Anderson et al., *this volume*, Haber and Wolfer, *this volume*, and Singer, *this volume*) concern possible alterations in basal ganglia 5-HT, subthalamic glutamate, striatal dopamine reuptake, and pallidal dynorphin. The data clearly warrant follow-up studies examining these particular neurochemical systems. In the future, the availability of increasingly sophisticated methodologies to apply to postmortem tissue will permit detailed examination of all potentially relevant neurotransmitter and neuroanatomical systems. Data from these direct studies on brain tissue will provide vital information for other approaches to studying living patients, including neuroimaging techniques focused on specific brain regions and neurochemical pathways.

Through the Tourette Syndrome Association, a brain-banking system has been put into place, including national dissemination of information about the importance of brain donations, methods for signing up individuals, and a central mechanism for collecting brains and then preparing and distributing samples. At present, however, only a small number of TS brains have become available for study. In the future, it will be important to try to obtain all available brains from patients with TS as well as from individuals who are likely to be carriers or genetically at risk (including grandparents, parents, and siblings). The optimal utilization of postmortem brain specimens also requires a far more rigorous approach to the retrospective collection of information about patients than has been available. The interpretation of neurochemical and structural data requires detailed knowledge of the natural history, medication usage, and associated problems of individuals whose brains become available for study.

BRAIN IMAGING

Sophisticated neuroimaging methodologies are now being used to provide preliminary answers to the question: How do changes in brain function affect the expression and severity of tic and obsessive–compulsive symptoms (see Demeter, *this volume*)?

Magnetic resonance imaging (MRI) is being used to assess the size of structures in the brain that are thought to play a role in the expression of TS symptoms. Preliminary findings suggest that children with TS may have slightly altered basal ganglia structures, specifically, larger caudate nuclei and smaller globus pallidi (18). A preliminary study by Peterson and colleagues (19) has suggested that adults with TS have smaller basal ganglia structures, particularly on the left side. Future neuroimaging studies can be expected to elucidate the size and shape of specific brain structures in individuals with TS across the developmental spectrum.

Preliminary studies with PET using 18-fluorodeoxyglucose (FDG) to assess metabolic activity in specific brain regions (20,21) have found alterations in the level of metabolic activity in various regions, particularly in basal ganglia and frontal cortical areas. Methodological differences between studies may explain discrepant findings and provide an incentive to investigators to apply more sophisticated techniques.

Regional cerebral blood flow (rCBF), which is highly correlated with regional cerebral metabolic activity, has been assessed using single photon emission computed tomography (SPECT) (Riddle et al., *this volume*). The major finding, decreased rCBF in the left lenticular nucleus (a subdivision of the basal ganglia), is provocative since it parallels the MRI finding reported by Peterson and colleagues (19) and the PET findings of Braun and colleagues (20). These results also point to the need to "coregister" structural scans (MRI) and functional scans (PET or SPECT) in the same individual so that differences due to changes in the size of a structure can be differentiated from differences in level of metabolism or blood flow per volume of tissue. Another important methodological concern is the mental state of the subject, which may affect functional dimensions measured by PET and SPECT, e.g., the degree to which the patient has been required to suppress tics actively.

PET studies on the density of neurotransmitter receptors or uptake sites in patients with TS are limited. Singer et al. (*this volume*) have shown increased density of striatal D_2 sites. However, using a different ligand and a different modeling procedure (equilibrium instead of kinetic modeling) Brooks and colleagues (*this volume*) found no difference in D_2 receptor density between adults with TS and matched controls.

Significant scientific advances can be expected over the next few years as new ligands are developed for assessing an ever-increasing array of receptors, uptake sites, and enzymes; as improvements in instrumentation lead to better quality images; and as more accurate methods for quantification of imaging data are developed.

TREATMENT APPROACHES

The decision whether to initiate specific treatment and the choice of treatments depend not only on the diagnosis of TS but on the extent of clinical impairment and the degree to which tics interfere with the individual's life and development. Most individuals with tic syndromes do not suffer serious morbidity, and even for those with some difficulties, tics tend to improve during the course of adolescence and young adulthood. Clinicians generally see patients when their symptoms are at a peak; usually with time there is some natural remission. When clinicians do intervene, there are several overarching principles of clinical care:

1. The primary emphasis in clinical care is helping the child, adolescent, or adult as a whole person, and not just focusing on the total elimination of tics as such.
2. The goal of care is to help the individual to navigate developmental tasks as successfully as possible—to relate well with parents, siblings, and family; develop friendships; feel competent in school and work; and experience the normal pleasures of life.
3. During the course of treatment, the child, family, and physicians must work together to assess the benefits and side effects of treatment.

The Decision to Initiate Treatment

The clinical problems presented by most patients who come for treatment are often complicated. In addition, clinical assessment has a broader scope than simply determining the presence of tics and associated problems. It includes understanding the impact of these symptoms on the individual's life and the way in which the individual is functioning in all spheres of development. Following careful evaluation, over the course of one or more sessions, it is generally useful for the clinician and patient to collaborate in a period of monitoring over

the course of months; during this process, it becomes possible to establish a baseline, define associated difficulties better, obtain medical tests, assess the fluctuations in symptoms, and establish a patient–physician relationship.

Evaluation and a period of monitoring may be therapeutic interventions in their own right. Patients and their families find it helpful to share their stories with experienced clinicians, sometimes for the very first time, and they may be reassured by being heard and being educated about TS. They may no longer feel as isolated, frightened, or uniquely burdened, and they will know where to turn when more help is needed. Indeed, many patients require no more than this type of evaluation and guidance. They can be reassured about their functioning and about the long-term prognosis. For these individuals, future treatment may be intermittent or *as needed* contact with a clinician over the next years. Other patients and their families may benefit from more specific treatment.

Psychosocial Treatments

Nonpharmacological treatments are often useful in the clinical care of individuals with TS.

Psychotherapeutic Approaches

Individuals with adjustment, affective, anxiety, or other psychiatric difficulties may benefit from individual or group psychotherapy, or other types of psychiatric/psychological therapy for these problems. While psychotherapy is not useful for the tics, psychosocial therapies can be quite useful in helping a child, adolescent, or adult cope better with chronic illness and the psychiatric consequences that may arise from symptoms and the social distress they cause. Families often require psychoeducational help: guidance in how to deal with the family member with TS and with their own emotional responses, including potential overinvolvement or negative patterns of interaction. Similarly, some families will experience considerable relief from family therapy or support groups.

School Interventions

Academic intervention may be a critical treatment approach for children and adolescents with learning disorders, ADHD, and other types of difficulties that interfere with academic performance (see Burd and Kerbeshian, *this volume*). Depending on their individual needs, children with TS may require tutoring, a learning laboratory, a self-contained classroom, or a special school. School performance may improve when children are allowed to type, use computers, do their work orally, and take untimed tests, or when they may leave the classroom when their tics, or their attempts at suppression, are too great an interference with their classroom functioning.

Behavioral Approaches

Behavioral methodologies have been used to help patients relax, to learn to inhibit tics, or to perform acts that are in opposition to emitting a tic. The use of operant conditioning methods has been reported to be helpful for some patients, but most clinicians have not been convinced that behavioral approaches lead to sustained and generalized tic improvement. Behavioral approaches may, however, be useful in relation to non-tic behavioral difficulties (such as oppositionality) and to improving areas of adaptive functioning, such as social skills. Also, behavioral methods clearly are beneficial for some patients with OCD, particularly those with well-defined compulsions (see Baer, *this volume*).

Research on Efficacy

While experienced clinicians generally make use of an array of nonspecific thera-

peutic approaches (such as educational guidance and reassurance) and more specific modalities (such as psychotherapy), there is a lack of rigorous data on the impact of these methods on tics or associated clinical difficulties. The evaluation of psychosocial methodologies is plagued by many methodological problems, including difficulties in defining suitable controls, utilizing well-defined treatment methods, and holding other interventions constant while only one psychosocial treatment is utilized. It is obviously hard to develop "placebo-controlled" methods. While it is clear that family dynamics may be profoundly upset by a child with TS and may, in turn, lead to a spiraling of the child's tics and behavioral problems, there is no systematic research on the benefits of family therapy (see Harper, *this volume* and Nomura et al., *this volume*), nor is there evidence about the ways in which school interventions may improve a child's development or tic status. This does not mean that these approaches are not useful. To the contrary, there is clinical agreement on their value for some patients and families. Rather, these clinical observations need to be put to rigorous testing to define the areas of improvement and the mechanisms and processes that may underlie clinical changes.

Pharmacotherapy for Tics

There are several effective medical treatments for TS and associated disorders. Unfortunately, there have been no major advances during the past decade in the pharmacological treatment of tic symptoms (see Erenberg, *this volume*).

For almost three decades, haloperidol has been the mainstay of pharmacological treatment for TS (22,23). Impressive benefits are seen at low doses, and patients may have almost complete remissions with few side effects. Some patients require higher doses, but results are generally not as good and side effects almost always limit the medication's overall clinical value. Although up to 70% of patients with TS initially benefit from haloperidol, long-term follow-up suggests that only a smaller proportion continue to use haloperidol for years, because of side effects. Also, haloperidol has been implicated in the onset of tardive dyskinesia (TD) in patients with TS. The long-term use of medication may lead to behavioral side effects, including phobias, memory difficulties, weight gain, lethargy, and personality changes, which have attracted a good deal of clinical attention over the past decade.

Pimozide, a diphenylbutylpiperidine derivative that is chemically distinctive from haloperidol and the phenothiazines, leads to blockade of postsynaptic dopamine receptors and blocks calcium channels. Studies and clinical experience suggest that pimozide is equivalent to haloperidol in the treatment of TS and perhaps less sedating. Because of its long half-life (55 hours), once a day dosage is feasible. The major side effects are similar to those of haloperidol. Even at low doses, electrocardiographic (EKG) changes have been observed in patients receiving pimozide, including T-wave inversion, U waves, QT interval prolongation, and bradycardia.

The first report in 1979 of the value of clonidine in treating TS has been followed by open and double-blind trials suggesting that some patients with TS benefit from its use. Not all studies have demonstrated efficacy, and in general about 40% of patients seem to be helped (see ref. 24 and Goetz, *this volume*). Clonidine reduces noradrenergic functioning by acting as an α-2 adrenergic agonist; thus its mode of action is quite different from the neuroleptics. Clonidine may indirectly affect central dopaminergic neurons. Clonidine seems especially useful in improving attentional problems and ameliorating complex motor and phonic symptoms and has been used in the treatment of ADHD without tics (25). Clonidine is started at low doses and slowly titrated over several weeks to maintenance levels. High doses are sometimes used but are more likely to lead to side effects, such as sedation.

Some patients respond to phenothiazines much as they do to haloperidol, when doses and side effects are equivalent. For the patient who cannot tolerate haloperidol or pimozide, a trial with a phenothiazine may be indicated. In the treatment of TS, dosages are generally much lower than those used in the treatment of psychosis.

Sulpiride and Tiapride, substituted dibenzylamines that inhibit dopamine receptors, particularly D_2 receptors, have been shown by double-blind studies and clinical experience in Europe and Israel to be useful for the treatment of TS. It is generally thought that drugs in this category are useful for "milder" TS and less likely to produce side effects than neuroleptics.

Selecting a Medication

There are few firm data to guide the choice of a first drug. While haloperidol has the longest history of use, and its efficacy is well established, many clinicians favor pimozide because they feel it has fewer side effects. The scientific evidence does not fully support this distinction. Clonidine is less likely to be dramatically effective, but is favored by many clinicians as the first drug because of its limited side effects, occasional efficacy in treating ADHD symptoms, and ease of discontinuation when it is gradually tapered over the course of a week or two.

The first medication chosen may be targeted at obsessive–compulsive symptoms or problems with ADHD, rather than tics. It is important to determine the symptom(s) that is causing the most functional impairment and to select a medication accordingly.

In certain respects, the past decade has been disappointing in relation to innovation in drug treatment for tic disorders. The major groups of medications have all been around for more than a decade. While they have proven benefit, there are many patients whose tic symptoms are not responsive or who cannot tolerate the side effects. All these medications seem to be rather distally involved in the pathobiology of the disorder, far from the primary biological dysfunction. The reduction in tics seen with neuroleptics is consistent with their effects in reducing symptoms of other movement disorders, indeed in reducing movement. Clonidine may be ameliorative but seems more to modulate—like toning down the carburetor—than to affect the neurobiology of tics specifically.

In the future, other treatment approaches may emerge based on a better understanding of the underlying pathobiology gained from the range of studies described earlier, including genetic and neurochemical research. Also, it is important for clinical researchers to investigate novel medications that may be helpful for individual patients or subgroups (see LeWitt, *this volume*).

Pharmacotherapy for ADHD in the Presence of TS

For children and adolescents with TS, it is often the symptoms of ADHD—hyperactivity, distractibility, and impulsivity—rather than tics that are the cause of the greatest impairment in school and at home. ADHD may precede the onset of TS; also, attentional problems, overactivity, and impulsivity may appear or increase along with tic symptoms. Clinical experience suggests that those individuals with TS who have preexisting or serious attentional and behavioral problems are most likely to have the most compromised long-term adjustment.

Several classes of medications are used to treat the symptoms of ADHD, including desipramine, clonidine, methylphenidate and dextroamphetamine.

A few studies suggest that clonidine is effective in children with ADHD without tics and in children with TS plus ADHD (25).

Desipramine, a tricyclic drug used in the treatment of children and adolescents with major depressive disorder and nocturnal enuresis, is also effective in the treatment of hyperactivity, impulsivity, and inattention (26,27). In children with TS plus ADHD, desipramine appears to reduce the ADHD symptoms without affecting the severity of tics (28,29). Side effects of low doses of desipramine are generally minimal, and desipramine has a low anticholinergic profile. The report of sudden death in several children who were receiving desipramine, however, has raised concerns about its use and suggests that careful monitoring of the EKG is important in identifying children with cardiac vulnerabilities (30). Clomipramine may also be useful for TS children with attentional problems, but there are no controlled studies as yet.

The stimulant medications methylphenidate and dextroamphetamine are the standard treatment for children with ADHD without tics. There is impressive scientific evidence for the efficacy and safety of stimulants for children with ADHD. For many years, clinicians have observed the emergence or exacerbation of tics during treatment with the stimulants (31). For this reason, many clinicians reserve stimulants for children with TS whose ADHD symptoms do not respond to clonidine or desipramine or who cannot tolerate these medications. More recently, however, some investigators have reported only rare exacerbations of tics or, surprisingly, actual decrease in tics in children with TS who are given stimulants.

The use of stimulant medications with children who have tic disorders or who have first-degree relatives with tics or TS remains an area of continuing difference of opinion among experienced clinicians. The evidence is not fully in on the association between stimulants and the triggering of full-blown TS in vulnerable children. Yet it seems clear that there are some children whose tics are worsened in a dose–response manner, while there are others who benefit from stimulants and whose tics are not worsened. Thus, the cautious use of stimulants, with monitoring for changes in tics and behavior, can probably be undertaken when there is careful clinical monitoring (see Sverd et al., *this volume*).

Future research is needed to clarify the precise relations between ADHD, seen in about 50% of TS patients who come for treatment, and the tic diathesis. While stimulant medications have been around for decades, and are the best studied of all drugs used in child psychiatry, we still do not understand their mode of action. Clarification of their biological functioning may provide interesting leads related to the underlying biological mechanisms involved in attentional disorders as well as tics.

Pharmacotherapy for OCD in the Presence of TS

The major area of advance in the past decade in the psychopharmacological treatment of TS has been in the treatment of associated obsessive–compulsive symptoms (OCS) and OCD (see ref. 32 and King et al., *this volume*). Serotonin reuptake inhibitors—including clomipramine, fluoxetine, and fluvoxamine—reduce the severity of OCS in patients with primary OCD, and an emerging body of data supports the efficacy of these medications in treating OCD in patients with TS.

Fluoxetine, which is used primarily to treat depression, has been available in the United States since 1988, and clinical trials have demonstrated its efficacy in treating OCD. Alone or in combination with a tic-reducing medication (such as pimozide), fluoxetine is effective in reducing OCD, but not tic symptoms in patients with TS. Children appear to be more sensitive to side effects of fluoxetine (33), and a liquid formulation makes it convenient to start with quite low doses (e.g., 5 mg/day). Suicidal ideation in adults and self-destructive phenomena in children have been described as possible

side effects of fluoxetine, but the clinical significance of these observations is not known (34).

Clomipramine, a tricyclic antidepressant, is effective in reducing the severity of OCS in children, adolescents, and adults with primary OCD. Clinical experience suggests that it is also helpful to some TS patients, with an efficacy profile comparable to that of fluoxetine. Although published reports of children treated for primary OCD suggest that side effects are minimal, clinicians often find that the dosage should be lowered, sometimes below the therapeutic range, to prevent intolerable side effects in many TS patients.

The current intense research and clinical interest in OCD is likely to generate both improved knowledge and treatment approaches over the next years. These findings will be of direct relevance to those patients with TS whose lives are often more burdened by incessant, meaningless, and intrusive thoughts and actions than by the tic symptoms of TS.

Depression and Anxiety in the Presence of TS

Antidepressant medications are not useful in the treatment of tics, but TS patients may develop depressive and anxiety disorders that respond to antidepressant medication. Antidepressants (such as imipramine) have been added to ongoing TS treatments (haloperidol, clonidine) with good results.

Various minor tranquilizers, including benzodiazepines, have been used in the treatment of TS with no apparent benefit to tic symptomatology. However, individual patients benefit from these medications when used to help alleviate anxiety or to improve sleep. Their prescription for TS patients should follow the usual guidelines, including careful monitoring for side effects and dependency (see Coffey, et al., *this volume* and Goetz, *this volume*).

Medication Combinations

Most patients with TS benefit sufficiently from a single medication, but combinations of two or more medications are on occasion necessary to minimize side effects or treat varied symptom clusters (comorbidity). For example, patients who require pharmacological treatment for tics and OCS may benefit from a combination of pimozide or haloperidol (for tic symptoms) with fluoxetine or clomipramine (for OCD). Also, some clinicians report good results in treating children with ADHD + TS with a combination of methylphenidate or desipramine (for attentional problems) and haloperidol (or pimozide) for tic control.

There remains a paucity of rigorous data on long-term, multimodal and multiple-drug treatment of children and adults with TS. Studies require large numbers of patients, long-term follow-up, and complex designs, and they may be quite costly. Research on treatment approaches would thus benefit from various strategies, including multicenter collaborative studies.

Discontinuing Medication

The decision to stop medication is complicated and not well studied. Clinicians must consider both the patient's tic status and his or her functioning in other areas of life, including school, work, and family. Most clinicians tend to consider dosage reduction or discontinuation after a year or two on medication if the individual has benefited and side effects are tolerable. After several years, medications often can be tapered and discontinued without any noticeable effect in many patients. It is wise to taper medications over a few weeks since cold-turkey withdrawal may lead to "rebound" exacerbation of symptoms.

"Alternative" Therapies

Various other pharmacological, biological, and dietary approaches have been attempted with TS, but results have yet to be rigorously demonstrated (see Wurtman, *this volume*). There are anecdotal reports of the benefit of megavitamins, elimination diets, nutritional supplements, and the use of amino acids and minerals. Similarly, there are anecdotal reports of the value of allergic desensitization and environmental decontagion for allergens. No systematic studies have been reported, and the use of these approaches is not based on available scientific data (Haslam, *this volume*).

CONCLUSIONS

The modern history of TS began during the middle 1960s when Arthur Shapiro demonstrated the efficacy of haloperidol. His pioneering studies of the clinical features and psychopharmacology of TS opened up a new era in modern psychiatry and neurology. The creation of the national Tourette Syndrome Association also established a new paradigm for a productive collaboration among clinicians, investigators, and patients and their families. Over the last two decades, the field of clinical care and research on TS has burgeoned and TS today is recognized as a model, neuropsychiatric disorder that reflects biological vulnerability and environmental modulation (see ref. 35 and Leckman et al., *this volume*).

Over the last two decades, clinical investigators have learned that while TS is often persistent or even lifelong, there are many cases of remission during adolescence or adulthood. Also, while tics may sometimes be quite severe, in many cases they interfere less with development than associated obsessive–compulsive, attentional, and behavioral problems. The phenomenology of TS remains an area of keen scientific interest and investigation. We still know far too little about the different pathways between genetic vulnerability and clinical expression, the biological and social factors that influence the range and severity of expression, and the reasons for amelioration or exacerbation with development (see Earls, *this volume*). We know virtually nothing about the origin of specific symptoms, the everchanging nature and replacement of symptoms, and the phenomenon of waxing and waning. Understanding issues such as these will provide knowledge relevant not only to TS but to many other conditions.

Research has contributed to the clinical care of patients, and general agreement has emerged among experienced clinicians about the importance of broad-based evaluation and long-term treatment planning. Clinical evaluation of individuals with TS must include concern for the individual's overall social, emotional, familial, and cognitive functioning, and not only the presence or severity of tics. Clinical management calls upon a range of approaches, such as education about the condition, reassurance, emotional support, guidance, and advocacy in relation to school, vocational and social issues. Today, there is an armamentarium of effective medications for tic syndromes and associated disorders. These can ameliorate major symptoms and improve an individual's symptomatic status and functioning, yet there are patients who remain very impaired. There is hope that basic advances in brain sciences and studies of TS will suggest new approaches to treatment.

Advances in genetics have clarified aspects of phenomenology, such as the relation between tic syndromes and OCD. Over the last decade, an international network of investigators has been collaborating in studies of the genetics of TS and the search for the genetic locus using linkage methods. When the gene is identified, it will be possible to clarify the areas in the brain in which it is expressed, the nature of the interference with brain functioning, and the steps involved in the progression from vulnerability to the unfolding, over the course of childhood, of a clinical condition.

One decade ago researchers dreamed of the possibility of studying TS brains neurochemically. We now have pilot studies on the neurochemistry of TS from postmortem brains. Remarkably, dopamine and its metabolites have not emerged as markedly abnormal, while there are intriguing suggestions about other neurochemical systems. The available brain tissue is quite limited, and the small number of brains restricts the power of current neurochemical research, yet the preliminary findings are provocative and promising. Perhaps as important as any specific finding is the creation of a mechanism for obtaining and sharing postmortem specimens and for demonstrating the feasibility of this approach.

Brain imaging has emerged as an exciting new field of psychiatric research over the past years, and the available technologies are now being extended in a rigorous fashion to studies of TS. The field of neuroimaging is progressing at such a rapid rate that only pilot studies are available using up-to-date methods with TS patients. PET, MRI, SPECT, and other methods, such as magnetic resonance spectroscopy (MRS), offer the promise of helping delineate underlying brain mechanisms involved in different aspects of TS and associated disorders. They may also allow investigators to follow the emergence of difficulties in genetically vulnerable individuals and to correlate brain mechanisms with clinical changes from the use of medications. Brain imaging is thus closely related to other areas of clinical research on natural history and phenomenology. In turn, brain imaging may help target new neurochemical research ideas and explain treatment response and resistance. Finally, brain imaging may be of profound importance in clarifying underlying neurobiological vulnerabilities, e.g., the involvement of corticothalamic pathways and other such circuits, and their expression in different phases of the disorder.

Research on TS has demonstrated the close relations between basic and clinical science: with new findings about genetics, pharmacology, natural history, and other areas, clinicians are able to provide patients and their families with more accurate knowledge and more thoughtful, effective care. Clinical researchers in the field of TS have been quick to exploit emerging new methodologies and, in some respects, the methods developed in relation to TS have set the standard for research in other fields. Over the next years, we can anticipate a more rapid pace of investigations, which will lead to a deeper understanding of TS and to the extension of basic research to clinical care. Such advances also are likely to be useful in relation to research and understanding of other disorders that emerge during the course of development and that span the domain between psychiatry and neurology. In this way, research on TS has implications far beyond the boundaries of this disorder.

REFERENCES

1. Friedhoff AJ, Chase TN (eds). *Gilles de la Tourette syndrome. Advances in neurology*, vol 35. New York: Raven Press, 1982.
2. Shapiro AK, Shapiro E, Bruun RD, Sweet RD. *Gilles de la Tourette's syndrome*. New York: Raven Press, 1976.
3. Shapiro AK, Shapiro E, Young JG, Feinberg TE (eds). *Gilles de la Tourette syndrome*, 2nd ed. New York: Raven Press, 1988.
4. Cohen DJ, Bruun RD, Leckman JF (eds). *Tourette's syndrome & tic disorders: Clinical understanding and treatment*. New York: John Wiley & Sons, 1988.
5. Bliss, J. Sensory experiences of Gilles de la Tourette syndrome. *Arch Gen Psychiatry* 1980; 37:1343–7.
6. Cohen DJ. The pathology of the self in primary childhood autism and Gilles de la Tourette syndrome. *Psychiatr Clin North Am* 1980;3:383–402.
7. Dykens E, Leckman JF, Riddle MA, Hardin MA, Schwartz S, Cohen DJ. Intellectual, academic, and adaptive functioning of Tourette syndrome children with and without attention deficit disorder. *J Abnorm Child Psychol* 1990;18:607–14.
8. Berkson J. Limitations of the application of fourfold table analysis to hospital data. *Biomet Bull* 1946;2:47–53.
9. Leckman JF, Knorr A, Rasmusson A, Cohen DJ. Basal ganglia research and Tourette's syndrome. *Trends Neurosci* 1991;14:94.
10. Cohen DJ, Detlor J, Shaywitz BA, Leckman JF. Interaction of biological and psychological factors in the natural history of Tourette's syndrome. In: Friedhoff AJ, Chase TN, eds. *Gilles de la Tourette syndrome. Advances in neurology*, vol 35. New York: Raven Press, 1982;31–40.
11. Friedhoff AJ. Receptor maturation in the pathogenesis and treatment of Tourette syndrome. In:

Friedhoff AJ, Chase TN, eds. *Gilles de la Tourette syndrome. Advances in neurology*, vol 35. New York: Raven Press, 1982;130–40.
12. Friedhoff AJ. A dopamine-dependent restitutive system for the maintenance of mental normalcy. In: Burrell CD, Strand FL, eds. *Second Colloquium in Biological Sciences. Ann NY Acad Sci* 1986;463:47–52.
13. Leckman JF, Riddle MA, Berrettini WH, et al. Elevated CSF levels of dynorphin A [1–8] in Tourette's syndrome. *Life Sci* 1988;43:2015–23.
14. Kurlan R, Majundar L, Deeley C, et al. A controlled trial of propoxyphene and naltrexone in patients with TS. *Ann Neurol* 1991;30:19–23.
15. Leckman JF, Scahill L. Possible exacerbation of tics by androgenic steroids [Letter]. *N Engl J Med* 1990;322:1674.
16. Peterson B, Leckman JF, Scahill L, et al. Steroid hormones and Tourette's syndrome: early experience with antiandrogen therapy. 1992 (*submitted*).
17. Casas M, Alvarez E, Duro P, Garcia-Ribera C, Udina A, Velat D, Rodriguez-Espinosa J, Salva P, Jane F. Antiandrogenic treatment of obsessive-compulsive neurosis. *Acta Psychiatr Scand* 1986; 73:221–2.
18. Denckla MB, Harris EL, Aylward EH, Singer HS, Reiss AL, Reader MJ, Bryan RN, Chase GA. Executive function and volume of the basal ganglia in children with Tourette syndrome and attention deficit hyperactivity disorder. *Ann Neurol* 1991; 30:476(abst).
19. Peterson B, Riddle MA, Cohen DJ, et al. Reduced basal ganglia volumes in Tourette's syndrome using 3-dimensional reconstruction techniques from magnetic resonance images. 1992 (*submitted*).
20. Braun AR, Hsiao J, Randolph C, Chase TN. Functional neuroanatomy of Tourette's syndrome studied with FDG PET. *Neurology* 1991;41:359(abst).
21. Stoetter B, Blin J, Blesa R, Miletich RS, Chase TN. Distribution of brain dysfunction in Tourette syndrome revealed by PET scanning. *Neurology* 1991;41:358(abst).
22. Shapiro AK, Shapiro E. Clinical efficacy of haloperidol, pimozide, penfluridol, and clonidine in the treatment of Tourette syndrome. In: Friedhoff AJ, Chase TN, eds. *Gilles de la Tourette syndrome. Advances in neurology*, vol 35. New York: Raven Press, 1982;383–6.
23. Shapiro E, Shapiro AK, Fulop G, et al. Controlled study of haloperidol, pimozide, and placebo for the treatment of Gilles de la Tourette's syndrome. *Arch Gen Psychiatry* 1989;46:722–30.
24. Leckman JF, Hardin MT, Riddle MA, Stevenson J, Ort SI, Cohen DJ. Clonidine treatment of Tourette's syndrome. *Arch Gen Psychiatry* 1991; 48:324–8.
25. Hunt RB, Minderaa RB, Cohen DJ. Clonidine benefits children with attention deficit disorder and hyperactivity: report of a double-blind placebo-crossover therapeutic trial. *J Am Acad Child Psychiatry* 1985;24:617–29.
26. Biederman J, Baldessarini RJ, Wright V, Knee D, Harmatz JS. A double-blind placebo controlled study of desipramine in the treatment of ADD: I.

Efficacy. *J Am Acad Child Adol Psychiatry* 1989; 28:777–84.

27. Biederman J, Baldessarini RJ, Wright V, Knee D, Harmatz JS, Goldblatt A. A double-blind placebo controlled study of desipramine in the treatment of ADD: II. Serum drug levels and cardiovascular findings. *J Am Acad Child Adol Psychiatry* 1989; 28:903–11.

28. Riddle MA, Hardin MT, Cho SC, Woolston JL, Leckman JF. Desipramine treatment of boys with attention-deficit hyperactivity disorder and tics: preliminary clinical experience. *J Am Acad Child Adol Psychiatry* 1988;27:811–4.

29. Singer HS, Brown J, Quaskey S, Mellits ED, Denckla MB, Rosenberg LA. The treatment of attention deficit hyperactivity disorder in Tourette syndrome: a double-blind placebo-controlled study with clonidine and desipramine. *Ann Neurol* 1992(abst) (*in press*).

30. Riddle MA, Nelson JC, Kleinman CS, et al. Sudden death in children receiving Norpramin: a re-view of three reported cases and commentary. *J Am Acad Child Adolesc Psychiatry* 1991;30:104–8.

31. Golden GS. Gilles de la Tourette's syndrome following methylphenidate administration. *Dev Med Child Neurol* 1974;16:76–8.

32. Leonard HL, Swedo SE, Rapoport JL, et al. Treatment of obsessive-compulsive disorder with clomipramine and desipramine in children and adolescents. *Arch Gen Psychiatry* 1989;46:1088–92.

33. Riddle MA, King RA, Hardin MT, et al. Behavioral side effects of fluoxetine in children and adolescents. *J Child Adolesc Psychopharm* 1991; 1:193–7.

34. King RA, Riddle MA, Chappel PB, et al. Emergence of self-destructive phenomena in children and adolescents during fluoxetine treatment. *J Am Acad Child Adol Psychiatry* 1991;30:79–86.

35. Cohen DJ. Tourette's syndrome: a model disorder for integrating psychoanalytic and biological perspectives. *Int Rev Psychoanalysis* 1991;18: 195–209.

Subject Index

A

Abbreviated Parent Rating Scale, 275
Abbreviated Teacher Rating Scale, 273
Academic intervention, 311–316, 355
Acetylcholine. *See also* Cholinergic system
  choline effects on, 300
Acetylcholinesterase, 145
Acquired Tourettism, 203–204
ACTH, and naloxone, 253–260
Adaptive model, family, 321
Adenylate cyclase, postmortem study, 138
Adolescence, tic development, 2
Adrenarche, 49
Affective spectrum disorder, 190
Affective symptoms, carbohydrate craving,
  296–297
Age of onset
  attention deficit disorder, 4
  tics, 2, 342
  trends, 57–58
Aggression
  incidence, 5
  obsessive-compulsive disorder, 39
Akathisia
  definition, 10
  propranolol treatment, 267
  subjective perceptions, 27
  suppressibility, 28
  voluntary nature of, 26–28
Alcoholism, 195
Alpha-methyl-para-tyrosine, 267
Alprazolam, 97–98
"Alternative" therapies, 303–310, 359
Alzheimer's disease, choline treatment, 301
Amantadine, 267
Amygdala
  motor tic role, 22
  postmortem studies, 125–130
  sexual dimorphism, 21
Anafranil. *See* Clomipramine
Androgenic steroids
  gender differences origin, 21–22
  research issues, 352
  and symptom exacerbation, 352
  Tourette syndrome cause, 17
Anhidrosis, 109

Anterolateral thalamus, 124–130
Anteromedial thalamus, 124–130
Anterior putamen, 218
Antiandrogens
  and neurobiological theories, 21–22
  in obsessive-compulsive disorder, 21, 352
Anxiety
  benzodiazepine treatment, 97–98, 358
  comorbidity, 95–104
  family history, 103
  incidence, 4
  in obsessive-compulsive disorder, 33–41
Arithmetic scores, 77
Arithromania, 4
Ascertainment bias
  alternative hypothesis, 192
  and epidemiologic methods, 47–48
  research issues, 344
Ascorbic acid
  in attention deficit disorder, 305–310
  side effects, 309
Aspartate
  postmortem study, 127
  precursor control, 298
Asperger syndrome
  definition, 69
  family history, 71–72
  North Dakota comorbidity study, 69, 71–72
Associative striatal territory
  chemospecific systems, monkeys, 116–117
  Parkinsonian monkeys, 119–120
Assortative mating, 164–165
Attention deficit hyperactivity disorder
  ascertainment bias assumption, 191
  clonidine treatment, 357
  comorbidity, 48–49, 190–192, 345
  dopamine D2 receptor gene, 195
  family studies, 48, 190–192
  management suggestions, 313–316
  megavitamin therapy, 303–310
  methylphenidate in, 271–280, 357–358
  natural history, 3–5
  school problems, 76
  as spectrum disorder, 190
  tic comorbidity, 345

Attention deficit hyperactivity disorder
  (*contd.*)
  tricyclic antidepressants, 357
  variant manifestations, 345
Autistic disorder
  California prevalence study, 70
  family history, 70–72
  North Dakota comorbidity study, 68–73
  prognosis with Tourette syndrome, 69–73
  self-injurious behavior, 108
"Autocannibalism," 300
Automatic movements
  classification, 7
  in motor tics, 31–32
Autosomal dominance
  alternative assumptions, 193–194, 347
  family history study, 155
  genetic model, 16, 154–155, 179, 347
  and phenotype range, 347

B

Bacteriophage M13, 184–186
Baltimore pedigree study, 46
Basal ganglia
  FDG-PET study, 218–224
  HMPAO uptake, SPECT, 209–210
  limbic-motor interactions, 148–149,
    223–224
  obsessive-compulsive disorder, 84
  parkinsonian monkeys, 115–121
  postmortem analysis, 139, 141
  structural imaging, 202–205
Behavior problems
  megavitamin effects, 308–310
  natural history, 4–5
Behavior therapy
  evaluation, 355
  misconceptions, 334
  obsessive-compulsive disorder, 333–339,
    355
  outcome studies, 334–335
  Tourette syndrome, 338–339
  treatment failure predictors, 335–336
  trichotillomania, 337–338
Benzodiazepines, 97–98, 358
Bereitschaft potential, 8
Berkson's bias, 47–48, 344
Beta-adrenergic blockers, 267
Beta-adrenergic receptors, 137–138
Beta-endorphin, 109
Black children, tics, 78

Blepharospasm
  as dystonic tics, 9
  and eyeblinking tics, 29
Block design, 77, 236
Borderline personality disorder, 108–109
Botulinum toxin
  dystonic tic treatment, 9, 30–31
  long-term benefit, 30–31
  pain relief, 30
Bradykinesia, 242
Brain banking system, 352
British National Child Development study, 78
Burd's prevalence study. *See* North Dakota
    study
Buspirone
  augmentation use, 287
  in obsessive-compulsive disorder, 286–287

C

Caine's study. *See* Monroe County, New
    York study
Calbindin, 119–120
Calcium channel blockers, 265–266
California prevalence study
  epidemiologic methods, 46, 61, 78
  special education estimates, 78–79
Canadian Mennonite Tourette kindred, 175
Candidate gene approach, 168, 182, 196
Cannabinoids, 265
Carbamazepine, 265
Carbohydrate craving, 296–297
Carbohydrate diet
  brain serotonin levels, 294–295
  and food choice, 296–297
Carbon monoxide poisoning, 203–204
Cardiotoxicity, clomipramine, 284
Case identification
  in epidemiological studies, 45, 49–50
  informant education, 49–50
Catecholamines
  postmortem study, 126–127, 129–130
  research issues, 350–351
  tyrosine control of, 298–300
    neuron firing effects, 299
Caudate nucleus
  brain imaging, 203, 357
  obsessive-compulsive disorder, 84, 203
Caudate region
  dopamine, 139–140
  postmortem study, 124–130, 136–143
Cavum septum pellucidum cavities
  head bangers, 110
  structured imaging, 202

Cerebral blood flow. *See* Regional cerebral
  blood flow
Cerebral cortex
  cyclic AMP, 138, 141–142
  motor system interactions, 148–149
  postmortem neurochemistry, 135–143
Cerebral peduncles, 203
Checking rituals
  behavior therapy response, 336–337
  natural history, 4
  NIMH study, 84
  in obsessive-compulsive disorder, 35–36
Choline
  as precursor, 300
  therapeutic use, 300–301
Choline acetyltransferase, 137
Choline chloride, 266
Cholinergic system
  postmortem analysis, 137–138
  and treatment strategies, 266–267
Chorea, subjective perceptions, 27
Chromosomal abnormalities, 167–172
Chromosome 4q31, 195
Chromosome 9, 177–178
Chromosome 18q22.1, 168
Chronic multiple tics
  Netherlands genetic study, 169–170
  and obsessive-compulsive disorder, 343
  prevalence assumption, 194
  Salt Lake City pedigree, 159–165
Classification, 7–13
Classroom performance. *See* School
  performance
Cleaning rituals
  behavior therapy response, 336–337
  NIMH study, 83–84
Clinic-based studies, 45–48
Clinician's illusion, 46–47
Clomiphene, 267–268
Clomipramine
  augmentation of, 287
  cardiotoxicity, 284
  in children, 289
  comparative efficacy, 288–289
  in obsessive-compulsive disorder, 283–285,
    287, 358
  response predictors, 284
  self-injurious behavior, 110
  side effects, 284, 289
  tic effects, 285
Clonazepam, 245–250
  as GABAergic drug, 267
  and habit reversal, 339

in obsessive-compulsive disorder, 286–287,
    289
  side effects, 249
  Tourette syndrome treatment, 247, 249
Clonic tics, 8–10
Clonidine, 245–250, 356
  in attention deficit disorder, 357
  biological markers of response, 246–247
  clinical trials, 246
  dosage, 247
  inconsistent response to, 245–247
  selection of, 356–357
  side effects, 247–248
  tic treatment, 245–250, 356
  transdermal patch formulations, 247
  withdrawal effects, 247
Clozapine, 267
CM&M inheritance, 196
Cocaine, 17
[11]C-Cocaine, 238
Cognitive challenges, 28
Cognitive performance, 236–237
Cognitive tics, 39
Colpocephaly, 202
Comings' study. *See* California prevalence
  study
Community-based studies
  advantages, 46–47, 79
  research needs, 51
Comorbidity, 43–52
  alternative hypotheses, inheritance,
    190–196
  Berkson's bias, 47–48
  California study, 70
  epidemiological methods, 43–52
  North Dakota study, 67–73
  obsessive-compulsive disorder, 83–92
  research issues, 344–345
Competing response training, 338
Complex tics
  classification, 8–9
  versus compulsive rituals, 10, 83–84
  differential diagnosis, 8–10
Compliance, behavior therapy, 335–336
Compulsive behavior. *See* Rituals
  definition, 40, 83
  behavior therapy, 333–337
  in obsessive-compulsive disorder, 35–39
  phenomenology and diagnosis, 10
Computerized tomography
  obsessive-compulsive disorder, 203
  versus PET scans, 233
  Tourette syndrome, 202–205

Conduct disorders, 5
Conners Parent Rating Scale, 273
Contamination fears, 336–337
Coprolalia
    frequency in Japan, 323
    natural history, 2
    Salt Lake City pedigree, 161, 164
    in signing tics, 31
Coprolalopraxia, 31
Copropraxia, 9
Corticosteroid treatment, 267
Corticostriatal loops, 223
Corticostriato-thalamo-cortical circuits
    inhibitory failure, 17–18, 20
    range of symptoms explanation, 346
    regional cerebral blood flow, 210
    "short-circuit" of, 224
Cortisol, and naloxone, 253–260
Counting games, 4, 160
Cultural factors, 55–59
    Japanese families, 323–332
    research needs, 58
Cyclic AMP, 138, 141–142
Cynomolgus monkeys, 115–121

D
Deanol, 266
deLange syndrome, 108
Delta receptors, 260
Depression
    and behavior therapy, 336
    carbohydrate craving, serotonin, 296–297
    incidence, 5
    in obsessive-compulsive disorder, 37
    self-injurious behavior, 108
Depression spectrum disorder, 190
Desipramine, 284, 357
Desmethylclomipramine, 284
Dextroamphetamine, 357
Diagnosis, 7–13, 342–343
Diagnostic criteria
    and genetic linkage studies, 348
    tic disorders, 12, 342–343
Diagnostic specificity-sensitivity, 348
Digit symbol, 77
3,4-Dihydroxyphenylacetic acid (DOPAC)
    postmortem analysis, 126–127, 137, 139
    tyrosine effects, 299
Diltiazem, 266
Discontinuation of medication, 359
Distraction maneuvers, 28
DNA fingerprint, 183–184

DNA polymorphisms. *See* Polymorphic DNA
    markers
^{18}F-Dopa PET, 227–231
Dopamine
    alternative hypothesis, 195
    postmortem analysis, 137–143
    research issues, 350–351
    tyrosine effects, diet, 298–299
        and neuron firing, 299
Dopamine beta-hydroxylase, 168
Dopamine D1 receptor
    genetic linkage study, 163, 168
    postmortem analysis, 139–140, 143
    supersensitivity hypothesis, 143
Dopamine D2 receptor
    age-related declines, 236
    alternative interpretation, gene, 194–195
    genetic linkage study, 163, 168, 194–195
    3-N-(^{11}C)methylspirone PET, 233–238
    positron emission tomography, 227–231,
        233–238
    postmortem analysis, 137, 139–140, 143
    ^{11}C-raclopride PET, 227–231
    supersensitivity hypothesis, 142, 234
Dopamine receptors. *See also* Dopamine D1
        receptor; Dopamine D2 receptor
    as candidate gene, 17
    positron emission tomography, 233–238
    supersensitivity hypothesis, 234
Dopaminergic system
    dynorphin interactions, 148
    hyperinnervation hypothesis, 142
    pallidal territories, monkeys, 119–120
    parkinsonian monkeys, 119–120
    positron emission tomography, 227–231,
        233–238
    postmortem analysis, 137–143
    research issues, 350–351
    self-injurious behavior, 109
    striatal territories, monkeys, 116–119
    tyrosine effects on, 298–299
Dorsomedial thalamus, 124–130
Drug combinations, 359
Drug therapy, 355–359. *See also specific*
        drugs
Duration of symptoms, 342
Dutch genetic study, 167–172
Dynorphin, 109
    basal ganglia staining, 145–149
    dopaminergic interactions, 149
    and obsessive-compulsive symptoms, 254
    postmortem study, 109
    receptor affinities, 260
    research issues, 351

Dystonia
  dystonic tic relationship, 28–32
  neuroleptic side effect, 242
Dystonic tics
  botulinum toxin treatment, 9, 30–31
  differential diagnosis, 8–10, 28–32
  dystonia relationship, 28–32
  geste antagonistique, 30
  sensory premonitory symptoms, 25–26
  subjective perceptions, 27

E
Echolalia
  definition, 9
  Salt Lake City pedigree, 161–164
  in signing tics, 31
Echolaliopraxia, 31
Echopraxia
  definition, 9
  Salt Lake City pedigree, 161
Educational management, 311–316, 355
Elderly, tic symptomatology, 3
Eltoprazine, 111
Emotional adaptation, family, 321
Employment, Japanese patients, 327–332
Endocrine factors, 21–22, 351–352
Endogenous opioids. *See* Opioid peptides
Endorphins, 109
Enkephalin
  basal ganglia staining, 145–149
  pallidal territories, monkeys, 118–120
  parkinsonian monkeys, 120
Environmental factors, 17
Epidemiological studies. *See also*
      Comorbidity; Prevalence
  fundamental considerations, 43–45
  methodology, 43–52
  research needs, 51–52
  school-age children, 78
Estradiol, 21
Estrogen treatment, 267
Etiology, 44–45
"Evening up" symptoms, 4
Exaggerated startle response, 8
Exertional pain, 29
Exposure
  in obsessive-compulsive disorder,
      333–337
  trichotillomania, 337
External pallidal segment
  immunohistochemistry, monkeys,
      118–120
  parkinsonian monkeys, 120

Eye blinking tics
  blepharospasm relationship, 29
  geste antagonistique, 30
  natural history, 2
Eye mutilation
  association with Tourette syndrome, 106
  obsessive-compulsive disorder, 110
  and psychosis, 106, 108
Eysenck Personality Questionnaire, 34

F
Facial tics
  as initial symptom, 2
  neurobiological substrate hypothesis, 18
False-positive diagnosis, 156, 348
Family history studies
  attention deficit disorder, 48
  disadvantages, 192–193
  and family structure, 348
  and genetic models, 155
  Israeli Defense Force study, 64–65
  North Dakota study, 70
  obsessive-compulsive symptoms, 48,
      86–92, 152–153
  pervasive developmental disorder, 70
  research needs, 52
  reverse ascertainment bias, 192–193
  and single gene hypothesis, 153
Family relationships, 319–322
  and adaptation, 321
  clinicians' role, 320–322
  interventions, 354–355
  in Japan, 323–332
  research methods, 57
  understanding of, 319–321
FDG-PET studies, 213–224, 353
Fear, 36
Fear of contamination, 4
Fenfluramine, 287
  affective symptom treatment, 297
  obsessive-compulsive disorder, 287
Finish prevalence study, 46
Five Minute Speech Sample, 57
Flunarizine, 266
Fluorodeoxyglucose-PET, 213–224, 353
Fluoxetine
  augmentation, 287
  in obsessive-compulsive disorder, 285–287,
      358
  self-injurious behavior, 110
  side effects, 285–286
  tic symptom effects, 285
Flutamide, 22, 352

Fluvoxamine, 286
  augmentation strategy, 287–288
  comparative efficacy, 288–289
  in obsessive-compulsive disorder, 286–287
  tic response, 288
Fnu4HI restriction enzyme, 186
Foods, brain effects, 293–301
Fragile X, 70–71
Freud, Sigmund, 95
Friendships, 327–332
Frontal cortex
  cyclic AMP, 138, 141–142
  HMPAO uptake, SPECT, 209–210
  postmortem neurochemistry, 136–143
Frontalis muscle, 30–31

G
GABA, postmortem analysis, 127–130, 137
GABAergic treatment strategies, 366
γ-vinyl-GABA, 267
Gastrin-releasing peptide, 168
Gender differences. *See* Sex differences
Gene frequency, 194
Gene selection hypothesis, 197
Generalized anxiety disorder, 96–104
  benzodiazepine treatment, 97–98
  comorbidity, 96–104
Genetic counseling, 349
Genetic heterogeneity, 170, 179, 182
Genetic linkage, 16–17
  alternative hypotheses, 195–196
  and diagnostic criteria, 348
  false-positives problem, 156, 348
  issues in studies of, 151–156, 347–348
  microsatellite DNA polymorphism study, 173–180, 183–186
  multigenic versus single gene hypothesis, 153–157
  Netherlands study, 167–172
  phenotype issue, 152–153, 347–348
  and prevalence, 348
  Salt Lake City pedigree, 163–164
  St. Louis study, 181–186
Genetic model, 151–156, 347–348
  alternative hypotheses, 193–194, 347
  family history studies, 155, 348
  research issues, 347–348
Genetic spectrum disorder. *See* Spectrum disorder concept
Geste antagonistique, 30
Global Assessment of Functioning Scale, 35, 37
Global Tic Rating Scale, 273–280

Globus pallidus
  and automatic movements, 7–8
  dynorphin staining, 145–149
  HMPAO uptake, 209
  immunohistochemistry, monkeys, 118–119
  limbic-motor interactions, 148–149
  magnetic resonance imaging, 203, 353
  parkinsonian monkeys, 119–120
  postmortem studies, 124–130, 145–149
Glutamate
  in medial globus pallidus, 127–128
  postmortem study, 127–130
  precursor control, 298
Glutamate decarboxylase, 137
Glutamine, postmortem study, 127
Gonadal hormones, 21–22, 352
Grieving model, 321
Gts gene frequency, 194
Gts gene selection, 196

H
Habit reversal
  major components, 338
  in Tourette syndrome, 339
  in trichotillomania, 337–338
HaeIII restriction enzyme, 184–186
Hairpulling. *See* Trichotillomania
Haloperidol, 241–242, 355–356
  dosage schedule, 241–242
  and Nicorette chewing gum, 265
  and nifedipine, 266
  versus pimozide, 241
  side effects, 242, 356
  tyrosine effects, 299
Handwriting problems, 312
Head banging
  associated symptoms, 106
  computerized tomography, 110
  Lesch-Nyhan syndrome, 107
  and Tourette syndrome, 105
Head rotation tics, 30
Hemiballismus, 130
Herpes encephalitis, 204
Heterogeneity assumption, 170, 179, 182
Hexamelthylpropylene amine oxime uptake, 208–210
5-HIAA
  and clomipramine response, 284
  postmortem analysis, 125–126, 137
HMPAO uptake, 208–209
Home assignments, 312
Homovanillic acid
  and clonidine response, 246

postmortem analysis, 125–126, 136, 139, 142
tyrosine effects, 299
Hormones, 21–22, 351–352
Hostility
    incidence, 5
    and self-injurious behavior, 106
Huntington's chorea
    GABAergic striatal neurons, 128
    obsessive-compulsive disorder, 84
5-Hydroxyindoleacetic acid. *See* 5-HIAA
5-Hydroxytryptophan, 267
Hyperactivity. *See* Attention deficit hyperactivity disorder
Hyperekplexia, 8
Hyperkinetic movement disorders, 10–11
Hyperlexia
    North Dakota comorbidity study, 69, 73
    prognosis, 73

I
Ideopathic dystonia, 29
Impulse control disorders
    definition, 41
    and obsessive-compulsive disorder, 33–39
Incomplete penetrance, 154, 163, 179
Infantile autism
    family history, 70–72
    North Dakota comorbidity study, 68–73
    prognosis with Tourette syndrome, 69–73
Inferior insular cortex, 218–223
Inferior rolandic cortex, 218–224
Informants
    education of, 50–51
    epidemiologic studies, 49–50
Inhibited personality traits, 34–41
Inosine, 267
Insular cortices, 218–223
Intelligence
    North Dakota comorbidity, study, 69
    and self-injurious behavior, 107–108
Intentional tics
    and movement classification, 7–8
    subjective perceptions, 10, 26–27
Intermittent tics, 28
Internal pallidal segment, 118–119
Interventions, children, 311–316, 354–359
Intralaminar thalamic nuclei, 21
Involuntary tics
    and movement classification, 7–8
    and premonitory symptoms, 343
    subjective perceptions, 10–11, 26–27
IOWA Conners Teacher's Rating Scale, 273

Israeli Defense Force study, 46–47, 61–65
    as population study, 61–65
    reporting bias, 47
    screening weakness, 64

J
Japanese families, 323–332
Jogging, 109

K
Kappa receptors, 260, 351
Kindred 159, 159–165
Klonopin. *See* Clonazepam

L
Language ability, 69
Large neutral amino acids, 295, 297
Lateral globus pallidus
    amino acids, 128
    postmortem studies, 124–130
Lateral ventricles, 202
Learning disorders
    educational management, 311–316
    incidence, 4, 75–77
    neuropsychological tests, 76–77
Lecithin, 266
Left lenticular nucleus, 353
Left thalamus, SPECT, 210
Leipzig prevalence, study, 46
Lenticular nucleus, 353
Lesch-Nyhan syndrome
    self-injurious behavior, 107, 110
    serotonergic system, 110
Levodopa-induced dyskinesias, 28
Leyton Obsessive-Compulsive Inventory, 34, 37–38
LH, and naloxone, 253–260
Life events, 58
Life style, Japanese patients, 327–332
Limbic system
    chemospecific systems, monkeys, 116–118
    FDG-PET study, 213–224
    motor interactions, 148–149, 213–224
    parkinsonian monkeys, 119–120
Linkage analysis. *See* Genetic linkage
Lip biting, 105
    association with Tourette syndrome, 105–106
    and obsessionality, 110

Lithium
    augmentation, 287
    therapeutic use, 264–265
Lod score, 348
Longitudinal studies, 51–52
Lorazepam withdrawal, 268
Luvox. *See* Fluvoxamine

M

M13 minisatellite, 184–186
Macaca fascicularis, 115–121
Magnetic resonance imaging
    basal ganglia, 17, 202–205
    obsessive-compulsive disorder, 203
    research issues, 353
    Tourette syndrome, 202–205
Male to female ratio. *See* Sex differences
Mannerisms, 9
Marijuana, 265
Mass media advertisements, 47–48
Math difficulties, 312
Medial globus pallidus
    glutamate levels, 127
    postmortem studies, 124–130
Medial preoptic area, 21
Medication combinations, 359
Megavitamin therapy, 359
    attention deficit hyperactivity disorder,
        303–310
    negative effects, 309–310
Mental arithmetic, 28
Mental coprolalia, 161, 164
Mental play, 35–37
Metenkephalin, 109
Methodology, epidemiology, 45–52
Methylphenidate
    behavioral effects, 276–280
    dose-response profile, 278–279
    double-blind study, 272–280
    hyperactive boys, 271–280
    mood effects, 278–279
    parents ratings, 278–280
    tic effects, 271, 357–358
3-N-(^{11}C)Methylspiperone-PET, 233–238
MHPG, and clonidine response, 246
MHPG-SO$_4$, 299
Microsatellite DNA polymorphism, 173–180,
    183–186
Minnesota prevalence study, 46
Minor tranquilizers, 97, 98, 358

MK-801, 268
Monkey model, parkinson's disease, 115–121
Monozygotic twins, 16
Monroe County, New York study, 46–47, 61,
    77
Mood effects, methylphenidate, 278–279
Mood swings, incidence of, 4–5
Motor challenges, 28
Motor circuit, limbic interactions, 148–149
Motor tics
    automaticity and purpose in, 31–32
    behavior therapy, 339
    block design correlation, 236
    cholinergic drugs, 266–267
    diagnostic criteria, 12, 342–343
    frequency of, 194
    gender differences, anatomy, 22
    HMPAO uptake, SPECT, 210
    methylphenidate effects, 277–280
    naloxone dose-response study, 257–260
    and obsessive-compulsive disorder, 87–92
    pain in relief of, 29–30
    phenomenology, 8–9, 25–32
    research needs, 51
    versus rituals, 83, 86
    school performance impairment, 76
    sensory premonitory symptoms, 25
Mourning, 321
Movements, classification, 7–8
MPTP, 120
Mu receptors, 260
Multifactorial models, 45
Multifactorial polygenic inheritance
    genetic models, 153–156
    Salt Lake City pedigree, 163
Muscarinic compounds, 267
Muscle pain, 29
Myoclonus
    subjective perceptions, 27
    and writing tasks, 28

N

Nail biting, 110
Naloxone
    behavioral effects, 253–260
    dose-response study, 254–260
    mu receptors, 260
    neuroendocrine effects, 253–260
    research issues, 351
    in self-injurious behavior, 109
    tic modulation, 268
    videotaped tic counts, 257–260

Naltrexone
  and propoxyphene, 351
  in self-injurious behavior 109, 268
  tic treatment, 254
Natural history
  and disease definition, 44, 50
  tics, 103
  variability in, 50
Netherlands genetic study, 167–172
Neuroacanthocytosis, 108
Neuroendocrine factors, 21–22, 351–352
Neuroleptic drugs, 241–242, 355–356
  augmentation use, 287–289
  dosage, 241–242
  limited usefulness, 242
  selection of, 356–357
  side effects, 242
  tic treatment, 241–242, 355–356
Neuropeptides. See Opioid peptides
Neuropsychological tests
  functional imaging correlation, 236
  school age children, 76–77
  tic severity correlation, 236–237
Neurotransmitters
  food effects, brain, 293–301
  precursor control, 297–298
  research issues, 350–351
  tyrosine effects, 298–300
Niacinamide
  in attention deficit hyperactivity disorder,
    305–310
  liver effects, 309
Nicorette chewing gum, 265
Nicotine, 265
Nicotine withdrawal, 297
Nifedipine, 265–266
NMDA antagonism, 268
11C-NMSP-PET, 233–238
Noncompliance, behavior therapy, 335–336
Norepinephrine
  postmortem analysis, 126–127, 137
  research issues, 350–351
  tyrosine effects, diet, 298–299
  and neuron firing, 299
North Dakota study
  comorbidity data, 67–73
  epidemiologic methods, 46–48, 61, 77
  physician reporting, 46–48, 61
Nutrients, brain effects, 293–301

O
"Obsessional psychoses," 336
Obsessions, 40, 83

Obsessive-compulsive disorder/symptoms
  antiandrogen treatment, 21
  behavior therapy, 333–339
  clomipramine treatment, 283–285, 358
  comorbidity, 48, 71–72, 83–92, 101–102,
    343
  definition, 41, 83–84
  drug augmentation strategies, 287
  dynorphin levels, CSF, 254
  eye mutilation, 110
  family history studies, 84–92, 152–153
  gender differences, 21
  genetics, 11–12, 48, 84, 86–92, 169
  HMPAO uptake, SPECT, 209–210
  incidence, 4
  natural history, 3–5
  Netherlands genetic study, 169
  NIMH study, 83–92
  North Dakota comorbidity study, 71–72
  overview, 83–84
  PET studies, dopamine, 227–231
  psychopharmacology, 283–289, 358
  and school problems, 76
  self-injurious behavior, 106, 109
  St. Louis pedigree, 182
  structural imaging, 203–204
  structural interview studies, 84–92,
    152–153
  subtyping by drug response, 287–288
  symptomatology, 35, 288
  and tics, 85–86, 288
  Tourette's syndrome comorbidity, 83–92,
    101–102, 343
  Tourette's syndrome differences, 33–41
  Tuft's study, 101–102
Occipital lobe
  cyclic AMP concentrations, 138
  postmortem neurochemistry, 136–143
Oculogyric deviations, 9
Olfactory tubercle, 124–130
Onychophagia, 110
Onset of symptoms. See Age of onset
Opioid peptides. See also specific peptides
  and endocrine function, 253–260
  mu receptor, 260
  research issues, 351
  self-injurious behavior, 109
  striatal staining, 148
  withdrawal effects, 260
Orbitofrontal cortices
  behavioral inhibition role, 222
  FDG-PET study, 218–223
  motor system connections, 223
  obsessive-compulsive disorder, 222

P

Pain, 29–30
Pain relief
  botulinum toxin, 30
  tic function, 29–30
Palilalia, 9, 31
Palilaliopraxia, 31
Pallidum. *See* Globus pallidus
Panic disorder
  benzodiazepine treatment, 97–98
  comorbidity, 95–104
Parahippocampal region
  FDG-PET study, 218–223
  motor responses role, 222–223
Parent-child relationship. *See* Family
    relationships
Parent ratings, methylphenidate, 278–280
Parkinsonian monkeys, 119–121
Parkinsonian tremor, 28
Paroxysmal dyskinesias, 28
Peer relationships
  Japanese patients, 327–332
  rankings of, 319–320
Penetrance
  alternative assumptions, 194
  and genetic models, 154, 169
  Netherlands study, 169–170
  Salt Lake City pedigree, 163
Peptides. *See* Opioid peptides
Perinatal events, 17
Persistent dystonia, 9–10
Personality characteristics, 58
Personality disorders
  self-injurious behavior, 108–109
  and Tourette syndrome, 37–38
Pervasive development disorders
  California prevalence study, 70
  DSM-III-R definition, 68
  family history, 70–72
  North Dakota comorbidity study, 67–73
  prognosis with Tourette syndrome, 69–73
Pharmacotherapy, 355–359
Phenocopies, 345–346
Phenomenology, 8–13, 341–347
Phenothiazines. *See* Neuroleptic drugs
Phenotype
  definition of, 345–347
  genetic linkage issue, 152–153, 347–348
  Salt Lake City pedigree, 164
Phobic disorders
  benzodiazepine treatment, 97, 98
  comorbidity, 96–104
Phonic tics. *See* Vocal tics

Phosphatidylcholine
  choline effects on, 300
  therapeutic use, 300–301
Phosphatidylethanolamine, 300
Phosphatidylserine, 300
Physician-family relationship, 321–322
Physostigmine injections, 266
Pimozide
  fluvoxamine augmentation, 287
  versus haloperidol, 241, 356
  side effects, 242, 356
Pleiotropic manifestations, 344–345
Polygenic inheritance. *See* Multifactorial
    polygenic inheritance
Polymorphic DNA markers
  microsatellite technique, 173–180
  Netherlands study, 167–172
Population-based studies
  epidemiologic methods, 46
  Israel Defense Force, 61–65
Positron emission tomography
  brain region correlations, 213–224
  distinguishing features, 213–214
  dopamine D-2 receptors, 227–231, 233–238
  dopaminergic system, 227–231
  limbic-motor interaction study, 213–224
  research issues, 353
  versus SPECT imaging, 207
Postencephalitic Parkinson's disease, 84
Postmortem studies, 123–130, 135–143,
    145–149, 352–353
Postsynaptic function
  overview, 135–137
  PET study, dopamine, 234–238
  postmortem analysis, 137–143
Posttraumatic stress disorder, 195
Prefrontal cortices, 218–224
Premenstrual syndrome, 296–297
Premonitory symptoms
  anatomical distribution, 19
  clinical description, 19–20, 343
  neurobiological origins, 20–21
  sensory tics, 25–27
  subjective perceptions, 26–27
  tic diagnosis, 10–11
Premotor cortices, 218–224
Prenatal stress, 49
Presynaptic function
  overview, 135–137
  postmortem analysis, 137–143
Prevalence
  alternative assumptions, 194
  case identification, 49–50

and disease definition, 50–52
and genetic linkage studies, 348
Israeli Defense Force study, 61–65
methodological aspects, 43–52, 77–78
North Dakota study, 67–73
population studies, 46, 61–65
and sample selection bias, 45–48
school-age children, 78
tics, 3
variations in, 12–13, 46
Primary Secondary Symptom Checklist, 273,
275
Primates, 115–121
Progabide, 267
Prognosis
Salt Lake City pedigree, 164
tic symptomatology, 3, 50
variability in, 50
Propoxyphene, 351
Propranolol, 267
Protective factors
epidemiologic studies, 49
psychosocial aspects, 56–57
Protein meal, 294–295
Prozac. *See* Fluoxetine
Psychoanalysis
and long-term adjustment, 49
obsessive-compulsive disorder, 334
Psychogenic abnormal movements, 28
Psychosis, self-injurious behavior, 108
Psychosocial factors, 55–59
Psychostimulants, 357–358. *See also*
Methylphenidate
Psychotherapy, 354–355. *See also* Behavior
therapy
Purine metabolism, 107
Putamen
cyclic AMP concentrations, 138
dopamine, 139–140
FDG-PET study, 218–224
limbic system coupling, 223–224
metabolic rates, 219–224
postmortem neurochemistry, 136–143
sensorimotor cortices relationship, 219
Pyridoxine
in attention deficit hyperactivity disorder,
305–310
toxicity, 309

Q

Questionnaire methods, 79
Quinolinic acid, 196

R

^{11}C-Raclopride PET, 227–231
"Random mapping," 182
Red-cell acid phosphatase, 181
Regional cerebral blood flow
HMPAO uptake validity, 208–209
neuronal activity correlation, 207–208
research issues, 353
SPECT imaging, 207–210
Relaxation, and tic diagnosis, 11
Relaxation training, 338
Remission, tics, 3
Repeating rituals, 84
Reporting bias, 47
Reserpine, 267
Response prevention
obsessive-compulsive disorder, 333–337
trichotillomania, 337
Responsive movements, 7–8
Restless legs syndrome, 10
Reverse ascertainment bias, 192–193
"Reverse genetics," 167–168
Risk
epidemiological methods, 49, 52
gender differences, 57
psychosocial factors, 56–57
Rituals
behavior therapy, 333–337
definition, 83
versus motor tics, 83, 86
NIMH study, 83–84
versus trichotillomania, 337
Road tracking test, 77
Rolandic cortices
FDG-PET study, 218–223
and ventral striatum, 223
Rotterdam linkage study, 167–172
RS–86, 267

S

Saccades, 128
Saimiri sciureus, 115–121
Salt Lake City pedigree, 159–165
Sample selection bias, 45, 344
Schizophrenia, 108
Schizotypal personality, 336
School behavior
megavitamin effects, 308–310
methylphenidate effect, 279
School performance
impairments, 74–76
interventions, 311–316
Japanese patients, 327–332

School performance (*contd.*)
  megavitamin effects, 308–309
  as risk factor, 57
SCID II, 35, 37–38
Scopolamine, 266
Scrupulosity, 84
Seasonal affective disorder, 296–297
Segregation analyses
  family history data, 155–157
  Netherlands study, 170
  Salt Lake City pedigree, 161–163
Seizures, and clomipramine, 284–285
Selection bias, 45, 344
Self-injurious behavior, 105–111
  biochemistry, 109–110
  incidence, 5, 107
  management, 111
  obsessive-compulsive disorder, 35, 38
"Semi-dominant, semi-recessive" hypothesis,
    154, 194, 347
Sensitivity-specificity tradeoff, 348
Sensorimotor striatal territory
  chemospecific systems, monkeys, 116–119
  parkinsonian monkeys, 119–120
Sensory neuropathies, 109
Sensory tics
  clinical phenomenology, 25–28
  obsessive-compulsive disorder, 39
  and pain, 29
  premonitory symptoms, 10, 25
  subjective perceptions, 26–27
Separation anxiety, 96–104
Serencis,   111
Serotonergic system
  pallidal territories, monkeys, 119
  postmortem study, 125–126, 129–130
  self-injurious behavior, 109–110
  striatal territories, monkeys, 118–119
Serotonin
  and clomipramine response, 284
  food effects, brain, 294–295
  and nutrient choice, 296–297
  postmortem study, 125–126, 129–130
  research issues, 350–351
  Tourette syndrome genetics, 195–196
Serotonin reuptake inhibitors
  augmentation of, 287
  in obsessive-compulsive disorder, 283–287,
    358
Sertraline
  comparative efficacy, 288
  in obsessive-compulsive disorder, 286

Sex differences
  clinical description, 21
  and culture, 58
  Israeli Defense Force study, 64
  North Dakota study, 68, 73
  neurobiological origins, 21–22, 351–352
  obsessive-compulsive disorder, 153
  prognosis, 73
  psychosocial factors, 57
  research issues, 351–352
  Salt Lake City pedigree, 161, 164
Sexual dimorphism, 21
Signing tics, 31–32
Simple tics, 8–9
Single gene hypothesis
  family history studies, 153, 347
  Salt Lake City pedigree, 163–164
SK&F 38393, 267
Sleep, tic persistence, 11
Social adaptation
  incidence of problems, 4–5
  intervention programs, 312
  Japanese families, 323–332
  as rescarch issue, 343–344
Social skills, 312
Soft signs, 4
Somatosensory cortex, 20–21
Spasmodic torticollis, 30
Special education population, 75–79
  survey needs, 79
  Tourette syndrome prevalence, 76, 78–79
Specificity-sensitivity tradeoff, 348
SPECT imaging
  advantages, 207
  cerebral blood flow, 207–210, 353
  research issues, 353
Spectrum disorder concept
  alternative hypothesis, 190
  family studies, 193
Spiradoline mesylate, 351
Spironolactone, 21
Spontaneous improvement, 3
Squirrel monkeys, 115–121
St. Louis linkage studies, 181–186
Stereotypies, 10
Steroid hormones. *See* Androgenic steroids
Stimulant drugs, 357–358. *See also*
    Methylphenidate
Stimulant Side Effects Checklist, 276,
    278–279
Stony Brook Child Psychiatric Checklist–3R,
    273

Stress model, family, 321
Stress sensitivity
 gender differences, 22
 and tic diagnosis, 10–11
Striatal brain region
 FDG-PET study, 218–224
 postmortem neurochemistry, 135–143
Striatopallidal neurons
 dynorphin deficiency, 148
 parkinsonian monkeys, 119–120
Striosomes, 116, 118, 120
Structural imaging, 201–205
Studies in Hysteria (Freud), 95
Stuttering, 160, 164
Subjective perceptions, 2, 26–27
Substance P
 basal ganglia staining, 145–149
 pallidal territories, monkeys, 118–120
 parkinsonian monkeys, 120
Substantia nigra pars compacta
 dopaminergic system, monkeys, 117, 119
 glutamate, 128
 parkinsonian monkeys, 119–120
 postmortem studies, 124–130
Substantia nigra pars reticulata
 glutamate, 128
 postmortem studies, 124, 130
 serotonergic neurons, monkeys, 118
Substitute symptoms, 334
Subthalamic nucleus
 glutamate, 128, 130
 hemiballismus, 130
 limbic-motor interactions, 148–149
Sudden death, and desipramine, 284, 357
Suffering, 36
Suicidality, and fluoxetine, 285–286
Sulpiride, 356
Superior lateral premotor cortex, 218
Superior parietal lobule, 218–223
superior rolandic cortex, 218–224
Superior sensorimotor regions
 attention deficit disorder, 224
 inferior limbic relationship, 223
 limbic interactions, PET, 218–224
 and ventral striatum, 223
Supplemental motor cortex
 cyclic AMP concentrations, 138
 FDG-PET study, 218–224
 limbic system interactions, PET,
  218–224
 postmortem neurochemistry, 136–143
 and ventral striatum, 223

Suppression of tics. See Tic suppressibility
Survey methods, 51. See also Prevalence
Sydenham's chorea, 84
Synaptic neurotransmission, 135–143
Syndrome definition, 45, 50–52

T

Tardive dyskinesia
 choline treatment, 300
 neuroleptic side effects, 242
 voluntary suppressibility, 28
Taurine, 127
Teasing by peers, 312
Temper outbursts, 4
Temporal lobe
 cyclic AMP concentrations, 138
 postmortem neurochemistry, 136–143
Testolactone, 21
Testosterone, 21, 352
Tetrabenazine, 130, 267
Thalamostriatal projections, 21
Thalamus, HMPAO uptake, SPECT,
  209–210
Thermal stress, 17, 22
Thumb opposition task, 28
Tiapride, 356
Tic counts
 methylphenidate effect, 275, 277–278
 naloxone effects, 257–260
Tic suppressibility
 classroom settings, 76
 and tic diagnosis, 10–11, 28
Tics. See also Motor tics; Vocal tics
 antiobsessional drug effects, 287–289
 and attention deficit disorder, 345
 behavior therapy, 338–339
 cholinergic drugs, 266–267
 classification, 7–13
 clinical phenomenology, 25–32
 diagnosis, 7–13
 diagnostic criteria, 12, 19–21
 differential diagnosis, 8–11, 27–29
 genetic linkage studies, 155–156
 HMPAO uptake, SPECT, 209–210
 methylphenidate effects, 271–280
 naloxone dose-response study, 257–260
 natural history, 1–3, 50, 164
 neuroleptics, 241–242, 355–356
 NIMH study, 86–92
 and obsessive-compulsive disorder, 84–85,
  155–156, 287–288

Tics (*contd.*)
  pathophysiology, 11–13
  phenomenology, 8–13
  phenotype issue, 152–153, 164
  premonitory symptoms, 10
  prognostic variability, 50, 164
  research needs, 51–52
  Salt Lake City pedigree, 159–165
  school-age children, 78
  subjective perceptions, 26–27
  tricyclic antidepressants, 285
Tongue biting, 105
Tonic tics, 8–10
Torsion dystonia, 9–10
Touching behavior
  as ritual versus motor tics, 83
  Tourette syndrome association, 86
Tourette Syndrome Association, 58, 341
Tourette syndrome-specific probes,
    182–186
Tourette Syndrome Unified Rating Scale,
    274–278
Transdermal patch formulations, 247
Treatment approaches, 354–359
Tremors, 27
Trichotillomania
  behavior therapy, 337–338
  and obsessive-compulsive disorder, 110,
    337
  versus obsessive rituals, 337
Tricyclic antidepressants. *See also*
    Clomipramine
  in depressive symptoms, 358
  tic effects, 285
Tryptophan
  food consumption, brain, 294–295
  postmortem study, 125–136, 129–130
Tryptophan oxygenase gene, 178,
    195–196
Tufts Medical Center study, 95–104
Twins, 16
  computerized tomography, 203
  concordance for Tourette syndrome, 16
Two-allele locus hypothesis, 154
Two-minute Tic count, 279
Tyrosine
  catecholamine synthesis, diet, 298–300
  haloperidol interactions, 299
  use as drug, 299–300
Tyrosine hydroxylase
  as candidate gene, 168
  catecholamine synthesis, diet, 298–300
  postmortem study, 127

U
Unvoluntary movements, 7–8
Unvoluntary tics, 26–27
Uric acid, 107

V
Variant manifestations, 344–345
Ventral pallidum
  dynorphin staining, 145–149
  immunohistochemistry, monkeys, 118–120
  limbic-motor interactions, 148–149
  parkinsonian monkeys, 120
Ventral striatum
  FDG-PET study, 218–224
  limbic system interactions, 148–149
  motor system interactions, PET, 223–224
Ventral tegmental area
  normal monkeys, dopamine, 117, 119
  parkinsonian monkeys, 119–120
Ventricular enlargement
  obsessive-compulsive disorder, 203
  Tourette syndrome, 202–203
Ventrolateral thalamus, 124–130
Verapamil, 265–266
Videotaped tic counts, 257–260
Vitamin C. *See* Ascorbic acid
Vitamins. *See* Megavitamin therapy
Vocal tics
  cholinergic drugs, 266–267
  diagnostic criteria, 8–9, 342–343
  DSM-III-R, 342
  methylphenidate effects, 277–280
  naloxone dose-response study, 257–260
  phenomenology, 8–9
  as presenting symptom, 2
  school performance impairment, 76
  sensory premonitory symptoms, 25
Voluntary suppressibility. *See* Tic
    suppressibility
Voluntary tics
  and movement classification, 7–8, 11
  premonitory sensory symptoms, 25–26, 343
  subjective perceptions, 26–27

W
Waxing and waning of symptoms, 342
[11]C-WIN 35, 238, 428
Wisconsin A pedigree, 175–179
Wisconsin Card Scoring Test, 236
Woolly fibers, 146
Work status, Japanese patients, 323–327

Wrist cutting
  and depression, 108
  personality disorders, 108–109
Writing tasks, 28

X
XY pseudoautosomal region, 181

Y
Yale Global Tic Severity Scale, 273–280
Yale-STSOBS, 62

Z
Zung Depression Rating Scale, 34, 37–38